Regional Therapy of Advanced Cancer

Regional Therapy of Advanced Cancer

Editors

Michael T. Lotze, M.D.
Professor of Surgery, Molecular Genetics and Biochemistry
University of Pittsburgh Cancer Institute
University of Pittsburgh
Pittsburgh, Pennsylvania

Joshua T. Rubin, M.D.
Associate Professor of Surgery
Department of Surgery
University of Pittsburgh
Pittsburgh, Pennsylvania

with 56 Contributors

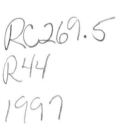 **Lippincott - Raven**
PUBLISHERS
Philadelphia • New York

Acquisitions Editor: Stuart Freeman
Developmental Editor: Mary Beth Murphy
Manufacturing Manager: Dennis Teston
Production Manager: Maxine Langweil
Production Editor: Kimberly Swan
Cover Designer: Karen Quigley
Compositor: Lippincott–Raven Electronic Production
Printer: Kingsport Press

9 8 7 6 5 4 3 2 1

Library of Congress Cataloging-in-Publication Data
Regional therapy of advanced cancer / editors, Michael T. Lotze,
    Joshua T. Rubin ; with 56 contributors.
        p.   cm.
    Includes bibliographical references and index.
    ISBN 0-397-51474-3
    1. Metastasis. 2. Cancer invasiveness. 3. Cancer—Treatment.
I. Lotze, Michael T. II. Rubin, Joshua T.
    [DNLM: 1. Neoplasms—therapy. 2. Neoplasm Metastasis.
3. Neoplasm Invasiveness—prevention & control. QZ 266 R336 1997]
RC269.5.R44 1997
616.99'406—dc21
DNLM/DLC
For Library of Congress

To our patients,
who inspire us;

our students and fellows,
from whom we continue to learn,
and with whom we test the application of these treatments;

and our families,
whose encouragement and emotional support
made this work possible.

Contents

Contributors xi

Preface xvii

Acknowledgments xix

Introduction xxi

Section I: Regional Therapy of Cancer

1. Biology of Cancer Metastases: Hematogenous Dissemination   1
    Ronald H. Goldfarb, Richard P. Kitson, and Kenneth W. Brunson

2. Biology of Cancer Metastases: Lymphatic Dissemination 11
    Michael T. Lotze

Section II: Thoracic Procedures

3. Diagnosis of Pulmonary Metastatic Disease 23
    Daphne J.Y. Mew, Jessica Donington, and Harvey I. Pass

4. Surgical Resection of Pulmonary Metastases 37
    Jeffrey L. Port and Michael Burt

5. The Role of Thoracoscopy in Thoracic Oncology 51
    Rodney J. Landreneau, Robert J. Keenan, Michael J. Mack,
    Lynda S. Fetterman, Stephen R. Hazelrigg, Peter F. Ferson,
    and Scott H. Hanan

6. Isolated Lung Perfusion for Pulmonary Metastases 63
    Harvey I. Pass

Section III. Hepatic Procedures

7. Imaging Liver Neoplasms 75
    Richard L. Baron

8. Surgical Treatment of Hepatic Metastases 99
    Kelly M. McMasters and Mark S. Roh

9. Infusional Chemotherapy of Hepatic-Metastatic Tumors 119
    Joshua T. Rubin and Keith A. Dookeran

10. Cryoablation of Hepatic Metastases 129
    Joshua T. Rubin

11. Isolated Perfusion of the Liver 141
Douglas L. Fraker and H. Richard Alexander, Jr.

Section IV: Intracranial Procedures

12. Diagnosis of Central Nervous System Metastases 151
Nicholas J. Patronas and Myles B. Koby

13. Surgical Treatment of Brain Metastases 175
Jeffrey W. Campbell, Ian F. Pollack, and Donald C. Wright

14. Radiosurgery of Brain Metastases 187
John C. Flickinger, Douglas Kondziolka, and
L. Dade Lunsford

15. Perfusional Therapy of Brain Metastases 195
William C. Welch and Paul L. Kornblith

Section V. Abdominal and Pelvic Procedures

16. Abdominopelvic Imaging in Cancer Patients 205
Michael P. Federle

17. Abdominal and Pelvic Procedures: Laparoscopic Resection 221
José M. Dominguez and Heidi Nelson

18. Surgical Treatment of Pelvic Recurrence 235
Michael P. Vezeridis and Harold J. Wanebo

19. Visceral and Parietal Peritonectomy Procedures 249
Paul H. Sugarbaker

20. Intraperitoneal Chemotherapy 259
Paul H. Sugarbaker

21. Shunting Procedures for Malignant Ascites and Pleural Effusions 271
H. Richard Alexander, Jr. and Douglas L. Fraker

22. Intraoperative Radiation Therapy 281
William F. Sindelar and Peter A. S. Johnstone

Section VI: Extremity Procedures

23. Diagnosis of Lymph Node Metastases 291
Richard Essner and Donald L. Morton

24. The Role of Lymph Node Dissection in the Treatment of Cancer 301
Sadiq S. Sikora and Michael T. Lotze

25. Isolated Perfusion of Extremity Tumors 333
Douglas L. Fraker and Daniel G. Coit

26. Surgical Treatment of Bone Metastases to the Axial Skeleton and Extremities 351
Kenneth M. Yaw and J. Scott Doyle

Section VII: Selected Topics

27. Metastasectomy for Islet Carcinoma 367
Sally E. Carty

28. Gene Therapy of Local Tumors 375
Gerard J. McGarrity and Yawen L. Chiang

29. Radioimmunoguided Surgery for Recurrent and Metastatic Colorectal Cancer 391
Julian A. Kim and Edward W. Martin, Jr.

30. Interventional and Ablative Procedures for Cancer Pain 401
Ricardo Segal and Anne Harris

31. Intraoperative Ultrasound in the Oncologic Setting: An Overview 417
Howard A. Zaren, Jeffrey H. Schwartz, Bernard Sigel, and
Junji Machi

Appendix: Manufacturers of Specialized Equipment 427

Subject Index 429

Contributors

H. Richard Alexander, Jr., M.D.
Head, Surgical Metabolism Section
Surgery Branch
National Cancer Institute
National Institutes of Health
Building 10, Room 2B07
Bethesda, Maryland 20854

Richard L. Baron, M.D.
Professor and Chairman
Department of Radiology
University of Pittsburgh School of Medicine
200 Lothrop Street
Pittsburgh, Pennsylvania 15213-2582

Kenneth W. Brunson, Ph.D.
Associate Professor of Pathology
Division of Basic Research
University of Pittsburgh Cancer Institute
200 Lothrop Street; and
Director, In Vivo Preclinical Research,
Health Sciences, University of Pittsburgh School
* of Medicine;*
Director, UPCI Tumor Model Facility
Pittsburgh, Pennsylvania 15213-2582

Michael Burt, M.D., Ph.D.
Attending Physician
Department of Surgery
Memorial Sloan-Kettering Cancer Center
1275 York Avenue
New York, New York 10021-6007

Jeffrey W. Campbell, M.D.
Resident of Neurosurgery
Department of Neurosurgery
University of Pittsburgh
Presbyterian Hospital
200 Lothrop Street, Suite B-400
Pittsburgh, Pennsylvania 15213-2582

Sally E. Carty, M.D.
Assistant Professor of Surgery/Endocrine Surgery
Department of Surgery
University of Pittsburgh Medical Center
497 Scaife Hall
3550 Terrace Street
Pittsburgh, Pennsylvania 15261

Yawen L. Chiang, Ph.D.
Vice President, Immunology
Genetic Therapy, Inc./Novartis
938 Clopper Road
Gaithersburg, Maryland 20878

Daniel G. Coit, M.D.
Associate Attending Surgeon
Department of Surgery
Memorial Sloan-Kettering Cancer Center
1275 York Avenue
New York, New York 10021

José M. Dominguez, M.D.
Fellow, Division of Colon and Rectal Surgery
Mayo Clinic and Foundation
200 First Street, S.W.
Rochester, Minnesota 55905

Jessica Donington, M.D.
Surgery Branch
National Cancer Institute
Building 10, Room 2B07
Bethesda, Maryland 20892

Keith A. Dookeran, M.D., F.R.C.S.
Director of Clinical Research and Protocols
The Mercy Cancer Institute
Codirector of Surgical Research
Department of Surgery
The Mercy Hospital of Pittsburgh
1400 Locust Street
Pittsburgh, Pennsylvania 15219

J. Scott Doyle, M.D.
Assistant Professor
Department of Orthopedic Surgery
University of Alabama Hospitals at Birmingham
1600 7th Avenue South
Birmingham, Alabama 35233

Richard Essner, M.D.
Assistant Director
Department of Surgical Oncology
John Wayne Cancer Institute
2200 Santa Monica Boulevard
Santa Monica, California 90404

Michael P. Federle, M.D.
Professor of Radiology
Department of Radiology
University of Pittsburgh Medical Center
200 Lothrop Street
Pittsburgh, Pennsylvania 15213-2582

Peter F. Ferson, M.D.
Professor of Surgery
Department of Thoracic Surgery
University of Pittsburgh Medical Center
Lilliane S. Kaufmann Building
3471 Fifth Avenue, Suite 201
Pittsburgh, Pennsylvania 15213

Lynda S. Fetterman, R.N.
Clinical Research Coordinator
Department of Thoracic Surgery
Allegheny General Hospital
Allegheny University of the Health
* Sciences–Allegheny Campus*
320 East North Avenue
Pittsburgh, Pennsylvania 15212-4772

John C. Flickinger, M.D.
Professor of Radiation Oncology and
* Neurological Surgery*
Department of Radiation Oncology
University of Pittsburgh Medical Center
200 Lothrop Street
Pittsburgh, Pennsylvania 15213-2582

Douglas L. Fraker, M.D.
Jonathan E. Rhoads Associate Professor of
* Surgery*
Chief, Division of Surgical Oncology
Endocrine Surgery/General Surgery
Department of Surgery
University of Pennsylvania
3400 Spruce Street
Philadelphia, Pennsylvania 19104

Ronald H. Goldfarb, Ph.D.
Professor of Pathology and Deputy Director
University of Pittsburgh Cancer Institute, Basic
* Research;*
Director, University of Pittsburgh Cancer
* Institute, Cancer Metastasis and Cell Biology*
* Program;*
Department of Pathology
University of Pittsburgh School of Medicine
200 Lothrop Street
Pittsburgh, Pennsylvania 15213-2582

Scott H. Hanan, M.D.
Fellow
Department of Surgical Oncology
University of Pittsburgh Medical Center
Lilliane S. Kaufmann Building
3471 Fifth Avenue, Suite 300
Pittsburgh, Pennsylvania 15219

Anne Harris, M.D.
Department of Anesthesiology/Critical Care
* Medicine*
University of Pittsburgh Medical Center and
* Department of Veterans Affairs Medical Center*
200 Lothrop Street
Pittsburgh, Pennsylvania 15213-2582

Stephen R. Hazelrigg, M.D.
Associate Professor and Chairman
Department of Cardiothoracic Surgery
Southern Illinois University School of Medicine
800 North Rutledge
Springfield, Illinois 62702

Peter A.S. Johnstone, M.A., M.D.
Assistant Clinical Professor
Department of Radiation Oncology
University of California
Naval Medical Center
San Diego, California 92134-5000

Robert J. Keenan, M.D.
Assistant Professor of Surgery
Department of Surgery
Division of Cardiothoracic Surgery
University of Pittsburgh Medical Center
200 Lothrop Street, Suite C-700
Pittsburgh, Pennsylvania 15213-2582

Julian A. Kim, M.D.
Assistant Professor of Surgery
Department of Surgery
Division of Surgical Oncology
Arthur G. James Cancer Hospital and Research
* Institute*
The Ohio State University College of Medicine
410 West 10th Avenue
Columbus, Ohio 43210

Richard P. Kitson, Ph.D.
Research Assistant Professor of Cell Biology and Physiology
Department of Cell Biology and Physiology
University of Pittsburgh School of Medicine
200 Lothrop Street
Pittsburgh, Pennsylvania 15213-2582

Myles B. Koby, D.D.S., M.D.
Clinical Assistant Professor
Diagnostic Radiology
Michigan State University
Michigan Capital Medical Center
401 West Greenlawn
Lansing, Michigan 48910

Douglas Kondziolka, M.D., M.Sc., F.R.C.S.(C), F.A.C.S.
Associate Professor of Neurological Surgery and Radiation Oncology
Departments of Neurological Surgery and Radiation Oncology
University of Pittsburgh Medical Center
200 Lothrop Street, Suite E-400
Pittsburgh, Pennsylvania 15213-2582

Paul L. Kornblith, M.D.
Director of Cancer Therapy Services
Institute for Transfusion Medicine
3636 Boulevard of the Allies
Pittsburgh, Pennsylvania 15213

Rodney J. Landreneau, M.D.
Professor of Surgery
Section Head, General Thoracic Surgery
Director, Allegheny Center for Lung and Thoracic Disease
Allegheny General Hospital
Allegheny University of the Health Sciences
320 East North Avenue
Pittsburgh, Pennsylvania 15212-4772

Michael T. Lotze, M.D.
Professor of Surgery, Molecular Genetics and Biochemistry
University of Pittsburgh Cancer Institute
University of Pittsburgh
200 Lothrop Street
Pittsburgh, Pennsylvania 15213-2582

L. Dade Lunsford, M.D.
Professor of Neurosurgery
Department of Neurosurgery
Presbyterian University Hospital
200 Lothrop Street, Suite B400
Pittsburgh, Pennsylvania 15213-2582

Junji Machi, M.D., Ph.D.
Associate Professor of Surgery
University of Hawaii at Manoa
320 Ward Avenue
Honolulu, Hawaii 96814

Michael J. Mack, M.D.
Clinical Assistant Professor
Department of Cardiothoracic Surgery
Columbia Hospital
Medical City Hospital
7777 Forest Lane, A-323
Dallas, Texas 75230

Edward W. Martin, Jr., M.D., F.A.C.S.
Professor of Surgery
Department of Surgery
Arthur G. James Cancer Hospital and Research Institute
Division of Surgical Oncology
The Ohio State University College of Medicine
410 West 10th Avenue
Columbus, Ohio 43210

Gerard J. McGarrity, Ph.D.
Senior Vice President
Research and Development
Genetic Therapy, Inc./Novartis
938 Clopper Road
Gaithersburg, Maryland 20878

Kelly M. McMasters, M.D., Ph.D.
Sam and Lolita Professor of Surgical Oncology
University of Lousiville-Brown Cancer Center
529 South Jackson Street
Louisville, Kentucky 40202

Daphne J.Y. Mew, M.D., Ph.D.
Assistant Professor of Surgery
Department of Surgery
University of Calgary, Foothills Hospital
1403 29th Street, N.W.
Calgary, Alberta, Canada T2N-2T9

Donald L. Morton, M.D.
Department of Surgical Oncology
John Wayne Cancer Institute
2200 Santa Monica Boulevard
Santa Monica, California 90404

Heidi Nelson, M.D., F.A.C.S.
Associate Professor of Surgery
Division of Colon and Rectal Surgery
Mayo Clinic and Foundation
200 First Street, S.W.
Rochester, Minnesota 55905

Harvey I. Pass, M.D.
Professor of Surgery and Oncology
Wayne State University
Karmanos Cancer Institute
Harper Hospital
3990 John Road, Suite 2102
Detroit, Michigan 48201

Nicholas J. Patronas, M.D.
Radiologist
Department of Radiology
National Institutes of Health, Clinical Center
Building 10, Room 1C660
Bethesda, Maryland 20892

Ian F. Pollack, M.D.
Associate Professor of Neurological Surgery
Co-Director, University of Pittsburgh
* Neurofibromatosis Clinic*
Co-Director, UPCI Brain Tumor Center
Department of Neurosurgery
University of Pittsburgh
Children's Hospital
3705 Fifth Avenue
Pittsburgh, Pennsylvania 15213

Jeffrey L. Port, M.D.
Fellow
Thoracic Oncology Laboratory
Memorial Sloan-Kettering Cancer Center
1275 York Avenue
New York, New York 10021

Mark S. Roh, M.D.
Professor of Surgery
Department of Surgical Oncology
Allegheny University Hospital
320 East North Avenue
Pittsburgh, Pennsylvania 15212

Joshua T. Rubin, M.D.
Associate Professor of Surgery
Department of Surgery
University of Pittsburgh
Lilliane S. Kaufmann Building
3471 Fifth Avenue, Suite 300
Pittsburgh, Pennsylvania 15213

Jeffrey H. Schwartz, M.D., F.A.C.S.
Assistant Director, Surgical Oncology
The Mercy Hospital of Pittsburgh
1400 Locust Street
Pittsburgh, Pennsylvania 15219

Ricardo Segal, M.D.
Associate Professor of Neurological Surgery
Department of Neurological Surgery
University of Pittsburgh Medical Center
V.A. Pittsburgh Health Care System
200 Lothrop Street
Pittsburgh, Pennsylvania 15213-2582

Bernard Sigel, M.D.
Senior Vice President
Cardiology Medical Director
Allegheny University of Health Sciences
Broad and Vine Streets
Philadelphia, Pennsylvania 19102

Sadiq S. Sikora, M.D.
Section of Surgical Oncology
University of Pittsburgh Medical Center
W1543, Biomedical Science Tower
Pittsburgh, Pennsylvania 15261

William F. Sindelar, M.D.,Ph.D.
Senior Investigator
Surgery Branch
National Cancer Institute
National Institutes of Health
Building 10, Room 2B42
Bethesda, Maryland 20892

Paul H. Sugarbaker, M.D.
Director of Surgical Oncology
The Washington Cancer Institute
Washington Hospital Center
110 Irving Street, N.W.
Washington, DC 20010

Michael P. Vezeridis, M.D.
Professor of Surgery
Department of Surgery
Brown University School of Medicine
Roger Williams Medical Center
825 Chalkstone Avenue
Providence, Rhode Island 02908

Harold J. Wanebo, M.D.
Director, Division of Surgical Oncology
Professor of Surgery
Brown University School of Medicine;
Chief of Surgery
Roger Williams Medical Center
825 Chalkstone Avenue
Providence, Rhode Island 02908

William C. Welch, M.D.
Assistant Professor
Department of Neurological Surgery, Orthopedic
  Surgery
University of Pittsburgh School of Medicine
Presbyterian University Hospital, Suite B-400
200 Lothrop Street
Pittsburgh, Pennsylvania 15213-2582

Donald C. Wright, M.D.
Associate Professor
Vice Chairman of Neurosurgery
Department of Neurosurgery
George Washington University Medical Center
2150 Pennsylvania Avenue N.W., Suite 7-420
Washington, DC 20037

Kenneth M. Yaw, M.D.
Assistant Professor
Department of Orthopaedic Surgery
University of Pittsburgh School of Medicine;
Chief, Division of Musculoskeletal Oncology
University of Pittsburgh Medical Center
3741 Fifth Avenue
Pittsburgh, Pennsylvania 15213

Howard A. Zaren, M.D., F.A.C.S.
Chairman, Department of Surgery
The Mercy Hospital of Pittsburgh
1400 Locust Street
Pittsburgh, Pennsylvania 15219

Preface

The patient with cancer deserves a hopeful physician.
—Jonathan Rhodes

The notion for this book arose a number of years ago with the realization that although local therapies were remarkably effective in approximately half of patients with cancer, the application of systemic therapies in practice, particularly for the most common epithelial malignancies, was difficult for the physician and morbid for the patient. This includes the use of systemic chemotherapies as well as the more recent systemic immunotherapies such as alpha-interferon and interleukin 2. Much of the basis for systemic therapies was predicated on the goal of cancer elimination. We have come to realize that cancer is a systemic disease and that cancer control may be a better operational strategy, given the great difficulty of elimination of the last tumor cell. Charged with increasing not only the quantity but also quality of life, regional therapies have evolved over the last 20 years to effectively treat both nodal and visceral metastatic disease. We recognize that tumors require an environment supportive for their continued growth, thus limiting the sites where we observe them. In fact, many patients will have tumors confined to a single site or organ for prolonged periods of time. This is frightening for the patient and frustrating for the caregiver.

We also recognize that changes in healthcare financing and administration will require that we provide evidence of efficacy and prolongation of survival. Our patients require not only effective therapies, but also a sense of hopefulness that their disease may be eliminated or checked. Organ-sparing procedures, both for primary resections as well as those involving metastatic disease, is becoming a widely applied principle throughout all cancer therapies. Recognition that larger, more ablative procedures are not more effective in general is now appreciated as is the fact that they limit the quality of life as well as future options. The recent advent of minimally invasive or video-assisted procedures using fiber optic devices has now made it possible to minimize the trauma, hospitalization, and recovery from many aggressive regional therapies involving metastasectomy, irradiation, application of cryotherapy, and regional chemotherapy. This is to be applauded and encouraged and we hope that this book will capture the major thrust in this area.

Cancer is clearly a genetic disorder characterized by its stepwise evolution in a host, which generally restricts its growth successfully. The acquisition of genetic mutations or alteration in their expression characterizes the three major genetic alterations associated with tumor progression. These include 1) acquisition of genetic mutations which allow continued growth (*ras, myc,* BRCA1) or tumor suppressor genes which usually limit tumor growth (p53, p16, RB); 2) genetic alterations which regulate cell death (*BCL-2*, Fas, p53); and 3) gene products which regulate immune recognition by immunologic effectors (ß2 microglobulin, Class I MHC, TAP, etc). Further understanding of these genetic alterations will allow for targeted strategies designed to limit tumor growth. Ultimately prevention strategies will likely obviate much of the necessity for many of the therapeutic modalities described here.

Michael T. Lotze
Joshua T. Rubin

Acknowledgments

We appreciate the patience and continued goodwill and support of our editor, Mr. Stuart Freeman and the editorial assistance of Margaret Corson, Kathy Rakow, and Maria Bond.

INTRODUCTION

The Role of Regional Therapy for Patients with Advanced Cancer (Regional Therapies for Regional Disease)

Local therapies for local disease, systemic therapies for systemic disease.

—*Edward Scanlon*

Cancer is a genetic disorder, and as such there are multiple pathways that regulate cell growth or death, the immune response, and, ultimately, the control of tumor. These vary from patient to patient. Many of the clinical trials in patients with various malignancies have failed to stratify for the molecular alterations associated with tumor growth, and these changes will probably be the basis for future clinical trials and observations. As such, individual therapies may very well have had only limited efficacy based on the patient's tumor or the inherent host response. As shown in Table 1, survival is improved in patients with localized disease and limited (but not nonexistent) in those with regional or distant disease (1). Improving the lot of these patients is the major goal and the daily task of most cancer clinicians.

Just as lymphomas are treated based on a difference in acquired or inherited mutations and relative aggressiveness, solid tumor treatment may in the future be distinguished by the role of local and regional approaches that reflect each tumor's aggressiveness. For example, in a recent article by Kirkwood and colleagues (2), it appears that patients with clinically and pathologically positive nodes did better when treated with adjuvant alpha-interferon after resection. When examined carefully, however, the survival of the treated group who had clinically and pathologically negative lymph nodes, even those with melanomas >4 mm, was, if anything, somewhat worse. Individualized treatments reflecting the biology of the patient's tumor appear warranted.

The patients who continue to come back to see us are those whose tumor growth is perhaps a bit less rapid and for whom selected therapies designed to limit disease progression and palliate symptoms are warranted. Patients often are surprised to find that they have hepatic or pulmonary metastatic disease when they feel quite well. This almost certainly reflects the lack of an effective immune response that is associated with the acute illnesses we observe with many viral or bacterial infections.

Recent advances in oncologic management—minimally invasive organ-sparing procedures, interoperative radiation therapy, gamma knife procedures, cryotherapy,

TABLE 1. *Cancer statistics 1996—5-year relative survival (%) by race and stage at diagnosis*

Organ	White			African-American		
	Local	Regional	Distant	Local	Regional	Distant
Lung	48	18	2	42	13	2
Breast	97	76	20	89	60	17
Prostate	99	93	31	90	77	25
Colon and Rectum	92	63	7	86	59	5
Pancreas	12	4	2	11	8	2
Ovary	91	49	23	83	47	22
Liver	14	8	2	11	5	0
Stomach	57	21	2	57	24	3
Melanoma	94	60	16	86	ID	ID
Bladder	94	50	7	79	38	4

From Parker SL, Tong T, Bolden S, Wingo PA. Cancer statistics, 1996. *CA Cancer J Clin* 1996;65:5–27.
ID, insufficient data.

TABLE 2. *Approach to the patient with advanced cancer*

I. Define nature of the malignancy
  A. Histology—special stains; define tissue of origin
  B. Molecular biology—genes mutated
  C. Angiogenesis
  D. Karyotype
  E. Tumor doubling time
II. Define extent of the malignancy
  A. Regional
    1. Selective node mapping; LN dissection; endoscopic ultrasound
    2. Negative margins to surgical resection
  B. Systemic
    1. CT/MRI
    2. CXR/routine labs
  C. Bone marrow aspirate/PCR on blood for informative markers/MRI of bone marrow
III. Define host reserve
  A. Pulmonary/cardiac
  B. Hepatic
  C. Renal
  D. Immunologic
IV. Outline plan of therapy
  A. Define goals
    1. Tumor control
    2. Immunologic reserve
    3. Palliation
  B. Limit injury to host

regional chemotherapy or immunotherapy—are described in this text. We are not advocating the global application of such regional approaches to all patients, but we suggest that for selected patients in whom systemic therapies have been largely ineffective, such approaches can both maintain organ and immunologic reserve and control tumor.

As shown in Table 2, there are four major issues in the approach to the patient with advanced cancer. The first is to define the nature of the malignancy, based on its histology and other clinical factors that affect outcome. These include defining, if possible, the precise mutations associated with the malignancy and defining the nature of the vascular or angiogenic response, the karyotype, and the tumor doubling time. The latter can vary considerably for various metastatic epithelial neoplasms and ranges from 30 to 120 days. The second issue is to define the extent of the malignancy—is it regionally limited? Recently, bone marrow aspirates, PCR evaluation of cells

circulating in the blood (3), and MRI of the long bones of the femur have been helpful in defining the extent of the malignancy (4). The third goal is to define the host factors important in tolerating regional or systemic therapies. In addition to the usual evaluation of organ function (eg, heart, lungs, liver, kidney) and the host immune response (including DTH to recall antigens), T-cell infiltrate within the tumor (5) has been defined in a wide range of malignancies (see Chap. 2). Infiltrate with dendritic cells has been noted to be clinically relevant in many tumors (6,7). Finally, one must outline the plan of therapy, defining carefully the goals of therapy and always considering aspects of limiting injury to the patient to increase the quality and quantity of life.

This book is organized into seven general sections. The basic principles of metastatic disease, both metastases to regional lymph nodes and systemic metastases, are found in Section I. Sections II–VI discusses organ- and region-specific therapies. Special topics—palliation of pain, development of gene therapies, and endocrine neoplasms—are considered in Section VII. We anticipate that this book will go into additional editions, and we would be pleased to receive any comments or criticisms about its organization or content.

REFERENCES

1. Parker SL, Tong T, Bolden S. Wingo PA. Cancer statistics, 1996. *CA Cancer J Clin* 1996;65:5–27.
2. Kirkwood JM, Strawderman MH, Ernstoff MS, Smith TJ, Borden EC, Blum RH. Interferon alpha-2b adjuvant therapy of high-risk resected cutaneous melanoma: The Eastern Cooperative Oncology Group Trial EST 1684. *J Clin Oncol* 1996;14(1):7–17.
3. Ghossein RA, Scher HI, Gerlad WL, et al. Detection of circulating tumor cells in patients with localized metastatic prostatic carcinoma. Clinical Implications. *J Clin Oncol* 1995;5:1195–1200.
4. Sanal SM, Flickinger FW, Caudell MJ, Sherry RM. Detection of bone marrow involvement in breast cancer with magnetic resonance imaging. *J Clin Oncol* 1994;12:1415–1421.
5. Pupa SM, Bufalino R, Invernizzi AM, et al. Macrophage infiltrate and prognosis in c-erbB-2-overexpressing breast carcinomas. *J Clin Oncol* 1996;14:85–94.
6. Tazi A, Bouchonnet F, Grandsaigne M, Boumsell L, Hance AJ, Soler P. Evidence that granulocyte macrophage-colony-stimulating factor regulates the distribution and differentiated state of dendritic cells/Langerhans cells in human lung and lung cancers. *J Clin Invest* 1993;91:566–576.
7. Zeid NA, Muller HK. S100 positive dendritic cells in human lung tumors associated with cell differentiation and enhanced survival. *Pathology* 1993;25:338–343.

CHAPTER 1

Biology of Cancer Metastases

Hematogenous Dissemination

Ronald H. Goldfarb, Richard P. Kitson, and Kenneth W. Brunson

Dramatic advances in patient care and cancer therapy have led to more favorable clinical results for many patients, but many others die from cancer metastases that are refractory to therapy. . . . Successful diagnosis and treatment of metastatic cancers can only advance with growing knowledge of the pathogenesis of metastasis and the unique properties of highly malignant cells and their host microenvironments, as well as the development of new approaches for the treatment of metastases.

—Nicolson and Fidler (14)

BACKGROUND

For more than a decade many reviews and even volumes have been devoted to various aspects of the history and clinical rationale for the importance of investigating the properties of metastatic tumor cells and the processes of cancer invasion and metastatic spread (1–20). For more detailed historical and comprehensive overviews pertaining to multiple aspects of cancer invasion and metastasis, the reader is referred to some of these earlier reviews, which are beyond the scope of the current chapter.

History

Investigations of cancer metastasis have been documented as early as 1889, when Paget proposed the "seed

and soil" hypothesis of metastatic cancer spread, suggesting that certain tumor cells ("seeds") grew best in certain favorable organ microenvironments ("soil") (21). Seminal studies in our understanding of cancer metastasis were made by Dr. Bernard Fisher and colleagues, who showed that regional lymph nodes do not function as effective barriers to tumor cell dissemination, that tumor cells can traverse regional lymph nodes to gain access to efferent lymph or the blood, that tumor cells do not necessarily lodge in the first organ capillary bed encountered during metastatic tumor dissemination, and that dormant tumor cells in animals could be stimulated to become manifest metastases (reviewed in 22). This led to important conceptual advances concerning metastatic spread and the relationship between primary and metastatic tumors that have had an impact on research to the current time.

Rationale and Clinical Significance

The invasive and metastatic properties of malignant tumor cells define the most serious clinical situations for patients with solid malignant neoplasms and are responsible for most of the morbidity and mortality that accompanies advanced cancer. Subpopulations of tumor cells can detach from the primary tumor site, undergo neovascularization, invade surrounding normal tissues, and successfully form widespread, disseminated colonies of tumor cells distant from the site of the primary tumor. These disseminated colonies are referred to as cancer metastases and arise following the sequence of events that define the cascade of tumor spread (Fig. 1) (1–4). At the time of diagnosis of patients who present with pri-

R. H. Goldfarb and K. W. Brunson: University of Pittsburgh Cancer Institute; Department of Pathology, University of Pittsburgh School of Medicine, Pittsburgh, Pennsylvania 15213-2582.

R. P. Kitson: Department of Cell Biology and Physiology, University of Pittsburgh School of Medicine, Pittsburgh, Pennsylvania, 15213-2582.

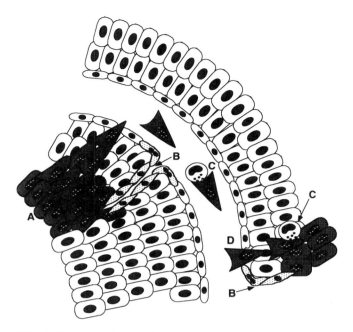

FIG. 1. Sequential steps in the process of cancer metastasis. Tumor cells (*shaded triangles*) are shown arising among normal cells to produce a primary tumor (**A**). Following growth and neovascularization, subpopulations of these cells can invade through vascular endothelial cells (**B**) and their subendothelial basement membranes to enter the vasculature. In the vasculature, tumor cells must survive biophysical shear of blood flow and attack by host effector cells of the immune response such as natural killer cells (**C**). Many tumor cells are destroyed in the vasculature, but subpopulations survive to extravasate through the endothelial cells (**B**) or exposed subendothelial basement membranes at the site of the secondary tumor (**D**). On entry into the stroma of the distant organ site, metastatic cells undergo angiogenesis and proliferation. There they must also evade immune attack by effector cells such as natural killer cells (**C**).

mary solid malignant neoplasms, more than half already have often undetectable microscopic metastases in organ sites distant from the primary lesion (5–7). The problem is complicated by the tumor cell heterogeneity that often occurs with malignant tumor growth and progression (1, 8–11). Investigation of the phenotypic properties of both primary and metastatic tumors has revealed heterogeneous subpopulations that differ in immunogenicity, biochemical and cell surface components, karyotype and growth behavior, and susceptibility to chemotherapy or radiotherapy, as well as to recognition and destruction by immune effector cells (8–11). The differing properties, including metastatic potential, of these phenotypically heterogeneous tumor cell subpopulations are important for determination of molecular properties of highly metastatic tumor cells and also have potential therapeutic implications, because the most metastatic subpopulations of tumor cells often appear to be the most resistant to therapy with many currently available antitumor agents (8–10). There is therefore a critical need for the develop-

ment of more effective approaches for the early diagnosis and the treatment of established cancer metastases.

This chapter will provide an overview of the cellular and molecular properties of malignant tumor cells that contribute to tumor cell invasiveness, metastatic spread, the initiation of metastasis formation at distant sites, and the properties of cancer cells, including their invasiveness and proliferation, within the microenvironment of established cancer metastases. This includes the interactions of invasive, metastatic tumor cells with the host microvasculature, the angiogenic properties of metastatic tumor cells, and the interactions of malignant cells with both endothelial cells and subendothelial extracellular matrices and with effector cells of the host immune response. We will also discuss how an understanding of the cellular properties of metastatic tumor cells can provide insights toward improved strategies for the earlier diagnosis of micrometastases and for treatment of established metastatic tumors.

METASTATIC CASCADE (INVASION, METASTASIS, ARREST, EXTRAVASATION, GROWTH)

Progressive steps in malignant neoplastic growth lead to tumor invasion and cancer metastasis. Following the neoplastic transformation of normal cells to form benign neoplastic cells, tumor progression ensues. When a tumor reaches a small mass of approximately 1 to 2 mm in diameter, angiogenesis factors are produced that induce new blood vessel formation within tumors, allowing for nutrient supply. Subpopulations of tumor cells in the primary tumor locally invade host stroma, penetrate the host microvasculature, and enter the circulation. This process appears to employ both degradative proteolytic enzymes and autocrine motility factors produced by invasive tumor cells. Single tumor cells or clumplike emboli of tumor cells that gain access to the vasculature are largely destroyed by elements of the host immune response or by physical shear forces of blood flow. Only a subpopulation of the cells that enter the vasculature can adhere to either the endothelial cells of host target organs or to exposed subendothelial extracellular matrix basement membranes. Tumor cells can extravasate out of the vasculature into the perivascular stroma by employing steps similar to those seen in initial tumor invasion. Following implantation within the parenchyma of the target organ, tumor cells proliferate during the formation and growth of secondary tumor metastases. To grow and survive, such micrometastases must again escape the attack of host effector cells of the immune response and maintain invasive and angiogenic functions within the metastatic microenvironment. This allows for continued growth and progression, which can lead to further metastatic spread and the formation of more metastases at additional sites—metastases arising from metastases. This process is reviewed in Fig. 1.

While the process of cancer metastasis represents a fascinating sequence of biochemical and molecular interactions, interest in this process is not restricted to academic curiosity with these dynamic and complex cellular events. Cancer metastases are known to be the predominant cause of treatment failure, morbidity, and death for patients or animals with solid malignancies (15). While the treatment modalities of chemotherapy, radiotherapy, and surgical intervention effectively treat about half the patients who have developed malignant tumors, most of the patients who are refractile to these therapeutic approaches yield to the direct or indirect effects of established tumor metastases or to the adverse sequelae associated with these therapeutic approaches. At the time of diagnosis of primary tumors, about half the patients with solid malignant tumors already have established micrometastases, which often with time expand and contribute to damage to the host organs. Indeed, a detected metastatic deposit in an organ may indicate the presence of additional undetected micrometastases (6). The heterogeneity of subpopulations of metastatic tumor cells, coupled with the widespread anatomic distribution of tumor metastases, often limits or prevents effective surgical or chemotherapeutic treatment approaches. Moreover, some of these treatment modalities can lead to immunosuppression and subsequent mortality arising from infectious disease. It is therefore quite important to employ tumor models that as much as possible mimic these critical aspects of the pathophysiology of human malignancy, including metastatic spread and the outgrowth of established tumor metastases (18).

In recent years significant insights into the progressive stages of malignant neoplastic growth, particularly tumor invasion and metastatic spread, have arisen from basic research dealing with molecular biology, biochemistry, cell biology, and immunology and the study of selective experimental therapeutic agents. Insights into the mechanisms of tumor progression leading to metastasis have emphasized biochemical and molecular mechanisms of tumor angiogenesis and tumor invasion, modes of tumor spread, and metastasis. Moreover, emphasis has been placed on the importance of tumor cell heterogeneity, host vasculature, and the immune response. As a result, significant progress has been made in understanding the biochemical mechanisms operative in tumor invasion and in understanding lymphatic and hematogenous tumor spread.

Recent studies have continued to elucidate the biochemical, cellular, and molecular mechanisms that underlie tumor invasiveness and cancer metastasis (15,23). During tumor invasiveness, malignant cells penetrate a number of barriers, including extracellular matrices. These extracellular matrices include dense, overarching lattices of collagen and elastin embedded within a net-work of glycoproteins and proteoglycans (6). One specialized extracellular matrix that is penetrated as metastatic tumor cells cross tissue boundaries is the basement membrane. The basement membrane is composed of type IV collagen and specific glycoproteins, including entactin, laminin, and heparan sulfate proteoglycans (24). Basement membranes and interstitial stroma separate tissue compartments from each other and must be traversed during tumor invasion.

Subpopulations of cells leave the primary tumor and interact with extracellular matrices at a number of stages during the metastatic process, including tumor cell entry into or exit from the vasculature, the invasion of muscle and nerve, and the penetration of epithelial barriers. During the invasion into or out of blood vessels (intravasation or extravasation), invasive tumor cells enter through areas they have degraded in the wall of a capillary or venule and must cross the perivascular interstitial stroma before the growth of metastatic colonies in the parenchyma of the organ seeded by the metastatic tumor cells. Aspects of the homing of metastatic tumor cells to target organs depends on the interaction of tumor cell surface molecules with the microvascular endothelial cells associated within these organs, as described above (24–26).

The degradation of extracellular matrices by invasive tumor cells has been shown to take place in several stages. The first step is tumor cell attachment to subendothelial extracellular matrices by cell surface receptors that bind to specific matrix components. The second step of matrix invasion is related to tumor cell protease-mediated degradation of the matrix. Considerable evidence exists in the literature that various degradative enzymes, including matrix metalloproteinases that degrade type IV collagen and neutral serine proteases that degrade noncollagenous components of extracellular matrices, play a key role in tumor invasiveness (15,23,27–29). The third step is tumor cell locomotion into areas of the matrix locally degraded by tumor cell-associated proteolytic enzymes. Migration of tumor cells employs movement along chemotactic or haptotactic gradients of components of extracellular matrices, including degradation products arising from limited proteolysis, as well as the use of tumor cell-associated autocrine motility factors. Continued invasion of the extracellular matrix may take place by repetition of these steps (24–28).

The steps of cancer metastasis are complex and selective and depend on both the properties of the tumor (eg, tumor invasiveness) and the properties of the host (eg, the immune response and host and tumor vasculature) (15,18,29). During the process of metastatic spread, tumor cells must overcome or evade systemic and locoregional host immune responses (eg, lymphoid effector cells that can infiltrate, accumulate within, and exhibit antitumor reactivity within tumor metastases). Moreover, following the establishment of tumor metastases in distant organs, the tumor cells can undergo neovascularization and colonial outgrowth, which is also under complex and dynamic regulation dependent on the host and tumor (15,18).

Much evidence exists that the immune response plays an important role in preventing metastatic spread; it may also be a potential therapeutic approach for the control of established tumor metastases (reviewed in 30). While a detailed survey of the immune response to cancer, including tumor metastases, is beyond the scope of this chapter, it is noteworthy that some components of the immune response have been shown to play important roles in protecting against the onset of tumor metastases and in the therapy of advanced tumors, including tumor metastases. Substantial knowledge exists regarding tumor-associated antigens and the role of antibodies and cellular immunity in cancer, the characteristics and basic mechanisms of antitumor effector cells, the role of immune effector cells within the tumor microenvironment, tumor-infiltrating lymphocytes in solid tumors, and the localization of effector cells of the immune response into tumor metastases (30). In recent years, a significant number of preclinical and clinical studies have shown the therapeutic potential for malignancies by immunomodulation for immunotherapy. The reader is directed toward a recent summary of immunity and cancer therapy that highlights major approaches in immune intervention, including tumor vaccines, immunoaugmenting and immunomodulating agents, antibodies, cytokines, and adoptive cell transfer (31). Natural killer (NK) cells and activated natural killer (A-NK) cells have been found to play a particularly important role in the prevention of metastases, and on activation with cytokines, including interleukin-2, have been found to accumulate within established metastases following their adoptive transfer (32,33).

It is also increasingly recognized that the progression of cancer cells to the invasive and malignant phenotype involves the response of metastatic tumor cells to mitogenic signals within the microenvironment of established cancer metastases (34). Indeed, the progression of cancer cells to an autonomous state of growth regulation leading to the proliferation of tumor cells within metastases appears to be under growth-control mechanisms distinct from tumor cells within primary neoplasms (34).

SELECTIVITY OF ORGAN DISTRIBUTION AND ROLE OF ORGAN MICROENVIRONMENT

Organ-specific colonization by metastatic tumor cells appears to be under the influence of various adhesive molecules, including those of endothelial cells (35). Such molecules are components of the organ-specific microvasculature and can be modulated through interactions with distinct extracellular matrix regulatory growth macromolecules. The heterogeneity of endothelial cells also affects the binding of metastatic tumor cells; more-

over, cytokines within the tumor microenvironment can also regulate the adhesion of tumor cells to the microvascular endothelium (35). Following their adherence to the endothelium by either specific or nonspecific mechanisms, tumor cells can then bind, often preferentially, to subendothelial extracellular matrices such as basement membranes.

It has been argued that the survival and growth of metastatic tumor cells is influenced by and dependent on the environment of the target organ (1,34,36,37). Microenvironmental stimuli, including growth factors, hormones, cytokines, adhesion molecule receptors, and degradative enzymes, might lead to modulation of the tumor cell phenotype to effect tumor cell survival, outgrowth, and expansion (37). Such microenvironmental issues, including the localization of tumor cells within growing, established metastases, can also affect how tumor cells respond to local fluctuations of blood flow rate, distribution of microvessels, pH, cellular waste accumulation, oxygen, and growth regulation in response to hypoxia. Considerable emphasis has recently been placed on both organ-specific growth factors and the influence of the target organ environment on the invasive potential of metastatic tumor cells and the effect of the organ environment on the response of metastases to therapeutic approaches, including chemotherapy (37). Interestingly, the extracellular matrix can also modulate the expression of adhesion molecules on the surface of endothelial cells. Moreover, the expression of integrins on tumor cells has been associated with site-specific metastatic spread and the surface phenotype of metastatic tumor cells (35,37,38). It has also recently been recognized that the properties of metastatic tumor cells, including sensitivity to chemotherapeutic drugs, can be strongly influenced by the microenvironment, especially whether or not the tumor is present in orthotopic or ectopic sites (39).

CELL–CELL INTERACTION/ADHESION

It is widely accepted that the modulation of cell surface adhesion molecules is critical to the process of tumor progression and of particular importance to tumor invasion and metastatic cancer spread to secondary organs (25). It is now also appreciated that endothelial cell adhesion molecules may also play a role in organ-specific colonization (35). Adhesive properties contribute to the capacity of tumor cells to move to distant sites and to disrupt their adhesive connections at primary sites before release into the circulation. Tumor cells also employ adhesion molecules for migration via the production and disruption of adhesive connections to various matrices and cell types. It has therefore been suggested that interference with cell adhesiveness should be able to lead to inhibition or regulation of tumor cell migration and invasiveness. A focus of research in cancer metastasis has therefore included the investigation of factors contributing to tumor cell lodgement, the interaction of tumor cells with platelets and with various organ-specific interactions that allow tumor cells to lodge selectively in target organs. These include interactions with vascular endothelial cells, subendothelial basement membranes, and other extracellular matrices (38).

TUMOR CELL INTERACTIONS WITH THE VASCULATURE

Cancer cells derived from primary tumors follow various routes of dissemination, including the veins, the lymphatics, and various body cavities. These routes often involve an invasive process characterized by degradation of the basement membrane-like extracellular matrices that act as barriers to separate the primary tumor from adjacent normal tissues, surround the vessels, and inhibit the invasive intravasation and extravasation of malignant tumor cells. The most frequent routes of tumor cell dissemination are by the bloodstream and the lymphatics.

As indicated in Fig. 1, the process of cancer metastasis can be classified into a number of discrete stages that must be completed before tumor cells can grow within the environment of the distant micrometastatic site. Following invasion and residence within the host vasculature, metastatic tumor cells must survive in the host bloodstream, enter and bind to endothelial cells within the vessel of the new host organ, and extravasate out of the vessel into the site of the host organ. While it is widely recognized that the vascular circulation is involved in the transport of tumor cells to distant sites, it is not always emphasized how important a role the vasculature plays in many of the steps of metastatic spread (40–44).

TUMOR ANGIOGENESIS

During tumor growth and progression, tumor cells are constantly in contact with vascular elements. Indeed, angiogenesis is a requirement for tumor growth, and vascular outgrowth is often proportional to tumor growth as sprouts migrating from pre-existing venules (39). Metastatic tumor cells interact with the vasculature at various steps during metastatic spread and in several ways, including:

Tumor cell shedding into the vasculature
The growth and function of tumor vasculature
The role of tumor blood vessels as a barrier to tumor cell release into the host vasculature
Vascular permeability
Intravasation of tumor cells
Transport of tumor cells in the bloodstream
The initial arrest of tumor cells

Adherence of tumor cells to components of the vasculature (including microvascular endothelial cells)
Extravasation of tumor cells
Motility of tumor cells
Degradation of vascular basement membranes and the growth of metastatic tumor cells
Angiogenesis within metastatic tumors
The function of the microvasculature of established metastatic tumors (24,40).

Tumor vessels are often thin-walled and leaky and lack a basement membrane. The entry of tumor cells into the bloodstream is an early and critical aspect of metastatic tumor spread and depends on the spatial relationship of tumor cells to tumor-induced blood vessels. These vessels are poor barriers to tumor cell passage and are not good barriers for the extravasation of tumor cells across the vessel wall into the circulation. Tumor cells that have entered the bloodstream have only a very short half-life, and the capacity of the cells to metastasize is highly dependent on their ability to arrest in the microvasculature at a secondary organ site, leave the bloodstream, and invade the host parenchymal tissue. These processes, in turn, are highly dependent on degradation of subendothelial basement membrane extracellular matrices, migration across the vessel wall into the parenchymal space, and proliferation at the secondary site of tumor growth (24,40). Such secondary growth of tumors is often site-specific and dependent on organ-specific vascular adhesion factors, growth factors, and chemoattractants. Lastly, solid tumor growth at the secondary site and further metastasis from metastases is also dependent on the growth of new blood vessels at the site of metastatic tumor growth.

TUMOR VASCULATURE

In recent years considerable effort has been placed on the investigation of how the tumor microvasculature is distinct from that of normal tissues. While the tumor vasculature originates from the host, the organization of the tumor vasculature may be very different from the host, depending on the tumor type, its location, and its growth rate. Moreover, tumor vasculature within peripheral and central areas of the tumor has been investigated. In tumors with peripheral vascularization, the center of the tumor often appears to be poorly perfused. Tumors often exhibit both types of vascular patterns (41). Microscopically, the tumor vasculature is heterogeneous and does not always exhibit the standard vascular organization of flow from artery to arteriole to capillaries to postcapillary venules to venules to veins. In contrast, ultrastructural studies have revealed that tumor vessels can include arteries and arterioles, nonfenestrated capillaries, fenestrated capillaries, discontinuous capillaries, blood channels without endothelial lining, capillary sprouts, post-capillary venules, venules and veins, and arteriovenous anastomoses/shunts (41). A key difference between normal and tumor vessels is that the latter are dilated, saccular, and tortuous and may contain tumor cells within the endothelial lining of the wall of the vessel. Moreover, in contrast to normal tissues, a tumor may have blood flowing from one venule to another or by an arteriovenous shunt. The branching patterns of blood vessels in a tumor are quite distinct from those in normal tissue, with many bi- or trifurcations, loops, and sprouts. Vascularization, therefore, plays a critical role in tumor biology and is central to angiogenesis.

TUMOR BLOOD FLOW

The tumor vasculature also affects the response to local therapy. One important component of the complex nature of tumor microcirculation is tumor blood flow. Many attempts have been made to control and reverse tumor growth based on the response of malignant tissue to pharmacologic agents. Some investigators have appreciated that blood flow plays a key role in this regard, both to transport active agents and to determine the response of tissue to their delivery. In other words, the control of tumor blood flow can be quite important in various strategies for the design of cancer treatments. In addition to pharmacologic approaches, emphasis has also been focused on various aspects of blood flow, including blood supply, pressure, viscosity, and vessel geometry. It has long been thought that the outcome of such approaches might lead to the increase or decrease of tumor blood flow, which might be helpful with delivering therapeutic agents or inhibiting tumor growth directly, respectively.

Tumor blood flow has been extensively investigated in several experimental tumors by various techniques (42). Heterogeneity in tumor blood flow has been noted and has been a challenge in identifying reproducible techniques for monitoring tumor blood flow. Considerable time and effort has therefore been devoted by many investigators to measure total blood flow, local tumor blood flow, intratumor blood flow distribution, and the influence of vasoactive drugs on tumor blood flow (42). Many investigators have measured the local blood flow rate of tumors based on the uptake or clearance of a tracer from a single region, or several regions, of the tumor. Spatial and temporal heterogeneity in tumor blood supply raises doubts as to whether such values are representative for the whole tumor. Some studies in which the blood flow rate of the whole tumor has been measured have shown that the average perfusion rate of the tumor (eg, carcinomas) is less than that of the host origin. Generally, as tumors grow to larger sizes, they often develop necrotic foci, with resultant decreases in perfusion rate with tumor size (41,42). Well-defined experimental sys-

tems of the angioarchitecture of tumors, including vascular density, vascular length, distance between tissues and their nearest blood vessel, and the length of microvascular network per unit area, have been used to investigate issues related to blood supply in tumors that increase in size (43). Low-flow and no-flow areas of tumors have been described during tumor progression that appear to confer resistance to the delivery of anticancer drugs.

A number of studies have revealed that blood flow in tumor vessels is intermittent, with random periods of flow reduction and stasis followed by resumption of flow, sometimes in opposite directions. Such fluctuations may be related to host arteriole vasomotor activity, the respiratory or cardiac cycle, low perfusion pressures in tumor vessels, elevated interstitial tumor pressure in tumors, or rheologic factors related to the passage of red blood cells, white blood cells, or cancer cells in a blood vessel (42). A number of studies have investigated tumor blood flow as a functional characteristic of tumor vessels (44). Some studies, for example, have employed angiotensin II to elevate blood pressure to yield an enhancement in tumor blood flow without increasing blood flow in normal tissue and uninvolved tissue in tumor-bearing animals. This type of study has suggested that the delivery of systemic anticancer drugs could be enhanced in tumor tissue by the induction of hypertension. Interestingly, at least one study found parallel increases in angiotensin II-induced hypertension on tumor interstitial tumor pressure and tumor blood flow, failing to support the view that elevated pressure leads to vascular collapse to decrease tumor blood flow (45).

Tumor blood flow has widely been considered to be an important determinant of the effectiveness of cancer chemotherapy, and the delivery of anticancer drugs to tumor tissues is thought to be dependent on the flow rate of circulating blood in the tumor (46). It has been suggested that anticancer therapy may be viewed as a direct local tumor blood flow microvascular event highly dependent on the features of the tumor microcirculation and highly specialized when compared to normal tissue. While this has been recognized for the delivery of anticancer agents, it has also been considered important for radiologic and hyperthermia-based approaches to treatment of cancer. Moreover, it has increasingly been appreciated that tumor blood flow itself can be modified to have effects on the destruction of tumor cells. For example, it has been suggested that agents such as interleukin-1, tumor necrosis factor, and flavone acetic acid might contribute to tumor cell destruction via hemorrhagic necrosis related to diminishment of blood flow (47–49).

While a number of approaches, including biologic therapies (eg, interleukin-1, TNF, and flavone acetic acid), hyperthermia, and photodynamic therapies, have attempted to target vascular effects in connection with anticancer therapies, and while some vasoactive agents may either enhance or decrease blood flow, there remains the need to define and identify agents that have significant effects on blood flow that can be characterized for their antitumor effects (50). In particular, the need remains to characterize the effects of such compounds on established cancer metastases and on the properties of the tumor vasculature, tumor angiogenesis, and tumor invasiveness.

Indeed, recent studies have described the location, morphologic appearance, origin, and density of microvessels of B16 melanoma metastases (51). This has led to the description of four types of B16 melanoma metastases: superficial or deep loose (microvessel-rich) or superficial or deep compact (devoid of microvessels or hypovascular) tumors. These insights into the distribution and connection of pre-existing and newly formed vessels in relation to B16 melanoma metastases in mouse lungs provide an important system for determining the effects of experimental antimetastatic therapeutic agents on blood flow to established tumors with varying degrees of vascularization. This in turn will allow for the resolution of whether such compounds function only on tumor blood flow or also exert antitumor activity in tumors devoid of or low in microvessels (51). This may be of particular importance for studies with microvascular endothelial cells, which for the first time were recently isolated from established tumors (52). Studies with such tumor-derived microvascular endothelial cells should soon allow for the investigation of the possible role of cytokine activation of microvascular endothelial cells. This is of interest because it has been reported that B16 melanoma-associated microvessel endothelial cells, on activation by cytokines, have the potential to lyse tumor cells (53). It has indeed been reported that nitric oxide plays a role in the lysis of tumor cells by cytokine-activated endothelial cells (54).

METASTATIC TUMOR CELLS INTERACT WITH BOTH EFFECTOR CELLS AND MICROVASCULAR ENDOTHELIAL CELLS

Recent studies have continued to explore effector cells of the immune response and their interaction with metastatic tumor cells and their reactivity within established cancer metastases (29–33). Studies with A-NK cells reflect progress in this area. It has recently been shown that fluorescently labeled, adoptively transferred A-NK cells selectively accumulate by 16 hours within pulmonary and hepatic metastases (55,56). Ultrastructural studies have revealed that A-NK cells can migrate out of tumor vessels and can establish direct contact with both tumor cells and microvascular endothelial cells (55). The significance of the observed in situ interactions of effector A-NK cells within metastases with both tumor cells and microvascular endothelial cells have been further investigated in an in vitro system that investigated the

binding of A-NK cells to microvascular endothelial cells (57). It is likely that such approaches will allow for the elucidation of candidate molecular mechanisms responsible for the findings observed in situ. It is also noteworthy that because adoptively transferred A-NK cells have the capacity to accumulate within tumor metastases, they might constitute excellent candidate vehicles for locoregionally transporting therapeutic anticancer drugs to the site of cancer metastases, in addition to functioning as potentially exciting vehicles for gene therapy (56,58).

INTERVENTION AGAINST METASTATIC SPREAD AND THERAPY OF ESTABLISHED METASTATIC CANCER

As our understanding of the properties of metastatic tumor cells and the complex interactions between tumor cells, effector cells of the immune response, and the vasculature becomes clarified, novel strategies for inhibiting metastatic spread and for treating established cancer metastases should emerge. These will probably include new therapeutic modalities as well as new uses for existing agents that might better be locoregionally employed for nontoxic and selective targeting of tumor metastases than has been possible to date. A better understanding of the tumor microenvironment is likely to provide insights for formulating new strategies for the discovery and development of new agents and approaches for enhanced efficacy for the therapy of metastatic cancer (1,37). A number of recent reviews have described agents that either inhibit metastatic spread or are used to treat established cancer metastases (15,18,29). Indeed, it is quite encouraging that a number of novel approaches for the treatment of cancer metastasis are emerging that exploit our current knowledge of tumor cell biology and the pathophysiology of metastatic spread. For example, monoclonal antibodies directed against tumor vessel fibronectin in the subendothelial extracellular matrix can be used to deliver vasoactive agents to tumors (59), and heretofore undescribed combination therapies for treatment of cancer metastases have been reported. These include the combination of matrix metalloproteinase inhibitors and cytotoxic anticancer drugs (60) and the use of chemotherapeutic agents followed by adoptive therapy with A-NK cells (61). The latter study provides an encouraging approach that can overcome the barriers to drug delivery to tumors that often limit the use of conventional anticancer agents (61,62). Indeed, it is likely that adoptively transferred A-NK cells, either alone or as a vehicle for locoregional drug delivery, might be effective in the orthotopic or in situ microenvironment of tumor metastases and reach metastatic tumor cells to allow for effective locoregional therapeutic effects with minimal toxicity to normal cells (61,62). In this manner, an understanding of cancer metastases might allow for the optimal delivery of molecular medicines to cancer metastases (62). It is likely that additional innovative approaches will continue to be developed as our understanding of the issues described in this chapter are elucidated.

REFERENCES

1. Fidler IJ. Modulation of the organ microenvironment for treatment of cancer metastasis. *J Natl Cancer Inst* 1995;87;1588.
2. Fidler IJ. Critical factors in the biology of human cancer metastasis: Twenty-eighth G.H.A. Clowes Memorial Award lecture. *Cancer Res* 1990;50:6130.
3. Nicolson GL, Brunson KW, Fidler IJ. Specificity of arrest, survival, and growth of selected metastatic variant cell lines. *Cancer Res* 1978;38:4105.
4. Grundmann E, ed. *Metastatic tumor growth*. Stuttgart: Gustav Fischer Verlag, 1980.
5. Nicolson GL, Poste G. Tumor cell diversity and host responses in cancer metastasis—Part 1. *Current Problems in Cancer* 1982;7:3.
6. Liotta LA, Hart IR, eds. *Tumor invasion and metastasis*. The Hague: Martinus Nijhoff Publishers, 1982.
7. Owens AH, Coffey DS, Baylin SB, eds. *Tumor cell heterogeneity: origins and implications*. New York: Academic Press, 1982.
8. Nicolson GL. Generation of phenotypic diversity and progression in metastatic tumor cells. *Cancer Metastasis Rev* 1984;3:25.
9. Schirrmacher V. Cancer metastasis; experimental approaches, theoretical concepts, and impacts for treatment strategies. *Adv Cancer Res* 1985;43:1.
10. Heppner GH. Problems posed for cancer treatment by tumor cell heterogeneity. In: Honn KV, Powers WE, Sloane BF, eds. *Mechanisms of cancer metastasis*: potential therapeutic implications. Boston: Martinus Nijhoff, 1986:69.
11. Poste G. Pathogenesis of metastatic disease; implications for current therapy and for the development of new therapeutic strategies. *Cancer Treat Rep* 1986;70:183.
12. Honn KV, Powers WE, Sloane BF, eds. *Mechanisms of cancer metastasis*. Boston: Martinus Nijhoff, 1986.
13. Welch DR, Bhuyan BK, Liotta LA, eds. *Cancer metastasis; experimental and clinical strategies*. New York: Alan R. Liss, Inc., 1986.
14. Nicolson GL, Fidler IJ, eds. *Tumor progression and metastasis*. New York: Alan R. Liss, 1988.
15. Goldfarb RH, Brunson KW. Overview of current understanding of tumor spread. In: Goldfarb RH, ed. *Fundamental aspects of cancer*. Dordrecht, Holland: Kluwer Academic Publishers, 1989:28.
16. Brunson KW, Goldfarb RH. Observations of primary and secondary lesions in the same patient. In: Levine AS, ed. *Fundamental aspects of cancer*. Dordrecht, Holland: Kluwer Academic Publishers, 1989:214.
17. Mareel MM, De Baetselier PD, Van Roy FM. *Mechanisms of invasion and metastasis*. Boca Raton: CRC Press, 1991.
18. Goldfarb RH, Brunson KW. Therapeutic agents for treatment of established metastases and inhibitors of metastatic spread; preclinical and clinical progress. *Curr Opin Oncol* 1992;4:1130.
19. Liotta LA, Stetler-Stevenson WG. Principles of molecular cell biology of cancer; cancer metastasis. In: DeVita VT, Hellman S, Rosenberg SA, eds. *Cancer: principles and practice of oncology*, 4th ed. Philadelphia: JB Lippincott, 1993:134.
20. Vile RG, ed. *Cancer metastasis; from mechanisms to therapies*. Chichester, United Kingdom: John Wiley & Sons, 1995.
21. Paget S. The distribution of secondary growths in cancer of the breast. *Lancet* 1889;1;571.
22. Fisher B. Contributions of clinical trials research to the understanding and treatment of breast cancer. In: Fortner JG, Rhoads JE, eds (General Motors Cancer Research Foundation). *Accomplishments in cancer research 1993*. Philadelphia: JB Lippincott, 1994;101.
23. Goldfarb RH, Kornblith PL. Tumor invasion and brain cancer. *J Neuro-Onc* 1994;18:5.
24. Liotta LA, Goldfarb RH. Interaction of tumor cells with the basement membrane of endothelium. In: Honn KV, Sloane BF, eds. *Hemostatic mechanisms and metastasis*. Boston: Martinus Nijhoff Publishing, Kluwer Academic Publishers Group, 1984;319.
25. Nicolson GL. Metastatic tumor interactions with endothelium, basement membrane and tissue. *Curr Opin Cell Biol* 1989;1:1009.
26. Liotta LA, Rao NC, Barsky SH, Turpeenniemi-Hujanen TM. Domains of laminin and basement membrane collagen which play a role in metastasis. In: Honn KV, Powers WE, Sloane BF, eds. *Mechanisms of cancer metastasis*. Boston: Martinus Nijhoff, 1986:299.
27. Goldfarb RH. Proteolytic enzymes in tumor invasion and degradation of host extracellular matrices. In: Honn KV, Powers WE, Sloane BF, eds. *Mechanisms of cancer metastasis*. Boston: Martinus Nijhoff, 1986:341.
28. Goldfarb RH, Liotta LA. Proteolytic enzymes in cancer invasion and metastasis. *Sem Thromb Hem* 1986;294.
29. Goldfarb RH, Brunson KW. Antimetastatic therapy. In: DeVita VT, Hellman S, Rosenberg SA, eds. *Biologic therapy of cancer*, 2d ed. Philadelphia: JB Lippincott, 1995;853.
30. Goldfarb RH, Whiteside TL, eds. *Tumor immunology and cancer therapy*. New York: Marcel Dekker, 1994.
31. Mihich E. Immunity and cancer therapy; present status and future projections. In: Goldfarb RH, Whiteside TL, eds. *Tumor immunology and cancer therapy*. New York: Marcel Dekker, 1994:293.
32. Goldfarb RH, Basse PH, Ohashi M, Kitson T, Brunson KW. Preclinical studies of IL-2 activated natural killer effector cells for locoregional therapy of metastatic cancer. *J Infus Chemo* 1994;4:77.
33. Goldfarb RH, Whiteside TL, Basse TL, Lin W-C, Vujanovic N, Herberman RB. Natural killer cells and gene therapy; potential of gene transfection for optimizing effector cell functions and for targeting gene products into tumor metastases. *Nat Immun* 1994;13:131.
34. Nicolson GL. Cancer progression and growth; relationship of paracrine and autocrine growth mechanisms to organ preference of metastasis. *Exp Cell Res* 1993;204:171.
35. Pauli BU, Augustin-Voss HG, El-Sabban ME, Johnson RC, Hammer DA. Organ preference of metastasis. *Cancer Metastasis Rev* 1990;9:175.
36. Moghaddam A, Bicknell R. The organ preference of metastasis—the journey from the circulation to the second site. In: Vile RG, ed. *Cancer metastasis, from mechanisms to therapies*. Chichester, United Kingdom: John Wiley & Sons Ltd., 1995:145.
37. Fidler IJ. Invasion and metastasis. In: Abeloff MD, Armitage JO, Lichter AS, Niederhuber JE, eds. *Clinical oncology*. New York: Churchill-Livingstone, 1995:55.
38. Rusciano D, Burger M. Why do cancer cells metastasize into particular organs? *Bioessays* 1992;14:185.
39. Folkman J. Clinical applications of research on angiogenesis. *N Engl J Med* 1995;333:1757.
40. Netland PA, Zetter BE. Tumor-cell interactions with blood vessels during cancer metastasis. In: Goldfarb RH, ed. *Cancer growth and progression; fundamental aspects of cancer*. Dordrecht, The Netherlands: Kluwer Academic Publishers, 1989:84.
41. Jain RK. Vascular and interstitial barriers to delivery of therapeutic agents in tumors. *Cancer Metastasis Rev* 1990;9:253.
42. Peterson H-I. The microcirculation of tumors. In: Orr FW, Buchanan MR, Weiss L, eds. *Microcirculation in tumor metastases*. Boca Raton: CRC Press, 1991:278.
43. Kaysuyoshi H, Suzuki M, Tanda S, Saiot T. Characterization of heterogeneous distribution of tumor blood flow in the rat. *Jpn J Cancer Res* 1991;82:109.
44. Suzuki M, Hori K, Saio S, et al. Functional characteristics of tumor vessels; selective increase in tumor blood flow. *Sci Rep Res Inst Tohoku U* 1989;36(C):1.
45. Zlotecki RA, Boucher Y, Lee I, Baxter LT, Jain RK. Effect of angiotensin II-induced hypertension on tumor blood flow and interstitial fluid pressure. *Cancer Res* 1993;53:2466.
46. Hori K, Suzuki M, Tanda S, Saito S. In vivo analysis of tumor vascularization in the rat. *Jpn J Cancer Res* 1990;81:279.
47. Braunschweiger PG, Johnson CS, Kumar N, Ord V, Furmanski P. Antitumor effects of recombinant human interleukin-1α in RIF-1 and Panc02 solid tumors. *Cancer Res* 1988;48:6011.
48. Johnson CS, Chang MJ, Braunschweiger PG, Furmanski P. Acute hemorrhagic necrosis of tumors induced by interleukin-1α; effects independent of tumor necrosis factor. *J Natl Cancer Inst* 1991;83:842.
49. Bibby MC, Double JA, Loadman PM, Duke CV. Reduction of tumor blood flow by flavone acetic acid; a possible component of therapy. *J Natl Cancer Inst* 1989;81:216.
50. Moore JV, West DC. Vasculature as a target for anti-cancer therapy. *Cancer Cells* 1991;3:100.

51. Nannmark U, Johansson BR, Bryant JL, et al. Microvessel origin and distribution in pulmonary metastases of B16 melanoma; implication for adoptive immunotherapy. *Cancer Res* 1995;55:4627.

52. Modlewski RA, Davies P, Watkins SC, Auerbach R, Chang M-J, Johnson CS. Isolation and identification of fresh tumor-derived endothelial cells from a murine RIF-1 fibrosarcoma. *Cancer Res* 1994;54:336.

53. Li L, Nicolson GL, Fidler IJ. Direct in vitro lysis of metastatic tumor cells by cytokine-activated murine vascular endothelial cells. *Cancer Res* 1991;51:245.

54. Li L, Kilbourn RG, Adams J, Fidler IJ. Role of nitric oxide in lysis of tumor cytokine-activated endothelial cells. *Cancer Res* 1991;51:2531.

55. Basse PH, Nannmark U, Johansson BR, Herberman RB, Goldfarb RH. Establishment of cell-to-cell contact by adoptively transferred adherent lymphokine-activated killer cells with metastatic murine melanoma cells. *J Natl Cancer Inst* 1991;83:944.

56. Basse P, Herberman RB, Nannmark U, et al. Accumulation of adoptively transferred adherent, lymphokine-activated killer cells in murine metastases. *J Exp Med* 1991;174:479.

57. Brunson KW, Ohashi M, Miller CA, Kitson RP, Basse PH, Goldfarb RH. Interleukin-2 (IL-2) activated natural killer (A-NK) cells; binding to microvascular endothelial cells and BRM enhancement of cytolytic activity. *In Vivo* 1994;8:71.

58. Goldfarb RH, Whiteside TL, Basse PH, Lin W-C, Vujanovic N, Herberman RB. Natural killer cells and gene therapy; potential of gene transfection for optimizing effector cell functions and for targeting gene products into tumor metastases. *Nat Immun* 1994;13:131.

59. Epstein AL, Khawli LA, Hornick JL, Taylor CR. Identification of a monoclonal antibody, TV-1, directed against the basement membrane of tumor vessels, and its use to enhance the delivery of macromolecules to tumors after conjugation with interleukin 2. *Cancer Res* 1995;55:2673.

60. Anderson IC, Shipp MA, Docherty AJP, Teicher BA. Combination therapy including a gelatinase inhibitor and cytotoxic agent reduces local invasion and metastasis of murine Lewis lung carcinoma. *Cancer Res* 1996;56:715.

61. Goldfarb RH, Ohashi M, Brunson KW, et al. Augmentation of IL-2 activated natural killer cell adoptive immunotherapy with cyclophosphamide. *Proc Am Assoc Cancer Res* 1996;37:480.

62. Jain RK. Delivery of molecular medicine to solid tumors. *Science* 1996;271:1079.

CHAPTER 2

Biology of Cancer Metastasis

Lymphatic Dissemination

Michael T. Lotze

It was indeed remarkable, then, in the majority of our experiments cancer did not extend beyond the popliteal node even after six weeks of intranodal growth. Removal of the cancerous lymph node was not followed by the development of cancer elsewhere. These results strongly emphasized the effectiveness of the lymph node as a temporary barrier to the further spread of cancer.

—*Zeidman and Buss (1)*

INTRODUCTION AND HISTORY

The term *lymph* comes from the Greek "nymph," a creature living by clear streams (2). Fabricius, the Italian anatomist, discovered valves and veins in 1578 (3). He had two equally famous pupils, Asellius and Harvey. Asellius (4) identified the lymphatic system in 1623 by demonstrating, both in the dog and human, that the intestinal lymphatic filled with chyle after meals. Five years later, Harvey (5,6) demonstrated that valves limited the reverse flow of human blood in his monograph, *De motu cordis*.

In 1650 Olaf Rudbeck, a Swede, and Thomas Bartholinus, a Dane, demonstrated that lymphatics drained into the thoracic duct (7). In 1778 William Hewson (8) demonstrated that the thymus and lymph nodes produced lymph, which was rich in "globules" (which we know as lymphocytes); at that time they were believed to be important for normal homeostasis. One hundred years later, in 1878, Claude Bernard (9,10) concluded that lymph arising in the tissue is the equivalent of plasma in the blood and that this was an important vehicle for the exchange of nutrients and gases in the body.

M. T. Lotze: University of Pittsburgh Cancer Institute, Pittsburgh, Pennsylvania 15213-2582.

By the early 20th century it had long been recognized that tumors could spread to nodal sites; in fact, in 1908, Moynihan stated, "A surgery of malignant disease is not the surgery of organs; it is the anatomy of the lymphatic system" (11). At that time it was emphasized that for effective treatment of malignant disease, it was important to remove not only the tumor but also lymph nodes draining this site. With the availability of histologic stains and the identification of cellular subsets, first in Germany (12–14) and then in the United States (15–18), it became clear that blood cells originated from the bone marrow and included lymphocytes. Lymphocytes were considered small, rather unimportant cells (19). In 1924 Alexis Carrel, a surgeon performing studies at the Rockefeller Institute, demonstrated that leukocytes produced substances called trephones, which we call lymphokines (20). Lymphocytes were subsequently shown to migrate into multiple body tissues, tremendously affected by steroids and radiation therapy and the two major subsets of lymphoid cells delineated: (1) the B-cell arising within the bone marrow and within the chicken in the bursa of Fabricius and (2) the T-cell requiring passage through the thymus gland, an embryologic derivative of the third gill pouch (15).

TUMOR-DRAINING LYMPH NODES IN CANCER

The literature related to lymph node metastases and cancer is extensive and cannot be totally reviewed here (Table 1). In the last century, the notion that the lymph nodes served as an effective barrier to the dissemination of cancer was widely held (1,21,22). It has now been

TABLE 1. *Literature relating to nodal metastases (1991–1995)*

	Total	Lymphatic metastases	Operation: lymph node metastases
Total/tumor	—	4,945	20,457
Breast	14,374	1,063	42
Colon	14,731	89	8
Lung	11,563	574	40
Melanoma	4,907	260	11
Prostate	5,162	277	9
Thyroid	2,323	150	10

appreciated that the lymph nodes serve an important immunologic function where T-cells and B-cells first encounter antigen from dendritic cells passing through tissues into the lymph and then into the nodes (23). Pioneering studies by Fisher and Fisher (24–26), however, suggested that the lymph node was not an impervious barrier to tumor cells, but rather that tumor cells could easily pass through such lymphatic channels directly into more distal lymph nodes and into the systemic circulation. In breast cancer, it was suggested that patients whose lymph nodes were left intact might actually do better than those who had had prophylactic nodal dissection (27,28): the survival rate of the group undergoing simple mastectomy was 17% higher than those treated by radical mastectomy. This observation was not subsequently confirmed, however, and it now appears from most studies that the presence of regional nodal metastasis actually is a fairly good indicator of the prognosis, with the number of lymph nodes involved with tumor affecting the likelihood of subsequent regional and systemic recurrence (29, 30). Similar studies performed in rectal cancer (31–34) found that extensive nodal dissection does not, in and of itself, confer a survival advantage. Some researchers (35, 36) have suggested that radical nodal dissection at the time of gastrectomy improves survival in nonrandomized studies. Elective lymphadenectomy has yet to be shown to be of benefit in melanoma (37,38). Although nodal dissection in head and neck cancer is frequently performed and can control local disease, its superiority over radiation therapy remains to be demonstrated (39–43).

We believe that the lymph nodes play an important role in immune responses to the tumor. Unfortunately, at the time of presentation, many of the important alterations in cancer have already occurred—escape from immune detection, tolerization of the requisite T-cells, and failure to mount an effective immune response (44–48).

ORGANIZATION OF THE LYMPHATICS

The lymphatics (49,50) generally drain most tissues throughout the body (Fig. 1, Table 2). The extracellular

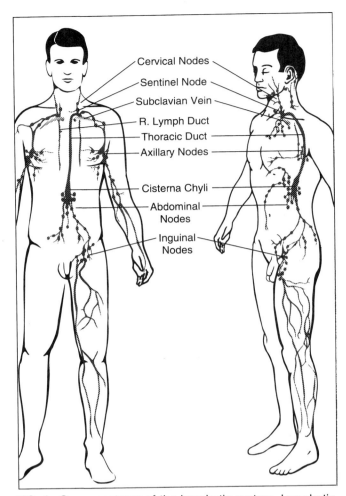

FIG. 1. Gross anatomy of the lymphatic system. Lymphatic channels course throughout the body except as noted in Table 2. These drain the tissues through a series of progressively larger channels that contain valves. For example, the lower legs drain into the inguinal lymph nodes and thence into the deeper pelvic and abdominal nodes. The abdominal viscera drain into the cisterna chyli, which sits behind the duodenum and on top of the anterior portions of the psoas. This in turn drains into the thoracic duct, usually into the left subclavian vein. A frequent site of tumor recurrence from abdominal viscera is the left supraclavicular sentinel node of Virchow. (From Guyton AC, Taylor AE, Granger HJ. *Circulatory physiology II: dynamics and control of the body fluids.* Philadelphia: WB Saunders, 1975.)

space is composed of an amorphous ground substance consisting of proteoglycans, hyaluronic acid, collagen, and other molecules. The tissue polysaccharides exert a high osmotic force (Table 3) that leads to a so-called "swelling pressure" that excludes large macromolecules but allows transport of small molecules and ions, largely by diffusion. The lymphatics arise within the tissues as completely endothelial-lined spaces (Fig. 2) in close topographic relation to end capillary venules (49–52). Although it has been difficult to stain these lymphatics

TABLE 2. *Tissues without blood vessels in the human body*

Without blood or lymph vessels
   Crystalline lens of the eye
   Cartilage
   Epidermis
   Cornea
   Intima/media of large arteries
Without lymph vessels (only "prelymphatics")
   Central nervous system (brain, retina)
   Bone and bone marrow
   Maternal portion of the placenta
   Endomysium surrounding muscle fibers

(Table 4), it is clear that they have some morphologic differences when compared with blood vessels (53–64). They appear to have a wider and more irregular lumen. They are not surrounded by a basement lamina. Cells within the wall of the vessel are easily separated and filaments attach the plasma membrane to the adjoining connective tissue, allowing swelling pressure to cause opening of the lymphatics. Lymphatics do not exist in the brain, retina, and bone marrow (see Table 2).

These small lymphatics give rise to collecting vessels called the collecting ducts, which in turn flow to regional lymph nodes. They are surrounded by elastin and collagen fibers and nonmyelinated nerve fibers. Efferent vessels from the lymph nodes finally drain into the major lymphatic trunks, which, like the arteries and veins, have an intima, media, and adventitia with a rich network of vasa vasorum. There are connections at multiple levels between the venous system and the lymph system, other than in the left and right thoracic ducts (see Fig. 1), particularly during periods of lymph blockage within lymph nodes at the inferior vena cava, at the level of the renal veins, and at multiple other venous sites. It is also thought that connections occur from the vasa vasorum in the large lymphatic channels to the lymph vessels themselves.

The lymph capillaries, but not blood capillaries, stain for 5^1 nucleotidase and guanylate cyclase (54). They weakly (see Table 4) express the endothelial markers

TABLE 3. *Interstitial pressure in the lymphatics*

Negative interstitial pressure (–6 mm Hg)
   Subcutaneous tissue
   Lung
   Skeletal muscle
Positive interstitial pressure
   Kidney
   Intestine
   Brain
   Liver
   Tumors

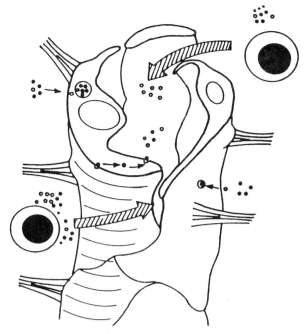

FIG. 2. Diagram of the initial lymphatic. Solute, water, and particulates, as well as proteins and other small molecules, pass through the clefts within cells of the terminal lymphatic *(large arrows)*. Large molecules can also transit the endothelial cells within vesicles *(small arrows)*. These vesicles can move through the cell to form phagocytic vacuoles within which digestion occurs. Others can pass directly into the lumen and discharge their contents into the lymph. It is thought that much of the lymph, as it passes into regional lymph nodes, contains a variety of different particulate debris, cell fragments, and tissue fluid and protein. (Olszewski WL. *Peripheral lymph: formation and immune function.* Boca Raton: CRC Press, 1985.)

(EN-4, von Willebrand factor/factor VIII-related antigen), mural markers (alpha-smooth muscle actin, heparan sulfate proteoglycan, collagen type IV) and do not express adhesion molecules (with the exception of PECAM-1). In other words, they are negative for E-Selectin, ICAM-1, and VCAM-1. The lymphatic endothelium does not have Weibel-Palade bodies or fenestrations or very many pinocytotic vesicles (52). Perhaps the best stain is PAL-E staining, the absence of which indicates that it is a lymphatic. Kaposi's sarcoma, which is widely thought to be of endothelial origin, may indeed be from lymphatics (64b). Particles up to 100 nanometers in diameter can be transported from interstitial spaces into the lymph capillaries, but larger particles (eg, those in dermal tattoos) are retained at the site. So-called "block copolymers" using synthetic polyoxyethylene can be used to enhance uptake in the lymphatic system. This is now being used for imaging lymph nodes in both MRI and CT scanning (see below). Particles coated with such materials might enhance vaccines and imaging modalities or could be used as a sustained-release system.

TABLE 4. *Staining results in normal skin: differences in the expression of microvascular markers between cutaneous blood and lymph vessels*

Antibody (marker)	Blood vessels	Lymph vessels	Reference
PAL-E	intense staining of the micropinocytotic vesicles and focal linear positivity of the luminal endothelial surface	no staining	55
EN-4	linear staining at the luminal endothelial surface, micropinocytotic vesicles positive	focal staining at endothelial interdigitations or overlaps, micropinocytotic vesicles partly positive	56
FVIII-RA	marked cytoplasmic staining of organelles, compatible with Weibel-Palade bodies, and of the subendothelial space	sporadically weak staining of the endothelial surface	57
ASMA (smooth muscle actin)	cytoplasmic staining of surrounding smooth muscle cells/pericytes	no staining of capillaries	58
COLL-IV (collagen type IV)	intense linear staining of basal lamina enclosing endothelium and smooth muscle cells at arterial side, multilaminated linear staining of the basal lamina at venous side	linear staining of subendothelial matrix encompassing the endothelium, interrupted at interendothelial gaps	59
HSPG (heparan sulfate proteoglycon)	staining pattern like collagen IV, but less intense	no staining	60
BBIG-E6 (SelectinLAM-1)	no staining	no staining	61
BBIG-I1 (ICAM-1)	linear staining at the luminal endothelial surface	no staining	62
BBIG-P1 (PECAM)	linear staining at the luminal endothelial surface, micropinocytotic vesicles positive	focal staining at interendothelial interdigitations or overlaps, micropinocytotic vesicles partly positive	63
BBIG-V1 (VCAM-1)	no staining	no staining	52
VEGF	no staining	no staining	64

ROLE OF THE LYMPH NODE IN IMMUNE RESPONSES

Initially the lymph node was considered a barrier to the passage of embolic tumor cells (65–69). It was thought that they arrested in the subcapsular sinus of the corresponding lymph nodes. Perhaps part of the mechanism by which tumors escape immune recognition is by first enlodging in a privileged site such as the lymph node, where lymphocytes are engaged by professional antigen-presenting cells such as the dendritic cell (Fig. 3). Encountering tumor cells during these critical periods of lymphocyte maturation may indeed inhibit induction of an effective immune response. It may even be an early event in tumor progression. A dynamic exchange of cells occurs at various mucosal and cutaneous sites. Dendritic cells of both lymphoid and myeloid origin migrate from bone marrow sites into tissues. This dynamic exchange is less pronounced in the skin, where epidermal Langerhans cells are believed to have a half-life of about 30 days. Hart and colleagues have suggested that the turnover at mucosal sites is much more rapid, with a half-life of about 3 days (70). Within the tissues, particulate antigen is captured, cytokines are released, and dendritic cells are stimulated to migrate across the dermal lymphatics (see Fig. 3).

There are about 500 lymph nodes in the body, each weighing about 1 g (total, 500 g). The spleen, rich in B-cells and T-cells, weighs (in a normal person) 150 g, and there are another 10 billion (10 g) lymphocytes circulating in the peripheral blood. Lymphocytes are richly present in Peyer's patches and at other mucosal sites, so that the total number of lymphocytes in the body is about 1 kg, or 10^{12} cells. Although multiple tissues do not have lymph vessels (see Table 2), these tissues have alternative strategies to remove tissue fluid (71). There is a negative interstitial pressure (see Table 3) in the subcutaneous tissue, lung, and skeletal muscle, whereas in most other sites there is a positive interstitial pressure (49,50).

Identification of lymphatics within tissues is difficult, as noted above. The flattened endothelium of the lymphatic can best be demonstrated by its usual lack of a muscular wall, which are usually not a collapsed formation. Other markers include staining for guanylate cyclase (54). In addition, various particulates are taken up into the lymphatics (72); their use allows visualization of the nodes and sometimes the lymphatic vessels themselves. Carbon suspensions of smaller size (72) are somewhat better than the larger (>200 nanometer) particles found in India ink.

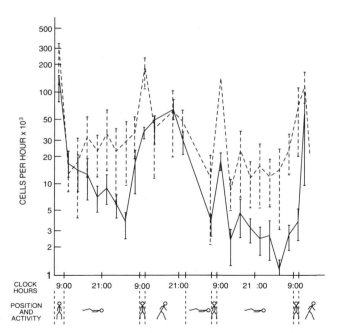

FIG. 3. Dendritic cell (DC) maturation: role of cytokines. One of the major roles of the lymphatic vessel is to ferry cells from the bloodstream into the tissue and from the tissue into the lymph nodes, where effector cells mature and expand. These in turn are exported into the bloodstream, where they again can migrate into tissue sites. From stem cells arising in the bone marrow come all the nucleated cells that circulate in the peripheral blood. These include the granulocyte macrophage/DC (myeloid) cells, which give rise to myeloid DCs, granulocytes, basophils, eosinophils, and macrophages (GM/DC), and the so-called lymphoid/DC (L/DC) cells, which, under the influence of various cytokines, give rise to T-cells within the thymus, B-cells within the bone marrow, NK cells within the bone marrow, and dendritic cells within the thymus and bone marrow (lymphoid DCs). These all circulate throughout the bloodstream, crossing vascular endothelial barriers into tissues. The dendritic cells and macrophages sit in tissue consuming effete, apoptotic cells, which, during injury, damage, or inflammation, are activated to assume an antigen-presenting function. These cells then ferry antigen in the form of bound particulates to the regional lymph nodes, where they encounter T-cells and B-cells in the so-called "menage à trois," exporting T-cells and antibody into the peripheral circulation as effector cells and molecules.

LYMPHATIC FLOW

Studies in different species have focused on lymphatic flow and clearance (65,73–81). In the gut of pigs, intercellular fluid between intestinal epithelial cells passes through pores in the basal lamina to enter intracellular channels and ultimately lacteals (73). These small lymphatics penetrate the muscularis mucosa and are in continuity with lymphatic vessels from the deep submucosa and the lymphatic sinuses coursing along the follicles. In the horse (74), the afferent lymphatic vessel spreads over the capsular surface of the lymph node by fusing with trabeculae entering the subcapsular sinuses, and the medulla

by sinuses coursing between the medullary cords. The efferent lymphatics coalesce between the medullary cords within the subcapsular sinus and within the trabeculae to exit the lymph node through sinuses measuring 5 to 30 microns across. Similar structures are found in the lung and pleural surfaces of rats, where lymphatics course around the blood vessels and bronchials (75). Although it was thought that immunologically privileged sites such as the testes might have a different drainage, there is apparently no direct conduit from the testes into the systemic circulation; rather, they drain directly into the appropriate regional lymph nodes (76).

In the skin (77), lymph flow velocities on the order of 1 to 20 microns per second are found within a rich network of interlacing lymphatics. Lymph is driven through both intrinsic and extrinsic mechanisms (78) based on myogenic activity in the more terminal lymphatics draining tissues, as well as local muscular motion. The intrinsic myogenic activity occurs with a contractile activity of about 4 to 8 mm per second (79) in the lymphatic, allowing forward propulsion of lymphatic fluid. Neurogenic control is mediated by various substances, including substance P and calcitonin gene–related peptide (80). Pressures within these vessels are sensed by baroreceptors, which cause increased pumping up to a pressure of 18 to 26 cm H_2O, decreasing after higher pressure is reached in the lymphatics (81). When a vessel is occluded or there is a marked increase in outflow pressure, flow rates rapidly decline (82). Thus, it appears that the lymphatics, like the blood vessels, have both intrinsic and extrinsic pumping capacity. This may be impeded by tumor cell invasion or blockage or surgical procedures to remove the lymph nodes.

The study of lymphatics and lymphatic vessels may be facilitated by the development of culture conditions using collagen type 1 as a matrix substance; this will allow further in vitro studies of lymphatic vessels (83). The output of lymphocytes and erythrocytes and volume from the lymphatics have been measured in normal persons (Fig. 4) and in the postoperative period (Fig. 5).

EFFECTS OF IMMUNIZATION ON LYMPH FLOW AND LYMPHOCYTE MIGRATION

Following antigen challenge, there is a marked increase in afferent and efferent lymph flow through the lymph node. In sheep (84), lymphocyte output initially goes through a shutdown phase, when there is an 80% decrease in the number of lymphocytes exiting the lymph node (primarily the naive type). During the recruitment phase, there is a marked increase in the number of CD4[+]-memory type T-cells migrating from the lymph node through a non-L-selectin mediated event. This may be due to expression of vascular cell adhesion molecule 1 (VCAM-1), which is also increased on blood vessels at

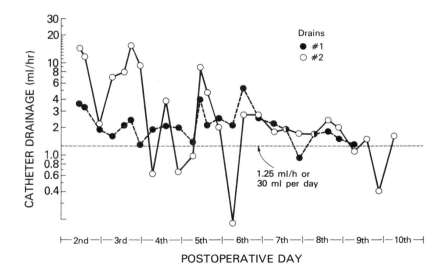

FIG. 4. The output of lymphocytes and erythrocytes in leg lymph vessels of healthy volunteers was studied over a period of 3 days during the night and during daily activity. The mean lymphocyte output in night lymph is 81 ± 19 × 10³ per hour. During activity, the highest output of lymphocytes, erythrocytes, and monocytes was found in early morning, amounting to 1.5 to 2 logs more cells when compared with the evening. Shown is the variation in counts, with means ±1 standard error. (Olszewski WL, Engeset A. Lymphatic circulation of humans. In: Johnston MG, ed. *Experimental biology of the lymphatic circulation.* Amsterdam: Elsevier, 1985.)

the site of antigen challenge. Thus, similar vascular changes are found in the lymph node and at the site of antigenic challenge.

The increased lymphocyte traffic through lymph nodes is thought to enhance the opportunity for interaction between antigen-presenting cells carried in the afferent lymph and naive T-cells entering the lymph node through the arterial vessel. The initial migration of these lymphocytes in the lymph node is L-selectin mediated (85). Two sulfated glycoprotein ligands of 50 and 90 kilodaltons have been identified as the mucinlike ligands on the high endothelial venules mediating extravasation of L-selectin-positive cells. The first of these has been termed glycosylation-dependent cell adhesion molecule 1 (Gly-CAM-1). Expression of this molecule is abolished by ligation of the afferent lymphatics, suggesting that a soluble

factor (eg, a cytokine) is responsible for the enhanced adhesiveness. This may be due to tissue release of factors such as interferon-alpha (86) or other smaller-molecular-weight species, including bradykinin or, more likely, histamine. Bacterial products such as N-formyl-methionyl-leucyl-phenylalanine (F-Met-Leu-Phe) causes increases in local fluid extravasation in tissue and increased lymphatic flow, which is paralleled by an increase in lymphatic pumping (87). Interferon-gamma appears to enhance the trafficking of naive but not memory T-cells into lymph nodes and their retention there and may be the factor selectively enhancing expression of the L-selectin ligands (88). Tumor necrosis factor (TNF)-alpha has also been shown to cause rapid migration of dendritic cells from tissue into the draining lymph nodes (89). This appears to be mediated by the p75 receptor for TNF because human TNF-alpha did not mediate these effects in mice (only the murine TNF-alpha did), nor did GM-CSF. TNF may cause loss of expression of the E-catherin molecule, which is important for retention of Langerhans cells in the skin, where they adhere to laminin and fibronectin beta-1 receptors. This also may be related to the enhanced alpha-4-integrin expression on dendritic cells that occurs with activation (see Fig. 3).

The variety of targeted deletions or transgenic overexpression of molecules in murine models (90–93) has led to rich insights into the normal maturation pathways and lymphatic traffic of lymphocytes and dendritic cells. It appears that in rel-b knockouts, migration of dermal dendrocytes, which are scant in such animals, limits the normal development of lymphoid architecture (90). Similarly, transgenic expression of the recombinases RAG1 and RAG2 leads to perivascular lymphoid accumulations and choking within lymphatics and lymph nodes because of their altered migratory capabilities (92). Failure to express the gamma common chain receptor of the IL-2, IL-4, IL-7, and IL-15 receptors causes a marked diminu-

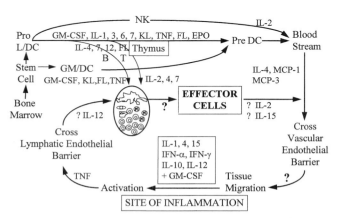

FIG. 5. Lymphatic flow in the postoperative period. Shown is the drainage in milliliter per hour from two separate drains placed in the inguinal space after a superficial nodal dissection. We generally remove drains when there is less than 30 ml/day. Notice the daily variations: peak lymph flow midday, falling during the evening.

TABLE 5. *Novel agents developed for imaging lymph node (LN) metastases*

Agent	Imaging	Results	Reference
CH40, CH1500AA Carbon suspensions (150,167NM)	Visual after subcutaneous injection	69% of LN with metastases seen at operation (gastric cancer)	72
Iodinated contrast	Spiral CT	Visualized normal hilar lymph nodes	94
Noncontrast 5-mm cuts	CT	5-mm sections of mediastinum revealed more LN than contrasted 10-mm sections	95
Ethiodol	Bipedal lymphangiography	Almost all normal pelvic LN <10 mm maximum short-axis diameter	96
Perflubron emulsion in tissue	CT	2 days later revealed involvement of LN in axilla	97,98
18F Fluorodeoxyglucose	PET scanning	Markedly increased uptake in metastatic lung cancer to LN	99
Carbon particle	Lymphangiography	96% of lymph nodes draining the rectum in 12 patients visualized	100
Pelvioscopy	Visual	101 patients with bladder and prostate cancer; 100% specificity and positive predictive value	101
Dextran-coated supramagnetic iron oxide	MRI	IV administration to 12 patients with 40/42 metastatic nodes and 41/49 benign nodes in head and neck cancer visualized	102

tion in the total numbers of T-cells and B-cells and an absence of NK cells (93). Although immune-privileged sites such as the testes and the brain were previously thought to lack connection with the immune system, we now know that these earlier conceptions were incomplete, with evidence of profound interactions, especially within the central nervous system (71).

IMAGING STUDIES OF THE LYMPHATICS

In Chapter 24, detailed information about lymph node metastases and their treatment is given. Several innovations in the imaging of lymphatics may lead to broader application of regional therapies for tumors metastatic to lymph nodes (76,94–106). Although CT and MRI have revolutionized the imaging of tumor in nodal and nonnodal sites, it is often difficult to differentiate a borderline-sized metastatic lymph node without central necrosis or extracapsular spread from a reactive lymph node, which is frequently seen in cancer patients.

Several classes of new agents allow enhanced detection of nodal metastases. These have largely been tested in experimental animals but are now moving into human clinical trials. Some of these novel imaging techniques are listed in Table 5. They include colloidal carbon suspensions of a discrete size (<200 nm) to visualize lymph nodes directly at the time of surgery, laparoscopic or "pelvioscopic" techniques to visualize lymph nodes directly (101), and the use of contrast material—perflubron emulsions (97,98) for CT scanning and Dextran-coated supramagnetic iron oxide (102–106) for MRI scanning. PET scanning has shown an increasing application, particularly in thoracic imaging (99). These new modalities will probably advance our knowledge of the

biology of lymphatic drainage and allow enhanced identification of metastases within lymph nodes.

TUMOR CHANGES ASSOCIATED WITH LYMPH NODE METASTASIS

Various agents can be applied in murine experimental models to alter the nature and quantity of nodal metastases. Several characteristics of both murine and human tumors have been examined (Table 6) that appear to enhance metastases to lymph nodes (107–115). Most of these involved enhanced adhesive characteristics: gener-

TABLE 6. *Tumor changes associated with lymph node metastases*

Characteristic	Tumor type	Effect	Reference
Halies pomatia binding	Gastric cancer	↑	107
Integrin αVβ3 expression	Melanoma	↑	108
Prostacyclin analogs	Rat mammary tumor	↓	109
Sphingomyelin	Prostate cancer	↑	110
Adhesion to lymph node sinus	Murine melanoma	↑	111
Cyclosporin A	Hamster cheek pouch tumors	↑	112
β1,β3 integrins	Murine, human tumor	↑	113
Hyperthermia, radiation	Murine melanoma	↑	114
EGFR expression	Melanoma	↑	115

TABLE 7. *Genetic alterations associated with lymphatic metastases*

Genetic finding	Tumor type	Reference
Allelic loss chromosome 1	Breast cancer	116
Decreased MHC class I	Carcinomas	117
c-erbB2	Breast cancer (p=0.001)	118
Deletions chromosome 16	Breast cancer	119
MUC 18 expression	Melanoma	120

ally, the number of adhesion molecules important for endothelial binding is increased on tumor cells. Prostacyclin analogs decrease metastases (109), and immunosuppressive agents (112) generally enhance them. Even some treatments, including hyperthermia and radiation, can enhance metastatic spread to lymph nodes (114). Whether specific genetic alterations are associated with lymphatic metastases is less clear. Expression of certain genes, such as c-erbB2 and MUC 18 (Table 7), has been associated with cancer progression and lymphatic metas-

tasis (116–120). For example, c-erbB2 (118) is associated with a markedly enhanced risk of nodal metastases when it is highly expressed (p=0.001). Other alterations include loss of class I molecules (117) and deletions on chromosomes 1 and 16 (116,119).

Perhaps most intriguing has been the finding, in various tumor types, that dendritic cell infiltration at the primary tumor site, as well as within the lymph node, is directly related to prognosis (Table 8). Many different tumors in humans have been examined, and most of them have an improved prognosis when dendritic cells are present. This suggests that critical interactions occur between the host immune system and the tumor. The poor prognosis associated with decreased dendritic cell number may be related to:

1. Decreased traffic of dendritic cells into the tumor due to immunosuppressive factors made by the tumor, or lack of effective immunity
2. Increased death of dendritic cells related to, again, factors made by the tumor that promote dendritic cell apoptosis

TABLE 8. *Relation between dendritic cell infiltration and prognosis in malignancy*

Tumor	Reference	DC infiltration
Arsenical skin	*Proc Nat Cl Ch* 1992;16:17	Less compared to normal skin
Basal cell	*Br J Derm* 1994;130:273	Less in tumors*
Basal cell	*Br J Derm* 1992;127:575	?Improved
Breast	*J Pathol* 1991;163:25	?Improved prognosis
Bronchoalveolar	*Eur J Ca* 1992;28A:1365	No effect
Cervix	*Am J Clin Path* 1993;99:200	Less in HPV+ tumors
Cervix	*Cancer* 1992;70:2839	Improved*
Cervix, stage III	*In Vivo* 1993;7:257	Markedly improved prognosis*
Cervix/Penile	*J Urol* 1992;147:1268	Less with HPV infection
Cervix/HIV	*Gynecol Oncol* 1993;48:210	Less in AIDS
Esophageal	*Virchow's Arch* 1992;61:409	Markedly improved prognosis
Esophageal	*In Vivo* 1993;7:239	Direct relation to grade
Gastric	*Int Surg* 1992;77:238	Markedly improved prognosis*
Gastric	*Cancer* 1995;75:1478	More in tumor-draining LNs
Gastric, stage III	*In Vivo* 1993;7:233	Markedly improved prognosis*
Head and neck	*Cancer Immunother* 1993;36:108	PBMC DC less functional
Head and neck	*Cancer Immunother* 1994;38:31	Present in some tumors
Hodgkin's disease	*Am J Cl Path* 1994;101:761	FDC improve prognosis*
Larynx	*Orl* 1991;53:349	Present in tumors
Larynx	*Chin J Otorhinol* 1992;27:297	Markedly improved prognosis
Larynx	*In Vivo* 1993;8:229	Improved prognosis
Lung	*Pathology* 1993;25:338	Markedly improved prognosis*
Lung	*J Clin Invest* 1993;91:566	Related GM-CSF production
Melanoma	*J Invest Derm* 1993;100:269	Inverse with tumor thickness
Mycosis fungoides/SS	*In Vivo* 1993;7:277	Markedly improved prognosis*
Nasopharyngeal	*Laryngoscope* 1991;101:487	Markedly improved prognosis
Oral	*J Oral Path Med* 1992;21:100	Less with smokeless tobacco
Oral	*J Cut Pathol* 1992;19:398	Less in tumors
Oral squamous	*J Oral Path Med* 1995;24:61	No relation to prognosis
Oropharynx	*In Vivo* 1994;8:543	Less in tumors
Prostate	*Prostate* 1991;19:73	Improved prognosis
Skin tumors	*Arch Dermatol* 1995;131:187	Less in tumors
Thyroid (papillary)	*Zent f Chir* 1992;117:603	No effect

DC, dendritic cell
* Statistically significant difference when compared to either normal or less DCs

3. Enhanced clearance of dendritic cells from the site of tumor because of endogenous production of factors such as TNF-alpha.

The precise mechanism is unclear, and this is a rich area for investigation.

SURGICAL EVALUATION OF LYMPH NODES

The presence of nodal metastases carries a particularly adverse prognosis in most neoplasms, and the ability to identify and treat those sites of disease in patients with occult lymphatic metastases is problematic. In part, this is related to the fact that inguinal lymphadenectomy is associated with both cosmetic and physiologic alterations. In a study (121) evaluating the effect of popliteal lymphadenectomy in dogs, markedly decreased lymphatic flow was observed, but no more than that occurring after simple ligation of the major lymphatic channels. A subsequent study performed in patients (122) suggested that the type of inguinal incision did not modify the incidence of alterations in lymphatic drainage, consistent with what was observed in the animal studies. Selective lymphadenectomy required the development of strategies to identify (123–127) the appropriate nodal drainage basins. This has been most often done using lymphoscintigraphy. In a feline model (128), it was suggested that a predictable pattern of drainage to individual lymph nodes was observed. Thus, various techniques using radionuclides and blue dye studies evolved in the setting of melanoma, breast cancer, and genitourinary malignancies (129–132). These allowed identification of a "sentinel node," which if positive on biopsy suggested the need for more extensive nodal dissection.

The consequences of such nodal dissection may or may not affect the long-term survival of patients, but the ability to identify patients who might benefit most from nodal dissection could lead to the performance of the procedure only in them. This question is being tested in a prospective randomized study by Don Morton and associates (see Chap. 23). Further evolution of this strategy will probably need to take into consideration the adverse consequences of nodal dissection, the immunologic implications, and the availability of additional adjuvant modalities. The recent identification of alpha-interferon as an adjuvant therapy for patients with metastatic melanoma (133) supports the vigorous evaluation of strategies to identify patients with suspected metastatic disease.

REFERENCES

1. Zeidman I, Buss JM. Experimental studies on the spread of cancer in the lymphatic system. I. Effectiveness of the lymph nodes as a barrier to the passage of embolic tumor cells. *Cancer Res* 1954;14:403–405.
2. Shields JW. Lymph, myphomania, lymphothrophy, and HIV lymphocytopathy: a historical perspective. *Lymphology* 1994;27:21–40.
3. Adelman HB. *The embryological treatises of Hieronymous Fabricius of Aquapendent.* Ithaca: Cornell University Press, 1942.
4. Aselli G. *De lactibus sine lacteis venis, quarto vasorum mesaraicorum genere, novo invento.* Nediolani, Bidellum JB, 1627.
5. Fulton JF. *Selected readings in the history of physiology.* Springfield, Ill.: Thomas, 1930.
6. Harvey W. *Exercitationes de generatione animalium,* 1651.
7. Mayerson JS. Three centuries of lymphatic history—an outline. *Lymphology* 1969;2:143–152.
8. Dameshek W. William Hewson, thymicologist: father of hematology? *Blood* 1963;21:513–516.
9. Bernard C. *Leçons sur les phénomènes de la vie communs aux animaux et aux vegetaux.* Paris, Bailliere, 1878.
10. Robin ED. Claude Bernard, pioneer of regulatory biology. *JAMA* 1979;242:1283–1284.
11. Moynihan BGA. The surgical treatment of cancer of the sigmoid flexure and rectum. *Surg Gynecol Obstet* 1908;6:463–466.
12. Metchnikoff E. Immunity in infective diseases. Cambridge University Press, 1905.
13. Ranvier L. Des clasmatocytes. *Compt Rend Acad Sci* 1890;110:165–169.
14. Downey HF, Weidenriech. Ueber die Bildung der Lymphocyten in Lymphdruesen und Milz. *Arch Mikr Anat Entw Mech* 1912;80:306–395.
15. McCutcheon M. Studies on the locomotion of lymphocytes III. The rate of locomotion of human lymphocytes in vitro. *Am J Physiol* 1931;69:279–282.
16. Kindred JE. A quantitative study of the haemopoietic organs of young albino rats. *Am J Anat* 1940;67:99–149; 1942;71:207–243.
17. White A, Dougherty TF. The role of lymphocytes in normal and immune globulin production and the mode of release of globulin from lymphocytes. *Ann NY Acad Sci* 1946;46:859–882.
18. Humble JG, Hayne WHW, Pulvertaft RJ. Biological action between lymphocytes and other cells. *Br J Haematol* 1956;2:283–294.
19. Trowell OA. The lymphocyte. *Internat Rev Cytol* 1958;7:235–293.
20. Carrel A. Leukocyte trephones. *JAMA* 1924;82:255–258.
21. Virchow R, translated by F Chance. Cellular pathology. New York: Dover Publications, 1971:218–222.
22. Zeidman I. The late fate of circulating tumor cells. I. Passage of cells through capillaries. *Cancer Res* 1961;21:38.
23. Heys SD, Eremin O. The relevance of tumor draining lymph nodes. *Surg Gynecol Obstet* 1992;174:533–540.
24. Fisher B, Fisher ER. Interrelationship of hematogenous and lymphatic tumor cell dissemination. *Surg Gynecol Obstet* 1966;122:791–798.
25. Fisher B, Fisher ER. Transmigration of lymph nodes by tumor cells. *Science* 1966;152:1397–1398.
26. Fisher B, Fisher ER. Role of the lymphatic system in the dissemination of tumor. In: Mayerson HS, ed. *Lymph and the lymphatic system.* Springfield, Ill.: Charles C. Thomas, 1968:324.
27. Crile G Jr. Possible role of uninvolved regional nodes in preventing metastasis from breast cancer: a first report of results from a prospective randomized clinical trial. *Cancer* 1977;39:2827–2839.
28. Langlands AO, Pocock SJ, Kerr GR, Gore SM. Long-term survival of patients with breast cancer: a study of the curability of the disease. *Br Med J* 1979;2:1247–1251.
29. Trojani M, de Mascarel I, Bonichon F, et al. Micrometastases to axillary lymph nodes from carcinoma of the breast. Detection by immunohistochemistry and prognostic significance. *Br J Cancer* 1987;55:303–306.
30. Trojani M, de Mascarel I, Coindre JM, Bonichon F. Micrometastases to axillary lymph nodes from invasive lobular carcinoma of breast: detection by immunohistochemistry and prognostic significance. *Br J Cancer* 1987;56:838–839.
31. Enker WE, Heilwell ML, Heriz REL, et al. En bloc pelvic lymphadenectomy and sphincter preservation in the surgical management of rectal cancer. *Ann Surg* 1986;203:426–433.
32. Grinnel RS. Results of ligation of inferior mesenteric artery at the aorta in resection of carcinoma of the descending and sigmoid colon and rectum. *Surg Gynecol Obstet* 1965;120:1031–1036.
33. Pezim ME, Nicholls RJ. Survival after high or low ligation of the inferior mesenteric artery during curative surgery for rectal cancer. *Ann Surg* 1984;200:729–733.
34. Glass RE, Ritchie JK, Phillips RK. High versus low ligation of the inferior mesenteric artery in rectal cancer. *Br J Surg* 1990;77:618–621.
35. Shiu MH, Moore E, Sanders M, et al. Influence of the extent of resec-

tion on survival after curative treatment of gastric carcinoma: a retrospective multivariate analysis. *Arch Surg* 1987;122:1347–1351.

36. Noguchi Y, Imada T, Matsumoto A, et al. Radical surgery for gastric cancer. A review of the Japanese experience. *Cancer* 1989;64: 2053–2062.

37. Sim FH, Taylor WF, Pritchard DJ, et al. Lymphadenectomy in management of stage 1 malignant melanoma: a prospective randomized study. *Mayo Clin Proc* 1986;61:697–705.

38. Cady B, Legg MA, Redfern AB. Contemporary treatment of malignant melanoma. *Am J Surg* 1975;129:472–482.

39. Jesse RH, Fletcher GH. Treatment of the neck in patients with squamous cell carcinoma of the head and neck. *Cancer* 1977;39:868–872.

40. Vikram MB, Strong EW, Shah J, Spiro R. Elective postoperative radiation therapy in stages III and IV epidermoid carcinoma of the head and neck. *Am J Surg* 1980;140:580–584.

41. Byers RM. Modified neck dissection. A study of 967 cases from 1970–1980. *Am J Surg* 1985;150:414–421.

42. O Brien CJ, Smith JW, Soong S-J, et al. Neck dissection with and without radiotherapy—prognostic factors, patterns of recurrence and survival. *Am J Surg* 1986;152:456–463.

43. Vandenbrouck C, Sancho-Garner J, Chassagne D, et al. Elective versus therapeutic radical neck dissection in epidermoid carcinoma of the oral cavity. *Cancer* 1980;46:386–390.

44. Eremin O, Roberts P, Plumb D, Stephen JP. Human regional tumor lymph nodes: alterations of micro-architecture and lymphocyte subpopulations. *Br J Cancer* 1980;41:62–72.

45. Steele RJC, Eremin O, Brown M. Blood monocytes and tumor infiltrating macrophages in human breast cancer: difference in activation levels as assessed by lysozyme content. *J Natl Cancer Inst* 1983;71: 941–945.

46. Vanky FT, Stjernsward J, Nilsonne U, Sundblad R. Differences in the tumor-associated reactivity of blood lymphocytes and tumor-draining lymph node cells in sarcoma patients. *J Natl Cancer Inst* 1973;51: 17–24.

47. Nakamura H, Ishigurd K, Mori T. Different immune functions of peripheral blood, regional lymph nodes, and tumor-infiltrating lymphocytes in lung cancer patients. *Cancer* 1988;62:2489–2497.

48. Mainou-Fowler T, Eremin O. Tumour-associated proliferative responses in vitro of regional lymph nodes draining solid cancers in man. *Cancer Immunol Immunother* 1989;30:300–306.

49. Johnston MG, ed. *Experimental biology of the lymphatic circulation.* New York: Elsevier, 1985.

50. Olszewski WL. *Peripheral lymph: formation and immune function.* New York: CRC Press, 1985.

51. Leak LV. Lymphatic removal of fluid and particles in the mammalian lung. *Envir Health Perspect* 1980;35:55.

52. Erhard H, Rietveld FJR, Bröcker EB, de Waal RMW, Ruiter DJ. Phenotype of normal cutaneous microvasculature. *J Invest Dermatol* 1996;106:135–140.

53. Ryan TJ. Structure and function of lymphatics. *J Invest Dermatol* 1989;93:18S–24S.

54. Nishida S, Ohkuma M. Enzyme-histochemical staining of dermal lymphatic capillaries by guanylate cyclase. *Lymphology* 1993;26:195–199.

55. Schlingemann RO, Dinghan GM, Emeis JJ, Blok J, Warnaar SO, Ruiter DJ. Monoclonal antibody PAL-E specific for endothelium. *Lab Invest* 1985;52:71.

56. Cui TC, Tai PC, Gatter KC, Mason DY, Spry CJ. A vascular endothelial cell antigen with restricted distribution in human foetal, adult and malignant tissues. *Immunology* 1983;49:183.

57. Hoyer LW, de los Santos RP, Hoyer JR. Antihemophilic factor antigen. Localization in endothelial cells by immunofluorescent microscopy. *J Clin Invest* 1973;52:2737

58. Laurie GW, Leblond CP, Martin GR. Localization of type IV collagen, laminin, heparan sulfate proteoglycan, and fibronectin to the basal lamina of basement membrane. *J Cell Biol* 1986;95:340.

59. Skalli O, Ropraz P, Treciac A, Benzonana G, Gillesen D, Gabbiani G. A monoclonal antibody against alpha-smooth muscle actin: a new probe for smooth muscle differentiation. *J Cell Biol* 1986;103:2787.

60. Horiguchi Y, Couchman JR, Ljubimov AV, Yamasaki H, Fine JD. Distribution, ultrastructural localization, and ontogeny of the core protein of a heparan sulfate proteoglycan in human skin and other basement membranes. *J Histochem Cytochem* 1989;37:961.

61. Bevilacqua MP, Pober JS, Mendrick DL, Cotran RS, Gimbrone MAJ. Identification of an inducible endothelial-leukocyte adhesion molecule. *Proc Natl Acad Sci USA* 1987;84:9238.

62. Dustin ML, Rothlein R, Bhan AK, Dinarello CA, Springer TA. Induc-

tion by IL 1 and interferon-gamma: tissue distribution, biochemistry, and function of a natural adherence molecule (ICAM-1). *J Immunol* 1986;137:245.

63. Stockinger H, Gadd SJ, Eher R, et al. Molecular characterization and functional analysis of the leukocyte surface protein CD31. *J Immunol* 1990;145:3889.

64a. Pötgens AJG, Lubsen NH, van Altena MC, Schoenmakers JGG, Tuiter DJ, de Waal RMW. Vascular permeability factor expression influences tumor angiogenesis in human melanoma lines xenografted to nude mice. *Am J Pathol* 1995;146:197.

64b. Beckstead JH, Wood GS, Fletcher V. Evidence for the origin of Kaposi's sarcoma from lymphatic endothelium. *Am J Pathol* 1985; 119:294–300.

65. Moghimi SM, Hawley AE, Christy NM, Gray T, Illum L, Davis SS. Surface engineered nanospheres with enhanced drainage into lymphatics and uptake by macrophages of the regional lymph nodes. *FEBS Lett* 1994;344:25–30.

66. Sokolowski J, Jacobsen E, Johannessen JV. *Lymphology* 1978;11:202.

67. Abe R, Taneichi N. Lymphatic metastases in experimental cecal carcinoma: effectiveness of lymph nodes as barriers to the spread of tumor cells. *Arch Surg* 1972;104:95.

68. Engeset A. Barrier function of lymph glands. *Lancet* 1962;1:324.

69. Fisher B, Fisher ER. Barrier function of lymph node to tumor cells and erythrocytes. I. Normal nodes. *Cancer* 1967;20:1907.

70. Holt PG, Oliver J, Bilyk N, et al. Downregulation of the antigen presenting cell function(s) of pulmonary dendritic cells in vivo by resident alveolar macrophages. *J Exp Med* 1993;177:397–407.

71. Cserr HF, Knopf PM. Cervical lymphatics, the blood-brain barrier and the immunoreactivity of the brain: a new view. *Immunology Today* 1992;13:507–512.

72. Hagiwara A, Takahashi T, Sawai K, et al. Lymph nodal vital staining with newer carbon particles suspensions compared with India ink: experimental and clinical observations. *Lymphology* 1992;25:84–89.

73. Lowden S, Heath T. Ileal Peyer's patches in pigs: intercellular and lymphatic pathways. *Anat Rec* 1994;239:297–305.

74. Nikles SA, Heath TJ. Pathways of lymph flow through intestinal lymph nodes in the horse. *Anat Rec* 1992;232:126–132.

75. Schraufnagel DE. Forms of lung lymphatics: a scanning electron microscopic study of casts. *Anat Rec* 1992;233:547–554.

76. Kazeem AA. Species variation in the extrinsic lymphatic drainage of the rodent testis: its role within the context of an immunologically privileged site. *Lymphology* 1991;24:140–144.

77. Leu AJ, Berk DA, Yuan F, Jain RK. Flow velocity in the superficial lymphatic network of the mouse tail. *Am J Physiol* 1994;267: H1507–1513.

78. Negrini D, Ballard ST, Benoit JN. Contribution of lymphatic myogenic activity and respiratory movements to pleural lymph flow. *J Appl Physiol* 1994;76:2267–2274.

79. Zawieja DC, Davis KL, Schuster R, Hinds WM, Granger HJ. Distribution, propagation, and coordination of contractile activity in lymphatics. *Am J Physiol* 1993;264:H1283–1291.

80. Sacchi G, Weber E, Agliano M, Comparini L. Subendothelial nerve fibers in bovine mesenteric lymphatics: an ultrastructural and immunohistochemical study. *Lymphology* 1994;27:90–96.

81. Eisenhoffer J, Lee S, Johnston MG. Pressure-flow relationships in isolated sheep prenodal lymphatic vessels. *Am J Physiol* 1994;267: H938–943.

82. Eisenhoffer J, Elias RM, Johnston MG. Effect of outflow pressure on lymphatic pumping in vitro. *Am J Physiol* 1993;265:R97–102.

83. Leak LV, Jones M. Lymphangiogenesis in vitro: formation of lymphatic capillary-like channels from confluent monolayers of lymphatic endothelial cells. *In Vitro Cellular & Developmental Biology Animal.* 1994;30A:512–518.

84. Mackay CR, Marston W, Dudler L. Altered patterns of T cell migration through lymph nodes and skin following antigen challenge. *Eur J Immunol* 1992;22:2205–2210.

85. Mebius RE, Dowbenko D, Williams A, Fennie C, Lasky LA, Watson SR. Expression of GlyCAM-1, an endothelial ligand for L-selectin, is affected by afferent lymphatic flow. *J Immunol* 1993;151:6769–6776.

86. Pessina GP, Bocci V, Carraro F, Naldini A, Paulesu L. The lymphatic route. IX. Distribution of recombinant interferon-alpha 2 administered subcutaneously with oedematogenic drugs. *Physiol Res* 1993;42: 243–250.

87. Benoit JN, Zawiewja DC. Effects of f-Met-Leu-Phe-induced inflammation on intestinal lymph flow and lymphatic pump behavior. *Am J Physiol* 1992;262:G199–202.

88. Westerman J, Persin S, Matyas J, van der Meide P, Pabst R. Migration of so-called naive and memory T lymphocytes from blood to lymph in the rat. The influence of IFN-gamma on the circulation pattern. *J Immunol* 1994;152:1744–1750.

89. Cumberbatch M, Fielding I, Kimber I. Modulation of epidermal Langerhans cells frequency by tumour necrosis factor-alpha. *Immunology* 1994;81:395–401.

90. Weih F, Carrasco D, Durham SK, et al. Multiorgan inflammation and hematopoietic abnormalities in mice with a targeted disruption of RelB, a member of the NF-kappa B/Rel family. *Cell* 1995;80: 331–340.

91. Georgopoulos K, Bigby M, Wang JH, et al. Phe Ikaros gene is required for the development of all lymphoid lineages. *Cell* 1994;79: 143–156.

92. Wayne J, Suh H, Sokol KA, et al. TCR selection and allelic exclusion in RAG transgenic mice that exhibit abnormal T cell localization in lymph nodes and lymphatics. *J Immunol* 1994;153:5491–5502.

93. DiSanto JP, Muller W, Guy-Grand D, Fischer A, Rajwesky K. Lymphoid development in mice with a targeted deletion of the interleukin 2 receptor gamma chain. *Proc Natl Acad Sci USA* 1995;92:377–381.

94. Remy-Jardin M, Duyck P, Remy J, et al. Hilar lymph nodes: identification with spiral CT and histologic correlation. *Radiology* 1995;196: 387–394.

95. Haramati LB, Caragena AM, Austin JH. CT evaluation of mediastinal lymphadenopathy: noncontrast 5 mm vs postcontrast 10 mm sections. *J Comp Assist Tomog* 1995;19:375–378.

96. Vinnicombe SJ, Normal AR, Nicolson V, Husband JE. Normal pelvic lymph nodes: evaluation with CT after bipedal lymphangiography. *Radiology* 1995;194:349–355.

97. Hanna G, Saewart D, Shorr J, et al. Preclinical and clinical studies on lymph node imaging using perflubron emulsion. *Artificial Cells, Blood Substitutes, & Immobilization Biotechnology* 1994;22: 1429–1439.

98. Wolf GL, Rogowska J, Hanna GK, Halpern EF. Percutaneous CT lymphography with perflubron: imaging efficacy in rabbits and monkeys. *Radiology* 1994;191:501–505.

99. Scott WJ, Schwabe JL, Gupta NC, Dewan NA, Reeb SD, Sugimoto JT. Positron emission tomography of lung tumors and mediastinal lymph nodes using [18F] fluorodeoxyglucose. The Members of the PET-Lung Tumor Study Group. *Ann Thorac Surg* 1994;58:698–703.

100. Kumashiro R, Sano C, Sakai T, et al. Radical lymphadenectomy for rectal cancer facilitated by a carbon particle infusion lymphangiography. *Surgery Today* 1992;22:512–516.

101. Mazemen E, Wurtz A, Gillict P, Biserte J. Extraperitoneal pelvioscopy in lymph node staging of bladder and prostatic cancer. *J Urol* 1992; 147:366–370.

102. Anzai Y, Blackwell KE, Hirschowitz SL, et al. Initial clinical experience with Dextran-coated superparamagnetic iron oxide for detection of lymph node metastases in patients with head and neck cancer. *Radiology* 1994;192:709–715.

103. Taupitz M, Wagner S, Hamm B, Binder A, Pfefferer D. Interstitial MR lymphography with iron oxide particles: results in tumor-free and VX2 tumor-bearing rabbits. *AJR* 1993;161:193–200.

104. Mountford CE, Lean CL, Hancock R, et al. Magnetic resonance spectroscopy detects cancer in draining lymph nodes. *Invasion & Metastasis* 1993;13:57–71.

105. Guimaraes R, Clement O, Bittoun J, Carnot F, Frija G. MR lymphography with superparamagnetic iron nanoparticles in rats: pathologic basis for contrast enhancement. *AJR* 1994;162:201–207.

106. Vassallo P, Matei C, Heston WD, McLachlan SJ, Koutcher JA, Castellino RA. AMI-227-enhanced MR lymphography: usefulness for differentiating reactive from tumor-bearing lymph nodes. *Radiology* 1994;193:501–506.

107. Kakeji Y, Maehara Y, Tsujitani S, et al. Helix pomatia agglutinin binding activity and lymph node metastasis in patients with gastric cancer. *Sem Surg Oncol* 1994;10:130–134.

108. Nip J, Shibata H, Loskutoff DJ, Cheresh DA, Brodt P. Human melanoma cells derived from lymphatic metastases use integrin alpha v beta 3 to adhere to lymph node vitronectin. *J Clin Invest* 1992;90: 1406–1413.

109. Schirner M, Lichtner RB, Schneider MR. The stable prostacyclin analogue Cicaprost inhibits metastasis to lungs and lymph nodes in the 13762NF MTLn3 rat mammary carcinoma. *Clin Exp Metastasis* 1994;12:24–30.

110. Dahiya R, Boyle B, Goldberg BC, et al. Metastasis-associated alter-ations in phospholipids and fatty acids of human prostatic adenocarcinoma cell lines. *Biochemistry Cell Biol* 1992;70:548–554.

111. Whalen GF, Sharif SF. Locally increased metastatic efficiency as a reason for preferential metastasis of solid tumors to lymph nodes. *Ann Surg* 1992;215:166–171.

112. Yamada T, Mogi M, Kage T, Ueda A, Nakajima J, Chino T. Enhancement by cyclosporin A of metastasis from hamster cheek pouch carcinoma. *Arch Oral Biol* 1992;37:593–596.

113. Brodt P. Adhesion mechanisms in lymphatic metastasis. *Cancer & Metastasis Reviews* 1991;10:23–32.

114. Nathanson SD, Nelson L, Anaya P, Havstad S, Hetzel FW. Development of lymph node and pulmonary metastases after local irradiation and hyperthermia of footpad melanomas. *Clin Exp Metastasis* 1991; 9:377–392.

115. Mueller BM, Romerdahl CA, Trent JM, Reisfeld RA. Suppression of spontaneous melanoma metastasis in scid mice with an antibody to the epidermal growth factor receptor. *Cancer Res* 1991;51:2193–2198.

116. Borg A, Zhang QX, Olsson H, Wenngren E. Chromosome 1 alterations in breast cancer: allelic loss on 1p and 1q is related to lymphogenic metastases and poor prognosis. *Genes, Chromosomes & Cancer* 1992;5:311–320.

117. Rubin JR, Eberline LB. The effect of inguinal lymphatic manipulation on regional lymph flow patterns. *J Vasc Surg* 1993;17:896–901.

118. Hartmann LC, Ingle JN, Wold LE, et al. Prognostic value of c-erbB2 overexpression in axillary lymph node positive breast cancer. Results from a randomized adjuvant treatment protocol. *Cancer* 1994;74: 2956–2963.

119. Lindblom A, Rotstein S, Skoog L, Nordenskjold M, Larsson C. Deletions on chromosome 16 in primary familial breast carcinomas are associated with development of distant metastases. *Cancer Res* 1993; 53:3707–3711.

120. Luca M, Hunt B, Bucana CD, Johnson JP, Fidler IJ, Bar-Eli M. Direct correlation between MUC18 expression and metastatic potential of human melanoma cells. *Melanoma Research* 1993;3:35–41.

121. Pantel K, Schlimok G, Kutter D, et al. Frequent down-regulation of major histocompatibility class I antigen expression on individual micrometastatic carcinoma cells. *Cancer Res* 1991;51:4712–4715.

122. Haaverstad R, Johnsen H, Saether OD, Myhre HO. Lymph drainage and the development of post-reconstructive leg oedema is not influenced by the type of inguinal incision. A prospective randomised study in patients undergoing femoropopliteal bypass surgery. *Eur J Vasc Endovasc Surg* 1995;10:316–322.

123. Wells KE, Cruse CW, Daniels S, Berman C, Norman J, Reintgen DS. The use of lymphoscintigraphy in melanoma of the head and neck. *Plast Reconstr Surg* 1994;93:757–761.

124. Cambria RA, Gloviczki P, Naessens JM, Wahner HW. Noninvasive evaluation of the lymphatic system with lymphoscintigraphy: a prospective, semiquantitative analysis in 386 extremities. *J Vasc Surg* 1993;18:773–782.

125. Uren RF, Howman-Giles RB, Shaw HM, Thompson JF, McCarthy WH. Lymphoscintigraphy in high-risk melanoma of the trunk: predicting draining node groups, defining lymphatic channels and locating the sentinel node. *J Nuclear Med* 1993;34:1435–1440.

126. Norman J, Wells K, Kearney R, Cruse CW, Berman C, Reintgen D. Identification of lymphatic drainage basins in patients with cutaneous melanoma. *Sem Surgical Oncol* 1993;9:224–227.

127. Taminiau AH, Arndt JW, van Bockel JH, Steenhoff JR, Pauwels EK. Evaluation of the lymph flow with lymphoscintigraphy after rotationplasty for the treatment of bone tumors. *J Bone Joint Surg [Am]* 1992; 74:101–105.

128. Wong JH, Cagle LA, Morton DL. Lymphatic drainage of skin to a sentinel lymph node in a feline model. *Ann Surg* 1991;214:637–641.

129. Reintgen D, Cruse CW, Wells K, et al. The orderly progression of melanoma nodal metastases. *Ann Surg* 1994;220:759–767.

130. Giuliano AE, Kirgan DM, Guenther JM, Morton DL. Lymphatic mapping and sentinel lymphadenectomy for breast cancer. *Ann Surg* 1994; 220:391–398.

131. Morton DL, Wen DR, Wong JH, et al. Technical details of intraoperative lymphatic mapping for early stage melanoma. *Arch Surg* 1992; 127:392–399.

132. Cabanas RM. Anatomy and biopsy of sentinel lymph nodes. *Urol Clin North Am* 1992;19:267–276.

133. Kirkwood JM, Strawderman MH, Ernstoff MS, Smith TJ, Borden EC, Blum RH. Interferon alpha-2b adjuvant therapy of high-risk resected cutaneous melanoma: the Eastern Cooperative Oncology Group Trial EST 1684. *J Clin Oncol* 1996;14(1):7–17.

CHAPTER 3

Diagnosis of Pulmonary Metastatic Disease

Daphne J. Y. Mew, Jessica Donington, and Harvey I. Pass

We know of no malignant growth the metastases of which occur in one form of tissue only.
— *Sir William Osler,* The Principles and Practice of Medicine (1909).

The most dreaded and defining aspect of cancer is its ability to metastasize. The search for occult spread is a critical factor in cancer management because the detection of metastatic disease significantly alters the prognosis and directs the potential treatment pathways. For many malignancies, the lungs are the most frequent site of metastatic disease. It is the only site of metastatic spread in 20% of autopsy cases (1). Lung metastases are frequently seen in breast, thyroid, and kidney cancers (>50% incidence), followed by melanoma, osteosarcomas, and chorionepitheliomas (2). This chapter reviews the pathogenesis and signs and symptoms of pulmonary metastases. Current diagnostic (nonsurgical) modalities are also discussed.

PATHOGENESIS OF PULMONARY METASTASIS

The distribution of metastases depends in part on the tumor's histologic type and primary anatomic location. However, many malignancies preferentially metastasize to the lungs. Two models have been proposed to explain the lungs' susceptibility for metastasis. The anatomic model views the lungs as a rich vascular sink that may be the first capillary bed encountered by circulating tumor cells exiting the venous drainage of the primary cancer.

In this model, the lungs act as the initial site of filtration to trap the disseminated malignant cells mechanically. Subsequent tumor growth in the lungs would, in this case, be due solely to the tumor's drainage pathways. The patterns of metastatic spread observed with head and neck cancer, thyroid cancer, sarcomas, and melanomas would be consistent with this model. The finding of hepatic metastases before lung involvement so typical with cancers of the pancreas and gastrointestinal tract is also in keeping with the anatomic model. The initial capillary bed entered by potential metastatic cells would be the liver via portal drainage. However, this model alone does not account for the pattern of all metastatic spread. The anatomic model would predict a high incidence of metastasis in tissues with rich capillary beds, such as the skin or skeletal muscle; clinically, secondary lesions in these tissues are infrequent.

Hence, investigators have proposed an organ tropism model in which tumor cells develop metastatic foci in tissues with microenvironments conducive to growth. In this model, potential metastatic cells distribute to all organs but grow only in specific tissues. Organ specificity may be due to the presence of local growth factors or hormones, specific organ endothelial adhesion interactions with tumor cells, chemotaxins secreted by target organs that attract tumor cells, or susceptible tissue matrices that are easily invaded by tumor cells.

Both models probably play a role in the mechanism of metastatic spread. The role of each model in the pathophysiology of metastatic spread also may vary with tumor histology and the location of the primary.

Regardless of the mechanism, the most common pathway for pulmonary metastasis is through hematogenous dissemination. Malignant emboli of single cells or tumor cell clusters reach the circulation after escaping from the primary tumor by erosion through thin-walled tumor vessels or pre-established normal host vasculature. The tumor emboli are then filtered or caught in the precapil-

D. J. Y. Mew: Department of Surgery, University of Calgary, Foothills Hospital, Calgary, Alberta, Canada T2N-2T9.

J. Donington: Surgery Branch, National Cancer Institute, National Institutes of Health, Bethesda, Maryland 20892.

H. I. Pass: Departments of Surgery and Oncology, Wayne State University, Karmanos Cancer Institute, Harper Hospital, Detroit, Michigan 48201.

lary venules of the lung by mechanical trapping or adherence. Most of these cells are either neutralized by host defenses (host macrophages, natural killer cells, activated T-cells) or fail to gain a foothold into susceptible tissue due to an inability to invade (3). To form a metastatic focus, the tumor cells must disrupt the host endothelial basement membrane before infiltrating the susceptible pulmonary stroma. Further proliferation of the malignant emboli is then determined by both tumor and local tissue factors. It is estimated that only a small number (<0.01%) of the circulating tumor cells can initiate metastasis (4).

Direct lymphatic or lymphangitic spread through hematogenous dissemination is another mechanism for pulmonary metastasis. Passage of tumor cells into lymphatic channels occurs at the tumor periphery, because in general tumors lack a well-developed lymphatic system. The tumor emboli are delivered to regional lymph nodes. The lymphangitic formation of metastatic foci in the lungs may also occur via retrograde lymphatic spread through involved lymph nodes to hilar or mediastinal nodes (5–7) or via circulation into the regional or systemic venous system through lymphatic hematogenous communications. Other pathways for pulmonary metastasis include transbronchial dissemination via aspiration, endobronchial metastasis through secondary bronchial invasion, or direct bronchial arterial seeding (6,7). Malignant pleural effusion may be associated with parietal pleural metastases due to increased pleural capillary permeability, decreased absorption, or tumor erosion of parietal vessels (8).

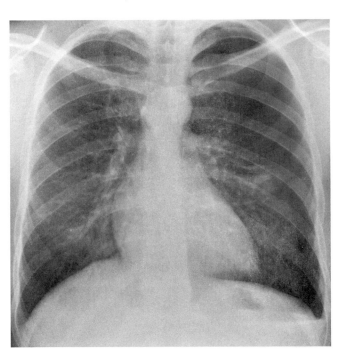

FIG. 2. Patient with a known history of metastatic sarcoma who suffered a left-sided pneumothorax.

SIGNS AND SYMPTOMS OF PULMONARY METASTASES

The most common physical finding of pulmonary metastatic disease is no sign or symptom at all. Because pulmonary metastatic lesions are generally located in the peripheral subpleura or lung parenchyma, it is not surprising that 85% to 95% of patients with metastases are asymptomatic (9–11). The slow, gradual development of dyspnea may be due to direct airway obstruction or to loss of lung capacity due to pleural effusion or tumor replacement of pulmonary parenchyma. The sudden onset of dyspnea may herald the development of a pneumothorax or hemorrhage into a pulmonary lesion or pleural effusion, with subsequent acute loss of lung capacity (Fig. 1). Metastatic pneumothorax may be due to subpleural bleb rupture secondary to tumor invasion and expansion (Fig. 2). Dyspnea in the presence of diminished diffusing capacity and arterial saturation and in the absence of (or minimal) chest radiographic findings may be caused by lymphangitic spread of tumor (12,13) or tumor emboli (14). Wheezing or cough may be secondary to obstructive pulmonary lesions or postobstructive pneumonia/pneumonitis. Patients with hemoptysis should undergo bronchoscopic examination to rule out potentially treatable endobronchial lesions. Chest pain may signify parietal pleural metastasis, invasion of the chest wall, or rib involvement.

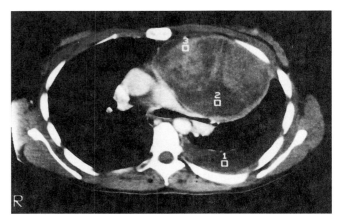

FIG. 1. CT in a patient with known synovial cell sarcoma who presented with acute dyspnea and chest pain. Note the extremely large pulmonary metastasis causing mediastinal shift and compression of the left main stem bronchus. The numbered squares depict areas of different densities: (1) an associated pleural effusion, (2) an area of liquefaction necrosis or hemorrhage in the metastasis; and (3) a more solid component of the metastasis.

TABLE 1. *Etiology of pulmonary nodules*

Multiple
  Benign processes
    Infectious
      Granulomas: histoplasmosis, coccidioidomycosis,
        tuberculosis
      Opportunistic infections: *Nocardia, Aspergillus,*
        Cryptococcus
      Parasitic lesions: hydatid cysts
      Septic emboli
      Pyogenic abscesses
    Drug-induced lesions
      Methotrexate
      Bleomycin
    Autoimmune
      Rheumatoid nodules
      Wegener's granulomatosis
      Sarcoidosis
    Benign tumors: papillomatosis, hamartomas,
      chondromas, leiomyomas
    Others: arteriovenous malformations, silicosis,
      pulmonary emboli
  Malignant processes
    Metastatic disease (most common)
    Lymphomas
Solitary
  Benign processes
    Infectious granulomas: tuberculosis, non-TB
      mycobacteria, coccidioidomas, histoplasmomas,
      mucormycosis, cryptococcosis, *Pneumocystis carinii*
    Noninfectious granulomas: sarcoidosis, rheumatoid
      nodule, Wegener's granulomatosis
    Tumors: hamartomas, chondromas
    Others: pulmonary infarct, vascular lesion,
      bronchogenic cyst
  Malignant processes
    Bronchogenic carcinoma, solitary metastatic nodule,
      carcinoid tumors, lymphoma

X-RAY CHARACTERISTICS OF PULMONARY METASTASES

The number and morphology of lung lesions are important considerations in the evaluation of the etiology of pulmonary metastases. The presence of multiple pulmonary lesions in the setting of established extrathoracic malignancy tends to be very suspicious for pulmonary metastases. However, other causes of multiple pulmonary lesions are possible, such as granulomas, opportunistic infections (eg, *Cryptococcus, Aspergillus*), sarcoidosis, drug-induced pulmonary changes (eg, bleomycin, methotrexate), and pulmonary emboli (Table 1). A solitary pulmonary nodule, on the other hand, may represent a new primary tumor, a benign lesion, or a metastatic focus. The discovery of such an incidental nodule may be the best opportunity for diagnosing primary lung cancer at a potentially curable stage.

Two radiographic criteria have been useful in predicting whether a solitary nodule is benign: rate of growth and patterns of calcification. The characteristic absence

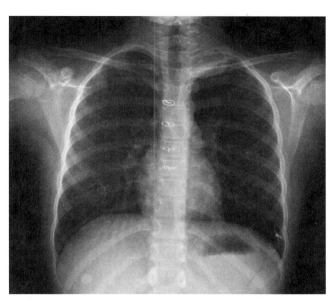

FIG. 3. Plain chest radiograph revealing a subtle apical lesion on the left in a 15-year-old with known osteogenic sarcoma.

of growth for two or more years is useful only if retrospective evaluation of older chest films revels the presence of a nodule that was not previously recognized. Clearly, it would be inappropriate to follow an indeterminate pulmonary lesion prospectively, especially because small size does not rule out malignancy. The presence of patterns of calcification (eg, central nidus, popcorn, lamination, or diffuse calcification) has been described in the diagnosis of benign pulmonary lesions. However, calcification has also been noted in metastatic disease (Figs. 3–5). Osteogenic sarcoma, chondrosarcoma, and synovial sarcoma are all associated with calcification. Pulmonary metastases from thyroid, ovarian, breast, or mucinous gastrointestinal cancers have also been found occasionally to be calcified. The degeneration of pulmonary metastatic lesions after chemotherapy or radiation therapy may also result in calcification (15–20). In the so-called "scar carcinoma," the eccentric calcic stippling is within

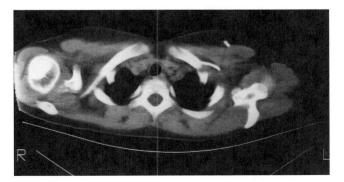

FIG. 4. Previous CT scan of the apex in the patient in Fig. 3 did not reveal an apical deformity.

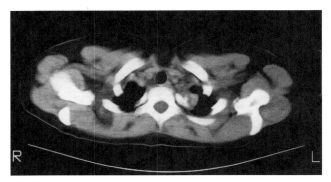

FIG. 5. Follow-up CT scan of the apex at the time of presentation of the apical lesion seen in Fig. 3. Note the calcification in the nodule that appears to be intimately associated with the first rib on the left.

the scar tissue; the noncalcic portion represents the engulfing tumor mass.

In a patient with an extrapulmonary cancer, a solitary malignant nodule is virtually always a metastasis if the primary was a melanoma or sarcoma. It may be either a new primary or a metastasis if the original primary was an adenocarcinoma. It is usually a new primary if the original cancer was squamous carcinoma (21).

A tissue diagnosis is mandatory for all solitary pulmonary nodules without the characteristic "benign" calcification, and those demonstrating any increase in size. A diagnosis of cancer was made in 40% of such nodules brought to thoracotomy (22). Although the size and mor-

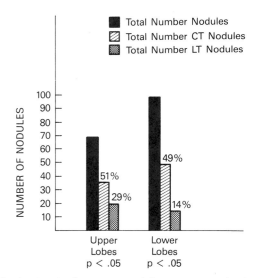

FIG. 6. Anatomically, more nodules are seen in the lower lobes than in the upper lobes, regardless of the examining study. More nodules are detected by CT than by linear tomography in all locations. (Pass HI, Dwyer A, Makuch R, Roth JA. Detection of pulmonary metastases in patients with osteogenic and soft tissue sarcoma: the superiority of CT scan compared with conventional linear tomograms using dynamic analyses. *J Clin Oncol* 1985;3:1261–1265, with permission.)

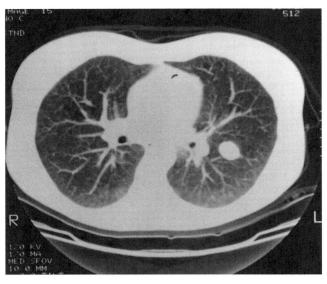

FIG. 7. A larger-than-average but typically shaped pulmonary metastasis to the left lower lobe from melanoma. Note the roughly spherical shape.

phology of a solitary pulmonary nodule are generally not predictive of malignancy, a lesion >3 cm in diameter is more likely to be cancerous (23). About one third of solitary pulmonary lesions initially noted on chest x-ray proved to be multiple lesions on computed tomography (CT). In up to 80% of these cases, the multiple nodules were metastatic in nature (24).

There is no predilection for laterality of pulmonary metastasis (25). Metastatic lesions tend to localize at the lung bases, reflecting the flow characteristics of the pulmonary circulation and the greater lung volume at the bases (Fig. 6) (26). A notable exception is the posterior upper lobe location of choriocarcinoma pulmonary meta-

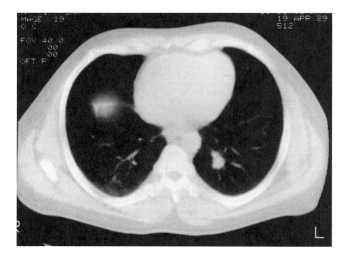

FIG. 8. A pulmonary metastasis in the left lower lobe with rougher, less well-demarcated margins. It arose from a renal cell cancer.

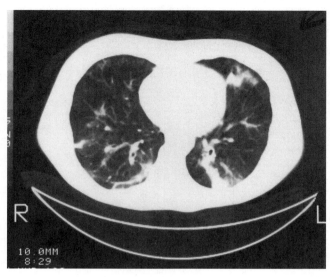

FIG. 9. This patient presented with new-onset dyspnea and a previous history of breast cancer. CT reveals patchy infiltrates anteriorly and at the bases.

static lesions. This is due to patient positioning and subsequent dissemination at the time of curettage (27,28).

The size and appearance of the pulmonary lesion may give clues to its benign or malignant nature. Pulmonary metastasis due to hematogenous tumor emboli give rise to nodular lesions, independent of histology (Figs. 7, 8). They appear as roughly spherical densities with sharply demarcated borders on plain chest radiographs. Pulmonary lesions with an irregular edge usually imply primary lung cancer, but factors such as age of the lesion, prior radiation therapy, chemotherapy and bleeding may alter the appearance. On high-resolution CT, different characteristics of benign and malignant lesions can be appreci-

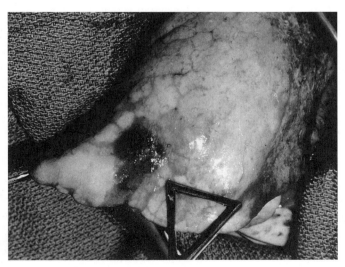

FIG. 10. Operative findings at thoracotomy in the patient in Fig. 9 revealed lymphangitic carcinomatosis.

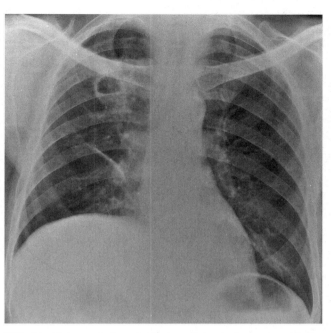

FIG. 11. This cavitating right upper lobe lesion proved to be metastatic bladder cancer.

ated. Benign lesions generally have smooth, well-demarcated margins. Nonspherical lesions are more likely to be benign (29). Malignant nodules may have lobulated or blurred edges on CT. The presence of spiculation is very suggestive of malignancy (30). Lymphangitic patterns of metastases are due to retrograde dissemination of tumor from lymphatic vessels leading from the mediastinum (Figs. 9, 10) (6,31). In early stages, lymphangitic metastases may have only minimal chest x-ray findings. They appear as an interstitial infiltrate indistinguishable from fibrosis or edema. At later stages, they may be distinguished by linear markings and enlarged hilar nodes. A diffuse miliary pattern of metastasis has been described for metastatic pulmonary lesions secondary to medullary cancer of the thyroid, ovarian carcinoma, and renal cell carcinoma (32).

Cavitation occurs in about 5% of pulmonary metastases. This may be associated with sarcoma or head and neck squamous carcinoma (Fig. 11). Central necrosis and liquefaction of the metastatic lesion, due either to rapid tumor growth or treatment-related cell death, leads to this characteristic appearance (5). Cancers from the upper gastrointestinal tract (eg, stomach, pancreas) are usually associated with lymphangitic pulmonary metastases. Colonic metastases are typically in the form of nodular lesions. Cancers of the genitourinary tract tend to form nodular pulmonary lesions. Pulmonary "cannonball" metastases are classically described with clear cell carcinoma of the kidney. Ovarian and prostatic cancer are an exception to the genitourinary nodular pulmonary pattern; they tend to be associated with pleural effusions and

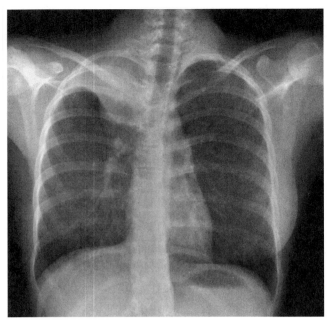

FIG. 12. Right upper lobe atelectasis in a patient with known osteogenic sarcoma.

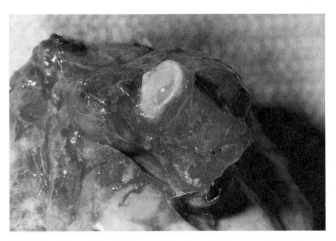

FIG. 14. Operative photograph after right upper lobe sleeve resection in the patient in Figs. 12 and 13. The bronchus has been transected and excised en bloc with the lobe, which was blocked by the endobronchial lesion.

lymphangitic spread (33). Pleural bleb formation can be associated with testicular metastases (34). Spontaneous malignant pneumothorax is a rare presentation of intrathoracic metastatic disease. In a 1973 review of >1,100 spontaneous pneumothoraces, only 10 cases were associated with metastatic disease (35). Spontaneous pneumothorax has been diagnosed after chemotherapy (36). Breast cancer is associated with nodular, miliary, or lymphangitic patterns of metastasis. Endobronchial metastasis is found in up to 28% of cancer patients (Figs. 12–14) (37–39). The most commonly reported primary cancers associated with this presentation are carcinomas of the breast, kidney, colon, and pancreas. Radiographic findings range from lobar or total lung collapse and postobstructive pneumonia/pneumonitis to no findings at all. Mediastinal and hilar adenopathy may also be observed in association with pulmonary metastasis; rarely, it is the only sign of intrathoracic metastatic disease.

Another uncommon form of intrathoracic adenopathy is the involvement of the internal mammary lymph nodes. This is most often associated with breast cancer (40). Pleural effusions in the presence or absence of parenchymal lesions are also part of the spectrum of radiologic findings in intrathoracic metastatic disease. They may be due directly to pleural metastatic lesions and subsequent exudative tumor-positive effusion, or to a serous transudate secondary to the impaired lymphatic drainage of tumor-laden mediastinal lymph nodes. Cancer-associated disease processes such as pulmonary embolism, pneumonia, atelectasis, and low plasma oncotic pressure secondary to cachexia may contribute to the development of pleural effusion in the absence of intrathoracic metastatic disease. Absent or minimal chest radiographic findings may also be associated with pulmonary metastasis, especially with lymphangitic lesions. In Goldsmith and associates' series of breast cancer patients with proven lymphangitic intrathoracic metastasis, up to 50% had a normal chest x-ray (41). Other radiologically occult pulmonary metastatic lesions include tumor emboli and, as previously mentioned, endobronchial masses.

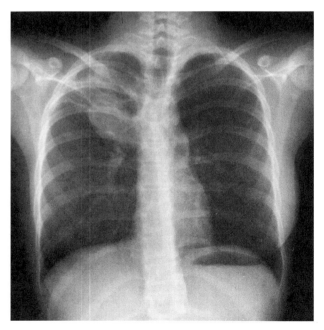

FIG. 13. Bronchoscopy revealed an endobronchial metastasis of osteogenic sarcoma in the patient in Fig. 12. Note the clearing of the atelectasis after bronchoscopy and the clear depiction of the large pulmonary nodule.

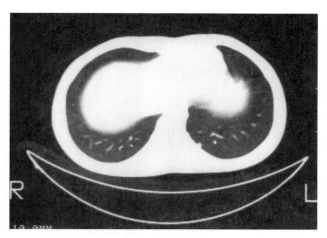

FIG. 15. CT scan reveals a posterior basal lesion in a patient with a soft-tissue sarcoma.

X-RAY EXAMINATION

The ideal imaging modality should be able to detect the smallest abnormality, should be specific for metastatic disease, should minimize radiation exposure to the patient, and should be cost-effective for initial diagnosis and follow-up screening.

Posteroanterior and lateral chest radiographs are routine techniques for pulmonary metastasis surveillance in both the initial staging and interval follow-up of some malignant diseases. The plain chest x-ray serves as a baseline evaluation and a possible diagnostic tool for detecting coexisting cardiopulmonary disease in the initial workup of cancer patients. A suspicious finding on initial chest radiography may be more accurately interpreted with a previous chest film for comparison to define the possibly malignant nature of the lesion. However, a CT scan of the chest is usually required to rule out the presence of other lesions and to define further the nature of the abnormality (Figs. 15, 16).

CT of the chest has become the standard of care for the initial evaluation, treatment planning, and interval follow-up of the cancer patient at risk for pulmonary metastasis, especially since the development of "fast CT" scanners. CT is superior to plain chest radiography in defining lesion morphology and detecting calcification. It is also more sensitive in detecting mediastinal disease. CT of the chest is more useful in the diagnosis of lymphangitic metastases than is conventional chest radiography. Characteristic CT findings suggestive of lymphangitic lesions include basilar and circumferential nodular septal thickening in the absence of architectural distortion. These findings may be identified even in patients with apparently normal or minimal findings on plain chest films (41). CT is superior to conventional linear tomography for detecting pulmonary metastasis because it eliminates structural overlap and shadows in the cross-sectional images (42). Subpleural abnormalities are easily identified. Contrast resolution exceeds conventional techniques by at least a factor of 10, allowing the identification of lesions as small as 3 mm in diameter (26). Pulmonary lesion size can be underestimated because of partial volume averaging, where the lesion is not fully viewed in the CT axial cut or when attenuation of the lesion is decreased because of abutting aerated lung. Small nodules adjacent to blood vessels can be difficult to identify, but resolution has been improved with the use of intravenous contrast (43–48). A typical CT of the chest involves 8- to 10-mm axial sections throughout the chest cavity with simultaneous intravenous administration of iodinated contrast material to detect or follow metastatic

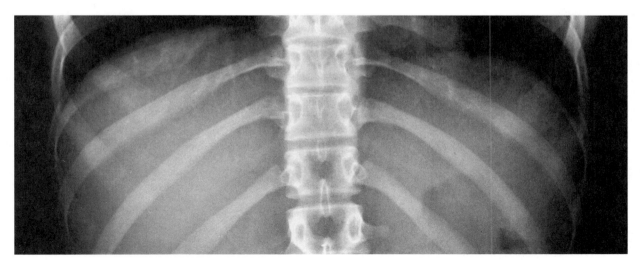

FIG. 16. The abdominal film on corresponding linear tomography in the patient seen in Fig. 15 fails to reveal the lesion. The bases and costophrenic angles are poor areas of visualization on linear tomography as compared to CT.

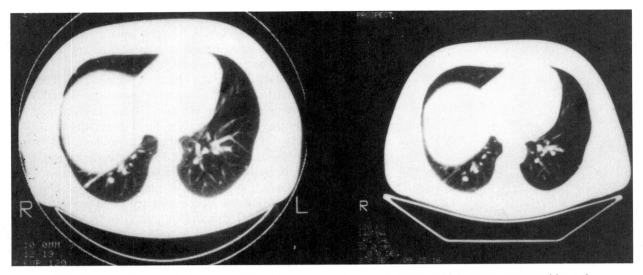

FIG. 17. A stable nodule is seen at the right base on these CT scans, which were separated by a 6-month interval.

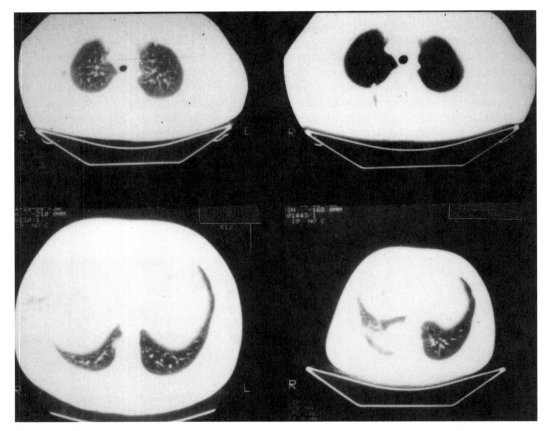

FIG. 18. *(Upper panel)* A newly developing nodule seen in the right lung in a patient with metastatic sarcoma. *(Lower panel)* A right-sided paravertebral nodule exhibited growth over a 4-month period and was subsequently resected.

iodinated contrast material to detect or follow metastatic disease.

The major advantage of CT is its ability to identify pulmonary nodules and define their behavior temporally. The appearance and development of pulmonary metastasis depend on many variables. The pattern of pulmonary lesions at any particular time is a cumulative phenomenon. It depends on the frequency and intensity of the embolic showers, the invasive/colonizing capacity of the metastases, the time course of the malignancy, and the histology of the disease. Individual metastatic lesions may grow at different rates, based on the original tumor clone growth characteristics. In the surveillance of pulmonary metastases, the problem is essentially to distinguish between benign and malignant processes. Usually the benign nodule is static in growth.

Serial CT scanning can determine the dynamic properties of the pulmonary lesions, specifically in a homogeneous patient population (Figs. 17, 18). Nodules can be classified as stable, new onset, or growing. The predictive value of CT in defining a nodule as malignant is not as high in nodules that demonstrate a stable size on sequential scans (26). However, the development of a new CT abnormality in the sarcoma patient, or the growth of a previous nodule, can be histologically documented as malignant with a 90% confidence level (26). Questionable abnormalities demand repeat CTs at 2- to 3-month intervals to document any biologic change that would justify exploration or a change in treatment pathways.

USE OF CT IN MONITORING SPECIFIC HISTOLOGIES

If a suspicious nodule is identified on a plain chest film, CT should be performed to verify the finding and to document the presence or absence of other lesions. The role of chest CT versus plain chest radiography in the diagnosis or follow-up of cancer patients depends on the natural history of the primary malignancy. In patients with malignancies that have a predilection for pulmonary metastasis (eg, testicular carcinoma, soft-tissue sarcoma, choriocarcinomas), chest CT should be performed initially as a baseline. This is especially important if aggressive early treatment of pulmonary metastasis has been found to improve survival significantly. Such is the case with sarcoma. In cancer patients with multiple nodules on chest radiography, CT scans may be useful to monitor therapeutic response. If active treatment is not an issue, repeat follow-up examination using plain chest radiography would be sufficient and considerably more cost-effective. In patients with malignancies that tend to seed other organs before metastasizing to the lung, plain chest radiography may be adequate if the potential sites of metastasis are negative for disease. For example, in the absence of laboratory evidence of hepatic metastasis and a normal

CT of the liver, patients with cancers of the colon, rectum, pancreas, or stomach are unlikely to have pulmonary metastases. Under these circumstances, a negative chest radiograph has a high probability of being a true-negative finding, and a diagnostic CT of the chest is unnecessary (49). Similarly, in patients with prostate cancer and other patients who have a high probability of initial metastatic spread to bone, in the face of a normal bone scan, the use of chest CT should be limited to patients with abnormalities diagnosed on the chest radiograph.

The schedule of surveillance for pulmonary metastasis should be tailored to the natural history of the primary cancer as well. For example, the natural course for sarcoma predicts a high probability of lung metastasis in the first two years after diagnosis. In these patients, chest CTs at 3-month intervals are recommended.

NEWER IMAGING METHODS

Because multiple doses of radiation are delivered to patients in an attempt to detect metastatic disease, a sensitive screening modality free of ionizing radiation would be valuable, especially in younger patients. Magnetic resonance imaging (MRI) has made considerable diagnostic strides in the diagnosis of chest diseases, but few studies have addressed its use in the detection of pulmonary metastases. A prospective trial at the National Cancer Institute compared the use of MRI, chest radiography, computed tomography, and surgical verification of disease in 12 patients (50). For nodules >5 mm, MRI was at least as sensitive as CT and significantly more sensitive than chest x-ray. MRI studies of the chest are not as diagnostic as CT scans. MRI is not useful in the evaluation of pulmonary nodules because it fails to detect calcification. The signal characteristics of MRI cannot distinguish between benign and malignant lesions or lymphadenopathy. It is inferior to CT in spatial resolution. CT allows superior evaluation of the bronchi, small lymph nodes, and lung parenchyma. The only imaging advantage of MRI over CT lies in its ability to evaluate the posterior mediastinum, lung apex, and diaphragmatic regions (51). Future studies with newer MRI scanners will be needed to define its role in comparison with CT as the gold standard for the detection and surveillance of pulmonary metastases.

Positron emission tomography (PET) is an imaging technique that uses the differences in biochemical processes in tissues to produce a three-dimensional picture. Malignancy can be distinguished biochemically from normal tissue by its accelerated rate of glycolysis. This characteristic can be exploited with the use of radiolabeled glucose analogs to image areas of potential tumor involvement. The role of PET scans relative to other imaging techniques in intrathoracic metastatic disease has yet to be fully defined. In one report of the use of PET scans in metastatic malignant melanoma, CT imaging of the chest was more sensitive than PET in detecting small pulmonary lesions (52). The application of PET imaging in pulmonary metastatic disease may lie in the ability to evaluate tumor metabolism rather than to detect new lung lesions. Recurrent tumor may be differentiated from posttreatment scarring, necrotic lesions, static or slow-growing metastases with the use of PET technology, as all these lesions should demonstrate markedly different metabolic characteristics.

The use of chest ultrasound and color flow Doppler imaging offers an intriguing alternate technique that does not involve radiation. Hypervascular tumors demonstrate tumor flow signals that appear as distinctive high-velocity patterns on Doppler studies (53). This imaging technique was used to identify metastatic pulmonary choriocarcinoma in a pregnant patient (54). Other metastatic lesions known to have tumor flow signals include breast cancer, primary hepatomas, and renal cell carcinomas (55–57). In the future, this technique may be used to identify lesions that have a high risk of bleeding after biopsy or to evaluate pulmonary lesions after therapy. Responding lesions after treatment may demonstrate decreased or no blood flow signals, suggestive of effective killing of the mass (54).

Ventilation/perfusion (V/Q) scanning is not a useful diagnostic tool for staging the chest for metastasis. Nonetheless, V/Q scans in combination with pulmonary function tests are useful in screening patients prethoracotomy to predict postoperative performance, especially if there is a possibility for pneumonectomy.

INVASIVE DIAGNOSTIC MEANS (EXCLUSIVE OF THORACOTOMY)

Factors such as equivocal imaging studies, the patient's physiologic status, the potential for cure, the histology of the original primary, and the location of the lesion must be considered in pursuing a tissue diagnosis of a suspicious pulmonary nodule. Certainly, any pleural effusion associated with nodules in the lungs requires cytologic verification of malignancy and possibly a pleural biopsy. Patients unable to tolerate thoracotomy due to decreased physiologic reserves may still require a histologic diagnosis for determining appropriate treatment pathways. The full extent of metastatic spread must be documented, especially if it will affect the magnitude or aggressiveness of treatment (eg, limb salvage versus amputation for possible cure in sarcomas).

Noninvasive diagnostic studies such as sputum cytology and bronchoscopy have been of limited value in the diagnosis of pulmonary metastatic disease. In one review, sputum cytologic examination revealed malignant cells in only 5% of patients with documented pulmonary metastases (58). Bronchoscopies were diagnostic in only 10% of patients with known pulmonary metastatic disease (58).

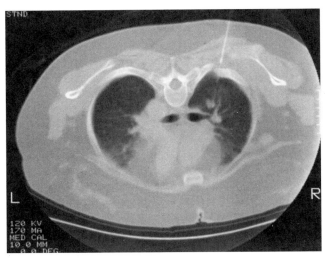

FIG. 19. Positioning of a Chiba needle under CT guidance for FNAB of a presumed lung metastasis.

However, with endobronchial metastasis, bronchoscopies should be performed to see if operative intervention is possible. In an isolated metastasis seen by bronchoscopy, lobectomy or sleeve lobectomy may be associated with a reasonable chance of survival. If resection is impossible, endobronchial management with or without laser ablation may be of great palliative interest.

One of the major indications for transthoracic fine-needle aspiration biopsy (FNAB) is the diagnosis of potential metastatic disease from an extrathoracic malignancy. In combination with CT or other imaging techniques, FNAB may be used to differentiate metastatic from benign lesions. If a specific benign diagnosis is made, thoracotomy may be avoided. FNAB is especially useful in patients who require histologic confirmation to guide treatment options but are unable to tolerate thoracotomy (Fig. 19) (59). FNAB of metastatic lesions reportedly has a high diagnostic sensitivity (88%) for melanoma, breast cancer, gastrointestinal cancer, germinal cell tumors (45, 46,60,61), and soft-tissue sarcomas (62–64). The most common complications of transthoracic FNAB are pneumothorax and minor hemoptysis. The risk of pneumothorax ranges from 25% to 35% (65), with chest tube placement being needed in only 4% (66). Minor hemoptysis occurs in 1% to 10% of transthoracic FNAB procedures; in the absence of coagulopathy, it seldom requires active treatment (67). Air embolism is a rare but potentially fatal complication. Malignant needle track implantation is mainly a theoretical consideration. Clinically, it is extremely rare: in Sinner's series of 2,726 FNAB cases, only one case of needle track implantation was identified (68). FNAB is contraindicated in patients with bleeding diathesis, compromised pulmonary function and pulmonary hypertension, and bullous disease surrounding the lesion or in the needle biopsy pathway (69).

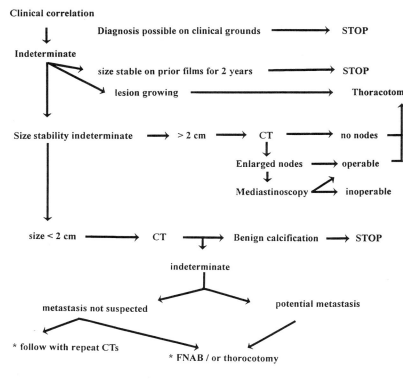

FIG. 20. Diagnostic algorithm for the roentgenographic evaluation of the solitary pulmonary nodule. (Modified from Lillington GA. Management of solitary pulmonary nodules. *Dis Mon* 1991;37:272–318.)

THORACOSCOPY

The use of thoracoscopy to diagnose pleural effusions and pulmonary metastases has increased and is now combined with video monitoring for documentation and ease of exploration. The multiple-trocar technique and new instruments for endoscopic surgery (including the Endo-GIA, US Surgical) have made this technique very popular for thoracic diseases. For lesions on the surface of the visceral pleura, resection can be performed. Deeper parenchymal lesions must be palpated to be found, and the capability of endoscopic instruments for resection is applicable in only the most superficial lesions (70–73). The major advantage of this technology is the ability to visualize suspicious lesions directly to allow adequate sampling.

ROENTGENOGRAPHIC MANAGEMENT OF PULMONARY LESIONS

A solitary pulmonary nodule ("coin lesion") refers to a single lung lesion in the absence of other pulmonary findings (ie, hilar adenopathy, atelectasis, or pneumonia on chest x-ray). About 40% to 50% of solitary lesions are malignant; most are bronchogenic carcinomas, 10% are single metastatic nodules, and <3% are carcinoid tumors (74). The primary objectives in the workup of the solitary pulmonary nodule are to diagnose any potentially curable malignancy and to reduce the number of thoracotomies

for surgically incurable disease or benign disease (Fig. 20). In general, the presence of calcification in a benign pattern, or stable size after retrospective review of previous films (especially in a patient <35 and with no risk factors) is enough for the diagnosis of benign disease. With a positive history of risk factors such as heavy smoking or previous malignancy or a suspicious calcification pattern (eg, spiculation), the diagnostic pathway should be directed toward a thoracotomy. The management pathway of the radiographically indeterminate lesion depends on its size on presentation. However, small size does not rule out malignancy: in a series of 431 nodules 2 cm or less in size, 43% were found to be malignant (75). If an indeterminate lesion is <2 cm and is not suspected to be malignant, it could be appropriate to do nothing and repeat the CT at 4- to 8-week intervals to monitor for any change. This is especially suitable if the patient is reluctant to undergo a thoracotomy. However, a FNAB or thoracotomy could also be appropriate if the patient is anxious about waiting for a diagnosis.

Multiple pulmonary lesions in most cases represent metastatic disease. With a known extrapulmonary malignancy, it may be appropriate to make the diagnosis on clinical grounds. However, in potentially treatable disease (ie, metastatic lesions from thyroid, breast, kidney, or prostate, lymphomas, or infectious processes) (see Table 1), a diagnosis may be accomplished by transthoracic or transbronchial FNAB.

REFERENCES

1. Viadana E, Irwin D, Bross J, Pickren JW. Cascade spread of blood-borne metastases in solid and nonsolid cancers of humans. In: Weiss L, Gilbert H, eds. *Pulmonary metastases*. Boston: GK Hall, 1978:142–167.
2. Mountain L. Comment: Pulmonary metastatic disease—progress in a neglected area. *Int J Radiat Oncol Biol Phys* 1976;1:755–757.
3. Vaage J. Humeral and cellular immune factors in the systemic control of artificially induced metastasis in C3H7 mice. *Cancer Res* 1973;33: 1957–1965.
4. Schirrmacher V. Experimental approaches, theoretical concepts, and impact for treatment strategies. *Adv Cancer Res* 1985;43:1–32.
5. Libshitz HI, North LB. Pulmonary metastases. *Radiol Clin North Am* 1982;20:437–451.
6. Janower ML, Blennerhassett HJB. Lymphangitic spread of metastatic cancer to the lung. *Radiology* 1971;101:267–273.
7. Heitzman ER, Markarian B, Raasch BN, et al. Pathways of tumor spread through the lung: Radiologic correlations with anatomy and pathology. *Radiology* 1982;144:3.
8. Naidich DP, Zerhouni EA, Siegelman SS, eds. *Computed tomography of the thorax*. New York: Raven Press, 1984:261.
9. Putnam JB Jr, Roth JA, Wesley MN, Johnston MR, Rosenberg SA. Survival following aggressive resection of pulmonary metastases from osteogenic sarcoma: analysis of prognostic factors. *Ann Thorac Surg* 1983;36:516–523.
10. Putnam JB, Roth JA, Wesley MN, Johnston MR, Rosenberg SA. Analysis of prognostic factors in patients undergoing resection of pulmonary metastases from soft tissue sarcomas. *J Thorac Cardiovasc Surg* 1984; 87:260–268.
11. D'Angio GJ, Iannoccone G. Spontaneous pneumothorax as a complication of pulmonary metastases in malignant tumors of childhood. *AJR* 1961;86:1092.
12. Lome LG, John T. Pulmonary manifestations of prostatic carcinoma. *J Urol* 1973;109:680.
13. Schwarz MI, Waddell LC, Dombeck DH, et al. Prolonged survival in lymphangitic carcinomatosis. *Ann Intern Med* 1969;71:779.
14. Cher CK, Hutcheson MA, Hyland RH, Walker Smith GJ, Patterson BJ, Mathey RA. Pulmonary tumor embolism: a critical review of clinical, imaging and hemodynamic features. *J Thorac Imaging* 1987;2:4–14.
15. Morse D, Reed JO, Bernstein J. Sclerosing osteogenic sarcoma. *AJR* 1963;88:491–495.
16. Fraser Rg, Pare JAP, eds. *Diagnosis of disease of the chest*. Philadelphia: WB Saunders, 1978:1132.
17. Zollikofer C, Castaneda-Zuniga W, Stenlund R, Sibley R. Lung metastases from synovial sarcoma simulating granulomas. *AJR* 1980;135: 161–163.
18. Rosenfield AT, Sanders RC, Custer LE. Widespread calcified metastases from adenocarcinoma of the jejunum. *Am J Dig Dis* 1975;20: 990–993.
19. Fraley EE, Lange PH, Kennedy BJ. Germ cell testicular cancer in adults. *N Engl J Med* 1979;301:1370–1377.
20. Panella J, Mintzer RA. Multiple calcified pulmonary nodules in an elderly man. *JAMA* 1980;244:2559–2560.
21. Cahan WG, Shah JP, Castro ELB. Benign solitary lung lesions in patients with cancer. *Ann Surg* 1978;187:241.
22. Trunk G, Gracey DR, Byrd RB. The management and evaluation of the solitary pulmonary nodule. *Chest* 66:236–239, 1974.
23. Luriyama K, Takeishi R, Doi O, et al. CT–pathologic correlation in small peripheral lung cancer. *AJR* 1987;149:1139–1143.
24. Penchot M, Libshitz HL. Pulmonary metastatic disease: Radiologic–surgical correlations. *Radiology* 1987;164:719.
25. Roth JA, Pass HI, Wesley MN, White D, Putnam JB, Seipp C. Comparison of median sternotomy and thoracotomy for resection of pulmonary metastases in patients with adult soft tissue sarcomas. *Ann Thorac Surg* 1986;42:134–138.
26. Pass HI, Dwyer A, Makuch R, Roth JA. Detection of pulmonary metastases in patients with osteogenic and soft tissue sarcoma: the superiority of CT scan compared with conventional linear tomograms using dynamic analyses. *J Clin Oncol* 1985;3:1261–1265.
27. Hendin AS. Gestational trophoblastic tumors metastatic to the lung. *Cancer* 1984;53:58–61.
28. Wagner D. Trophoblastic cells in the blood stream in normal and abnormal pregnancy. *Acta Cytol* 1968;12:137–139.
29. Huston J III, Muhm JR. Solitary pulmonary opacities: plain tomography. *Radiology* 1987;165:481–485.
30. Zwirewich CV, Vidal S, Miller RR, et al. Solitary pulmonary nodule: high-resolution CT and radiologic–pathologic correlation. *Radiology* 1991;179:469–476.
31. Dwyer AJ, Reichert CM, Woltering EA, Flye MW. Diffuse pulmonary metastasis in melanoma: radiographic–pathologic correlation. *AJR* 1984;143:983–984.
32. Fraser RG, Páre JAP, Páre PD, Fraser RS, Geneveux GP. *Diagnosis and diseases of the chest*. Philadelphia: WB Saunders, 1989:1623.
33. Berman CG, Clark RA. Diagnostic imaging in cancer. *Prim Care* 1992; 19:677–713.
34. Sarno RC, Carter BL. Bullous change by CT heralding metastatic sarcoma. *Comput Radiol* 1985;9:115.
35. Dines DE, Cortese DA, Brennan MD, Hahn RG, Payne WS. Malignant pulmonary neoplasms predisposing to spontaneous pneumothorax. *Mayo Clin Proc* 1973;48:541–544.
36. Biran H, Dgari R, Wassermen JP, Weissberg D, Shari F. Pneumothorax following induction chemotherapy in patients with lung metastases: a case report and literature review. *Ann Oncol* 1992;3:297–300.
37. King DS, Castleman B. Bronchial involvement in metastatic pulmonary malignancy. *J Thorac Surg* 1943;12:305–315.
38. Braman SS, Whitcomb ME. Endobronchial metastases. *Arch Intern Med* 1975;135:543–547.
39. Shepherd MP. Endobronchial metastatic disease. *Thorax* 1982;37: 362–370.
40. McCloud TC, Meyer JE. Mediastinal metastases. *Radiol Clin North Am* 1982;20:453–468.
41. Goldsmith HS, Baily HD, Callahan EL, Beattie EJ Jr. Pulmonary lymphangitic metastasis from breast carcinoma. *Arch Surg* 1967;94: 483–488.
42. Pass HI, Roth JA. Diagnosis of pulmonary metastases. In: Rosenberg SA, ed. *Surgical treatment of metastatic cancer*. Philadelphia: JB Lippincott Co., 1987:37–67.
43. Cohen M, Grosfeld J, Baehner R, Weetman R. Lung CT for detection of metastases: solid tissue neoplasms in children. *AJR* 1982;139: 895–898.
44. Piekarski JD, Schlumberger M, Leclere J, et al. Chest computed tomography in patients with micronodular lung metastases of differentiated thyroid carcinoma *Int J Radiat Oncol Biol Phys* 1985;11:1023.
45. Lund G, Heilo A. Computed tomography of pulmonary metastases. *Acta Radiol Diag* 1982;23:617–620.
46. Sones PJ, Torres WE, Colvin RS, Meier WL, Sprawls P, Rogers JV. Effectiveness of CT in evaluating intrathoracic masses. *AJR* 1982;139: 469–475.
47. Krudy AG, Doppman JL, Herdt JR. Failure to detect a 1.5-cm lung nodule by chest computed tomography. *J Comp Assist Tomog* 1982;6:1178.
48. Kuhns LR, Borlaza G. The "twinkling star" sign: an aid in differentiating pulmonary vessels from pulmonary nodules on computed tomograms. *Radiology* 1980;135:763–764.
49. Chiles C, Ravin CE. Intrathoracic metastasis from an extrathoracic malignancy: a radiographic approach to patient evaluation. *Radiol Clin North Am* 1985;23:427–438.
50. Feuerstein IM, Jicha DL, Pass HI, et al. Pulmonary metastases: MR imaging with surgical correlation—a prospective study. *Radiology* 1992;182:123–129.
51. Grover FL. The role of CT and MRI in staging of the mediastinum. *Chest* 1994;106:391S–396S.
52. Gritters LS, Francis IR, Zasadry KR, Wahl RL. Initial assessment of positron emission tomography using 2-fluorine-18-fluoro-2-dioxy-D-glucose in the imaging of malignant melanoma. *J Nucl Med* 1993;34: 1420–1427.
53. Taylor KJ, Ramos I, Carter D, et al. Correlation of Doppler US tumor signals with neovascular morphologic features. *Radiology* 1988;166: 57–62.
54. Liaw YS, Yang PC, Yuan A. Ultrasonography and color Doppler imaging of metastatic pulmonary choriocarcinoma. *Chest* 1993;104: 1600–1601.
55. Cosgrove DO, Banks JC, Davey JB, McKinna JA, Sinnet HD. Color Doppler signals from breast tumors. *Radiology* 1990;176:175–180.
56. Tanaka S, Kitamura T, Lajita M, Nakanishi K, Okuda S. Color Doppler imaging of liver tumors. *AJR* 1990;154:509–514.

57. Kuijpers D, Jasper R. Renal mass: differential diagnosis with pulsed Doppler US. *Radiology* 1989;170:59–60.
58. Vincent RG, Choksi LB, Takita H, Guiterrez AL. Surgical resection of the solitary pulmonary metastases. In: Weiss L, Gilbert HA, eds. *Pulmonary metastases*. Boston: GK Hall, 1978:224.
59. Johnston WW. Percutaneous fine-needle aspiration biopsy of the lung: a study of 1,015 patients. *Acta Cytol* 1984;28:218–224.
60. Poellein S, Rothenberg J, Penkava RR. Metastatic malignant melanoma in the lung: diagnosis by thin-needle aspiration biopsy. *Arch Pathol Lab Med* 1982;106:119.
61. Pilotti S, Rilke F, Gribaudi G, et al. Transthoracic fine-needle aspiration biopsy in pulmonary lesions, updated results. *Acta Cytol* 1984;28:225.
62. Silverman JF, Weaver MD, Gardner EW, et al. Aspiration biopsy cytology of malignant schwannoma metastatic to the lung. *Acta Cytol* 1984;29:15.
63. Nieberg RK. Fine-needle aspiration cytology of alveolar soft-part sarcoma. *Acta Cytol* 1984;228:198.
64. Nguyen GK, Jeannot A. Cytopathologic aspects of pulmonary metastasis of malignant fibrous histiocytoma, myxoid variant. *Acta Cytol* 1982;26:349.
65. Saunders C. Transthoracic needle aspiration. *Clin Chest Med* 1992;13:11–16.
66. Crosby JH, Hager B, Hoeg K. Transthoracic fine-needle aspiration. *Cancer* 1985;56:2504–2507.
67. Greene R. Transthoracic needle aspiration biopsy. In: Athanasoutis CA, Pfister RC, Grane RE, et al, eds. *Interventional radiology*. Philadelphia: WB Saunders, 1982:587–633.
68. Sinner WN. Complications of percutaneous transthoracic needle aspiration biopsy. *Acta Radiol Diag* 1976;17:813–827.
69. Khouri NF, Meziane MA, Zerhouni EA, Fishman EK, Siegelman SJ. The solitary pulmonary nodule: assessment, diagnosis and management. *Chest* 1987;91:128–133.
70. Page RD, Jeffrey RR, Donnelly RJ. Thoracoscopy: a review of 121 consecutive surgical procedures. *Ann Thorac Surg* 1989;48:66–68.
71. Bonniot JP, Homasson JF, Roden SL, Angebault ML, Renault PC. Pleural and lung cryobiopsies during thoracoscopy. *Chest* 1989;95:492–493.
72. Lewis RJ, Caccavale RJ, Sisler GE. Special report: video-endoscopic thoracic surgery. *NJ Med* 1991;88:473–475.
73. Inderbitzi R. Molnar J. Experiences in the diagnostic and surgical video-endoscopy of the thoracic cavity. *Schweiz Med Wochenschr* 1990;120:51–52.
74. Lillington GA, Caskey CI. Evaluation and management of solitary and multiple pulmonary nodules. *Clin Chest Med* 1993;14:111–119.
75. Siegelman SS, Khouri NF, Scott WW, et al. Solitary pulmonary nodules: CT assessment. *Radiology* 1986;160:307–312.
76. Lillington GA. Management of solitary pulmonary nodules. *Dis Mon* 1991;37:272–318.

CHAPTER 4

Surgical Resection of Pulmonary Metastases

Jeffrey L. Port and Michael Burt

If a metastasis is apparently solitary and accessible to surgical removal, it is definitely worthwhile to undertake removal of the metastasis as well as the primary growth.
—*Barney (1)*

Over the past 20 years, pulmonary metastasectomy has become one of the most common indications for pulmonary resection. The notion that we should attempt to render patients free of distant metastases may sound like misplaced enthusiasm, but many metastatic lesions can indeed be resected for cure. Although most patients never attain a cure, at present surgical resection is often the best therapy we can offer. Chemotherapy has decreased but not eliminated the occurrence of pulmonary metastases in tumors such as testicular carcinoma and osteosarcoma. Moreover, the surgeon is now often called on to resect pulmonary metastases not only for cure, but also for pathologic confirmation to guide further treatment.

Many tumor types have a strong propensity for thoracic metastases. Of patients with melanomas, sarcomas, and choriocarcinomas who succumb to their disease, 80% to 100% demonstrate pulmonary metastatic involvement (2). When one considers that, overall, the lung is the second most common site of metastatic involvement and that up to 20% of patients dying of pulmonary metastases have no other evidence of disease, the magnitude of the problem can be appreciated. With a consistent 20% to 30% 5-year survival now appreciated after pulmonary metastasectomy in selected patients, the presence of pulmonary metastases can no longer be considered evidence of an absolute fatal outcome.

HISTORY

In 1882 Weinlechner successfully resected the first pulmonary metastasis (3). The lesion was resected en bloc with a primary chest wall sarcoma. In 1884 Kroenlin published a case report documenting resection of a peripheral lung nodule that was recognized after resection of a recurrent chest wall sarcoma. Divis in 1926 was the first to perform a pulmonary metastasectomy as a separate procedure (3,4). The Prague surgeon removed a pulmonary metastasis from the right lower lobe 1 year after the resection of a soft-tissue sarcoma. In 1939, Barney and Churchill reported a patient who initially had only x-ray evidence of a metastatic pulmonary lesion (1). The patient underwent a nephrectomy 5 months later for a hypernephroma, and 15 months after the nephrectomy underwent pulmonary resection of the metastatic lesion. The patient survived 23 years without recurrence, finally succumbing to coronary disease. The first series recording pulmonary metastasectomy was by Alexander and Haight in 1947 (5). The series reviewed the outcome of 24 patients after resection and documented the apparent cure of 3 patients with various histologies.

In these early reports, patients were selected with long disease-free intervals (DFIs) and solitary lesions. These reports served as an impetus for and a validation of pulmonary metastasectomy. However, although these cases hinted at a survival benefit, it was not until the advent of modern surgical and anesthetic techniques that larger series of patients undergoing pulmonary metastasectomy were reported (6).

The development of effective chemotherapeutic regimens bolstered the use of more aggressive surgical approaches to pulmonary metastases (7,8). The treatment of osteosarcomas was revolutionized in the early 1970s by the introduction of high-dose methotrexate and leucovorin (9). These regimens could achieve considerable regression of the primary tumor. However, despite the best

J. L. Port: Thoracic Oncology Laboratory, Memorial Sloan-Kettering Cancer Center, New York, New York 10021.

M. Burt: Department of Surgery, Memorial Sloan-Kettering Cancer Center, New York, New York 10021.

chemotherapy available, 30% to 40% of patients still develop metastatic disease, at least 70% of whom experience failure only in the lung (10). Resection of these lesions led to 5-year survival rates of 30%; previously, there were no 5-year survivors. Subsequently, the guidelines for pulmonary metastasectomy were expanded. Martini and associates demonstrated that there were long-term survivors after resection of multiple lesions, even when they were bilateral (11). It also became apparent that the operation could be performed with low morbidity and negligible mortality (12). This led to the application of a more aggressive surgical approach to numerous histologic types of tumors, as well as multiple lesions, and to the report of large surgical series documenting long-term survival after resection of pulmonary metastases (1,13,14).

PULMONARY METASTASES

Incidence

The lungs are the most common site of extranodal metastases for many tumors. About 30% of patients with cancer develop pulmonary metastases (3). There is a high incidence of pulmonary metastases at clinical presentation for patients with renal cell carcinoma, choriocarcinoma, Wilms' tumor, and osteosarcoma (Table 1). The incidence of pulmonary metastasis at autopsy is as high as 80% for lesions such as melanoma or sarcoma. Overall, lesions that are isolated to the lung and amenable to resection are less common. Malignancies such as sarcomas often have pulmonary metastases, but they account for only 1% of all malignancies. Therefore, more common malignancies such as colon and breast cancer actually account for a significant number of isolated lung metastases, even though the incidence of pulmonary metastases in these diseases is only 1% to 2%.

TABLE 1. *Incidence of pulmonary metastases from extrathoracic tumors*

Primary lesion	Presentation (%)	Autopsy (%)
Melanoma	5	80
Thyroid	5–10	65
Breast	5	60
Colorectal	5	40
Head and neck	5	40
Bladder	5–10	30
Prostate	5	53
Choriocarcinoma	60	70–100
Kidney	5–30	50–75
Rhabdomyosarcoma	21	55
Wilm's tumor	20	60
Ewing's sarcoma	18	77
Osteosarcoma	15	75
Testicular (germinal)	12	70–80

Mechanism of Metastasis

Tumors have an increased propensity to metastasize preferentially to certain tissues. Numerous explanations have been proposed. In 1889, Paget collected the autopsy records of 735 patients who died of breast cancer and noted that most of these patients' metastases were to the liver and brain (15). Paget deduced that different tumors were predisposed to metastasize to certain organs, based on the organ's ability to support the tumor's growth. Paget drew an analogy between the development of metastases and the dispersal of plant seedlings and their later growth. He hypothesized that further study into the elements of the tissue ("soil") and the properties of the tumor ("seed") might be enlightening (15,16).

This "seed and soil" theory was challenged by Ewing, who attributed the preferential growth of certain metastases to routes of blood flow (16). The first tissue bed encountered by tumor cells would be the site of most metastases. This theory could explain the pattern of metastasis for some malignancies such as melanoma, sarcoma, thyroid carcinoma, and testicular carcinoma. Carcinomas of the pancreas, colon, and stomach, which drain via the portal circulation, would therefore be expected to metastasize to the lungs only infrequently. However, this anatomic or mechanical theory of metastasis fails to explain the rare involvement of richly vascularized organs such as the skin, skeletal muscle, and heart.

In essence, both theories play a role in the pattern and development of metastases. Pulmonary metastases most frequently occur through hematogenous delivery via the pulmonary artery. Lymphatic and endobronchial spread is much less common (17). Recently, emphasis has been placed on the cellular and biochemical properties of tumor cells and their interactions with target cells, as well as angiogenesis at the primary tumor site. Research has focused on chemoattractants for tumor cells, cellular adhesion molecules, organ-specific growth factors, and site-specific invasion of tissue matrices (15,16). For tumor cells to establish a metastatic colony, they must complete five steps:

1. Growth at the primary site
2. Escape into the vascular or lymphatic system or transbronchial aspiration
3. Adherence to the endothelium or basement membrane at a secondary site
4. Invasion into the parenchyma
5. Proliferation.

It has been estimated that over 99% of escaped tumor cells are destroyed; however, some tumor cells survive, and pulmonary micrometastases develop (18). At some point, these metastases themselves disseminate to other distant sites.

Vascular Supply

Primary bronchogenic malignancies have a bronchial blood supply (19–21). However, the more peripheral the tumor is within the lung parenchyma, the greater is the contribution from the pulmonary circulation. Similarly, pulmonary metastases in the central third of the lung have a bronchial blood supply, and lesions located peripherally have a predominantly pulmonary artery contribution. In one series of experimental pulmonary metastases, 48% were supplied by the pulmonary circulation, 36% by mixed pulmonary and bronchial, and 16% by the bronchial circulation alone (20). Evidence for extensive pulmonary artery vascular supply for pulmonary metastases lends support for isolated lung, pulmonary artery perfusion with anti-neoplastic therapy.

Distribution and Appearance

Pulmonary metastases vary in radiologic appearance (Table 2). Lesions are often bilateral and well defined, with smooth edges, and are located predominantly in the periphery of the lung (19,22–25). Autopsy reports in patients with advanced stages of metastatic spread show a preference for metastatic involvement of the middle and lower lung zones rather than the apices, which correlates with the pulmonary arterial supply. However, evaluation of 100 patients with 344 surgically resected pulmonary metastases revealed the upper lobes to be involved in 41%, the lower lobes in 41%, and the right middle lobe in

6% (22). Metastatic lesions often show no radiologic signs of lung invasion; this helps distinguish them from primary lung nodules, which are often spiculated and irregular in radiologic appearance (2). In one autopsy series that examined the location, size, and appearance of multiple histologic types of metastases, 82% of lesions were seen peripherally, 59% were pleural- or subpleural-based, and 59% were less than 5 mm in diameter (25). The combination of peripheral location and small size helps explain why many additional pulmonary metastases are not identified by preoperative radiologic screening. Also, there is no typical shape to a lesion, especially when it is in close proximity to the pleura. Lesions can appear as "hairy" or even star-shaped and can mimic areas of pneumonia or infarction.

The presence of a calcification in a pulmonary nodule often indicates that the lesion is a hamartoma or granuloma. However, calcification is often noted in pulmonary metastases derived from osteosarcomas and less frequently in synovial cell sarcoma, chondrosarcoma, and carcinomas of the thyroid, breast, and colon. Calcification may also occur in lesions after irradiation or chemotherapy, especially in lesions such as choriocarcinoma or testicular carcinoma (26).

Cavitation and occasionally pneumothorax have been described in patients with pulmonary metastases (2,26). Cavitation has been reported in metastatic squamous cell carcinoma from head and neck origin, as well as from genitourinary tract primary tumors. Chemotherapy may increase the occurrence of cavitation associated with pulmonary metastases. A patient with a known primary tumor who presents with a pneumothorax should make one consider the possibility of occult pulmonary spread.

Pulmonary metastases can also manifest a lymphangitic pattern (2,23,26). Most lymphangitic metastases result from hematogenous spread with extension from the capillaries to the lymphatics. Rarely, these metastases are due to retrograde lymphatic spread from celiac nodes to posterior mediastinal and paraesophageal nodes, and then further spread to hilar nodes and peripheral lymphatics. This course of spread may be more common in upper gastrointestinal primary malignancies. The earliest radiographic finding in pulmonary lymphangitic carcinomatosis is an interstitial process similar to Kerley's B lines in patients with pulmonary edema. There are fine septal lines in the interstitium with a preponderance for the lower lung. Pleural effusions may develop and hilar nodal enlargement may be present, but it is not necessary. The process may be unilateral or bilateral, and there is often no radiographic evidence of disease. Clinically, patients may present with dyspnea out of proportion to radiologic findings.

Pleural effusions are the most common manifestation of pleural involvement by pulmonary metastases and have been ascribed to breast carcinoma metastases in as many as 33% of cases (2,26). A bloody, exudative effusion with

TABLE 2. *Radiographic patterns of pulmonary metastatic lesions*

Radiographic pattern	Most common histology
Multiple nodules	
Calcified	Osteogenic sarcoma, chondrosarcoma, thyroid, ovarian breast
Miliary	Thyroid, melanoma, renal cell, ovarian
Cannonball	Sarcoma, colorectal, renal cell, melanoma
Slow growing	Adenoid cystic (salivary gland), thyroid
Cavitary	Squamous cell, melanoma, sarcoma, germ cell, transitional cell (bladder)
Poorly defined	Choriocarcinoma, liposarcoma, laryngeal, pancreatic, gastric postchemotherapy
Solitary nodules	Nonspecific
Lymphangitic features	Adenoma of breast, lung, prostate, stomach, pancreas
Hilar or mediastinal adenopathy	GU, head and neck, melanoma, seminoma
Endobronchial disease	breast, colorectal, pancreas, renal cell
Pleural effusion	Lung, breast, lymphoma

TABLE 3. *Diagnostic probability of a solitary lesion in patients with known cancer*

Primary cancer	New primary lung cancer (%)
Sarcoma	10
Melanoma	10
Genitourinary, gastrointestinal, gynecologic	50
Head and neck/breast	66

positive cytology is often noted when the pleural surfaces are directly involved with tumor. When the effusion results from impaired lymphatic drainage, as occurs in mediastinal nodal infiltration, the effusion may be a transudate without positive cytology. Metastatic pleural involvement may also lead to discrete pleural-based nodules. The differential diagnosis for the presence of a pleural effusion in a patient with a malignancy includes tuberculosis, fungal disease, pulmonary infarction, and heart failure. Thoracentesis in this setting is often helpful for diagnosis.

Endobronchial metastases are infrequent and are most commonly associated with carcinomas of the breast, pancreas, colon, and kidney (2,17,26). Segmental atelectasis may be seen radiographically, and patients may present clinically with dyspnea or even hemoptysis. Mediastinal or hilar nodal involvement in association with pulmonary metastases is infrequent but does occur, especially in patients with melanoma, seminoma, or breast carcinoma. In a study of 65 patients with pulmonary metastatic melanoma, 43% had radiologic evidence of nodal involvement (27). In over 90% of cases, there was parenchymal involvement as well. Breast carcinoma also has the potential for involving the internal mammary nodes (2).

It is often difficult to differentiate a solitary nodule in a patient with a known malignancy. Numerous benign processes, as well as primary bronchogenic carcinoma, can mimic metastatic disease. In a study of 800 patients with a previously diagnosed malignancy who presented with solitary pulmonary nodules, 500 (63%) of these nodules were a second primary tumor, 196 were solitary metastases, and 11 were benign lesions (28). The probability that a solitary pulmonary nodule is a metastasis varies according to the known primary tumor (Table 3). This contrasts with a study of 955 patients without a previous history of malignancy who underwent resection of solitary lesions (29). Here, 49% of the lesions were malignant (38% bronchogenic carcinoma, 9% metastatic carcinoma) and 51% were benign. These data underscore the diagnostic dilemma with patients who present with solitary nodules and stress the importance of preoperative tissue biopsy in dictating therapy.

DIAGNOSIS OF PULMONARY METASTASES

Fine-Needle Aspiration Biopsy

In light of the overall specificity of computed tomography (CT), a definitive preoperative diagnosis may be important in designing treatment options. Fine-needle aspiration biopsy (FNAB) has become the diagnostic procedure of choice because of its ease and safety (30–32). FNAB may prove useful in patients who cannot tolerate an open thoracotomy, those with solitary nodules that must be differentiated preoperatively from primary bronchogenic carcinoma, and candidates enrolled in preoperative treatment protocols. FNAB is most easily performed under fluoroscopic guidance for large lesions (5–10 mm). FNAB performed under CT guidance is also an option for smaller lesions, but it is associated with a higher frequency of complications of pneumothorax and is more time-consuming (33,34). Overall, FNAB has almost 100% specificity and about 80% sensitivity. The risk of pneumothorax requiring thoracostomy tube drainage approaches 4%, and associated minor bleeding complications occur in <2% of cases (30,32,35).

Bronchoscopy

Flexible fiberoptic bronchoscopy has been successful in obtaining a tissue diagnosis in bronchogenic carcinoma. The procedure can confirm the diagnosis in 80% of cases (36). However, fiberoptic bronchoscopy does not provide as high a diagnostic yield for nodular pulmonary metastases: in only 30% of cases is a positive histology obtained. The lower diagnostic yield with bronchoscopy may be related to the hematogenous origin of metastases and their lack of continuity with bronchial epithelium, as well as their peripheral location. However, when there are clinical findings and radiologic findings consistent with endobronchial disease (hemoptysis or wheezing) or lymphangitic carcinomatosis, bronchoscopy provides higher yields (36).

PREOPERATIVE ASSESSMENT

The preoperative assessment of a patient undergoing resection of pulmonary metastases should include a general evaluation of the patient's medical condition, with specific attention to cardiac and pulmonary function. Pulmonary function tests, arterial blood gas analysis, and when necessary ventilation/perfusion scanning are required to ensure that the patient will have adequate pulmonary reserve after resection. Pulmonary resection can usually be tolerated if the postresection FEV_1 is 800 mL or greater. Underlying coronary artery disease may necessitate special perioperative monitoring or even treatment. These patients should be appropriately evaluated with stress tests, echocardiograms, and coronary angiography if indicated.

Many patients have previously received systemic therapy that might compromise pulmonary and cardiac function. Bleomycin and mitomycin are both associated with a decrease in the pulmonary diffusion capacity (37). Patients previously treated with doxorubicin may also suffer impaired cardiac function (38). These patients should have their cardiac status evaluated preoperatively as well.

Preoperative evaluation should be tailored to the patient's primary tumor type and its propensity and pattern of spread. Extremity soft-tissue sarcomas more frequently present with isolated pulmonary metastases, so a routine preoperative evaluation and a radionuclide bone scan are all that are necessary. In contrast, carcinomas and melanomas with a propensity for multiple sites of metastatic spread, including the liver, brain, and bone, necessitate a thorough assessment of all sites; CT imaging of the abdomen, pelvis, and brain are justified with these tumors.

SURGICAL RESECTION OF PULMONARY METASTASES

Eligibility Criteria

Only a few patients will benefit from pulmonary metastasectomy. The following criteria can be used to determine which patients will benefit from surgical intervention:

1. Local control, or the ability to gain control of the primary tumor after pulmonary resection
2. Absence of extrathoracic metastases
3. Radiologic features consistent with pulmonary metastases
4. Pulmonary metastases that appear to be completely resectable
5. Adequate pulmonary reserve to allow complete resection
6. General medical condition that permits thoracotomy
7. Absence of more effective systemic therapy.

However, even with patients who meet these criteria, only a few will derive benefit from surgical resection. Other prognostic factors that define the characteristics of a tumor and its behavior allow the surgeon to select patients who will most likely derive benefit from surgical resection.

Prognostic Factors Affecting Survival

Numerous prognostic factors have been analyzed to define which patients will benefit from pulmonary metastasectomy (Table 4). A prolonged disease free interval (DFI), longer tumor doubling time, and three or fewer metastatic nodules are most frequently associated with a positive outcome (39–42). Sex, age, histopathol-

TABLE 4. *Prognostic factors for pulmonary metastasectomy*

Prognostic factor	Tumor type	Author (ref.)	No. of patients	Correlation with survival
DFI	Sarcoma	Gadd (46)	78	None
	Sarcoma	Jablons (14)	74	Neg. < 1 yr vs. > 1 yr
	Sarcoma	Casson (39)	58	None
	Osteosarcoma	Skinner (7)	75	None
	Osteosarcoma	Putnam (44)	39	Neg. < 6 m. vs. >6 m.
	Colorectal	McCormack (47)	144	None
	Colorectal	McAfee (52)	139	None
	Renal	Pogrebniak (87)	23	None
	Breast	Lanza (45)	44	Neg. <1 yr vs. >1 yr
	Breast	Staren (53)	33	None
TDT	Sarcoma	Gadd (46)	78	None
	Sarcoma	Casson (39)	58	Neg. <40 d. vs. >40 d.
	Osteosarcoma	Skinner (7)	75	None
	Osteosarcoma	Putnam (44)	39	None
Nodules resected	Sarcoma	Gadd (46)	78	None
	Sarcoma	Jablons (14)	74	None
	Sarcoma	Casson (39)	58	Neg. >2 vs. <2
	Osteosarcoma	Skinner (7)	75	None
	Osteosarcoma	Putnam (44)	39	Neg. >4 vs. <4
	Colorectal	McCormack (47)	144	None
	Colorectal	McAfee (52)	139	Neg >1 vs. 1
	Renal	Pogrebniak (87)	23	None
	Breast	Lanza (45)	44	None
	Breast	Staren (53)	33	None

DFI, disease free interval; TDT, tumor doubling time.

ogy of the primary tumor, and unilateral versus bilateral pulmonary involvement have little effect on outcome. No single factor is discriminating enough to allow selection of a group of patients that will clearly benefit from resection.

Disease-Free Interval

The DFI is the period from the time of resection of the primary tumor to the time of diagnosis of pulmonary metastases. Numerous studies have demonstrated a correlation between a long DFI (>1 year) and prolonged long-term survival (43–45). However, this correlation does not hold for all histologic tumor types—the DFI appears to be significant only in soft-tissue sarcomas and osteosarcomas. A review by Gadd and colleagues failed to demonstrate a significant correlation between DFI and survival in 135 patients with metastatic pulmonary sarcoma (46). Overall, it appears that the DFI should not be used as a primary criterion for excluding patients from resection.

Tumor Doubling Time

Tumor growth kinetics have been analyzed as a possible predictor of clinical outcome. The tumor doubling time is calculated from the measurement of a single nodule from serial radiologic studies. Multiple authors have demonstrated that a longer tumor doubling time is associated with prolonged survival (13,39,41). Serial radiologic examination should be reserved for patients with lesions that are not suspected of being metastases and should be used only if resolution of the ambiguity is possible. Although some authors have shown that a tumor's doubling time has prognostic significance, many have not. We do not select patients for surgical resection based on their tumor's doubling time.

Number of Metastases Resected

Initially, pulmonary metastasectomy was performed in patients with solitary lesions. However, numerous reports have documented equivalent survivals for patients with multiple metastases that were completely resected, as well as patients with bilateral disease (7,14,46,47). In a study from Memorial Sloan-Kettering Cancer Center reviewing metastatic pulmonary sarcoma, the number of nodules resected and the presence of bilateral disease had no bearing on survival when all disease was resected (46). Similarly, McCormack and coworkers observed equivalent survival in patients with solitary or multiple bilateral pulmonary colonic metastases that were completely resected (47). This has led most authors to conclude that survival is related more closely to complete resection, regardless of the number of lesions resected (14,44,46,47).

Technique of Surgical Resection

Resection of pulmonary metastases requires adherence to two guidelines: complete resection of all disease, and maximum sparing of pulmonary parenchyma. Because most metastases are located peripherally and subpleurally, they are usually easily palpated and resected by wedge resection. A 1-cm margin is adequate for resection and spares the maximal amount of functioning lung tissue. Wedge resection can be performed with automatic staplers, electrocautery, or even laser. A more extensive resection requiring lobectomy or even pneumonectomy is reserved for patients with lesions that cannot be completely resected by wedge resection.

Pulmonary metastasectomy previously required either a lateral thoracotomy or median sternotomy. Complete exploration of the lung routinely requires collapse of the lung with assistance from double-lumen endotracheal intubation. The lung is palpated while deflated. The entire thoracic cavity is explored, paying particular attention to the mediastinum and chest wall. With peripheral lesions, the adjacent lung is grasped with Duval clamps and a TA automatic stapler (US Surgical, New York, New York) is used for resection (Fig. 1). Deeper lesions require that the visceral pleura be scored 1 cm from the lesion; using electrocautery or a scalpel, the incision is carried to 1 cm below the lesion to allow adequate resection. This cone is then grasped and completely excised (Fig. 2). Vessels are clipped as detected. Most importantly, the visceral pleura must be carefully reapproximated with interrupted suture. This is helpful in reducing adhesion formation and assists future reexplorations if needed.

Controversy exists over the best surgical approach in pulmonary metastasectomy (12,48). Studies have shown that 45% of patients with metastatic pulmonary sarcoma who had unilateral disease diagnosed on preoperative CT had bilateral disease at the time of median sternotomy (49). Therefore, many surgeons argue that median sternotomy will detect a significant number of occult metastases and thus eliminate the need for reexploration. However, when reviewed, median sternotomy offered no survival advantage over lateral thoracotomy in these patients. Presumably, metastases that recur in the contralateral lung can be re-resected without compromising the patient's survival.

Controversy also exists over the best surgical approach for known bilateral disease. In the past, patients with documented bilateral metastases underwent bilateral staged thoracotomies. However, median sternotomy has recently been popularized in this group of patients (50,51). The theoretical advantages to staged thoracotomies are the ability to resect all disease completely, regardless of location, and the avoidance of bilateral pulmonary contusions, which might necessitate prolonged ventilatory dependence. Lateral thoracotomy allows better exposure of large posterior or central lesions. Advantages of

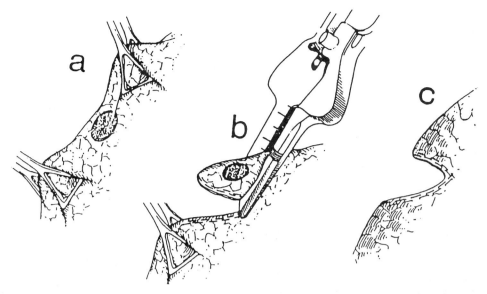

FIG. 1. Wedge resection performed using an automatic stapler for a peripheral and superficial lesion. **(a)** The edges of the lung are grasped 1 cm from the nodule with Duval clamps. **(b)** Wedge resection is performed with adequate margins. **(c)** The lung after resection.

median sternotomy include the need for a single operation, reduced postoperative discomfort, and possibly improved postoperative pulmonary function. However, comparisons have demonstrated similar complication rates with equally low morbidity and mortality (49). At Memorial Sloan-Kettering Cancer Center, we also use a bilateral anterior thoracotomy in the fourth intercostal space with transverse division of the sternum ("clamshell incision") for bilateral disease, especially when the lower lobes are involved.

Operative morbidity and mortality after pulmonary metastasectomy is consistently very low. Mortality rates for most series are reported to be 1% with operative complication rates of 10% (1,41,52–54). Complications include hemorrhage, infection, arrhythmias, and prolonged thoracostomy tube drainage.

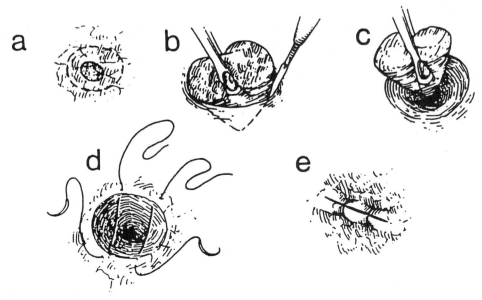

FIG. 2. Wedge resection performed using cautery technique for deeper lesions. **(a)** The visceral pleura is scored 1 cm from the lesion. **(b)** Cautery is used to extend the incision to 1 cm below the nodule. **(c)** The specimen is grasped with forceps and the core is completely excised. **(d,e)** The visceral pleura is reapproximated.

Thoracoscopy

Thoracoscopy has found many applications, both diagnostic and therapeutic, since it was first described in 1910 by Jacobeus (55). It has been used routinely to diagnose pleural effusions, to perform pleural biopsies, and to biopsy peripheral parenchymal lesions. However, the role of thoracoscopy in the management of pulmonary metastases has yet to be fully defined. There has recently been tremendous interest in expanding the role of thoracoscopy for therapeutic wedge resection, including resection of pulmonary metastases. Video-assisted thoracoscopy (VATS) offers the potential for therapeutic metastasectomy with less pain and a decreased hospital stay. However, there is concern that VATS does not allow bimanual palpation of the lungs, and with this loss of tactile sensation, multiple metastatic lesions not delineated on preoperative diagnostic studies might be missed (56). The surgeon becomes dependent on CT imaging for guidance, and this detects only 70% of metastatic lesions.

Proponents of thoracoscopy can argue that if a lateral thoracotomy is performed for unilateral disease, 43% of patients will have disease in the contralateral lung that was not detected by preoperative CT scanning. However, this has not translated into decreased survival. Therefore, if lesions are missed by thoracoscopy, these patients can present for re-resection without compromising their survival.

Prospective randomized studies comparing thoracoscopy with standard surgical approaches for pulmonary metastasectomy must be performed before an adequate judgment can be rendered as to the proper role for this technique.

Repeated Metastasectomy

There is evidence that patients who undergo repeated resections for recurrent metastatic pulmonary sarcoma can achieve prolonged survival (41,57,58). In one series, 43 patients underwent two or more resections for pulmonary metastatic sarcoma. There were no operative deaths, and 31 of 43 patients were rendered disease-free at the second thoracotomy (57). The complication rate of the series was 6%. The postresection survival rate was similar to that of patients undergoing a single resection.

RESULTS OF SURGICAL PULMONARY METASTASECTOMY FOR SPECIFIC HISTOLOGIES

Soft-Tissue Sarcoma

The incidence of soft-tissue sarcomas approaches 5,000 cases per year (59). Although improvements have been made in the treatment of patients with soft-tissue sarcoma, the major cause of death remains pulmonary

TABLE 5. *Pulmonary metastasectomy results for soft tissue sarcoma*

Author (ref.)	No. of patients	% 5-yr survival (unless otherwise indicated)
Putnam, 1984 (13)	63	30 (3 yr)
Mountain, 1984 (88)	49	33
Jablons, 1989 (14)	68	28
Casson, 1991 (39)	58	25
Ueda, 1993 (64)	23	25
Gadd, 1993 (46)	65	23 (3 yr)
Van Geel, 1994 (115)	67	39

metastases. The lungs are the most common site of initial recurrence as well as distant metastases, accounting for 80% of all metastases in most series. The primary site of origin, tumor grade, size, and histology are important factors predicting the incidence of pulmonary metastases. Lower-extremity lesions of high-grade histology and >5 cm have the greatest propensity for the development of pulmonary metastases (46). Spindle cell, extraskeletal osteosarcomas, and tenosynovial subtypes are most commonly associated with pulmonary metastatic disease.

About 19% of patients with extremity soft-tissue sarcomas present with isolated pulmonary metastases (46). Pulmonary metastases are usually observed within the first 2 years after treatment of the primary tumor (59). Systemic chemotherapy holds little promise for long-term survival (60). Pulmonary metastasectomy for soft-tissue sarcomas offers a potentially curative therapy, with 5-year survival approaching 25% (Table 5) (13,39,40,46, 50,61–64). However, most patients succumb to subsequent pulmonary recurrences and eventually die of their disease. Attempts have been made to determine prognostic indicators that may better predict the patients who will benefit from resection (48,51,65–67). There has been general agreement that the size, grade, site, or histology of the primary tumor, the patient's age or sex, multicentricity, the number of pulmonary nodules, and the thoracic surgical approach have no predictive value in determining survival after resection of pulmonary metastases. Other factors, such as a prolonged DFI and long tumor doubling time, have been associated with a favorable effect on survival (39–41,51). However, even these factors have not been consistent. The only factor consistently shown to affect overall survival is the ability to resect all disease completely.

Osteogenic Sarcoma

The treatment of osteogenic sarcoma is constantly evolving. Multimodal therapy, including adjuvant and neoadjuvant chemotherapy, limb-sparing surgery, and salvage therapy for relapse, has translated into an improved survival rate (10,11,38,42,44,68–73). The devel-

TABLE 6. *Pulmonary metastasectomy results for osteosarcoma*

Author (ref.)	No. of patients	% 5-yr survival (unless otherwise indicated)
Putnam, 1983 (44)	39	40
Mountain, 1984 (88)	56	51
Meyer, 1986 (68)	39	38
Carter, 1991 (69)	25	20
Skinner, 1992 (7)	25	37
Pastorino, 1992 (10)	27	47

opment of effective chemotherapy using methotrexate, doxorubicin, and cisplatin has apparently improved survival (7). However, lung metastases still account for the majority of failures and occur in up to 50% of patients (69). Patients in the past who died from pulmonary metastases often had no other evidence of disseminated disease. Before resection of pulmonary metastases from osteogenic sarcoma, 3-year survival was 5% from the time of diagnosis. Overall, about 40% of patients with metastatic pulmonary osteosarcoma enjoy prolonged survival with aggressive surgical treatment (Table 6).

Colorectal Metastases

Colorectal cancer remains the second most common visceral tumor in both incidence and death (74). There will be about 150,000 new cases and 50,000 related deaths in 1995. About 20% of patients with colorectal cancer develop pulmonary metastases (75); however, in only 2% to 4% of cases are these isolated pulmonary metastases. There is no significant 5-year survival for patients with pulmonary colorectal metastases with any treatment modality other than surgery (76,77). Colorectal carcinoma metastases to the lung usually are few in number and have long tumor doubling times, which makes these lesions more amenable to resection. The search for other metastatic sites must be thorough and must include CT of the chest and abdomen. Bone and brain scans are reserved for symptomatic patients. Pulmonary resection

TABLE 7. *Pulmonary metastasectomy results for colorectal cancer*

Author (ref.)	No. of patients	% 5-yr survival (unless otherwise indicated)
Mountain, 1984 (88)	28	28
Mansel, 1986 (81)	66	38
Brister, 1987 (79)	27	21
Goya, 1989 (80)	62	42
Saclarides, 1993 (74)	23	16
McAfee, 1991 (52)	139	30
McCormack, 1992 (47)	144	40

TABLE 8. *Pulmonary metastasectomy results for renal cell carcinoma*

Author (ref.)	No. of patients	% 5-yr survival (unless otherwise indicated)
Mountain, 1984 (88)	20	54
Dernevik, 1985 (89)	33	21
Pogrebniak, 1991 (87)	23	43 months (mean)
Cerfolio, 1993 (54)	96	36

in selected patients has led consistently in several series to 30% 5-year survival (Table 7) (47,52,74,78–83). Some authors have argued that the presence of resectable extrapulmonary disease (eg, at hepatic sites) should not be a contraindication to pulmonary metastasectomy, and that repeat thoracotomy for recurrent colorectal pulmonary metastases is also warranted (52,84). It is important to remember that solitary pulmonary lesions on preoperative radiologic studies have an equal chance of being primary bronchogenic carcinomas (85). If the lesion cannot be histologically confirmed as colorectal in origin preoperatively, then lobectomy with mediastinal staging is required. Analysis of prognostic indicators demonstrates no survival advantages for the patient except complete resection.

Urinary Tract Cancer

There are about 25,000 cases of renal cell carcinoma annually. The lung is the most common site of distant metastases (86): about half the patients with renal cell carcinoma develop pulmonary metastases (87). The 5-year survival after unresected metastatic disease is 2.7% (54). Chemotherapy and radiation therapy have not proven to be effective in the treatment of metastatic disease. The first resection for metastatic renal cell carcinoma was reported in 1938 (1), and since then numerous resections have been carried out (Table 8). However, pulmonary metastasectomy remains controversial, and the factors that predict survival are not well defined. Multiple studies have reported a survival benefit after metastasectomy, with 5-year survivals between 20% and 40% (54,87—91). Resectable extrapulmonary disease does not necessarily contraindicate pulmonary metastasectomy, and repeat thoracotomy may also be warranted in select patients.

Testicular Cancer

A multimodal approach is the cornerstone of treatment for germ cell tumors (8,92–96). Cisplatin-based chemotherapy has dramatically improved the survival of patients with disseminated germ cell tumors (8). Germ

TABLE 9. *Pulmonary metastasectomy results for testicular cancer*

Author (ref.)	No. of patients	% 5-yr survival (unless otherwise indicated)
Callery, 1982 (115)	25	59
Mandelbaum, 1983 (98)	72	74 (3 yr)
Mountain, 1984 (88)	20	54

cell tumors have a propensity to metastasize to the retroperitoneum and mediastinum. About 80% of patients with disseminated testicular cancer are cured (97,98). Thoracic surgical intervention can be performed to eradicate limited thoracic disease and to allow diagnosis of the pulmonary lesions (Table 9). Due to the pluripotential nature of nonseminomatous germ cell tumors, all lesions should be resected. At our institution and others, the three indications for pulmonary resection after intensive cisplatin-based chemotherapy for germ cell carcinoma metastases to the lung are elevated serum markers (beta-HCG, AFP), a residual mass on CT scan, and a physiologically fit patient (97–99). In this setting, after complete resection of all pulmonary nodules, about 40% will have benign teratoma, 40% necrosis or fibrosis, and 20% viable carcinoma. The prognosis for patients who have necrotic, fibrotic tissue or teratoma resected is excellent, with long-term survival approaching 90%. However, in patients with residual, viable carcinoma, only 27% will enjoy disease-free survival (98).

Melanoma

Excluding the skin and lymph nodes, the lungs are the most common site for metastatic melanoma (100,101). Autopsy series have shown up to an 80% incidence of lung involvement. Melanoma often has a metastatic pattern of spread involving multiple organs. However, some authors suggest that appropriately selected patients may

TABLE 10. *Pulmonary metastasectomy results for melanoma*

Author (ref.)	No. of patients	% 5-yr survival (unless otherwise indicated)
Overett, 1984 (55)	17	23
Pogrebniak, 1988 (102)	33	13-mo median
Wong, 1988 (104)	38	31
Gorenstein, 1990 (103)	56	25
Harpole, 1992 (110)	84	20
Karakousis, 1994 (107)	39	14

benefit from pulmonary metastasectomy (Table 10) (55, 100,102–107). In a study of 200 patients with distant metastases, Balch and associates noted that the first evidence of disseminated disease was an asymptomatic pulmonary nodule in 38% of patients (108). It has been estimated from radiologic studies that about 20% of these patients will have resectable disease (100). Predictors for pulmonary metastases are a higher Clark level, nodular or acral lentiginous histology, central location (trunk or head and neck), and regional positive lymph node metastases (98). The results in the literature for resection of isolated pulmonary melanoma metastases are disappointing: the best 5-year survival ranges between 19% and 30%, and many studies show no long-term survivors (109). In general, survival after resection does not correlate with Clark level, nodal status, or DFI. Patients with resected solitary nodules have somewhat longer survival. However, Harpole and colleagues, in a multivariate analysis of Duke's 20-year experience with 945 cases of pulmonary metastatic melanoma, found that survival correlated with complete resection, number of nodules, lymph nodes negative for metastasis, and histologic type (110). No form of chemotherapy, immunotherapy, or radiation therapy has been shown to extend survival. With the advent of modern immunotherapies such as interleukin-2 and interleukin-12, resection of residual disease could play a greater role.

Head and Neck Cancer

About 20% of patients with squamous carcinoma of head and neck origin present with distant metastases (111). Most of these metastases are to the lungs. In addition, many of these patients develop a second primary of

TABLE 11. *Pulmonary metastasectomy results for patients with tumors of other histology*

Histology	Author (ref.)	No. of patients	% 5-yr survival (unless otherwise indicated)
Head and neck	Mountain, 1984 (88)	48	41
	Mazer, 1988 (111)	44	43
	Finley, 1992 (110)	18	29
Breast	Lanza, 1992 (45)	37	49
	Staren, 1992 (53)	33	36
Uterine-Cervical	Mountain, 1984 (88)	34	24
	Seki, 1992 (119)	32	52

head and neck, esophagus, or lung origin. Resection of pulmonary metastases from patients with squamous cell carcinoma of the head and neck can be associated with a 5-year survival of up to 40% (Table 11) (88,111,112). Locoregional control is the most significant prognostic factor.

Breast Cancer

Breast cancer is the most prevalent cancer among women in the United States and accounts for about 30,000 deaths per year (43,45). Although an estimated 20% of patients will succumb to isolated pulmonary metastases, few cases of pulmonary resections appear in the literature. Five-year survival after metastasectomy has been reported to be 14% to 50% (Table 11) (45,53,88,113). Recent reports of improved survival may be related to more stringent patient selection based on the current routine use of bone scans, CT, and magnetic resonance imaging to identify patients with limited disease. Patients with solitary lesions must be evaluated for primary lung carcinomas: Cahan and coworkers demonstrated that in this setting only 32% of patients had breast metastases and the rest had new lung primaries or benign disease (85).

CONCLUSION

The rationale for pulmonary metastasectomy stems from evidence demonstrating that up to 20% of patients with a malignancy will die with isolated pulmonary metastases and that some patients who undergo pulmonary metastasectomy will enjoy a prolonged survival. The selection of a patient for metastasectomy must take into account the extent of disease and the patient's functional status. The most important predictor of survival is the ability to resect all disease completely. Although pulmonary resection should be complete, as much functioning lung tissue as possible should be preserved, particularly because repeat resections for recurrent disease can be anticipated. Surgical debulking plays no role in the management of patients with pulmonary metastases. Current radiologic screening significantly underestimates the number of metastases, so significantly more disease is often found on exploration. Pulmonary metastasectomy is believed to be beneficial in selected patients with sarcoma, renal cell cancer, testicular cancer, and colorectal cancer and occasionally in those with other tumor types.

Surgical resection is the best treatment we have to offer, so pulmonary metastasectomy is therefore justified in carefully selected patients. However, surgery has obvious limitations in the treatment of pulmonary metastases. Future considerations must be based on a multimodal approach, with the needs of each patient taken into consideration.

REFERENCES

1. Barney J, Churchill E. Adenocarcinoma of the kidney with metastasis to the lung. *J Urol* 1939;42:269.
2. Whitesell P, Peters S. Pulmonary manifestations of extrathoracic malignant lesions. *Mayo Clinic Proc* 1993;68:483.
3. VanDongen J, VanSlooten E. The surgical treatment of pulmonary metastases. *Cancer Treat Rev* 1978;5:29.
4. Kern K, Pass H, Roth J. Surgical treatment of pulmonary metastases. In: Rosenberg S, ed. *Treatment of metastatic cancer.* Philadelphia: Lippincott, 1987;69.
5. Alexander J, Haight C. Pulmonary resection for solitary metastatic sarcoma and carcinomas. *Surg Gynecol Obstet* 1947;85:129.
6. Thomford N, Woolner L, Clagett O. The surgical treatment of metastatic tumors in the lungs. *J Thoracic Cardiovasc Surg* 1965;49:357.
7. Skinner K, Eilber F, Holmes E, Eckardt J, Rosen G. Surgical treatment and chemotherapy for pulmonary metastases from osteosarcoma. *Arch Surg* 1992;127:1065.
8. Israel A, Bosl G, Golbey R, Whitmore Jr W, Martini N. The results of chemotherapy for extragonadal germ-cell tumors in the cisplatin era: the Memorial Sloan-Kettering Cancer Center experience (1975–1982). *J Clin Oncol* 1985;3:1073.
9. Jaffe N. Recent advances in the chemotherapy of metastatic osteogenic sarcoma. *Cancer* 1972;30:1627.
10. Pastorino U, Gasparini M, Valente M, et al. Primary childhood osteosarcoma: the role of salvage surgery. *Ann Oncol* 1992;3:43.
11. Martini N, Huvos A, Mike V, Marcove R, Beattie Jr E. Multiple pulmonary resections in the treatment of osteogenic sarcoma. *Ann Thorac Surg* 1971;12:271.
12. McCormack P, Martini N. The changing role of surgery for pulmonary metastases. *Ann Thorac Surg* 1979;28:139.
13. Putnam J, Roth J, Wesley M, Johnston M, Rosenberg S. Analysis of prognostic factors in patients undergoing resection of pulmonary metastases from soft tissue sarcomas. *J Thorac Cardiovasc Surg* 1984;87:260.
14. Jablons D, Steinberg S, Roth J, Pittaluga S, Rosenberg S, Pass H. Metastasectomy for soft tissue sarcoma, further evidence for efficacy and prognostic indicators. *J Thorac Cardiovasc Surg* 1989;97:695.
15. Zetter B. The cellular basis of site-specific tumor metastasis. *N Engl J Med* 1990;322:605.
16. Nicholson G. Molecular mechanisms of cancer metastasis: tumor and host properties and the role of oncogenes and suppression genes. *Curr Op Oncol* 1991;3:75.
17. Sheperd M. Endobronchial metastatic disease. *Thorax* 1982;37:362–365.
18. Davis S. CT evaluation for pulmonary metastases in patients with extrathoracic malignancy. *Radiology* 1991;180:1.
19. Miller B, Rosenbaum A. The vascular supply to metastatic tumors of the lung. *Surg Gynecol Obstet* 1967;1009.
20. Milne E, Noonan C, Margulis A, Stoughton R. Vascular supply of pulmonary metastases. *Invest Radiol* 1969;4:215.
21. Milne E. Circulation of primary and metastatic pulmonary neoplasms. *Am J Radiol* 1967;100:603.
22. Muller K, Respondek M. Pulmonary metastases: pathologic anatomy. *Lung* 1990;1137.
23. Munk P, Muller N, Miller R, Ostrow D. Pulmonary lymphangitic carcinomatosis: CT and pathologic findings. *Radiology* 1988;166:705.
24. Dinkel E, Mundinger A, Schopp D, Grosser G, Hauenstein K. Diagnostic imaging in metastatic lung disease. *Lung* 1990;1129.
25. Crow J, Slavin G, Kreel L. Pulmonary metastasis: a pathologic and radiologic study. *Cancer* 1981;47:2595.
26. Libshitz H, North L. Pulmonary metastases. *Radiol Clin North Am* 1982;20:437.
27. Webb W, Gamsu G. Thoracic metastasis in malignant melanoma. *Chest* 1977;71:176.
28. Cahan W, Shah J, Castro E. Benign solitary lesions in patients with cancer. *Ann Surg* 1978;187:241.
29. Toomes H, Delphendahl A, Manke H, Vogt-Moykopf I. The coin lesion of the lung. *Cancer* 1983;51:534.
30. Johnston W. Percutaneous fine needle aspiration biopsy of the lung. *Acta Cytol* 1984;28:218.
31. Crosby J, Hager B, Hoeg K. Transthoracic fine-needle aspiration. *Cancer* 1985;56:2504.

32. Pilotti S, Rilke F, Gribaudi G. Transthoracic fine needle aspiration biopsy in pulmonary lesions. *Acta Cytol* 1984;28:225.

33. Gobien R, Stanley J, Vujic I, Gobien B. Thoracic biopsy: CT guidance of thin-needle aspiration. *Am J Radiol* 1984;142:827.

34. VanSonnenberg E, Casola G, Ho M, et al. Difficult thoracic lesions: CT-guided biopsy experience in 150 cases. *Radiology* 1988;167:457.

35. Nordenstrom B. Technical aspects of obtaining cellular material from lesions deep in the lung. *Acta Cytol* 1984;28:233.

36. Poe R, Ortiz C, Israel R, et al. Sensitivity, specificity, and predictive values of bronchoscopy in neoplasm metastatic to lung. *Chest* 1985; 88:84.

37. Dresdale A, Bonow R, Wesley R. Prospective evaluation of doxorubicin-induced cardiomyopathy resulting from post-surgical adjuvant therapy of patients with soft tissue sarcomas. *Cancer* 1983;52:51.

38. McCrea E, Diaconis J, Wade J, Johnston C. Bleomycin toxicity simulating metastatic nodules to the lungs. *Cancer* 1981;48:1096.

39. Casson A, Putnam J, Natarajan G, et al. Five-year survival after pulmonary metastasectomy for adult soft tissue sarcoma. *Cancer* 1992; 69:662.

40. Verazin G, Warneke J, Driscoll D, Karakousis C, Petrelli N, Takita H. Resection of lung metastases from soft-tissue sarcomas. *Arch Surg* 1992;127:1407.

41. Rizzoni W, Pass H, Wesley M, Rosenberg S, Roth J. Resection of recurrent pulmonary metastases in patients with soft-tissue sarcomas. *J Thorac Card Surg* 1986;87:490.

42. Roth J, Putnam J, Wesley M, Rosenberg S. Differing determinants of prognosis following resection of pulmonary metastases from osteogenic and soft tissue sarcoma patients. *Cancer* 1985;55:1361.

43. Jardines L, Callans L, Torosian M. Recurrent breast cancer: presentation, diagnosis, and treatment. *Semin Oncol* 1993;20:538.

44. Putnam Jr J, Roth J, Wesley M, Johnston M, Rosenberg S. Survival following aggressive resection of pulmonary metastases from osteogenic sarcoma: analysis of prognostic factors. *Ann Thorac Surg* 1983; 36:516.

45. Lanza L, Natarajan G, Roth J, Putnam J. Long-term survival after resection of pulmonary metastases from carcinoma of the breast. *Ann Thorac Surg* 1992;54:244.

46. Gadd M, Casper E, Woodruff J, McCormack P, Brennan M. Development and treatment of pulmonary metastases in adult patients with extremity soft tissue sarcoma. *Ann Surg* 1993;218:705.

47. McCormack P, Burt M, Bains M, Martini N, Rusch V, Ginsberg R. Lung resections for colorectal metastases. *Arch Surg* 1992;127:1403.

48. Johnston M. Median sternotomy for resection of pulmonary metastases. *J Thorac Cardiovasc Surg* 1983;85:516.

49. Roth J, Pass H, Wesley M, White D, Putnam J, Seipp C. Comparison of median sternotomy and thoracotomy for resection of pulmonary metastases in patients with adult soft tissue sarcomas. *Ann Thorac Surg* 1986;42:134.

50. Meng R, Jensik R, Kittle C, Faber L. Median sternotomy for synchronous bilateral pulmonary operations. *J Thorac Cardiovasc Surg* 1980; 8:1.

51. Regal A, Reese P, Antkowiak J, Hart T, Takita H. Median sternotomy for metastatic lung lesions in 131 patients. *Cancer* 1985;55:1334.

52. McAfee M, Allen M, Trastek V, Ilstrup D, Deschamps C, Pairolero P. Colorectal lung metastases: results of surgical excision. *Ann Thorac Surg* 1992;53:780.

53. Staren E, Salerno C, Rongione A, Witt T, Faber P. Pulmonary resection for metastatic breast cancer. *Arch Surg* 1992;127:1282.

54. Carfolio R, Allen M, Deschamps C, et al. Pulmonary resection of metastatic renal cell carcinoma. *Ann Thorac Surg* 1994;57:339.

55. Overett T, Shiu M. Surg treatment of distant metastatic melanoma. *Cancer* 1985;56:1222.

56. McCormack P, Ginsberg K, Bains M, et al. Accuracy of lung imaging in metastases with implications for the role of thoracoscopy. *Ann Thorac Surg* 1993;56:863.

57. Pogrebniak H, Roth J, Steinberg S, Rosenberg S, Pass H. Reoperative pulmonary resection in patients with metastatic soft tissue sarcoma. *Ann Thorac Surg* 1991;52:197.

58. VanGeel A, Hoekstra H, VanCoevorden F, Meyer S, Bruggink E, Blankensteijn J. Repeated resection of recurrent pulmonary metastatic soft tissue sarcoma. *Eur J Surg Oncol* 1994;20:436.

59. Potter D, Glenn J, Kinsella T, et al. Patterns of recurrence in patients with high-grade soft-tissue sarcomas. *J Clin Oncol* 1985;3:353.

60. Lanza L, Putnam Jr J, Benjamin R, Roth J. Response to chemotherapy

61. Robinson M, Sheppard M, Moskovic E, Fisher C. Lung metastasectomy in patients with soft tissue sarcoma. *Br J Radiol* 1994;67:129.

62. Huth J, Holmes E, Vernon S, Callery C, Ramming K, Morton D. Pulmonary resection for metastatic sarcoma. *Am J Surg* 1980;140:9.

63. Flye M, Woltering G, Rosenberg S. Aggressive pulmonary resection for metastatic osteogenic and soft tissue sarcomas. *Ann Thorac Surg* 1984;37:123.

64. Ueda T, Uchida A, Kodama K, et al. Aggressive pulmonary metastasectomy for soft tissue sarcomas. *Cancer* 1993;72:1919.

65. Wright III J, Brandt III B, Ehrenhaft J. Results of pulmonary resection for metastatic lesions. *J Thorac Cardiovasc Surg* 1982;83:94.

66. Stewart J, Carey J, Merrill W, Frist W, Hammon Jr J, Bender Jr H. Twenty years' experience with pulmonary metastasectomy. *Am Surgeon* 1991;58:100.

67. Wilkins Jr E, Head J, Burke J. Pulmonary resection for metastatic neoplasms in the lung. *Am J Surg* 1978;135:480.

68. Meyer W, Schell M, Kumar A, et al. Thoracotomy for pulmonary metastatic osteosarcoma. *Cancer* 1987;59:374.

69. Carter S, Grimer R, Sneath R, Matthews H. Results of thoracotomy in osteogenic sarcoma with pulmonary metastases. *Thorax* 1991;46:727.

70. Beattie E, Harvey J, Marcove R, Martini N. Results of multiple pulmonary resections for metastatic osteogenic sarcoma after two decades. *J Surg Oncol* 1991;46:154.

71. Rosen G, Huvos A, Mosende C, et al. Chemotherapy and thoracotomy for metastatic osteogenic sarcoma. *Cancer* 1978;41:841.

72. Heij H, Vos A, deKraker J, Voute P. Prognostic factors in surgery for pulmonary metastases in children. *Surgery* 1994;115:687.

73. Marina N, Pratt C, Rao B, Shema S, Meyer W. Improved prognosis of children with osteosarcoma metastatic to the lung(s) at the time of diagnosis. *Cancer* 1992;70:2722.

74. Saclarides T, Krueger B, Szeluga D, Warren W, Faber L, Economou S. Thoracotomy for colon and rectal cancer metastases. *Dis Colon Rectum* 1993;36:425.

75. August D, Ottow R, Sugarbaker P. Clinical perspective of human colorectal cancer metastasis. *Cancer Metast Rev* 1984;3:303.

76. Abbruzzese J, Levin B. Treatment of advanced colorectal cancer. *Hematol/Oncol Clin North Am* 1989;3:135.

77. Moertel C. Clinical management of advanced gastrointestinal cancer. *Cancer* 1975;36:675.

78. Yano T, Hara N, Ichinose Y, Yokoyama H, Miura T, Ohta M. Results of pulmonary resection of metastatic colorectal cancer and its application. *J Thorac Cardiovasc Surg* 1993;106:875.

79. Brister S, DeVarennes B, Gordon P, Sheiner N, Pym J. Contemporary operative management of pulmonary metastases of colorectal origin. *Dis Colon Rectum* 1988;31:786.

80. Goya T, Miyazawa N, Kondo H, Tsuchiya R, Naruke T, Suemasu K. Surg resection of pulmonary metastases from colorectal cancer. *Cancer* 1989;64:1418.

81. Mansel J, Zinsmeister A, Pairolero P, Jett J. Pulmonary resection of metastatic colorectal adenocarcinoma. *Chest* 1986;89:109.

82. Mountain C, Khalil K, Hermes K, Frazier O. The contribution of surgery to the management of carcinomatous pulmonary metastases. *Cancer* 1978;41:833.

83. Wilking N, Petrelli N, Herrera L, Regal A, Mittelman A. Surg resection of pulmonary metastases from colorectal adenocarcinoma. *Dis Colon Rectum* 1985;28:562.

84. Smith J, Fortner J, Burt M. Resection of hepatic and pulmonary metastases from colorectal cancer. *Surg Oncol* 1992;1:399.

85. Cahan W, Castro E, Hadju S. The significance of a solitary lung shadow in patients with colon carcinoma. *Cancer* 1974;33:414.

86. Rabinovitch R, Zelefsky M, Gaynor J, Fuks Z. Patterns of failure following surgical resection of renal cell carcinoma: implications for adjuvant local and systemic therapy. *J Clin Oncol* 1994;12:206.

87. Pogrebniak H, Haas G, Linehan W, Rosenberg S, Pass H. Renal cell carcinoma: resection of solitary and multiple metastases. *Ann Thorac Surg* 1992;54:33.

88. Mountain C, McMurtrey M, Hermes K. Surgery for pulmonary metastasis: a 20-year experience. *Ann Thorac Surg* 1984;38:323.

89. Dernevik L, Berggren H, Larsson S, Roberts D. Surg removal of pulmonary metastases from renal cell carcinoma. *Scand J Urol Nephrol* 1985;19:133.

90. Sherry R, Pass H, Rosenberg S, Yang J. Surgical resection of meta-

does not predict survival after resection of sarcomatous pulmonary metastases. *Ann Thorac Surg* 1991;51:219.

static renal cell carcinoma and melanoma after response to inter-leukin-2-based immunotherapy. *Cancer* 1992;69:1850.

91. Kim B, Louie A. Surg resection following interleukin 2 therapy for metastatic renal cell carcinoma prolongs remission. *Arch Surg* 1992; 127:1343.

92. Wood D, Her H, Motzer R, et al. Surg resection of solitary metastases after chemotherapy in patients with nonseminomatous germ cell tumors and elevated serum tumor markers. *Cancer* 1992;70:2354.

93. Prenger K, Eysman L, VanderHeide J, et al. Thoracotomy as a staging procedure after chemotherapy in the treatment of stage III nonsemi-nomatous carcinoma of the testis. *Ann Thorac Surg* 1984;38:444.

94. Bajorin D, Herr H, Motzer R, Bosl G. Current perspectives on the role of adjunctive surgery in combined modality treatment for patients with germ cell tumors. *Semin Oncol* 1992;19:148.

95. Greenberg R, Charles R, Samaha A, Chelsky M, Rosen S. Surg man-agement of recurrent genitourinary malignancies. *Semin Oncol* 1993; 20:473.

96. Martini N, McCormack P, Bains M. Indications for surgery for intra-thoracic metastases in testicular carcinoma. *Semin Oncol* 1979;6:99.

97. Murphy B, Breeden E, Donohue J, et al. Surgical salvage of chemore-fractory germ cell tumors. *J Clin Oncol* 1993;11:324.

98. Mandelbaum I, Yaw P, Einhorn L, Williams S, Rowland R, Donohue J. The importance of one-stage median sternotomy and retroperitoneal node dissection in disseminated testicular cancer. *Ann Thorac Surg* 1983;36:524.

99. Loehrer P, Mandelbaum I, Hui S, et al. Resection of thoracic and abdominal teratoma in patients after cisplatin-based chemotherapy for germ cell tumor. *J Thorac Cardiovasc Surg* 1986;92:676.

100. Gromet M, Ominsky S, Epstein W, Blois M. The thorax as the initial site for systemic relapse in malignant melanoma. *Cancer* 1979;44:776.

101. Sirott M, Bajorin D, Wong G, et al. Prognostic factors in patients with metastatic malignant melanoma. *Cancer* 1993;72:3091.

102. Pogrebniak H, Stovroff M, Roth J, Pass H. Resection of pulmonary metastases from malignant melanoma: results of a 16-year experience. *Ann Thorac Surg* 1988;46:20.

103. Gorenstein L, Putnam Jr J, Natarajan G, Balch C, Roth J. Improved survival after resection of pulmonary metastases from malignant melanoma. *Ann Thorac Surg* 1991;52:204.

104. Wong J, Euhus D, Morton D. Surg resection for metastatic melanoma to the lung. *Arch Surg* 1988;123:1091.

105. Thayer Jr J, Overholt R. Metastatic melanoma to the lung: long-term results of surgical excision. *Am J Surg* 1985;149:558.

106. Lejeune F, Lienard D, Sales F, Badr-el-din H. Surgical management of distant melanoma metastases. *Semin Surg Oncol* 1992;8:381.

107. Karakousis C, Velez A, Driscoll D, Takita H. Metastasectomy in malignant melanoma. *Surgery* 1994;115:295.

108. Balch C, Soong S, Murad T. A multifactorial analysis of melanoma: prognostic factors in 200 melanoma patients with distant metastases. *J Clin Oncol* 1983;1:126.

109. Mathisen D, Flye M, Peabody J. The role of thoracotomy in the man-agement of pulmonary metastases from malignant melanoma. *Ann Thorac Surg* 1979;27:295.

110. Harpole D, Johnson C, Wolfe W, George S, Seigler H. Analysis of 945 cases of pulmonary metastatic melanoma. *J Thorac Cardiovasc Surg* 1992;103:743.

111. Finley III R, Verazin G, Driscoll D, et al. Results of surgical resection of pulmonary metastases of squamous cell carcinoma of the head and neck. *Am J Surg* 1992;164:594.

112. Mazer T, Robbins K, McMurtrey M, Byers R. Resection of pulmonary metastases from squamous carcinoma of the head and neck. *Am J Surg* 1988;156:238.

113. Morrow C, Vassilopoulos P, Grage T. Surgical resection for metastatic neoplasms of the lung. *Cancer* 1980;45:2981.

114. VanGeel A, VanCoevorden F, Blankensteijn J, et al. Surgical treatment of pulmonary metastases from soft tissue sarcomas: a retrospective study in the Netherlands. *J Surg Oncol* 1994;56:172.

115. Callery C, Holmes E, Vernon S, Huth J, Coulson W, Skinner D. Resec-tion of pulmonary metastases from nonseminomatous testicular tumors. *Cancer* 1983;51:1152.

116. Seki M, Nakagawa K, Tsuchiya S, et al. Surg treatment of pulmonary metastases from uterine cervical cancer. *J Thorac Cardiovasc Surg* 1992;104:876.

CHAPTER 5

The Role of Thoracoscopy
in Thoracic Oncology

Rodney J. Landreneau, Robert J. Keenan, Michael J. Mack, Lynda S. Fetterman,
Stephen R. Hazelrigg, Peter F. Ferson, and Scott H. Hanan

> Most of the change we think we see in life is due to truths
> being in and out of favor.
>   *—Robert Frost (1874–1963)*

HISTORICAL PERSPECTIVE

The history of any surgical procedure generally involves the concomitant development of many fields, and this holds true for video-assisted thoracic surgery (VATS). The development of the cystoscope in 1806 by Phillip Bozzini heralded the beginning of endoscopy (1). This instrument, which Bozzini named the Lichtleiter, was reportedly used to examine various body cavities. Improvements in optics and illumination over the ensuing years led to more modern rigid endoscopes, which could be better tolerated by patients.

The first thoracoscopic procedure is generally credited to the Swedish physician Hans Christian Jacobaeus. Using the cystoscope of his era, the pleural space could be explored. In the early 1920s, Jacobaeus reported on his experience using this technique in the setting of pulmonary tuberculosis to facilitate "collapse therapy." With the aid of fluoroscopy, adhesions to the chest wall were cauterized, allowing the formation of a pneumothorax. He also reported on the use of thoracoscopy in the localization and diagnosis of pleural and pulmonary disease, including malignant processes (2–4).

This procedure was popularized in the European literature over the next 30 years, primarily in the treatment of tuberculosis. With the advent of effective antitubercular agents and the development of more modern open thoracic surgical techniques, interest in thoracoscopy waned.

The parallel development of fiberoptics in the late 1950s, along with positive-pressure and single-lung ventilation, helped renew enthusiasm for thoracoscopy and VATS (5,6). The concurrent popularization of laparoscopic surgery aided in the development of specialized instruments, allowing more complex procedures to be performed. All these advances, coupled with the ability to perform what some consider a less traumatic operation, have led to the widespread application of VATS in the diagnosis and treatment of diseases of the lung, pleura, and mediastinum. This chapter presents current experience with these techniques as they relate to thoracic oncology.

R. J. Landreneau and L. S. Fetterman: Allegheny General Hospital, Allegheny University of the Health Sciences, Pittsburgh, Pennsylvania 15212-4772.
R. J. Keenan: Department of Surgery, University of Pittsburgh Medical Center, Pittsburgh, Pennsylvania 15213-2582.
M. J. Mack: Department of Cardiothoracic Surgery, Columbia Hospital, Medical City Hospital, Dallas, Texas 75230.
S. R. Hazelrigg: Department of Cardiothoracic Surgery, Southern Illinois University School of Medicine, Springfield, Illinois 62702.
P. F. Ferson: Department of Thoracic Surgery, University of Pittsburgh Medical Center, Pittsburgh, Pennsylvania 15213-2582.
S. H. Hanan: Department of Surgical Oncology, University of Pittsburgh Medical Center, Pittsburgh, Pennsylvania 15219.

VATS AND METASTASECTOMY

Pulmonary lesions identified in patients with synchronous remote malignancy, or a history of malignancy, require careful attention: a finding of metastatic disease has prognostic significance and can dictate the nature of subsequent systemic therapy (7–13). Metastasectomy may also have therapeutic value for selected patients with a long disease-free interval, slow tumor doubling time, limited metastatic burden, and favorable tumor histologies (13,14).

TABLE 1. *Histology of metastatic pulmonary lesions approached by VATS*

Histology	No. (n=135)
Renal cell	25
Colon	24
Head and neck	24
Hepatocellular	22
Breast	15
Soft-tissue sarcoma	9
Melanoma	9
Cervical/uterine	5
Pancreatic	2

TABLE 2. *Candidate pulmonary nodules*

Noncalcified, <3 cm in diameter
Indeterminate etiology after appropriate workup
Location in the outer third of the lung
Absence of endobronchial extension

The usual surgical approach to pulmonary metastasectomy has been a standard lateral thoracotomy (7–17). The median sternotomy approach has been advocated by some investigators studying the utility of therapeutic metastasectomy so that synchronous metastatic disease in the contralateral hemithorax can be simultaneously excised (18,19). The development of effective VATS techniques allows thoracic surgeons to perform pulmonary wedge resection of many peripheral pulmonary nodules equivalent to that achieved through these open surgical approaches (20–24). We describe our experience with the VATS approach to wedge resection of metastatic pulmonary nodules with the aim of identifying the most appropriate use of this technology in the management of patients with this pulmonary manifestation of their systemic disease.

PATIENT PROFILE AND PULMONARY LESIONAL CHARACTERISTICS

Over the last 5 years, we have used the VATS approach to accomplish wedge resection of new, noncalcified pulmonary nodules identified in 179 patients with a history of remote malignancy or concomitant malignant processes. We were able to perform VATS wedge resection in 167 of these patients (Table 1). Twelve patients required conversion to muscle-sparing thoracotomy to accomplish lesional resection because an unfavorable location or size of the lesion prohibited successful VATS wedge resection. All the lesions approached by VATS were identified during the preoperative metastatic workup of remote primary malignancy or during posttreatment surveillance examinations with routine chest roentgenography or computed tomographic (CT) scanning of the chest (Fig. 1). High-resolution, thin-cut CT of the chest was routinely obtained before VATS metastasectomy. In general, lesions approachable for VATS excision by stapled or laser wedge resection are small and located in the periphery of the lung. The unifying characteristics of lesions approached by VATS are noted in Table 2.

Of the 167 patients undergoing wedge resection, 135 were found to have evidence of metastatic disease on frozen-section histologic analysis. Ninety-three of these patients were identified by CT scan analysis to have multiple bilateral pulmonary lesions (Fig. 2). The goal of the VATS wedge resection for these patients was diagnosis only. A small lesional size, an unfavorable location for percutaneous biopsy, or a previous failure of endobronchial or percutaneous needle biopsy were the reasons for this diagnostic VATS intervention (25,26).

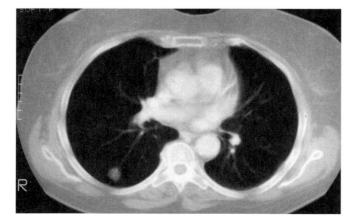

FIG. 1. Computed tomogram of solitary peripheral pulmonary nodule consistent with metastasis (note the arterial feeder into the lesion) in a patient with a history of colon cancer. This nodule is ideally suited for VATS excisional biopsy.

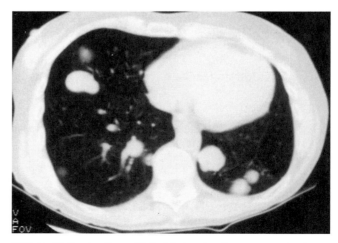

FIG. 2. Patient with multiple bilateral pulmonary metastases from renal carcinoma. In such a patient, VATS wedge resection biopsy is used for diagnosis only when less invasive diagnostic methods have failed.

Solitary pulmonary nodules consistent with metastasis were identified by CT scan analysis in 58 patients. Twenty-five of these patients were found to have benign lesions on frozen-section histologic examination of the resected specimen. The thoracoscopic resection was the definitive diagnostic maneuver for these patients. Seven patients were identified at frozen-section histologic analysis to have lesions consistent with primary lung cancers. Immediate conversion to open muscle-sparing thoracotomy was performed in these instances to accomplish formal lobar resection and mediastinal nodal staging. Twenty-three patients with peripheral solitary pulmonary metastases underwent successful VATS wedge resection. Three other patients with presumed solitary metastatic nodules by preoperative roentgenographic assessment were found to have other metastatic pulmonary lesions at thoracoscopic exploration. One patient who had four lesions identified thoracoscopically required conversion to thoracotomy to excise one of the more centrally located nodules. One other patient had numerous small lesions, along with sites of pleural metastatic implants. In this patient, diagnostic wedge resection and pleural biopsy were performed. The final patient had the two other peripheral lesions identified by the VATS approach; these were excised.

Finally, 16 patients with a limited number of pulmonary nodules (three or fewer) identified at preoperative roentgenographic analysis were managed with thoracoscopic excision of all lesions. All the metastatic sites of disease identified by CT scan were found and resected. Nine of these patients had bilateral disease. Two of these patients were managed with bilateral thoracoscopic resection under the same anesthetic. Sequential thoracoscopic resection was performed for the remaining 7 patients with bilateral disease, with 2 to 3 weeks between surgical interventions.

PREOPERATIVE STRATEGIES AND OPERATIVE PROCEDURE FOR VATS METASTASECTOMY

Because of the relative loss of tactile discrimination with the VATS approach compared to open thoracotomy, careful review of the preoperative chest roentgenogram and CT scan is mandatory to determine the best sites of intercostal access needed for VATS exploration of the lung and resection of the lesions (20–26). Lesions identified deep within the lung parenchyma are not suited for VATS excision; instead, plans for muscle-sparing thoracotomy must be made to approach the lesion or lesions (Fig. 3). Sometimes the peripheral pulmonary lesion identified roentgenographically is too small or in a relatively subpleural location, which can make timely or reliable nodular identification by VATS exploration questionable. In these circumstances, we have found CT-guided needle localization and staining of the lesion and

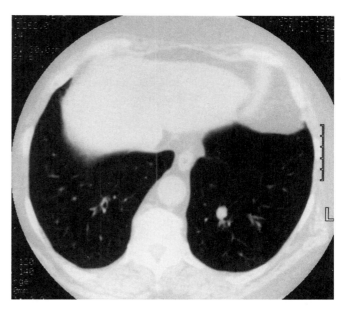

FIG. 3. Small deep pulmonary lesion inappropriate for VATS. Muscle-sparing thoracotomy and excisional biopsy using precision electrocautery or Nd:YAG laser resection techniques would be indicated. (Landreneau RJ, Hazelrigg SR, Johnson JA, Boley TM, Nawarawong W, Curtis JJ. Neodymium:yttrium–aluminum garnet laser–assisted pulmonary resections. *Ann Thorac Surg* 1991;51:973–8.)

proximate pulmonary parenchyma with methylene blue (0.1 mL) to be valuable aids in lesional identification (Fig. 4) (26–28). We have used this CT-guided needle localization technique in over 70 cases. Wire dislodgement has occurred in 15% to 20% of cases; however, the

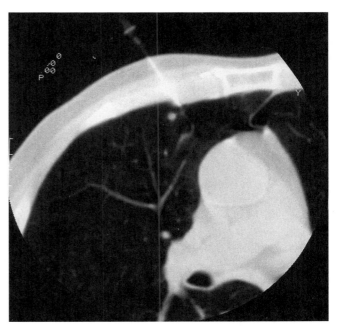

FIG. 4. Computed tomogram of chest demonstrating the wire needle localization technique used to assist identification of small subpleural pulmonary parenchymal lesions targeted for VATS resection.

concomitant methylene blue staining of the lung paren-chyma in the area of the lesion has allowed for identifi-cation and resection of the target pathology in all instances. There have been no adverse consequences from these CT-directed needle localization procedures, which are routinely scheduled immediately before the planned surgical intervention.

After induction of general anesthesia, the operative procedure begins with a careful bronchoscopic examina-tion of the airways for possible endobronchial metas-tases. This is performed through a single-lumen endotra-cheal tube. In the absence of endobronchial metastases (29), preparation is made for exploratory thoracoscopy. Conversion to a left-sided double-lumen endotracheal tube is performed to allow for contralateral single-lung ventilation and collapse of the ipsilateral lung. After institution of single-lung ventilation, the patient is placed in a full lateral position. The chest is prepared and draped for the VATS intervention and the possible need to convert to thoracotomy. The initial intercostal access site is determined by the anatomic location of the lesion and our intention to perform an adequate thoracoscopic exploration of the thoracic cavity (Fig. 5). We prefer to use a wide-angle, 0° operative thoracoscope (operating wide-angle 0° Hopkin's telescope, #26040A, Karl Storz Endoscopic America Inc., Culver City, CA) for these VATS procedures. The thoracoscope is introduced through a reusable 12-mm-diameter metal trocar (Snow-den Pencer, Inc., Tucker, GA) that is routinely used to protect the thoracoscope lens from smudging at its tip during operative manipulation. Two additional inter-costal access sites are established to introduce instru-mentation to examine the entire lung and to accomplish VATS wedge resection of the pulmonary lesions (Fig. 6). The lung is examined visually and by palpation with a blunt endoscopic probe and endoscopic forceps (Fig. 7). Effective collapse of the lung facilitates identification of lesions that will become effaced against the atelectatic pulmonary parenchyma. Slight enlargement of one of the trocar sites allows the introduction of a palpating finger to identify lesions that were not found with the other techniques.

Lesions found on the edge of the lung are resected with an endoscopic stapling device (EndoGIA, United States Surgical Corporation, Norwalk, CT, or Endo-scopic Linear Cutter, Ethicon Endoscopic, Cincinnati, OH) (Fig. 8). Occasionally, lesions on the edge of the lung cannot be completely resected with the stapler due to the thickness of the pulmonary tissue. For these lesions, resection across the base of the specimen is com-pleted with the Nd:YAG laser (Heraeus Lasersonics Inc., Milpitas, CA) (Fig. 9). For smoke evacuation during laser resections, a 28F chest tube is placed through one of the trocar sites and connected to a smoke evacuation system (LASE System II, LASE Inc., Model #SE-11111-BII, Cincinnati, OH).

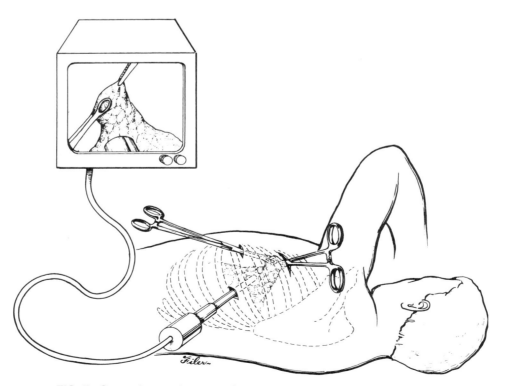

FIG. 5. General operative setup for thoracoscopic surgical interventions.

monly needed for larger lesions, those on the flat surface of the lung, and those relatively deep within the lung parenchyma.

RESULTS

VATS wedge resection was successfully accomplished in 167 of the 179 patients (93%) with peripheral pulmonary lesions thought to represent metastatic disease in this series. As mentioned earlier, 12 patients had lesions that could not be resected by VATS because of the technical limitations of VATS (ie, deep location preventing endoscopic wedge resection); these patients required conversion to an open thoracotomy to accomplish the nodular resection. Conversion to thoracotomy for formal anatomic resection was also performed for 7 patients in whom VATS excisional biopsy identified pulmonary nodules consistent with primary bronchogenic carcinoma.

Successful localization and diagnosis of the lesion or lesions in question was obtained with the VATS approach in all 167 patients undergoing VATS wedge excision. Nine of the 41 patients who underwent VATS resection with a potential therapeutic intent remain free of disease at a mean interval from their primary resection of 15 months. Three patients have undergone re-resection of a limited number of recurrent pulmonary nodules using the VATS approach. Two other patients have been re-resected through an open thoracotomy approach. Fourteen patients remaining alive have evidence of diffuse metastatic lung disease. The remaining 13 patients have all died of progressive metastatic disease from their primary malignancy.

There have been no operative deaths among the 167 patients undergoing VATS pulmonary nodular excision. The postoperative hospital stay among patients undergoing VATS wedge resection alone was 3.3±0.1 days. This

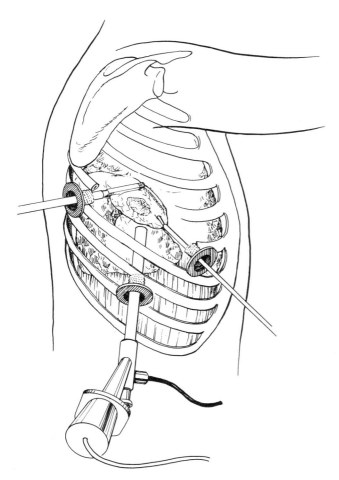

FIG. 6. A technique involving three intercostal access sites is routinely used for thoracoscopic exploration and VATS excisional biopsy.

After completion of the wedge resection, the specimen is removed from the thoracic cavity in a surgical retrieval bag (Pleatman sac, Cabbott Endoscopic Instruments) that is introduced into the chest through one of the intercostal access sites. The use of this retrieval system permits intact specimen removal and also prevents tumor seeding of the chest wall at the intercostal access site used for specimen removal (Fig. 10) (20–26,30,31). When frozen-section analysis reveals metastatic disease and the resection margins are free of tumor, thoracoscopic resection constitutes definitive operative therapy. A single 28F chest tube is placed through one of the intercostal access sites and is guided under direct visualization to the apex of the pleural cavity. The remaining incisional sites are closed with absorbable suture. The procedure is terminated after establishing a –20 cm H_2O suction to the chest tube evacuation system.

Conversion to a lateral thoracotomy is performed without delay if there is any concern that continuation with the attempted VATS wedge resection will compromise the surgical margins of resection. This is more com-

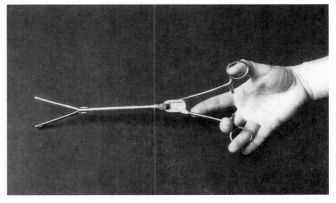

FIG. 7. The coaxial instrument design for endoscopic forceps our group is using for VATS avoids the awkwardness of pistol-grip tools and allows full working end excursion without limitation at the narrow rib interspaces.

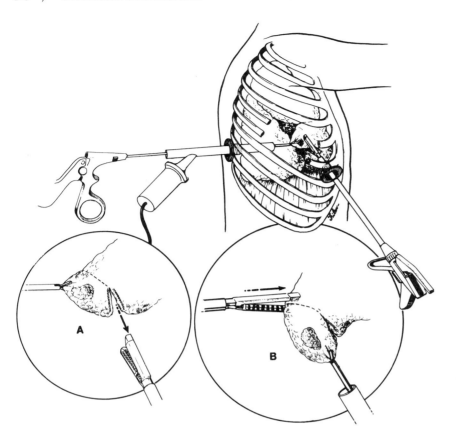

FIG. 8. Sequence of events in a standard VATS wedge resection using the endoscopic stapling device. The VATS approach using two intercostal access sites is demonstrated.

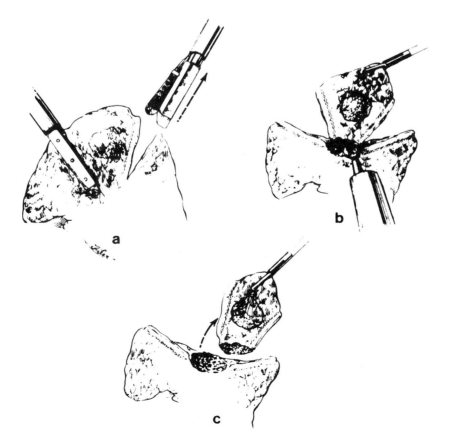

FIG. 9. Technique of combined endoscopic stapler and Nd:YAG laser wedge resection of a pulmonary nodule.

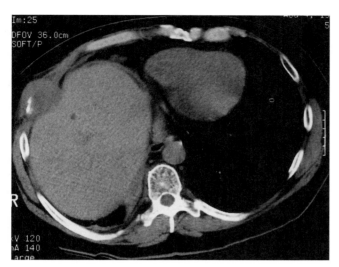

FIG. 10. Computed tomogram of the chest demonstrating a site of intercostal access seeding in the right chest wall that occurred during unprotected removal of a wedge resection specimen of metastatic head and neck cancer. Although the site of seeding was excised, the patient succumbed to systemic metastatic disease 5 months after the initial VATS resection.

compared favorably with the 6.7±1.3 days of hospitalization required for patients converted to thoracotomy to accomplish wedge resection and with the 8- to 10-day postoperative stay reported by us for open resection of peripheral lung lesions in earlier clinical studies (32,33).

DISCUSSION

Two patient populations are considered for metastasectomy of parenchymal lung lesions. The first group consists of patients who will not achieve a survival benefit from metastasectomy but for whom a diagnosis is required to estimate prognosis and to determine the course of further therapy. This group is primarily made up of patients with pulmonary lesions that preclude complete resection, multiple bilateral metastases, unfavorable tumor histology, and coexistent extrathoracic sites of metastases.

The second group of patients consists of those with a perceived limited pulmonary metastatic tumor burden and favorable primary tumor histologies who may achieve a survival benefit from metastasectomy (Table 3).

TABLE 3. *Criteria for "therapeutic" resection of pulmonary metastases*

Primary neoplasm controlled or controllable
Metastatic burden limited and isolated to the lung
Adequate cardiopulmonary reserve to undergo surgery *and* the extent of pulmonary resection contemplated

Other investigators have identified a potential survival benefit when a limited pulmonary disease burden is present in patients with favorable primary tumor histologies (15,17,34–41). Local control of the primary tumor is mandatory and no other site of metastasis can be present if a suggestion of therapeutic benefit will result from the resection of the pulmonary metastatic disease. Complete resection of the identifiable pulmonary metastatic disease must also be accomplished for any therapeutic benefit to be achieved. This latter concept has led some investigators to assume that radical resection of any and all pulmonary parenchymal lesions identified preoperatively or intraoperatively must be performed. However, careful review of the data from many reports reveals that the actual effect on survival related to incomplete resection was the inability to clear patients of an extensive disease burden (8,12–18,35–42). These findings support the concept that the extent of the patient's disease burden, rather than inattention of the thoracic surgeon toward resecting all demonstrable disease, is the true factor governing prognosis for most of these patients (see Figs. 1 and 2).

Other investigators have attempted to improve survival by performing median sternotomy with bilateral, bimanual palpation of the lung and extensive parenchymal-sparing resection of all pulmonary lesions (18,19). At sternotomy, 45% to 66% of patients with unilateral disease on preoperative studies are found to have bilateral metastases (18,19,37,43,44). Confounding data in a report by Roth and coworkers (44) leads us to question the utility of this approach. These investigators compared the results of therapeutic pulmonary metastasectomy in patients with extremity soft-tissue sarcoma undergoing either median sternotomy or lateral thoracotomy. These approach groups were equivalent with respect to tumor doubling time, disease-free interval, and number of nodules resected. Forty-five percent of patients with unilateral disease on CT were found to have bilateral metastases at sternotomy. However, resection of these occult metastases resulted in no survival advantage for their patients. It is therefore reasonable to conclude that the type of incision used to resect pulmonary metastases does not affect survival. It has also been noted that the recurrence of ipsilateral disease after metastasectomy is as common as the occurrence of contralateral metastases, despite the use of full thoracotomy with complete palpation of the lung and resection of all palpable lesions (37). In many respects, these findings reaffirm the importance of the biology of the metastatic process rather than the extent of the surgical intervention used for metastasectomy (45–47). These findings have led us to conclude that attempting to remove any and all pulmonary nodules identified on roentgenographic studies can lead only to the unnecessary sacrifice of normal pulmonary parenchyma surrounding many coincidentally found benign lesions and adds nothing to the patient's overall survival. Such a sacrifice of normal pulmonary tissue is also a lot to ask of patients who have a high likelihood of developing even further pulmonary functional impairment over time as a consequence of progressive metastatic involvement of the lung.

A literature review reveals that most patients undergoing resection of metastatic disease had very limited pulmonary disease burdens (8,12–18,35–42). In fact, most resections for nonsarcomatous malignancies in any series are wedge excisions for solitary pulmonary nodules. In many clinical series of pulmonary metastasectomy, the overall survival calculated to support this intervention is a compilation of the patient survival after resection of solitary nodules *and* the survival after resection of multiple metastatic nodules. Unfortunately, most series have very few long-term survivors when multiple nodules were resected. Using statistical manipulation, some reports have extrapolated a number of nodules below which a favorable prognosis is seen with metastasectomy. This takes advantage of the statistical biases resulting from the relatively large percentage of patients with solitary nodules and the relatively few patients with multiple nodules in any series of therapeutic metastasectomy reported. This is a major flaw in many metastasectomy series in the literature.

In attempting to analyze the survival data after pulmonary metastasectomy from any clinical report, it is important to realize that the absolute 5-year survival does not necessarily reflect any benefit from the metastasectomy. One must take into account the natural history of patients who develop pulmonary metastases. Basically, the 5-year survival for patients developing pulmonary metastases is in the 1% to 3% range. This percentage parallels the likelihood that a patient developing metastases will meet the basic criteria for therapeutic metastasectomy (see Table 3). Furthermore, if the patient is alive with metastatic disease at a given time interval from metastasectomy, one can attribute his or her survival only to the relatively indolent biologic nature of the metastatic disease. Certainly, we cannot consider metastasectomy as having had an important impact on survival in such patients who remain alive with recurrence or who die with later pulmonary metastases or distant disease. The biology of the tumor is the primary determinant of survival in these circumstances. A disease-free survival of over 5 years and an absolute survival of 10 years is therefore a more valid predictor of the true benefit of metastasectomy for any particular tumor type (48–52).

The role of improved systemic therapies for various metastatic malignant processes must also be considered when we investigate the evolving role of therapeutic pulmonary metastasectomy. This is particularly true with the advances in the systemic management of germ cell tumors and soft-tissue sarcomas. Although pulmonary metastasectomy appears to have an adjunctive role in the management of these diseases, the relative contribution to long-term survival provided by pulmonary metastasectomy versus systemic therapy is difficult to determine.

When surgical diagnosis of potential pulmonary metastases is the objective, the VATS approach offers an obvious advantage over thoracotomy with regard to reduced operative morbidity (20–24,33,53,54). However, the fear that some surgeons have regarding the VATS approach to therapeutic metastasectomy is that metastatic foci will be missed due to the restricted palpation of the lung available with VATS techniques (55). Careful examination of an adequately performed modern CT scan image of the pulmonary parenchyma makes this a moot clinical point under most circumstances. Nodules of 2 mm are consistently identified by such scanning methods (particularly the newer-generation spiral CT scanners). More importantly, lesions of this size are usually impossible to discern even at the time of open thoracotomy. As mentioned earlier, lesions identified by these CT scanning methods can be strategically found using wire needle localization techniques and successfully resected using the VATS approach (27,28).

Our bottom line regarding "therapeutic" pulmonary metastasectomy is influenced by the fact that if more than two or three lesions are found on thoracic exploration (open or VATS), the intervention takes on a diagnostic role only. We believe that the VATS approach is a valid alternative to thoracotomy for the "therapeutic" resection of limited metastatic disease (less than four lesions) identified as small, peripheral nodules by modern CT scanning techniques. If the targeted lesion or lesions cannot be localized during VATS, conversion to an open thoracotomy may be helpful. If more extensive metastatic disease is identified, we consider the procedure to have been of diagnostic utility only.

Our experience with VATS resection of peripheral pulmonary nodules has changed our approach to the management of patients with lung lesions presumed to be metastases. A thorough preoperative evaluation for the presence of extrathoracic metastases is performed. Our initial surgical approach is now VATS resection for those carefully selected patients with lesions in the outer third of the lung parenchyma. Among patients with favorable tumor histology, complete control of the primary malignancy, and minimal tumor burden located in the periphery of the lung, metastasectomy is performed both for diagnosis and in an attempt to provide a survival benefit. The use of the VATS approach in these circumstances does not close any options for subsequent pulmonary resection should sites of metastatic disease amenable to surgical resection be identified at a later time. Indeed, we have been able to perform repeated VATS excision of subsequent metastatic foci in several patients. Open thoracotomy approaches are still required for lesions deeper within the pulmonary parenchyma to avoid compromise of surgical resection margins and possible physiologic distortion of the remaining pulmonary lobar tissue (see Fig. 3) (56). In patients with unfavorable primary tumor histology or multiple unresectable metastases, thoracoscopic resection is used solely as a diagnostic maneuver. Protected retrieval of the wedge resection specimen is important. Although the occurrence of local and chest wall recurrence is in large part a function of an aggressive phenotype of the malignancy itself, technical errors in resection and manipulation of the tumor and seeding of the pleural space and chest wall should obviously be avoided.

VATS AND MALIGNANT PLEURAL PROCESSES

Managing malignant pleural effusions continues to be a difficult and common oncologic problem. Multi-institutional data from the Video-Assisted Thoracic Surgery Study Group (VATSSG) has shown pleural disease to be the second most common manifestation of thoracic disease treated by VATS (57). Thoracentesis and appropriate laboratory and cytologic examinations remain the initial tests of choice on pleural fluid. However, this approach is unsuccessful in diagnosing 20% to 40% of effusions encountered (58,59), and in these patients VATS technology can be helpful. As a diagnostic procedure, VATS has a reported accuracy of about 90% in collected series (Table 4) (60–65).

Besides this diagnostic utility, pleural disease can also be treated using the thoracoscope. Pleurodesis is an effective method of palliating the symptoms of pleural effusions, but the best method of producing pleurodesis in this setting is unknown. Retrospective data are available regarding the morbidity, mortality, and effectiveness of thoracoscopic talc pleurodesis. A study by Perrault and colleagues (66) addressed the operative morbidity and mortality of VATS in patients with malignant effusions. These investigators reported a 30-day operative morbidity of 32% and operative mortality of 13.6%. The mean survival from time of treatment in this group was 4 months. Based on these findings, we urge the use of stringent selection criteria when treating these patients.

Larger studies (67) report lower morbidity and mortality figures (3.7% and 2.3%, respectively); these again are retrospective in design. A prospective study from the Indiana University School of Medicine compared thoracoscopic talc pleurodesis with tetracycline and bleomycin pleurodesis via a thoracostomy tube (68). Although morbidity and mortality were not primary end points, no deaths were attributed to either procedure. In this study, the success rate in patients surviving their disease was 97% at 30 days and 95% at 90 days in the VATS group. This was significantly better than in the bleomycin group (69% at 30 days [$p=0.003$]) or the tetracycline group (33% at 30 days [$p<0.001$]). Other studies report similar success rates of 90% or better in the treatment of malignant pleural effusions (67,69). Whether this treatment is superior to tube thoracostomy and poudrage is currently being addressed in a prospective randomized study. The theoretical advantages of VATS in this setting are that the pleural space can be completely drained, adhesions can be lysed to allow full expansion of the lung, and under direct visualization pleurodesing agents can be uniformly applied to both parietal and visceral pleura. As current studies mature, subsets of patients will be identified who can most appropriately be treated by this technique. In patients with complex effusions identified by radiographic or ultrasonic means, we think that VATS technology offers an acceptable palliative approach.

VATS AND MEDIASTINAL NEOPLASTIC DISEASE

We have previously published our experience with the use of VATS for mediastinal pathology (Table 5) (70). These cases made up a minority of the procedures performed according to the VATSSG data (57). Our most common mediastinal application of VATS is as an alternative to the Chamberlain anterior mediastinotomy procedure in the evaluation of suspicious mediastinal adenopathy out of the reach of cervical mediastinoscopy.

Besides its possible role in the staging of lung cancer, the use of mediastinal VATS remains less well defined. Posterior mediastinal masses can be approached directly with this technique. Most of these tumors are benign and can be easily removed with the aid of an endoscopic bag (71).

TABLE 4. *Diagnostic accuracy of VATS*

Author (year)	No. of pt.	Dx	Accuracy (%)
Rusch and Mountain (1987)	25	25	100
Boutin et al. (1990)	215	206	96
Menzies et al. (1991)	102	95	96
Sharma and D'Cruz (1991)	27	24	89
Mack et al. (1992)	11	11	100

TABLE 5. *Use of VATS for mediastinal pathology*

Procedure	No. (n=113)
Mediastinal mass resection	
Anterior (thymectomy/cyst)	17
Cysts	4
Posterior (neurogenic tumors)	7
Mediastinal mass biopsy	
Staging lung CA	46
Biopsy mass/adenopathy	14
Pericardial disease	
Pericardiectomy	37
Cyst resection	3
Thoracic splanchnicectomy	5

We have also described the approach to anterior mediastinal masses (72). We think this is a reasonable application of VATS in early-stage thymomas and in the surgical treatment of myasthenia. The need for sternotomy is obviated; however, adequate videoscopic visualization is mandatory to avoid injury to the phrenic nerves or the innominate vein. This approach is technically feasible, but there are no long-term follow-up data and no comparisons to standard operative therapies in a prospective randomized fashion.

FUTURE DIRECTIONS

As with all new technologies, early enthusiasm leads to widespread application. The effects of this enthusiasm can be ascertained only by careful analysis of well-designed studies and long-term follow-up. VATS has been applied in many settings. Other interesting avenues of investigation include the use of VATS technology in the staging and treatment of esophageal cancers (73). There have been few prospective randomized studies with long-term data. Through efforts by groups such as VATSSG, questions related to procedure costs, complications, and long-term benefits can be addressed. It is only through this process that the true utility of VATS can be found.

REFERENCES

1. Braimbridge MV. The history of thoracoscopic surgery. *Ann Thorac Surg* 1993;56:610–614.
2. Jacobaeus HC. The practical importance of thoracoscopy in surgery of the chest. *Surg Gynecol Obstet* 1922;34:289.
3. Jacobaeus HC. Die Thorakoskopie und Ihre Praktische Bedeutung. *Ergebn Ges Med* 1925;7:112.
4. Jacobaeus HC. The cauterization of adhesions in pneumothorax treatment of tuberculosis. *Surg Gynecol Obstet* 1921;32:493.
5. Kapany NS. *Fiberoptics: principles and applications.* New York: Academic Press, 1967.
6. Carlens E. A new flexible double-lumen catheter for bronchospirometry. *J Thoracic Cardiovasc Surg* 1949;18:742.
7. Kern KA, Pass HI, Roth JA. Treatment of metastatic cancer to lung. In: Rosenberg SA, ed. *Surgical treatment of pulmonary metastases.* Philadelphia: JB Lippincott, 1987:69–100.
8. van Dongen JA, van Slooten EA. The surgical treatment of pulmonary metastases. *Cancer Treat Rev* 1978;4:29–48.
9. Roth JA. Treatment of metastatic cancer to lung. In: DeVita VT, Hellman S, Rosenberg SA, eds. *Cancer: principles and practice of oncology.* Philadelphia: JB Lippincott, 1989:2261–2275.
10. Pass HI. Resection of pulmonary metastases. In: Roth JA, Ruckdeschel JC, Weisenburger TH, eds. *Thoracic oncology.* Philadelphia: WB Saunders, 1989:619–629.
11. Miller SJ, Moores DWO, McKneally MF. Indications for resection of pulmonary metastasis. In: Baue AE, Geha AS, Hammond GL, Laks H, Naunheim KS, eds. *Glenn's thoracic and cardiovascular surgery,* 5th ed. Norwalk, CT: Appleton & Lange, 1991.
12. Harvey JC, Lee K, Beattie EJ. Surgical management of pulmonary metastases. *Chest Surg Clin North Am* 1994;4:55–66.
13. Joseph WL, Morton DL, Adkins PC. Prognostic significance of tumor doubling time in evaluating operability in pulmonary metastatic disease. *J Thorac Cardiovasc Surg* 1971;61:23–27.
14. Putnam JB, Roth JA, Wesley MN, Johnston MR, Rosenberg SA. Analysis of prognostic factors in patients undergoing resection of pulmonary metastases from soft tissue sarcoma. *J Thorac Cardiovasc Surg* 1984; 87:260–267.
15. Vogt-Moykopt I, Sabine K, Bulzebruck H, Schirren J. Surgery for pulmonary metastases: the Heidelberg experience. *Chest Surg Clin North Am* 1994;4:85–112.
16. Rosen G, Holmes EC, Forscher CA, Lowenbraun S, Eckardt JJ, Eilber FR. The role of thoracic surgery in the management of metastatic osteogenic sarcoma. *Chest Surg Clin North Am* 1994;4:75–83.
17. Mountain CF, McMurtey MJ, Hermes KE. Surgery for pulmonary metastases: a 20-year experience. *Ann Thorac Surg* 1984;38:323–330.
18. Johnston MR. Median sternotomy for resection of pulmonary metastases. *J Thorac Cardiovasc Surg* 1983;85:516.
19. Pogrebniak HW, Pass HI. Initial and reoperative pulmonary metastasectomy: indications, technique and results. *Semin Surg Oncol* 1993;9: 142–147.
20. Dowling RD, Ferson PF, Landreneau RJ. Thoracoscopic resection of pulmonary metastases. *Chest* 1992;102:1450–1454.
21. Landreneau RJ, Mack MJ, Keenan RJ, Dowling RD, Hazelrigg SR, Ferson PF. Strategic planning for video-assisted thoracic surgery (VATS). *Ann Thorac Surg* 1993;56:615–619.
22. Dowling RD, Keenan RJ, Ferson PF, Landreneau RJ. Video-assisted thoracoscopic surgery for pulmonary metastases. *Ann Thorac Surg* 1993;56:772–775.
23. Landreneau RJ, Mack MJ, Hazelrigg SR, Dowling RD, Keenan RJ, Ferson PF. The role of thoracoscopy in the management of intrathoracic neoplastic processes. *Semin Thorac Cardiovasc Surg* 1993;5:219–228.
24. Landreneau RJ, Mack MJ, Hazelrigg SR, Naunheim KS, Keenan RJ, Ferson PF. Video-assisted thoracic surgery: a minimally invasive approach to thoracic oncology. In: DeVita VT, Hellman S, Rosenberg SA, eds. *Cancer: principles and practice* (update series), 1994;8:1–14.
25. Mack MJ, Hazelrigg SR, Landreneau RJ, Acuff TE. Thoracoscopy for the diagnosis of the indeterminate solitary pulmonary nodule. *Ann Thorac Surg* 1993;56:825–832.
26. Mitruka S, Landreneau RJ, Mack MJ, et al. Diagnosing the indeterminate pulmonary nodule: percutaneous biopsy vs. thoracoscopy. *Surgery* 1995;113:676–684.
27. Mack MJ, Shennib H, Landreneau RJ, Hazelrigg SR. Techniques for localization of pulmonary nodules for thoracoscopic resection. *J Thorac Cardiovasc Surg* 1993;106:550–553.
28. Plunkett MB, Peterson MS, Landreneau RJ, Ferson PF, Posner MC. CT-guided preoperative percutaneous needle localization of peripheral pulmonary nodules. *Radiology* 1992;185:274–276.
29. Sheperd M. Endobronchial metastatic disease. *Thorax* 1982;37: 362–365.
30. Fry WJ. Thoracoscopic implantation of cancer with a fatal outcome. *Ann Thorac Surg* 1995;59:42–45.
31. Walsh GL, Nesbitt JC. Tumor implants after thoracoscopic resection of a metastatic sarcoma. *Ann Thorac Surg* 1995;59:215–216.
32. Landreneau RJ, Hazelrigg SR, Johnson JA, Boley TM, Nawarawong W, Curtis JJ. Neodymium:yttrium-aluminum garnet laser–assisted pulmonary resections. *Ann Thorac Surg* 1991;51:973–978.
33. Landreneau RJ, Hazelrigg SR, Mack MJ, et al. Postoperative pain-related morbidity: video-assisted thoracic surgery vs. thoracotomy. *Ann Thorac Surg* 1993;56:1285–1289.
34. Barney JD, Churchill ED. Adenocarcinoma of the kidney with metastases to the lung treated by pulmonary resection. *J Urol* 1939;42: 269–273.
35. Martini N, Huvos AG, Mike V. Multiple pulmonary resection in the treatment of osteogenic sarcoma. *Ann Thorac Surg* 1971;12:271–280.
36. McCormack PM, Burt ME, Bains MS, Martini N, Rusch VM, Ginsberg RJ. Lung resection for colorectal metastases: 10-year results. *Arch Surg* 1992;127:1403–1406.
37. Gorenstein LA, Putnam JB, Natarajan MA, Balch CA, Roth JA. Improved survival after resection of pulmonary metastases from malignant melanoma. *Ann Thorac Surg* 1991;52:204–210.
38. Harpole DH, Johnson CM, Wolfe WG, George SL, Seigler HF. An analysis of 945 cases of pulmonary metastatic melanoma. *J Thorac Cardiovasc Surg* 1992;103:743–748.
39. McAfee MK, Allen MS, Trastek VF, Ilstrup DM, Deschamps C, Pairolero PC. Colorectal lung metastases: results of surgical excision. *Ann Thorac Surg* 1992;53:780–786.
40. Lanza LA, Natarajan G, Roth JA, Putnam JB. Long-term survival after resection of pulmonary metastases from carcinoma of the breast. *Ann Thorac Surg* 1992;54:244–248.

41. Cerfolio RJ, Allen MS, Deschamps C, et al. Pulmonary resection of metastatic hypernephroma. *Ann Thorac Surg* 1994;57:339–344.
42. McCormack PM, Martini N. The changing role of surgery for pulmonary metastases. *Ann Thorac Surg* 1979;28:139–145.
43. Freidman B, Bohndorf K, Kruga J. Radiology of pulmonary metastases: comparison of imaging techniques with operative findings. *Thorac Cardiovasc Surg* 1986;34:120–124.
44. Roth JA, Pass HI, Wesely MN, White D, Putnam JB, Seipp C. Comparison of median sternotomy and thoracotomy for resection of pulmonary metastases in patients with soft tissue sarcoma. *Ann Thorac Surg* 1986;42:138–143.
45. Fidler IJ, Hart IR. Biologic diversity in metastatic neoplasms. Origins and implications. *Science* 1982;217:998–1002.
46. Fidler IJ. Recent concepts of cancer metastasis and their implications for therapy. *Cancer Treat Rep* 1984;68:193–199.
47. Fidler IJ, Balch CM. The biology of cancer metastasis and implications for therapy. *Curr Prob Surg* 1987;24:129.
48. Aberg T, Malmberg KA, Nilsson B, Nou E. The effect of metastasectomy: fact or fiction? *Ann Thorac Surg* 1980;30:378–384.
49. Roberts DG, Cardillo G, Dernevik L, et al. Long-term follow-up of operative treatment for pulmonary metastases. *Eur J Cardiothorac Surg* 1989;3:292–296.
50. Goya T, Miyazawa N, Kondo H, et al. Sugical resection of pulmonary metastases from colorectal cancer. 10 years followup. *Cancer* 1989;64:1418–1421.
51. Gastrointestinal Tumor Study Group. Adjuvant therapy of colon cancer. Results of a prospective randomized trial. *N Engl J Med* 1984;310:737–745.
52. Mansel JK, Zinseeister AR, Pairolero PC, Jett JR. Pulmonary resection of metastatic colorectal adenocarcinoma: A ten-year experience. *Chest* 1986;89:109–114.
53. Landreneau RJ, Herlan DB, Johnson JA, Boley TM, Nawarawong W, Ferson PF. Thoracoscopic Nd:YAG laser pulmonary resection. *Ann Thorac Surg* 1991;52:1176–1178.
54. Landreneau RJ, Hazelrigg SR, Ferson PF, et al. Thoracoscopic resection of 85 pulmonary lesion. *Ann Thorac Surg* 1992;54:415–420.
55. McCormack PM, Ginsberg KB, Bains MS, et al. Accuracy of lung imaging in metastases with implications for the role of thoracoscopy. *Ann Thorac Surg* 1993;56:863–866.
56. Landreneau RJ, Hazelrigg SR, Johnson JA, Boley TM, Nawarawong W, Curtis JJ. Neodymium:Yttrium-aluminum garnet laser–assisted pulmonary resections. *Ann Thorac Surg* 1991;51:973–978.
57. Hazelrigg SR, Nunchuck SK, LoCicero J 3d. Video-Assisted Thoracic Surgery Study Group data. *Ann Thorac Surg* 1993;56(5):1039–1043.
58. Canto A, Biasco E, Casillas M, et al. Thoracoscopy in the diagnosis of pleural effusion. *Thorax* 1977;32:550–554.
59. Rao NV, Jones PO, Greensburg SD, et al. Needle biopsy of the parietal pleura in 124 cases. *Arch Intern Med* 1965;115:34–41.
60. Boutin C, Astroul P, Seitz B. The role of thoracoscopy in the evaluation and management of pleural effusion. *Lung* 1990;168:1113–1121.
61. Menzies R, Charbonneau M. Thoracoscopy for the diagnosis of pleural disease. *Ann Intern Med* 1991;114:271–276.
62. Sharma S, D'Cruz A. Thoracoscopy in the diagnosis of pleural effusions of ambiguous etiology. *J Surg Oncol* 1991;48:133–135.
63. Rusch VM, Mountain C. Thoracoscopy under regional anesthesia for the diagnosis and management of pleural disease. *Am J Surg* 1987;154:264–268.
64. Mack MJ, Arnoff RJ, Acuff TE, Douthit MB, Bowman RT, Ryan WH. Present role of thoracoscopy in the diagnosis and treatment of diseases of the chest. *Ann Thorac Surg* 1992;54:403.
65. Kaiser LR. Diagnostic and therapeutic use of pleuroscopy in lung cancer. *Surg Clin North Am* 1987;67:1081.
66. Perrault LP, Page A, Gregoire J. Palliative treatment of malignant effusions by thoracoscopy under video assistance: morbidity and survival. *Annales de Chirurgie* 1994;48(8):768–772.
67. Bal S, Hasan SS. Thoracoscopic management of malignant pleural effusions. *Intl Surg* 1993;78(4):324–327.
68. Hartman DL, Gaither JM, Kesler KA, Mylet DM, Brown JW, Mathur PN. Comparison of insufflated talc under thoracoscopic guidance with standard tetracycline and bleomycin pleurodesis for control of malignant pleural effusions. *J Thorac Cardiovasc Surg* 1993;105(4):743–747.
69. Colt HG. Thoracoscopy. A prospective study of safety and outcome. *Chest* 1995;108(2):324–329.
70. Landreneau RJ, Mack MJ, Hazelrigg SR, Naunheim KS, Keenan RJ, Ferson PF. The role of video-assisted thoracic surgery in thoracic oncological practice. *Cancer Invest* 1995;13(5):526–539.
71. Mack MJ. Thoracoscopy and its role in mediastinal disease and sympathectomy. *Semin Thorac Cardiovasc Surg* 1993;5(4):332–336.
72. Landreneau RJ, Dowling RD, Castillo W, et al. Thoracoscopic resection of an anterior mediastinal tumor. *Ann Thorac Surg* 1992;54:142–144.
73. McKenna RJ Jr. Minimally invasive surgery for pulmonary and esophageal tumors. *Semin in Surg Oncol* 1994;10(6):411–416.

CHAPTER 6

Isolated Lung Perfusion
for Pulmonary Metastases

Harvey I. Pass

The ability to perfuse one lung without interrupting the general circulation is a distinct advantage . . . and the capacity of lung tissue to withstand such a chemical insult offers a new technique for administering chemotherapeutic agents.
—*Pierpont and Blades (6)*

BACKGROUND AND MAGNITUDE OF THE PROBLEM

The lung is the site of many neoplasms that due to location, size, or multiplicity cannot be resected. A few examples are metastatic lesions to the lung, including sarcoma, melanoma, renal cell cancer, and metastatic gastrointestinal disease (1). Although uncommon with the latter histologies, the first site of recurrence of sarcomas is the lung. In most patients with unresectable pulmonary metastases from soft-tissue sarcoma, the lung is the only site of disease and leads to their demise within 6 months. Even with complete resection of the pulmonary metastases, only a 25% 3-year survival is possible (2). Moreover, this is in a select group of patients; most of these patients will recur with nodules that cannot be resected, eventually leading to their demise from pulmonary failure. Despite various regimens, response rates of only 25% to 50% are noted for the chemotherapy of pulmonary metastases, and these responses are usually short-lived.

Most of these lung metastases are supplied by the pulmonary arterial circulation (3–5). Although there is debate on this issue, it is believed that 84% of all lung metastases are supplied by the pulmonary arteries alone or by a combination of the bronchial and pulmonary arteries. Because the pulmonary arterial circulation in a

H. I. Pass: Wayne State University, Karmanos Cancer Institute, Harper Hospital, Detroit, Michigan 48201.

normal person drains exclusively to the pulmonary veins, a complete isolation of the lungs for selective perfusion of cytotoxic agents should be theoretically possible. Balanced against this locoregional treatment would be the possible short- and long-term toxicity of the agent or other components of the therapy on the lung, as well as the ability to prevent systemic exposure to the agent (ie, a leak).

EARLY EXPERIMENTAL WORK

This concept of isolated lung perfusion (ILP) for the delivery of high doses of chemotherapeutic or biologic agents is not new. The agents used depended on the availability of chemotherapeutic drugs as well as the histologic type of tumor. Pierpont and Blades (6) reported that a dog's lung could be isolated from its pulmonary and bronchial blood supply for 30 minutes, and the animal could still withstand contralateral pneumonectomy. A method for isolation/perfusion of the left lung of a dog was described using closed suction drainage to empty blood from an isolated atrial segment into a collecting venous reservoir (Fig. 1). Nitrogen mustard (0.4 mg), one of the few agents available in the 1960s, was infused into the lung using this circuit and 10 of 23 animals survived. Jacobs and colleagues (7) used gravity drainage of an isolated atrial segment, allowing the collecting reservoir to increase due to bronchial flow. He reported surviving animals at doses of 1.7 mg/kg nitrogen mustard.

Johnston and associates expanded these studies of ILP using single-lung perfusion with doxorubicin (Adriamycin) (8,9) in hopes of using the drug in unresectable pulmonary metastases from sarcoma primary tumors (Fig. 2). Canines were perfused with 0.5 μg/mL Adriamycin perfusate for 45 minutes. Peak pulmonary artery pressures during the perfusion were 12 to 15 mm Hg, and flow rates were 100 to 200 mL/min. All the animals survived contralateral pneumonectomy. Follow-up studies with modification of the perfusion apparatus and using higher flow rates resulted in more even distribution of flow and higher tissue levels of Adriamycin compared to perfusate levels. Rickaby and associates (10), using isolated dog lungs perfused with autologous blood or salt solution, reported that these lungs tolerated hyperthermia to 44.4°C for 2 hours with no changes in lung weight, extravascular water, vascular volume, serotonin uptake urea permeability surface area product, perfusion pressure, or lung compliance. In a similar set of experiments, Baciewicz and colleagues (11) found that animals would survive isolated hyperthermic (39°C) lung perfusion and would tolerate contralateral pneumonectomy with perfusate doses up to 5.79 μg/mL.

In the earliest report of human ILP, Johnston and coworkers (8–10) used these perfusion techniques, under normothermic conditions, in 3 patients without complication, thus establishing the feasibility of the procedure. Johnston also established the in vivo feasibility of even more novel approaches for lung perfusion by describing

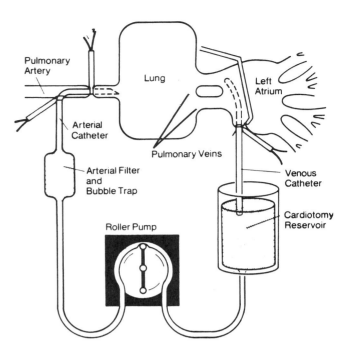

FIG. 2. Perfusion system described in Johnston's experimental work. (With permission from Johnston MR, Minchin R, Shull JH, et al. Isolated lung perfusion with Adriamycin. A preclinical study. *Cancer* 1983;52:404–409.)

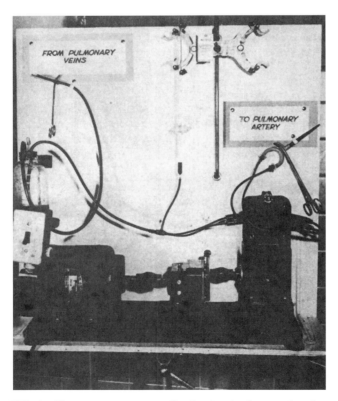

FIG. 1. Sigmamotor pump, collecting bottle, burette for chemotherapeutic agent, and disposable Tygon tubing described by Pierpont and Blades for their canine lung perfusion experiments. (With permission from Pierpont H, Blades B. Lung perfusion with chemotherapeutic agents. *J Thorac Cardiovasc Surg* 1960;39:159–165.)

successful total lung perfusion of dogs for 50 minutes using separate circuits for the systemic and pulmonic circuits, under cardioplegic arrest (9). Minimal leak was recorded, no significant changes in pulmonary or systemic physiologic parameters were recorded, and minimal changes were seen in the lungs on histopathologic examination.

RECENT EXPERIMENTAL WORK

Little work was devoted to experimental or human studies of the feasibility of ILP between 1985 and 1993. Benchwork activities then were started at the Memorial Sloan-Kettering Institute and the National Cancer Institute (NCI), using two different approaches.

To evaluate isolated single-lung perfusion with chemotherapy in a rat lung metastasis model, a model of in vivo isolated single-lung perfusion was developed at Memorial Sloan-Kettering. A left thoracotomy was performed with an operating microscope (×16 magnification), the left pulmonary artery was cannulated, and a left pulmonary venotomy was performed (Fig. 3). Isolated left lung perfusion was performed for 10 minutes at 0.5 mL/min with heparinized whole blood (n=10) or 0.9% normal saline (n=10). Pulmonary vein effluent was collected by suction. Ninety-five percent of the animals survived isolated left single-lung perfusion, and 78% survived subsequent right pneumonectomy 3 weeks later.

These data demonstrated that in vivo isolated single-lung perfusion in rats was feasible and led to multiple studies of isolated perfusion with diverse agents (12).

ILP with doxorubicin in the treatment of experimental pulmonary metastases in F344 rats was initially reported using this model (13). After randomization, rats received isolated left lung perfusion with doxorubicin 320 mcg/mL, left isolated lung perfusion with doxorubicin 480 mcg/mL, or doxorubicin 640 mcg/mL in an attempt to define the maximal tolerated dose. In a second experiment, two groups of F344 rats were injected intravenously with 10^7 viable methylcholanthrene-induced sarcoma cells and received either left isolated lung perfusion with saline or isolated lung perfusion with doxorubicin 320 micrograms/mL 7 days later. There were no survivors after left ILP with >320 mcg/mL. In the treatment of the pulmonary metastases model, animals had massive tumor replacement of the left (treated) lung in the control group; animals receiving isolated ILP had eradication of metastases in nine of 10 cases (Fig. 4).

In a similar experiment of ILP, tumor necrosis factor (TNF) was used in an experimental sarcoma lung metastasis model (14). F344 rats were injected with 10^7 methylcholanthrene-induced sarcoma cells. On day 7, four animals were perfused with 210 mcg of murine TNF, five animals were perfused with 420 mcg of murine TNF, 10 animals underwent ILP with 420 mcg of human TNF, and four animals were injected systemically with 420 mcg of human TNF. Animals perfused with 210 mcg/mL of murine TNF and animals treated by systemically administered human TNF showed no tumor response. Animals perfused with 420 mcg/mL of murine TNF had 7.8 ± 14.2 nodules on the left lung and 58.5 ± 66.0 nodules on the right lung ($p=0.07$). Animals perfused with 420 mcg/mL

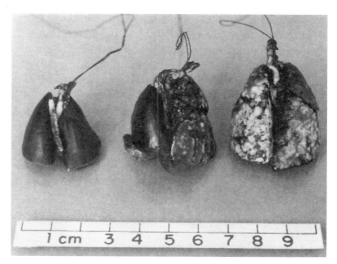

FIG. 4. Posterior view of rat lungs treated with doxorubicin ILP. *Left*, normal untreated lungs; *middle*, lungs after left ILP with doxorubicin; *right*, lungs after left lung perfusion with saline solution. Tumor areas are white. Note the decreased number of metastases in the left lung in the middle panel. (With permission from Weksler B, Lenert J, Ng B, Burt M. Isolated single lung perfusion with doxorubicin is effective in eradicating soft tissue sarcoma lung metastases in a rat model. *J Thorac Cardiovasc Surg* 1994;107:50–54.)

of human TNF had 21.7 ± 18.3 nodules on the left lung and 91.7 ± 66.2 nodules on the right lung ($p<0.01$). These studies complement the large-animal experiments of ILP with TNF performed at the NCI, which are discussed later in this chapter.

FUDR (2'-deoxy-5-fluorouridine) was also evaluated using the model of isolated single-lung perfusion in the rat (15). BDIX rats were inoculated intravenously with 10^6 viable Sp-5 colorectal adenocarcinoma cells. On day 10 after tumor inoculation, animals were randomized to receive continuous intravenous infusion of FUDR (1 mg/kg-1.d-1), isolated left lung perfusion with a buffered Hespan solution, or ILP with 3.5, 7, and 14 mg of FUDR per milliliter of the buffered Hespan solution. On day 26 after tumor inoculation, the animals in all groups were sacrificed and their lungs were stained and counted. Animals that underwent ILP with 14 mg of FUDR per milliliter of the buffered Hespan solution showed a significant decrease in the number of tumor nodules on the treated side versus the number on the untreated side (455.2 ± 87.3 versus 11 ± 6.4; $p< 0.0001$).

Large-animal work has also been performed recently in preparation for human trials of ILP with chemotherapy. Ratto and associates (16) randomly divided swine into four groups receiving cisplatin (2.5 mg/kg) through the pulmonary artery using one of the following techniques: stop-flow (group 1), stop-flow/outflow occlusion (group 2), lung perfusion (group 3), or lung perfusion with 5 mg/kg of infused drug (group 4). The animals were killed and

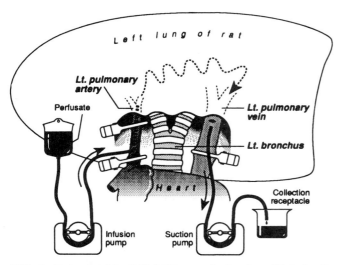

FIG. 3. Rat model for ILP. (With permission from Weksler B, Schneider A, Ng B, Burt M. Isolated single lung perfusion in the rat: an experimental model. *J Appl Physiol* 1993;74:2736–2739.)

platinum concentrations in plasma, plasma ultrafiltrate (free platinum), urine, and tissues were determined by flameless atomic absorption spectroscopy. Greater systemic plasma and lower pulmonary plasma and tissue platinum levels were detected when cisplatin was given using the stop-flow technique with respect to the other administration modalities. No significant difference in regional and systemic platinum exposure was found between groups 2 and 3. Lung perfusion resulted in higher mediastinal node and lower bone marrow platinum values. Morphologic alterations and impairment of gas exchanges in the treated lung were not dependent on the applied infusion technique.

CLINICAL USE OF ILP WITH CHEMOTHERAPY

Besides the early work performed at the NCI by Johnston, no other concentrated effort has been made to develop phase I or II studies using ILP and chemotherapy for human pulmonary metastases. This may change, of course, now that the groundwork has been laid by the Memorial Sloan-Kettering group. As of this writing, at least two groups in the United States are attempting to have protocols approved through their institutional review boards for this project. The true worth of these efforts will be realized only if sufficient numbers of patients can have a perfusion, if the perfusion technique is standardized from patient to patient, if toxicity trials define the maximal tolerated dose of the agent that can be delivered to the lung, and if there is roentgenographic follow-up to document any responses, even in the phase I setting.

Ratto's group, after completing their pharmacokinetic study in swine as detailed above, administered ILP with 5 mg/kg cisplatin to 4 patients intraoperatively after pulmonary metastasectomy. Their rationale for this adjuvant use of ILP was twofold: surgery could remove all recognized tumor, whereas chemotherapy could destroy the remaining microscopic foci; and sarcoma relapse even after metastasectomy is usually intrathoracic. Their approach, which involved thoracotomy, atrial clamping with a Satinsky clamp, and a 1-hour perfusion using an extracorporeal circuit, was completed by washing out the lung and metastasectomy. According to their data, published in abstract form, the morbidity observed included transient edema in one case. There were no systemic side effects of the cisplatin, and high cisplatin levels were obtained in the pulmonary plasma and in lung and tumor tissue (17). This bold approach is exciting but probably is premature in its use of ILP in the adjuvant setting. A phase I/II trial of cisplatin ILP to define the maximal tolerated dose in patients with unresectable metastases, however, would ensure the logic of their hypotheses.

POSSIBLE USE OF CYTOKINES IN ILP

The use of biologic agents such as TNF in the management of systemic cancer has been prevented by dose-limiting toxicity. TNF is a protein that derives its name from the activity demonstrated against subcutaneous methylcholanthrene-induced tumors in mice (18). Although preclinical murine studies demonstrated excellent antitumor activity against a variety of subcutaneous tumors (19), phase I trials of recombinant TNF in patients have been discouraging. The overall response rate in 251 patients given intravenous TNF in phase I studies was 4%, even with dose escalations where considerable toxicity was seen (20). The difference in efficacy of TNF between murine and human studies may be related to the dose intensity that can be delivered to these two species. The maximal tolerated dose in most human trials ranges from 150 to 300 mcg/m^2 of TNF, or 5 to 10 mcg/kg. The dose of TNF required for antitumor effects in the murine studies was in the range of 5 to 8 mcg per 20-g mouse, or 200 to 400 mcg/kg (19), approximately a 40-fold increase over the tolerable dose in humans. This interspecies difference in toxicity of TNF allows higher levels of TNF to be achieved in the murine tumors and may account for the dramatic difference in efficacy as an antineoplastic agent between mice and humans.

Further evidence for the potential efficacy of TNF, when it can be administered to tumors in high concentrations, comes from a series of reports using TNF, interferon (IFN)-gamma, and melphalan in isolated limb perfusions for extremity melanomas or sarcomas (21–23). For each of these histologies, 100% overall response rates with >90% complete response rates have been reported on patients from several European groups.

A theoretical basis for the use of TNF with IFN-gamma and hyperthermia for regional therapy is founded on several preclinical observations. First, TNF clearly has significant toxicity in high concentrations, and there is a definite dose response to TNF with inability to achieve effective antitumor concentrations in human trials. Therefore, the major benefit of an isolated perfusion—achieving high local concentrations of an agent while limiting systemic toxicity—is applicable to TNF. Also, the antitumor effect of TNF is very rapid, with histologic changes in the tumor occurring as early as 30 minutes. This short time to onset of action obviates the major disadvantage of isolated perfusion: limited exposure of the tumor to the active agent. Third, the combination of TNF with IFN-gamma and hyperthermia has shown augmented cytotoxicity compared to TNF alone. Theoretical reasons for the combination with IFN-gamma include up-regulation of TNF receptors and MHC antigens by IFN (24,25). Hyperthermia augments the activity of TNF both in vitro and in vivo (26).

A major component of TNF toxicity, besides reversible cardiac, renal, and hepatic dysfunction, has been a pulmonary response that is similar to endotoxemia (27–32). Intravenous administration of TNF injures pulmonary arterioles, venules, and capillaries, resulting in alveolar epithelial injury, alveolar exudation, alveolar neutrophil accumulation, and capillary endothelial injury (27–31, 33). Changes compatible with pulmonary edema and adult respiratory distress syndrome have been described with large-dose intravenous administration of TNF to rats. Thrombosis of small and medium-sized pulmonary blood vessels occurs, and wet lung weight ratios are increased with time. There are increases in pulmonary vascular permeability and vasoconstriction, probably mediated through platelet activating factor and thromboxane.

ANIMAL STUDIES (35)

As previously described, there is evidence for the potential efficacy of TNF when it can be administered to tumors in high concentrations in conjunction with IFN-gamma and melphalan in isolated limb perfusions for extremity melanomas or sarcomas (34). At the NCI/National Institute of Health, ILP has been investigated using naturally occurring cytokines—IFN and TNF. Large-animal experiments were performed to attempt to familiarize the perfusion team with the isolated lung circuit and to attempt to define the tolerance of normal lung to high-dose TNF doses, with and without hyperthermia. Pigs were chosen because of the similarities to the human in cardiac physiology and anatomic positioning of the great vessels, including the pulmonary veins and coronary arteries.

Technique

The animal was positioned and the skin prepared for a left thoracotomy after placing a Swan-Ganz catheter via the jugular approach, along with a carotid arterial line. On entering the chest, the Swan-Ganz catheter was manipulated so that the tip was in the right pulmonary artery. The left hemizygous vein was divided and ligated, and the left pulmonary artery, superior and inferior pulmonary veins, and left mainstem bronchus were isolated and encircled with tapes. The animal was then systemically heparinized, and purse-string sutures were placed in the pulmonary artery and the left atrium at the confluence of the pulmonary veins. An angled Satinsky clamp was placed on the atrial side of the venous purse-string, and a DLP 12-mm metal angled cannula (DLP Inc., Grand Rapids, MI) was placed in the excluded atrial pouch and connected to the circuit. A small Satinsky clamp was placed on the proximal pulmonary artery, and a second DLP 12-mm metal angled cannula was placed through the arterial purse-string and connected to the pump circuit.

The perfusion circuit consisted of a roller pump (Sarns 3M Health Care, Ann Arbor, MI), an oxygenator-reservoir (SciMed, Minneapolis, MN), a heat exchanger, and a blood filter. The circuit was primed with a 1-L volume of dextrose and saline. Perfusion was performed via the left pulmonary artery, with gravity drainage through the excluded left atrium. The tape around the left bronchus was tightened to occlude bronchial flow but not to collapse the left lung. Perfusion was maintained at flow rates of 200 to 400 mL/min. Once the perfusion was stable, hemodynamic parameters were obtained, and a baseline lung biopsy was performed, the TNF was delivered directly into the circuit as a bolus. The perfusion with TNF was continued for 60 to 90 minutes. Selected animals had hyperthermic (40°C) perfusion. Blood (10 mL) was sampled from the systemic and perfusion circuit at 15-minute intervals, and arterial blood gas measurements were determined. At the end of the perfusion, the circuit was flushed with 1,000 mL of dextran-crystalloid solution over a 10-minute period, followed by removal of the cannulae. The Satinsky clamps were removed, the cannulation sites were checked for hemostasis, and the chest was closed in layers. A chest x-ray was performed and the animal was allowed to recuperate. Animals were observed for evidence of fever, respiratory distress, or acute toxicity. Once animals were afebrile and eating normally, they were followed at a remote facility for 6 months, after which they were sacrificed and autopsies performed.

Results of Large Animal TNF-ILP

ILP was associated with a mild increase in pulmonary artery pressure, a decrease in cardiac output, an increase in heart rate, and no significant changes in the systemic arterial pressure (Fig. 5). Before, during, and after the perfusion, arterial oxygen saturations were always 100%, with pO2 levels >300 torr.

Systemic TNF levels (Fig. 6) during the perfusion period, as well as the concentration of TNF used in the pulmonary perfusion, correlated with the subsequent development of immediate life-threatening complications. Animals having the highest leak rates (those receiving 80 µg/kg) had the highest systemic levels (285 and 758 ng/mL). A single 80-µg/kg survivor had a peak level of 13 ng/mL. The mean peak TNF level for the five animals receiving 40 µg/kg TNF was 17±10 ng/mL.

The TNF concentration in the 40-µg/kg perfusion circuit ranged from 3.5 to 5.5 µg/mL; it was 10.1 to 13.6 µg/mL in the 80-µg/kg group (Fig. 7). The washout significantly reduced the TNF levels in the perfusate; however, in one of the 40-µg/kg animals with hyperthermia, the washout level just before releasing the pulmonary veins was 211 ng/mL. This animal exhibited signs of car-

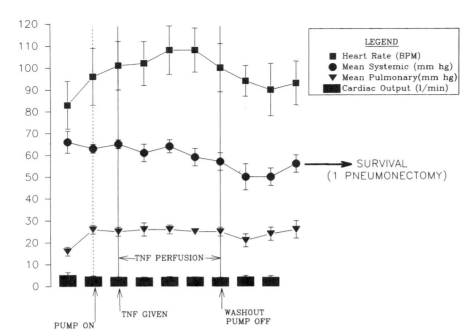

FIG. 5. Hemodynamic changes with TNF-ILP in swine. (With permission from Pogrebniak HW, Witt CJ, Terrill R, et al. Isolated lung perfusion with tumor necrosis factor: a swine model in preparation of human trials. *Ann Thorac Surg* 1994;57:1477–1483.)

diotoxicity that improved only after pneumonectomy. Because the systemic TNF levels measured shortly after the washout in this animal were low (12 ng/mL), we hypothesize that the cardiotoxicity may have been due to high local TNF levels until the lung was removed.

Immediately after ILP, mild pulmonary congestion was seen on the perfused side. This cleared rapidly; the appearance of both hemithoraces was equivalent by 1 week after operation. More severe immediate changes were appreciated in the animals receiving moderate hyperthermia; nevertheless, the congestion was gone within a week. Acutely, animals receiving 40 μg/kg TNF

with hyperthermia had mild subpleural and peribronchial edema along with neutrophilic infiltration during the ILP. No long-term sequelae were seen, as the histologic and roentgenographic pictures of the perfused and nonperfused lungs were identical at elective sacrifice. There was no evidence of focal fibrosis in the perfused, heated lung.

No short- or long-term sequelae were seen clinically in the animals who survived ILP-TNF. All gained weight after the initial operative insult, and there were no aberrations in the clinical chemistries or hematologic values compared to sham perfused animals.

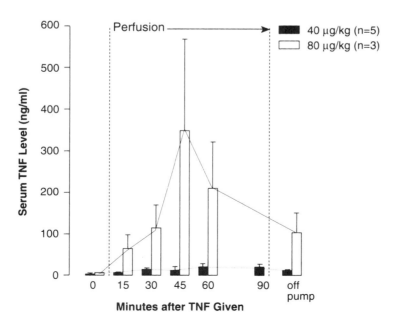

FIG. 6. Low systemic TNF levels during TNF-ILP indicate the absence of significant leak from the circuit. (With permission from Pogrebniak HW, Witt CJ, Terrill R, et al. Isolated lung perfusion with tumor necrosis factor: a swine model in preparation of human trials. *Ann Thorac Surg* 1994;57:1477–1483.)

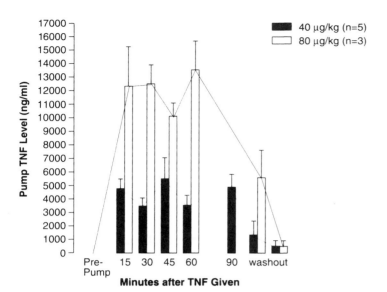

FIG. 7. Persistently high levels of TNF were recorded in the perfusate in the swine receiving TNF-ILP. (With permission from Pogrebniak HW, Witt CJ, Terrill R, et al. Isolated lung perfusion with tumor necrosis factor: a swine model in preparation of human trials. *Ann Thorac Surg* 1994;57:1477–1483.)

Observations from the Animal Studies

The method of perfusion, using standard cardiopulmonary bypass equipment and cannulae, lends itself readily to human trials. No animal model can precisely define the human tolerance to any drug. The goal of these experiments, however, was to pinpoint potentially life-threatening problems if ILP-TNF were used in humans. When there was incomplete isolation, either during the perfusion or at its completion, severe systemic toxicity led to life-threatening complications. This may be related to the peak TNF levels achieved during the perfusion, or to a level that leads to toxicity due to chronic exposure by sensitive organs. Conversely, if the leak from the perfusion circuit is controlled, humans may be able to tolerate >80 μg/kg.

TNF may be releasing other cytokines, vasoactive peptides, oxygen free radicals, or nitric oxide that potentiates the hemodynamic instability. The life-threatening complications seen acutely in the higher-dose animals were probably related to a significant leak of TNF into the systemic circuit during the perfusion. Acutely, however, at the end of the perfusion, acute cardiac injury was appreciated. Recently TNF and other inflammatory cytokines (eg, IL-6) have been implicated as mediators of "stunned myocardium" (36,37). These mediators, which cause negative inotropic effects, may do so by enhancing nitric oxide formation.

The conclusion is that human trials must include a mechanism for monitoring the quantity of leak from the pulmonary to the systemic circuit after isolation of the lung, and appropriate measures must be taken to minimize such a leak or abort the procedure. Due to the synergistic effects of TNF and hyperthermia (38), and the reported effects on endothelial cells of this combination, a human trial could incorporate both aspects of treatment if no untoward increase in toxicity was noted. Combined toxicity of the regimen, however, has been suggested in the literature (39).

HUMAN STUDIES OF TNF-ILP

Population

The initial use of this therapy in an ongoing, dose-escalating phase I trial has been limited to patients who have isolated pulmonary disease and are in relatively good functional class. The ideal population has been young patients with pulmonary metastases from soft-tissue or osteogenic sarcomas, or epithelial neoplasms metastatic solely to the lung. Patients with bronchoalveolar carcinoma with multicentricity could potentially avoid repeated pulmonary resection, with loss of lung function, if their tumor was responsive. A phase I trial was initiated to define the feasibility and safety of ILP with TNF-α (Knoll Pharmaceuticals), IFN-gamma, and moderate hyperthermia for patients with unresectable pulmonary metastases. Nineteen patients with lung metastases (Ewing's, 2; sarcoma, 7; melanoma, 6; other, 4) were considered for ILP.

Technique

Patients are primed with IFN before the resection, and a Swan-Ganz catheter is placed in the pulmonary artery contralateral to the ILP. Patients receive 1 g cefazolin (Ancef) or other appropriate antibiotics in the operating room before the skin incision. The incision used is either a standard posterolateral thoracotomy or median sternotomy. Once the chest is opened, the Swan-Ganz catheter is confirmed by palpation to be in the opposite

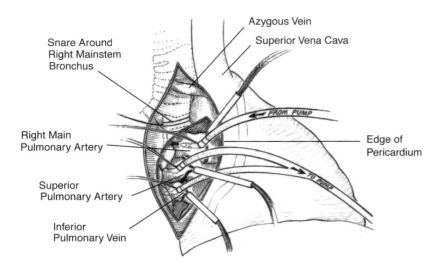

FIG. 8. Cannulation technique for a right-sided human ILP.

lung to the tumor, or the catheter is manipulated into that position. The pericardium is opened and a pericardial well constructed. The main pulmonary artery to the lung with the unresectable tumor is dissected free such that it can be encircled with a vascular tape. A purse-string is placed in the pulmonary artery. The superior and inferior pulmonary veins are isolated intra- or extrapericardially. If there is involvement of the pulmonary artery or either pulmonary vein with tumor such that purse-string sutures cannot be safely placed toward the lung side, or the atrial side of the veins cannot be clamped with the appropriate vascular clamp or Rommel tourniquet for pulmonary systemic isolation, the case is terminated. An alternate technique for hemithorax vein isolation entails the placement of a purse-string suture in the left atrial

appendage and the placement of a large Satinsky clamp across the atrium, dividing the right and left lung venous return.

The patient is systemically heparinized with 200 U/kg heparin. An appropriately sized arterial cannula is then placed in the isolated pulmonary artery and secured to the extracorporeal circuit. The superior and inferior pulmonary veins are then cannulated, either individually or via a left atrial vent in the excluded atrial segment, and secured to the extracorporeal circuit to drain into the venous reservoir (Figs. 8 and 9). Temperature probes are secured to the lung. ILP then proceeds for 90 minutes. After the perfusion, the pulmonary veins are released by removing the Rommel clamps or Satinsky clamp, and the venous cannula is removed, with tying of the purse-strings. The pulmonary artery cannula is removed, air is removed from the pulmonary artery, and the purse-string is tied. The proximal Rommel or occluding clamp on the pulmonary artery is then released.

The Isolated Perfusion Circuit

The extracorporeal circuit consists of a roller pump, membrane oxygenator, and heat exchanger, analogous to the extracorporeal circuit used in cardiac procedures (Fig. 10). The initial perfusate is a balanced salt solution (1,000 mL) prime. Flow rates are determined by the perfusion pressure, which is kept at levels compatible with physiologic pulmonary artery pressures (<20 mm Hg). Perfusate is initially heated to 42°C using a Hematherm cooler/heater (Model #400, Cincinnati SubZero Products, Cincinnati, OH). Lung temperature is monitored by 22-gauge thermistor probes placed into the lung parenchyma. The target tissue temperature for the perfusion is 38° to 39.5°C. After establishing a stable baseline, 400 µCi of I^{131} human albumin is injected into the perfusion circuit. An aliquot of blood (2 cc) from the circuit is

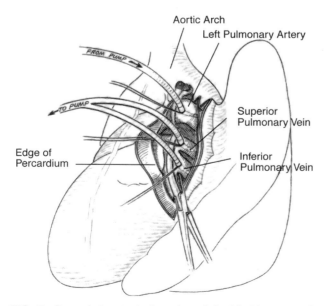

FIG. 9. Cannulation technique for a left-sided human ILP.

removed and counted in a gamma counter for 1 minute; at the same time, 2 cc of blood is removed from the systemic circulation from the arterial line (Fig. 11). The ratio of counts represents a first-order approximation of the leak rate. This leak is monitored for 10 minutes. If there is >1% leak over 10 minutes, adjustments are made to identify the source of the leak before administering TNF. This ensures that for a 90-minute TNF perfusion, no more than 10% of the total drug dose will leak into the systemic circulation. When the leak rate is <1% for 10 minutes, the TNF and IFN-gamma are injected into the perfusate circuit. The leak rate is monitored for the duration of the perfusion; if the cumulative leak is >10%, the perfusion is halted and the perfusate flushed from the circuit. Blood samples are taken from the systemic circulation and the perfusion circuit at 0, 10, 30, 60, and 90 minutes after isotope injection. Serum is counted in a gamma counter to verify the accuracy of the leak-monitoring equipment. After TNF and IFN-gamma are injected into the perfusate circuit, the perfusion is continued for 90 minutes. The perfusion is then halted and the perfusate flushed from the circuit. The serum is analyzed for cytokine and possibly nitrate levels.

Conduct of the Human TNF-ILP Trial

Patients receive 0.2 mg of recombinant IFN-gamma subcutaneously on each of the 2 days before the operation. The dose of IFN given during ILP is 0.2 mg. The dose of TNF is escalated after every third patient, according to our protocol. After ILP is established and the tissue

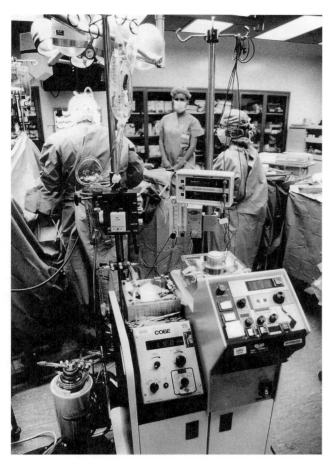

FIG. 10. Extracorporeal circuit using two pump heads (one used as a suction return back to the circuit), oxygenator, lung temperature monitoring, and gas-mix valves.

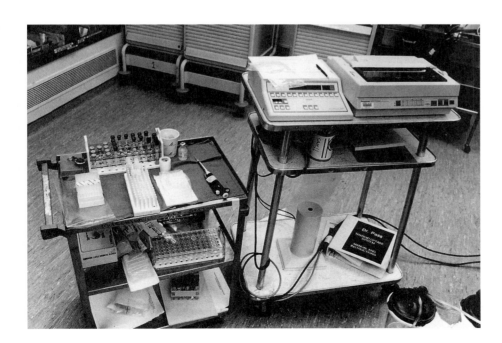

FIG. 11. Well-scintillation gamma counter used in the operating room to calculate TNF leakage from the circuit.

temperature has reached 38°C, the IFN and TNF are given as slow injections into the pulmonary arterial line over a period of one complete circulation of the perfusate to allow adequate mixing. Perfusion with IFN-gamma and TNF continues for 90 minutes. At 5, 15, 30, 60, and 90 minutes after TNF and IFN-gamma infusion, samples are taken from the venous return reservoir and from the systemic circulation to assay for TNF and IFN-gamma levels. The lung temperature, as measured by the thermistor probes, is kept between 38° and 39.5°C during the perfusion. After 90 minutes of perfusion, the lung is flushed with 2 L of saline and 1 L of albumin solution. Samples during the washout period are taken from the venous return line to assess whether the volume of washout is adequate. The cannulae are removed and the vessels closed.

Postoperative Care

Patients are monitored in an intensive care unit to evaluate for evidence of systemic toxicity due to TNF and to recover from this major thoracic surgery. Lung function and blood chemistries are followed closely during the postoperative period. Volume, dopamine, and possibly phenylephrine (Neo-Synephrine) are used to treat hypotension after the TNF lung perfusion. Pulmonary complications such as pulmonary edema and the adult respiratory distress syndrome are treated with standard intensive care techniques, including positive-pressure ventilation, positive end-expiratory pressure, and high FIO_2, as needed.

Results

Flow rates of 300 to 1,200 cc/min, with temperatures of 37° to 45.3°C, have been obtained. When the pulmonary to systemic leak (measured using I^{131} albumin) was <10% (as described above), 0.3 to 6.0 mg TNF and 0.2 mg IFN were delivered in the oxygenated pump circuit. Of 20 explorations thus far, 15 perfusions were performed in 14 patients (one was bilateral). Metastases were completely resected (no ILP) in 3 patients, 1 patient had extrapulmonic disease, and 1 ILP was aborted for mechanical reasons. Ten of the 15 patients had 0% leak. There were no significant changes in systemic arterial blood pressure or cardiac output during perfusion. Systolic pulmonary artery pressure increased from 32±2 to 44±4 mm Hg with isolation and returned to pre-ILP levels (35±3 mm Hg) after clamp release. The maximal systemic TNF level was 3 ng/mL; pump circuit TNF levels ranged from 200 to 5,200 ng/mL. There were no deaths, and the mean hospitalization was 9 days (range 5 to 34 days). A short-term (5- to 6-month) unilateral decrease in ILP nodules was noted in 3 patients (melanoma, 1; ade-

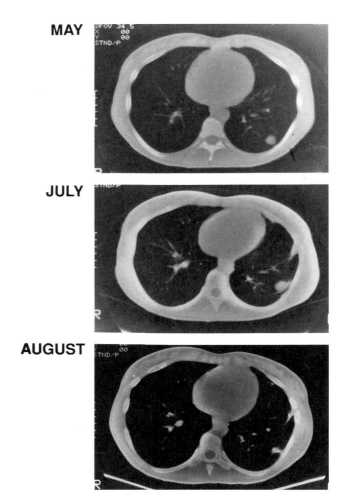

FIG. 12. Computed tomograms of left lower lobe melanoma nodule before TNF-ILP (May), 1 month after ILP (July), and 2 months after ILP (August). The nodule regressed completely and did not recur.

noid cystic carcinoma, 1; renal cell carcinoma, 1) (Fig. 12).

This phase I trial demonstrates that techniques are available for safe single-lung ILP in selected patients, but the agent of choice is unknown and may depend on histology.

FUTURE DEVELOPMENTS

With the aim of expanding the utility of TNF or other cytokines in ILP, future studies must concentrate on techniques to perfuse both lungs simultaneously and safely, as well as the development of antidotes that would have an immediate action after the cytokine septic cascade occurs in case of systemic leak. Candidates for such agents include neutralizing antibodies to the cytokines, receptor antagonists, and compounds that counteract the hypotensive and vasodilatory effects of generated nitric oxide.

REFERENCES

1. Pass HI. Management of metastatic disease to the lung. In: DeVita V, Hellman S, Rosenberg S, eds. *Cancer: principles and practice of oncology.* Philadelphia: JB Lippincott, 1992:2186.

2. Jablons D, Steinberg SM, Roth J, Pittaluga S, Rosenberg SA, Pass HI. Metastasectomy for soft tissue sarcoma. *J Thorac Cardiovasc Surg* 1989;97:695–705.

3. Cudlowica C, Armstrong JR. The blood supply of malignant pulmonary neoplasms. *Thorax Lund* 1951;8:152–155.

4. Wood DA, Miller M. Role of the dual pulmonary circulation in various pathologic conditions of the lungs. *J Thorac Surg* 1938;7:649–656.

5. Miller BJ, Rosenbaum AS. The vascular supply to metastatic tumors of the lung. *Surg Gynecol Obstet* 1967;1009–1115.

6. Pierpont H, Blades B. Lung perfusion with chemotherapeutic agents. *J Thorac Cardiovasc Surg* 1960;39:159–165.

7. Jacobs JK, Flexner JM, Scott HW Jr. Selective isolated perfusion of the right lung. *J Thorac Cardiovasc Surg* 1961;42:546–552.

8. Johnston MR, Minchin R, Shull JH, et al. Isolated lung perfusion with Adriamycin. A preclinical study. *Cancer* 1983;52:404–409.

9. Johnston MR, Christensen CW, Minchin RF, et al. Isolated total lung perfusion as a means to deliver organ-specific chemotherapy: long-term studies in animals. *Surgery* 1985;98:35–44.

10. Rickaby DA, Fehring JF, Johnston MR, Dawson CA. Tolerance of the isolated perfused lung to hyperthermia. *J Thorac Cardiovasc Surg* 1991;101:732–739.

11. Baciewicz FA, Arredondo M, Chaudhuri B, et al. Pharmacokinetics and toxicity of isolated perfusion of lung with doxorubicin. *J Surg Res* 1991;50:124–128.

12. Weksler B, Schneider A, Ng B, Burt M. Isolated single lung perfusion in the rat: an experimental model. *J Appl Physiol* 1993;74:2736–2739.

13. Weksler B, Lenert J, Ng B, Burt M. Isolated single lung perfusion with doxorubicin is effective in eradicating soft tissue sarcoma lung metastases in a rat model. *J Thorac Cardiovasc Surg* 1994;107:50–54.

14. Weksler B, Blumberg D, Lenert JT, Ng B, Fong Y, Burt ME. Isolated single-lung perfusion with TNF-alpha in a rat sarcoma lung metastases model. *Ann Thorac Surg* 1994;58:328–331.

15. Ng B, Lenert JT, Weksler B, Port JL, Ellis JL, Burt ME. Isolated lung perfusion with FUDR is an effective treatment for colorectal adenocarcinoma lung metastases in rats. *Ann Thorac Surg* 1995;59:205–208.

16. Ratto GB, Esposito M, Leprini A, et al. In situ lung perfusion with cisplatin. An experimental study. *Cancer* 1993;71:2962–2970.

17. Ratto BG, Tassara E, Fantino G, et al. A new approach in the treatment of lung metastases. *Lung Cancer* 1994;11:164.

18. Carswell EA, Old LJ, Kassel RL, Green S, Fiore N, Williamson B. An endotoxin-induced serum factor that causes necrosis of tumors. *Proc Natl Acad Sci USA* 1975;72:3666–3670.

19. Asher A, Mulé JJ, Reichert CM, Shiloni A, Rosenberg SA. Studies on the anti-tumor efficacy of systemically administered recombinant tumor necrosis factor against several murine tumors in vivo. *J Immunol* 1987;138:963–974.

20. Alexander RB, Rosenberg SA. Tumor necrosis factor: clinical applications. In: DeVita VT, Hellman S, Rosenberg SA, eds. *Biologic therapy of cancer.* Philadelphia: JB Lippincott, 1991:378.

21. Lienard D, Lejeune F, Delmotte J, et al. High doses of rTNFα in combination with IFN-gamma and melphalan in isolation perfusion of the limbs for melanoma and sarcoma. *J Clin Oncol* 1992;10:52–60.

22. Lienard D, Lejeune F, Evvalenko I. In transit metastases of malignant melanoma treated by high dose rTNFα in combination with interferon-gamma and melphalan in isolation perfusion. *World J Surg* 1992;16:234–240.

23. Eggermont AMM, Koops HS, Lienard D, et al. Limb salvage by isolated limb perfusion (ILP) with high-dose tumor necrosis factor-alpha (TNF) gamma-interferon(IFN) and melphalan in patients with irresectable soft tissue sarcomas. *J Clin Oncol* 1996;14:2653–2665.

24. Aggarwal BB, Eessalu TE, Hass PE. Characterization of receptors for tumor necrosis factor and their regulation by gamma-interferon. *Nature* 1985;318:665–667.

25. Wedgwood JF, Hatam L, Benagora VR. Effect of interferon-gamma and tumor necrosis factor on the expression of Class I and Class II major histocompatibility molecules by cultured human umbilical vein endothelial cells. *Cell Immunol* 1988;111:1–9.

26. Niitsu Y, Watanabe N, Umeno H, et al . Synergistic effects of recombinant human tumor necrosis factor and hyperthermia on in vitro cytotoxicity and artificial metastases. *Cancer Res* 1988;48:654–657.

27. Lo SK, Everitt J, Gu J, Malik AB. Tumor necrosis factor mediates experimental pulmonary edema by ICAM-1 and CD18-dependent mechanisms. *J Clin Invest* 1992;89:981–988.

28. Dawson CA, Christensen CW, Rickaby DA, Linehan JH, Johnston MR. Lung damage and pulmonary uptake of serotonin in intact dogs. *J Appl Physiol* 1985;58:1761–1766.

29. Hocking DC, Phillips PG, Ferro TJ, Johnson A. Mechanisms of pulmonary edema induced by tumor necrosis factor-α. *Circ Res* 1990;67:68–77.

30. Meyrick B, Christman B, Jesmok G. Effects of recombinant tumor necrosis factor-alpha on cultured pulmonary artery and lung microvascular endothelial monolayers. *Am J Pathol* 1991;138:93–101.

31. Fuchs HJ, Debs R, Patton JS, Liggitt HD. The pattern of lung injury induced after pulmonary exposure to tumor necrosis factor-α depends on the route of administration. *Diagn Microbiol Infect Dis* 1990;13:397–404.

32. Johnson J, Meyrick B, Jesmok G, Brigham KL. Human recombinant tumor necrosis factor alpha infusion mimics endotoxemia in awake sheep. *J Appl Physiol* 1989;66:1448–1454.

33. Yang SC, Owen-Schaub L, Mendiguren-Rodriguez A, Grimm EA, Hong WK, Roth JA. Combination immunotherapy for non-small cell lung cancer. *J Thorac Cardiovasc Surg* 1990;99:8–13.

34. Lienard D, Ewalenko P, Delmotti JJ, Renard N, Lejeune FJ. High-dose recombinant tumor necrosis factor alpha in combination with interferon gamma and melphalan in isolation perfusion of the limbs for melanoma and sarcoma. *J Clin Oncol* 1992;10:52–60.

35. Pogrebniak HW, Witt CJ, Terrill R, et al. Isolated lung perfusion with tumor necrosis factor: a swine model in preparation of human trials. *Ann Thorac Surg* 1994;57:1477–1483.

36. Finkel MS, Hoffman RA, Shen L, Oddis CV, Simmons RL, Hattler BG. Interleukin-6 (IL-6) as a mediator of stunned myocardium. *Am J Cardiol* 1993;71:1231–1232.

37. Finkel MS, Oddis CV, Jacob TD, Watkins SC, Hattler BG, Simmons RL. Negative inotropic effects of cytokines on the heart mediated by nitric oxide. *Science* 1992;256:387–389.

38. Hirako M, Li YP, Tsutsui K, Abe M, Miyachi Y. Effects of tumor necrosis factor and hyperthermia on Meth-A tumors. *Jpn J Cancer Res* 1991;82:1171–1174.

39. van den Aardweg GMJM, van der Zee J, van Rhoon GC, de Wit R. Thermal enhancement of TNF-α induced systemic toxicity in tumor bearing animals. *Proc AACR* 1993;34:457.

Manufacturers of Specialized ILP Equipment
Cobe Cardiovascular, Arvada, CA (perfusion pump)
Biodex Medical Systems, Shirley, NY (Atomlab 900 medical spectrometer)
Knoll Pharmaceuticals, Whippany, NJ (tumor necrosis factor)
DLP, Grand Rapids, MI (cannulae)
Baxter Bentley, Irvine, CA (perfusion packs)

CHAPTER 7

Imaging Liver Neoplasms

Richard L. Baron

"Nature is often hidden; sometimes overcome; seldom extinguished."

—Francis Bacon (1561–1626)
Essays, "Of Nature in Men"

Because of the high propensity for metastases to occur in the liver, as well as the high incidence of primary liver neoplasms in certain populations and risk conditions, imaging of the liver is an important aspect of the treatment of patients with neoplastic disease. The focus of this chapter is to review the appearances of liver neoplasms on computed tomography (CT), magnetic resonance imaging (MRI), and ultrasound, detailing relative accuracies and roles of these imaging techniques. A greater emphasis is placed on describing CT of the liver because CT is the imaging modality with widest general use in imaging the oncology patient. There is a particular emphasis on understanding appropriate imaging techniques that allow physicians treating liver oncology patients to appreciate the subtle differences that may exist between tumors and normal liver parenchyma in various clinical settings, as well as the limitations of each imaging method.

HISTORICAL CONTEXT

Before the modern computer era, the diagnosis of liver neoplasms was not possible to any clinically useful extent with imaging techniques. With the advent of new technologies, the ability to image the liver and detect neoplasms has dramatically increased over the past 20 years. Initially, the first clinical tool to image the liver for neoplasia was nuclear scintigraphy, using sulfur colloid agents taken up by normal reticuloendothelial structures in the liver. Neoplasms of significant size (generally greater than 2 cm) could often be appreciated as a hypo-

intense focus. The advent of cross-sectional tomographic imaging with ultrasound, CT, and MRI rapidly replaced scintigraphy as the screening method of choice for detecting liver neoplasms because of their ability to detect smaller neoplasms, avoid false-positive results, and provide better anatomic delineation. Comparative studies in the 1970s and early 1980s lacked good pathologic correlation and relied on intraoperative surgical palpation or follow-up imaging for confirmation or exclusion of lesions, both techniques having large numbers of false-positive and false-negative results. Comparison of numerous studies comparing imaging techniques is also problematic because of wide variations in quality of imaging equipment and techniques. Nonetheless, it quickly became clear that these newer modalities had higher accuracies in evaluating the liver for neoplastic disease (1,2). Although at one time hepatic scintigraphy was the most used method of detecting liver neoplasms, the advent of ultrasound, CT, and MRI has virtually eliminated the role of conventional nuclear medicine techniques for detecting liver tumors. It is not possible to compare the accuracies of older studies with poor pathologic correlation (and usually reporting higher tumor detection sensitivities) with more recent studies correlating with sectioned livers after hepatectomies (and detecting small lesions missed by the prior standards of surgical palpation). Nonetheless, for each study, the relative accuracies of each modality can be assessed and are presented throughout this chapter. Tables 1 and 2 present comparative data on sensitivities of imaging modalities for detecting patients with liver neoplastic disease (Table 1) and detecting the specific number of liver neoplastic lesions (Table 2) from multiple large studies. It can be seen in these tables that tumor detection sensitivity has been decreasing over the past decade despite the improved imaging technology and better understanding of contrast use, which would be expected to improve tumor detection. This discrepancy is due to the fact that the earlier studies used a poor standard, that of clinical and

R. L. Baron: Department of Radiology, University of Pittsburgh School of Medicine, Pittsburgh, Pennsylvania 15213-2582.

TABLE 1. *Sensitivity of imaging methods for detecting patients with neoplastic liver disease*

Study	Standard	US	CT	MR
Alderson et al, 1983 (1)	Imaging follow-up	82%	93%	NA
Stark et al., 1987 (3)	Imaging follow-up	NA	80%	82%
Chezmar et al., 1988 (4)	Imaging follow-up	NA	93%	96%
Vassiliades et al., 1991 (5)	Imaging follow-up	NA	89%	86%

US, ultrasound; CT, contrast-enhanced computed tomography; MR, magnetic resonance; NA, not applicable.

imaging follow-up or surgical palpation, whereas the more recent studies used resected liver specimens with serial sectioning as the standard (3–13).

IMAGING MODALITIES

Computed Tomography

The ability of CT to demonstrate liver neoplasms depends on tumors having a different CT attenuation from that of the normal liver. Although in some cases inherent differences in density exist between normal liver and tumors that allow visualization of tumors on non–contrast-enhanced CT, more often there is a lack of inherent tissue contrast, requiring the use of exogenous contrast material for adequate tumor detection. When using standard iodinated intravenous contrast agents, there are a number of ways to administer the contrast coupled with numerous CT scan techniques. The ability to visualize liver tumors with CT can change dramatically depending on the techniques chosen. Further complicating these issues is the fact that capabilities of CT scanners vary, particularly in time requirements to obtain images,

which, when using contrast, can also dramatically affect the ability to demonstrate liver tumors.

CT Contrast Techniques

The ability of liver CT to demonstrate hepatic tumors is both benefited and confounded by the dual blood supply to the liver. The liver is different from most abdominal organs in its dual blood supply, with the hepatic artery normally delivering 20% to 30% of blood flow and the portal vein 70% to 80% (14,15). In contrast, most liver neoplasms for functional purposes have only a hepatic arterial blood supply and receive little or no flow from the portal vein. By selectively providing contrast flow to either the hepatic artery or the portal vein, detection of hypervascular or hypovascular tumors can be optimized (16). Truly selective contrast delivery requires patients first to undergo angiographic placement of a catheter into the appropriate arterial source. These invasive techniques, as is described later, achieve the highest tumor detection rates because of this ability selectively to deliver contrast, but because they are invasive tests, they are typically reserved for patients being evaluated for potential surgical resection.

Intravenous Contrast-Enhanced CT

It is now well accepted that optimal CT detection of liver neoplasms requires the use of intravenous iodinated contrast agents using a rapid, sustained infusion of contrast, best delivered with a mechanical power injector (17, 18). The advent of electron beam CT and helical CT, able to scan the entire liver in 20 to 30 seconds, has dramatically affected the ability of CT to maximize information from contrast CT. These fast scanners can scan the entire liver during the two early and fleeting phases of enhancement after intravenous administration of contrast (16). The first phase, the arterial phase, occurs 20 to 30 sec-

TABLE 2. *Sensitivity of imaging methods for detecting liver neoplasms (sensitivity for predicting specific number of lesions)*

Study	Standard	US	IOUS	CT	MR	CTAP
Stark et al., 1987 (3)	Imaging follow-up	NA	NA	51%	64%	NA
Nelson et al., 1989 (6)	Liver sectioning	NA	NA	NA	67%	87%
Heiken et al., 1989 (7)	Liver sectioning	NA	NA	NA	57%	81%
Vassiliades et al., 1991 (5)	Imaging follow-up	NA	NA	71%	78%	NA
Soyer et al., 1992 (9)	Liver sectioning	NA	96%	NA	NA	91%
Soyer et al., 1994 (10)	Liver sectioning	NA	NA	NA	NA	87%
Soyer et al., 1994 (11)	Liver sectioning	NA	NA	NA	NA	94%[a]
Leen et al., 1995 (8)	Surgical palpation	48%	NA	80%	NA	NA
Hagspiel et al., 1995 (12)	Liver sectioning	39%	80%	41%	44%	NA
Kuszyk et al., 1996 (13)	Surgical palpation	NA	NA	81%[a]	NA	NA

[a]Helical computed tomography technology.
US, ultrasound; IOUS, intraoperative ultrasound; CT, contrast-enhanced computed tomography; MR, magnetic resonance; CTAP, computed tomography-arterial portography; NA, not applicable.

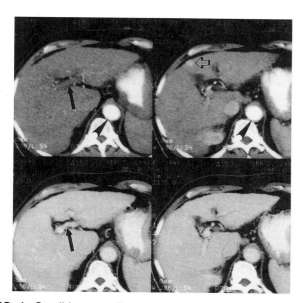

FIG. 1. Small hepatocellular carcinoma in a patient with cirrhosis. Arterial-phase images *(top two images)* demonstrate typical findings during the arterial phase of contrast enhancement. The aorta *(arrowheads)* is densely opacified, whereas the portal vein *(arrow)* is not significantly enhanced. The hepatocellular carcinoma nodule *(open arrow)* is densely enhancing during the arterial phase against the minimal enhancement of liver parenchyma. The portal venous phase images *(bottom two images)*, obtained 30 seconds later at the same levels as the arterial-phase images, show marked enhancement of the portal vein *(arrow)* as well as liver parenchyma. The tumor nodule is no longer detectable because the liver and nodule are enhanced to the same degree. (Reproduced with permission from Baron RL. Understanding and optimizing use of contrast material for CT of the liver. *AJR Am J Roentgenol* 1994;163:323.)

results in obscuration of some hypervascular masses that may have been well seen earlier, during the arterial phase. Fibrosis or necrosis within hypovascular lesions further aids in making these lesions appear hypodense compared with the enhanced liver parenchyma. Some helical CT scanners have the ability to scan during both the arterial and portal venous phases of contrast enhancement, and this approach has been shown to increase the detection of highly vascular metastases (19) and hepatocellular carcinoma (20,21). These studies have shown that the addition of arterial-phase imaging to more conventional portal venous-phase imaging detects approximately 40% more hepatocellular carcinoma nodules and is the only technique to detect tumor in 8% to 10% of such patients (21). Although very helpful in detecting hypervascular neoplastic foci in the liver, as seen with hepatocellular carcinoma and metastases from hypervascular tumors such as renal cell carcinoma and neuroendocrine tumors, in most other situations CT scanning is useful only during the portal venous phase of enhancement because hypovascular liver metastases (from, eg, colon, pancreas, lung) are optimally visualized during the portal venous phase, with little, if any incremental detection gained by adding arterial-phase imaging. The optimal contrast technique for CT detection of breast carcinoma metastases in the liver remains uncertain. Most such lesions are well seen on portal venous-phase imaging, but in a small percentage of cases metastases may be seen only on arterial-phase imaging (see Fig. 2).

Some controversy has existed over the optimal contrast administration rates, contrast volumes, and time required before initiating CT scanning after contrast infusion for optimal detection of liver neoplasms (22). Although some centers are reducing the volume of contrast material used, particularly when using high-cost, low-osmolarity agents, in general it is agreed that 150 to 180 mL of a 60% concentration agent is required to optimize liver enhancement (23–26); this should optimize tumor detection in all but very thin patients (27). It also is accepted that imaging should be completed before the onset of equilibrium, at which time even hypovascular tumors may become isodense with liver parenchyma. The time to the onset of equilibrium varies with the rate and dose of contrast administration, but with current accepted protocols (150 to 180 mL at 2 to 5 mL/second), equilibrium can occur as early as 100 seconds after administration (28), so scanning must be completed in a timely fashion. Several reports have shown that imaging the liver during the mid-to-late equilibrium phase of enhancement can obscure many lesions such that unenhanced CT will have a higher sensitivity for detecting tumors (17,29).

Liver Cysts and Cavernous Hemangiomas

The appearance of certain lesions on contrast-enhanced CT can be characteristic in some instances,

onds after initiating contrast infusion (depending on the rate of contrast administration), and reflects the time when the contrast material first reaches the hepatic artery in significant concentrations. At this time, the portal venous system carries unenhanced blood because of the longer circulation time required to deliver the contrast through the spleen or mesentery. This period of delivering predominantly enhanced arterial flow and unenhanced portal venous flow results in little or no enhancement of liver parenchyma (Figs. 1 and 2), but provides an excellent opportunity to visualize enhancing hypervascular neoplasms such as hepatocellular carcinoma (see Fig. 1) and vascular metastases such as from renal cell carcinoma, neuroendocrine tumors, breast carcinoma (see Fig. 2) and others (16,19). Approximately 25 to 30 seconds later (again, depending on the rate of contrast administration), contrast reaches the portal venous system in large concentrations, with resulting liver parenchymal enhancement; this is termed the portal venous phase. This phase is the optimal period for detecting hypovascular neoplasms (Fig. 3), such as most metastases, and conversely

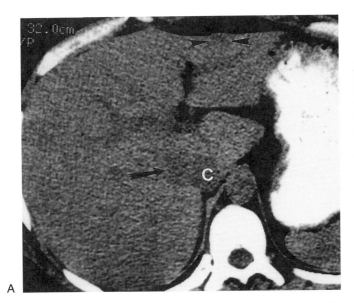

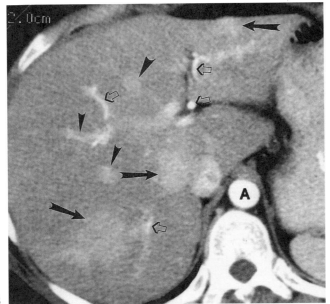

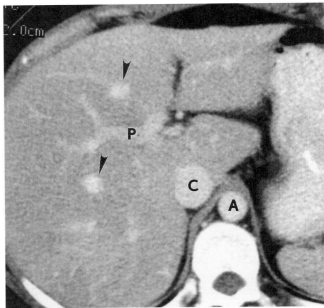

FIG. 2. Liver metastases from breast carcinoma. **A:** Liver metastases are difficult to see on unenhanced CT. One lesion *(arrow)* can be seen adjacent to the inferior vena cava (C) and, in retrospect, a small lesion *(arrowheads)* can be seen in the left lobe. **B:** Intravenous contrast-enhanced CT during the arterial phase shows three lesions *(arrows)* as enhancing masses against a background of minimally enhanced liver parenchyma. Note the dense enhancement of the aorta (A) and hepatic arterial branches *(open arrows)* and only faint enhancement of the portal venous branches *(arrowheads)* and hepatic venous branches *(arrow)*. **C:** CT 30 seconds later during the portal venous phase at the same level as (B) fails to visualize any of the tumor seen during the arterial phase. Note the denser enhancement of the right portal vein (P), hepatic vein branches *(arrowheads)*, and inferior vena cava (C) typical of portal venous-phase contrast images. Also note the lesser enhancement of the aorta (A) compared with the arterial-phase image.

highly suggestive in others, and unfortunately in many instances nonspecific. Liver cysts, when of sufficient size to avoid volume averaging (in general, lesions of 1 cm or more in diameter), have a characteristic CT appearance. These lesions have a homogeneous near-water density (0 to 15 Hounsfield units [HU]), sharp margins with an imperceptible wall, and demonstrate no enhancement after contrast (Fig. 4). Early studies with older CT scanners suggested some liver neoplasms could have a low attenuation similar to cysts (30,31). Although no formal investigation has been undertaken, it is thought that the current fast scanners allowing maximal contrast enhancement and image resolution do not result in an overlap in appearance between necrotic or cystic liver tumors and

benign cysts, with mural irregularity or internal septations being seen in such liver tumors (Figs. 5 and 6). Small benign cysts (<1 cm) remain a problem for CT because volume averaging with adjacent tissues in the CT slice raises the averaged CT density above that of water. In such cases, use of thin (3 mm) CT slices or ultrasound can clarify a lesion as a cyst, but small lesions (<5 mm) are usually too small to characterize with either modality.

Cavernous hemangiomas have a typical appearance when imaged with dynamic contrast CT techniques (Fig. 7). Earlier studies had suggested that CT could accurately characterize only approximately 55% of hemangiomas using the criteria of lesions being hypodense to liver precontrast, showing peripheral nodular contrast enhance-

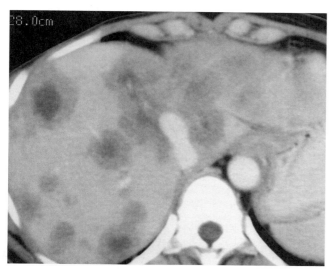

FIG. 3. Metastases to the liver from a leiomyosarcoma. A contrast-enhanced CT scan during the portal venous phase shows a typical hypodense appearance to the lesions compared with surrounding enhanced liver. The central portions of the lesions are less dense due to necrosis.

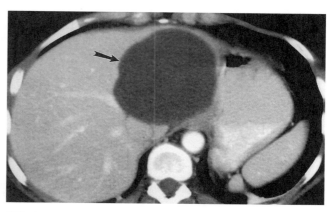

FIG. 4. Hepatic cyst. Contrast-enhanced CT shows the large cyst as a homogeneous, low-attenuation (approximately 0 to 10 HU) mass *(arrow)* with a sharp zone of transition and no perceptible wall or mural irregularity.

ment, and becoming totally isodense with liver on delayed (3 to 30 minutes) contrast images (32,33). More recent studies and experience with faster, higher-resolution equipment have shown that with proper attention to characteristics, approximately 90% of hemangiomas can

be clearly classified as such and not mistaken for malignancy. The key feature that allows for a higher specificity is recognition that hemangioma enhancement is of the same CT density as that of other liver vessels at two to three different imaging times, including precontrast (34, 35). Malignant lesions rarely, if ever, demonstrate this feature (Fig. 8). Small hemangiomas (<1.5 cm) often cannot be differentiated with as high an accuracy, and may be a diagnostic problem for CT when these features cannot be discerned because the lesion too rapidly becomes iso-

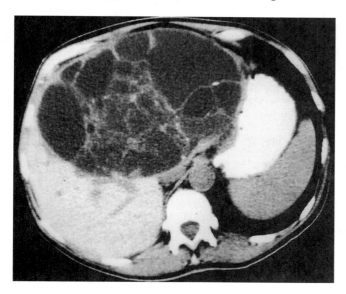

FIG. 5. Biliary cystadenocarcinoma. Unenhanced CT scan shows the malignant mass as having predominantly near-water attenuation, similar to a cyst. However, the presence of numerous septations and a thicker, perceptible wall excludes the diagnosis of simple cyst. (Reproduced with permission from Baron RL, Freeny PC, Moss AA. The liver. In: Moss AA, Gamsu G, Genant HK, eds. *Computed tomography of the body with magnetic resonance imaging.* 2nd ed. Philadelphia: WB Saunders, 1992:781.)

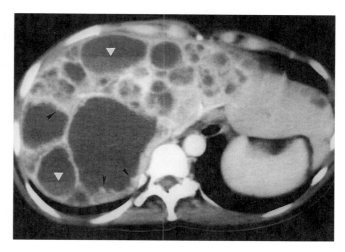

FIG. 6. Cystic islet cell metastases to the liver. Contrast-enhanced CT scan shows numerous low-attenuation lesions of near-water attenuation, simulating simple cysts. However, the mural irregularity *(black arrowheads)* and fluid–fluid levels *(white arrowheads)* in the larger lesions exclude the diagnosis of simple cysts. Further, the smaller lesions show areas of solid tumor that are of intermediate attenuation between that of the cystic tumor portions and surrounding liver parenchyma. (Reproduced with permission from Baron RL, Freeny PC, Moss AA. The liver. In: Moss AA, Gamsu G, Genant HK, eds. *Computed tomography of the body with magnetic resonance imaging.* 2nd ed. Philadelphia: WB Saunders 1992: 764.)

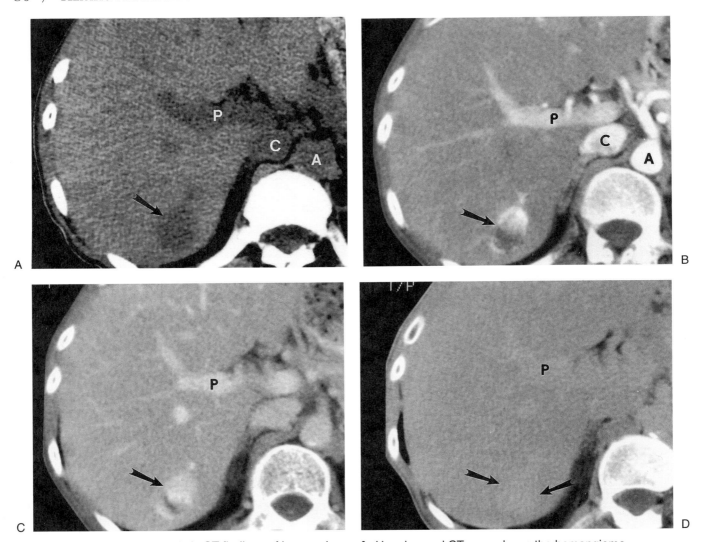

FIG. 7. Characteristic CT findings of hemangioma. **A:** Unenhanced CT scan shows the hemangioma *(arrow)* as hypodense to liver and with similar attenuation as vessels. C, inferior vena cava; A, aorta; P, portal vein. **B:** Arterial-phase contrast CT image shows the hemangioma *(arrow)* to demonstrate peripheral nodular enhancement, with the enhancement equal to that of other vessels seen in the liver. P, portal vein; C, inferior vena cava; A, aorta. **C:** Portal venous-phase contrast CT obtained 30 seconds after (B) shows the hemangioma *(arrow)* to demonstrate progressive fill-in of the enhancement into the lesion. The enhancement of the lesion has decreased in intensity compared with (B), but still matches the attenuation of other vessels. P, portal vein. **D:** Delayed image obtained 25 minutes later shows the hemangioma *(arrows)* to be homogeneously mildly enhanced. The lesion enhancement has continued to decrease, but still is identical to that of other vessels in the liver. This pattern of peripheral nodular enhancement with progressive fill-in of the lesion over time, with the enhancement attenuation matching that of liver vessels at all times evaluated, is diagnostic of cavernous hemangioma. P, portal vein.

dense with liver and vessels. Although some hemangiomas have an atypical appearance and can simulate neoplasm (Fig. 9), recent studies show that 89% to 94% of hemangiomas demonstrate characteristic appearances (34,35).

When encountering a small lesion at CT deemed too small to characterize (in general, <1 cm), delineation of the clinical setting can dramatically affect the prevalence of neoplastic disease versus benign disease. In the study by Jones et al. (36) of 45 patients with such small hepatic lesions seen at CT without a history of known underlying malignancy, in no case was a lesion subsequently determined to be malignant. Even in the presence of a known malignancy elsewhere, small lesions seen in the liver were subsequently shown to be malignant in only approximately 50% of patients. The fact that small lesions seen

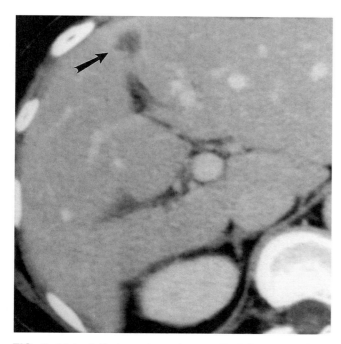

FIG. 8. Metastatic breast carcinoma. Portal venous-phase contrast-enhanced CT shows the metastasis *(arrow)* as a rounded, hypodense lesion with peripheral enhancement. Although peripheral enhancement can also be a feature of hemangiomas, note that the enhancement in this case is less intense than in other vessels throughout the liver, and is confluent and smooth rather than nodular and intermittent, as would be expected of a hemangioma.

at CT have such a high incidence of being benign can have a dramatic impact on patient care in patients with a known malignancy. Conversely, in the absence of such a history, this study suggests that little follow-up and medical effort should be made for small, incidentally detected lesions.

Liver Metastases

Metastases have varied CT appearances, none of which is diagnostic on CT. When such lesions are seen on CT, the diagnosis is usually made based on the clinical situation in conjunction with the imaging findings in the liver and elsewhere. The spectrum of appearances of metastases overlaps that of primary malignant lesions, as well as benign lesions such as atypical hemangiomas, abscesses, and benign neoplasms. Definitive diagnosis requires a biopsy, although in the proper clinical setting, the diagnosis of metastatic disease can usually be accurately determined. Many physicians are under the mistaken impression that biochemical liver function tests, rather than imaging tests such as CT or MRI, can be used as preliminary screening for metastatic disease. One study showed that one third of all patients with proven liver metastases had normal liver function test results

(37). CT sensitivities for detecting patients with liver neoplasms that have provided strong pathologic standards have reported detection rates of 80% to 93% of patients (see Table 1), although studies with the newer helical scanners have not yet been reported. In the presence of cirrhosis, CT fares worse because of a combination of poor portal venous contrast flow and distorted liver anatomy. In these situations, CT has been reported to detect only approximately 60% of patients with malignancy (38). These figures should improve with the advent of helical, biphasic (arterial- and portal venous-phase imaging) contrast CT techniques because in cirrhosis the suspected tumor is often hepatocellular carcinoma, a hypervascular tumor.

Accuracy in detecting the specific number of lesions within a liver is poorer, however (see Table 2). Such information is essential before consideration of surgical resection of isolated lesions, or in patients undergoing intraarterial chemotherapy, where the surgeon may wish to deliver the concentrated agent only to the lobe of tumor involvement. Dynamic incremental contrast CT has been reported to detect between 50% and 80% of liver lesions (5–7,9,38), although, again, these studies took place before the recent introduction of faster, helical CT scanners. One recent report with helical CT showed a liver lesion detection rate of 81% (13).

The CT appearance of liver neoplasms usually correlates with the degree of tumor vascularity. Most metastatic lesions are hypovascular and thus appear hypodense to adjacent enhanced liver parenchyma (see Fig. 3). Central low attenuation may be prominent either from central necrosis or as a result of cystic changes. Large tumors and sarcomas have a propensity for necrosis, and cystic primaries such as ovarian or pancreatic cystic malignancies typically develop cystic metastases in the liver. In such situations, however, typical characteristics (thick or nodular wall, internal heterogeneity, or CT density greater than water) are present and lead to the diagnosis of a potentially malignant liver lesion (see Fig. 6). Calcifications (usually best seen on noncontrast images) within metastases are most commonly seen in metastases from colon (Fig. 10) and ovarian cancer, although infrequently can be seen in other metastases and in primary hepatocellular carcinoma (39).

Malignant tumors with increased vascularity are less common and include hepatocellular carcinoma, metastases from renal cell carcinoma, islet cell carcinoma and other neuroendocrine tumors, sarcomas, and breast carcinoma; enhancement during the arterial phase of contrast enhancement excludes the diagnosis of hypovascular lesions such as metastases from colon cancer, pancreatic cancer, and so forth. Unfortunately, some benign lesions can be hypervascular, including focal nodular hyperplasia and liver cell adenoma, requiring biopsy in certain clinical situations to confirm malignant disease.

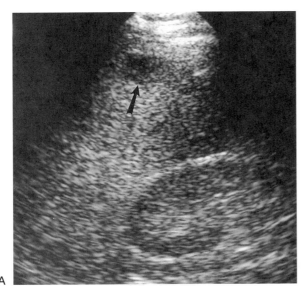

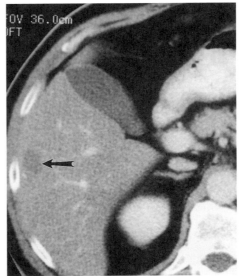

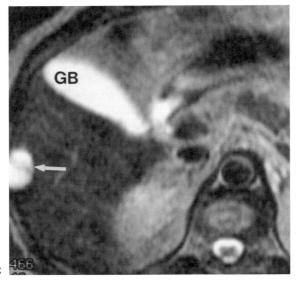

FIG. 9. Hemangioma with atypical imaging appearances at CT and ultrasound, and typical appearance at MRI. **A:** Longitudinal ultrasound image shows the hemangioma *(arrow)* as appearing hypoechoic to liver parenchyma. This is in part due to the increased echogenicity of the liver from fatty infiltration. **B:** Portal venous-phase contrast-enhanced CT shows the hemangioma *(arrow)* as hypodense compared with surrounding liver parenchyma, simulating neoplasm, lacking the peripheral enhancement of most hemangiomas. **C:** T2-weighted MRI shows the typical MR appearance of hemangioma *(arrow)* with a homogeneous, well circumscribed lesion of extreme high signal intensity matching the intensity of fluid structures, such as the gallbladder (GB).

Hepatocellular Carcinoma

The CT appearance of hepatocellular carcinoma is varied, reflecting differences in extent, differentiation, vascularity, necrosis, and venous occlusion. Often the tumors demonstrate marked heterogeneity within individual lesions, termed the mosaic sign, which is very suggestive of hepatocellular carcinoma (40) (Fig. 11). Typically, hepatocellular carcinoma is a heterogeneous mass, often hypervascular, that can appear as a solitary lesion or with multiple, discrete hepatic masses. Most hepatocellular carcinoma lesions are hypervascular, and small lesions may appear as homogeneously enhancing masses seen only during arterial-phase CT (see Fig. 1). Baron et al. reported that in 66 patients with hepatocellular carcinoma, the addition of arterial-phase images to conventional portal venous-phase imaging detected additional tumor lesions in 33% of patients, and, perhaps more important, in 11% of patients the diagnosis of hepatocellular carcinoma would have been missed if arterial-phase images had not been performed (21). Rarely, the tumor can be infiltrative and cause only diffuse liver heterogeneity at CT (41). Fatty metamorphosis within the tumors can result in very low attenuation (<-10 HU), an uncommon finding in all tumors except hepatocellular carcinoma and liver cell adenoma (42) (see Fig. 11; see also Fig. 25). Tumor encapsulation is seen in approximately 33% of cases (40) and can suggest the diagnosis because this finding is not present in metastatic disease at CT. Central portal vein thrombosis from tumor invasion can be seen on CT (see Fig. 11) and has been reported in 11% to 40% of cases (40,41,43) and, similarly, invasion of the hepatic venous system and biliary tree can be seen with CT. In all of

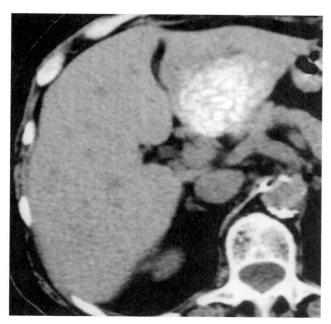

FIG. 10. Colon carcinoma metastasis to the liver. Unenhanced CT shows the metastasis as a high-attenuation lesion because of diffuse calcification in this mucinous adenocarcinoma metastasis.

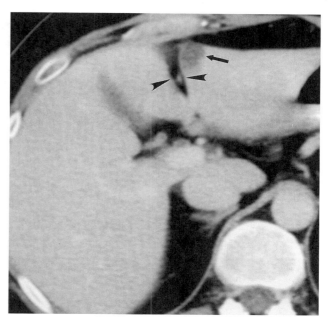

FIG. 12. Focal fat deposition in the liver. Contrast-enhanced CT shows a focal, well demarcated hypodensity *(arrow)* in the left lobe of the liver adjacent to the fissure for the ligamentum teres *(arrowheads)*. This is a characteristic location for focal fat deposition, which was proven by biopsy in this case.

these cases, such invasion strongly suggests the diagnosis of hepatocellular carcinoma, although rarely colon carcinoma can invade the venous system.

Because of the nonspecificity of many neoplastic lesions at CT, there are many benign entities that can simulate neoplasm at CT. Focal fatty infiltration can

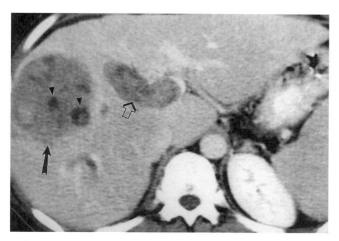

FIG. 11. Hepatocellular carcinoma (HCC) with portal venous invasion. Contrast-enhanced CT shows the large HCC lesion *(arrow)* as a heterogeneous mass with a peripheral enhancing capsule, findings typical of HCC. The low-attenuation regions *(arrowheads)* are of very low attenuation, lower than seen with necrosis and indicative of fat within the lesion, typical of HCC. Note the portal venous invasion with tumor thrombus *(open arrows)*.

appear as hypodense lesions, simulating neoplasm. In many such cases, the lesions are lobar in distribution (often with straight-line margins), without displacing vessels that can provide a clue to the diagnosis. Certain characteristic locations have a propensity for focal fatty infiltration that can provide a further clue (Fig. 12). MRI, with its capabilities of differentiating signal from protons rich in fat content, can be used with high sensitivity to detect fat (44). In some instances, particularly when rounded, focal fat deposition can be difficult to distinguish from neoplasm, and a biopsy may be necessary.

Other Benign Liver Lesions

Focal confluent fibrosis is a benign process occurring in advanced cirrhosis that often simulates neoplasm. In this entity, liver parenchyma is focally replaced by confluent masses of fibrosis that, if unrecognized, can lead to unnecessary and potentially dangerous biopsies or other interventions. Fortunately, this process often has a characteristic location and appearance, almost always associated with parenchymal volume loss and overlying capsular retraction, as well as a characteristic location in the anterior right and medial segments of the liver (45) (Fig. 13).

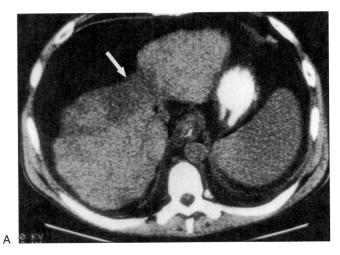

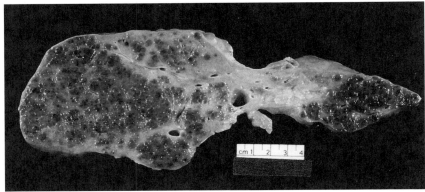

FIG. 13. Focal confluent fibrosis in a patient with cirrhosis. **A:** Unenhanced CT shows the focal fibrosis as a hypodense lesion in segments 8 and 4. The characteristic location of this lesion, as well as the associated capsular retraction *(arrow)*, aids in the diagnosis and differentiates this from neoplastic disease in the proper clinical setting. **B:** Pathologic specimen after liver transplantation shows the capsular retraction with underlying replacement of liver parenchyma by homogeneous yellow fibrous tissue, corresponding to the findings on the CT scan shown in (A). (See also Color Plate 1).

Delayed High-Dose Contrast CT (Delayed CT)

Scanning the liver 4 to 6 hours after a high dose of iodinated contrast can be a helpful technique to detect liver metastases. This technique is occasionally used in conjunction with a conventional contrast-enhanced CT or after CT-arterial portography to clarify confusing imaging findings. It has been shown to detect additional lesions in 28% of patients with colon carcinoma metastases and has been advocated as a tool in the presurgical screening of such patients (46,47). The technique is effective because 1% to 2% of iodine contrast is excreted by the liver and in the process is retained within hepatocytes, resulting in an approximately 20-HU increase in liver attenuation at 4 to 6 hours when 60 g of iodine is used initially (48). At 4 to 6 hours, while the liver is enhanced, there is virtually no iodine left in the circulating blood for delivery to tumors, maximizing lesion conspicuousness by preferentially retaining contrast in normal liver (Fig. 14). Although helpful in selected instances, it is a cumbersome technique, requiring patients to return 4 to 6 hours after a prior CT examination for a repeat series of images, and thus has not received wide acceptance. It cannot be used without first undergoing a conventional, contrast-enhanced CT to differentiate small lesions from

vessels as well as evaluate enhancement characteristics of liver parenchyma and lesions. It can be of help in determining exact tumor size and thus the potential for obtaining tumor-free surgical margins, if hepatic resection is being considered (49).

Noncontrast CT

It is well accepted that unenhanced liver CT alone is inferior to properly performed contrast-enhanced CT for detecting most liver neoplasms. There are certain situations, however, that may require limiting CT to noncontrast imaging. Significant allergies to iodinated contrast material or renal failure may preclude administering contrast agents to patients, although in these situations, ultrasound or MRI should be used if detection of liver neoplasms is important. If prior CT has shown that lesions are well demonstrated on unenhanced CT, the disease could be assessed at future examinations with unenhanced imaging.

Somewhat controversial is the role of unenhanced CT in patients with highly vascular liver tumors, such as hepatocellular carcinoma and metastases from renal cell carcinoma, pancreatic islet cell tumors, carcinoid tumors,

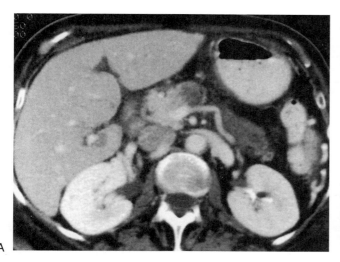 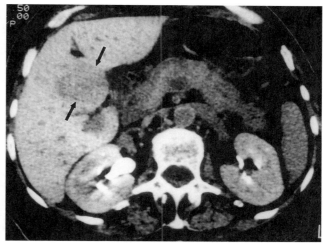

FIG. 14. Metastasis from pancreatic carcinoma demonstrated on delayed, high-dose, contrast-enhanced CT examination. **A:** Portal venous phase contrast CT fails to identify metastasis in the liver. **B:** Delayed, high-dose contrast-enhanced CT examination done 4 hours after image (A) shows a 5-cm hypodensity in segment 4 *(arrows)*, subsequently sampled for biopsy and shown to be a metastasis.

and breast carcinoma. Because of the vascular nature of these lesions, they may rapidly enhance and become iso-dense with the surrounding liver when imaged on conventional CT during the portal venous phase of contrast enhancement. Using unenhanced images in conjunction with enhanced CT aids in the detection of tumor nodules in these patients, with additional tumor nodules seen in up to 39% of patients (38,50,51). Other investigators have found that although additional nodules may be seen, this

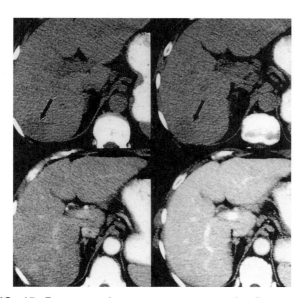

FIG. 15. Breast carcinoma metastases to the liver, seen best on unenhanced CT. Two unenhanced images *(top)* demonstrate the hypodense metastasis seen posteriorly in the liver *(arrows)*, which is not discernible on the arterial-phase *(lower left)* or portal venous-phase *(lower right)* contrast-enhanced images.

results in significant additional information that would affect patient management in only a small percentage of patients (52). Further, the role of helical CT scanning in providing the ability to screen the liver during the arterial and portal venous phases of enhancement after intra-venous contrast administration has not been clarified, but early experience suggests that arterial-phase imaging detects nearly all of the nodules previously only identi-fied on unenhanced images (53). There still exist, how-ever, vascular neoplasms that are best identified on unen-hanced CT (Fig. 15). With the altered portal venous and arterial flow to the liver in cirrhosis, my experience has been that unenhanced images are not infrequently the only sequence to demonstrate neoplasms.

When first visualized on unenhanced CT, accurate follow-up of such vascular tumors for response to therapy may best be determined on unenhanced images. Because of the dynamic nature of contrast enhancement in these lesions, vascular tumors may have isodense portions. Accurate comparison of tumor size between two different contrast-enhanced examinations may be difficult because the exact liver location will not be imaged at the same time relative to contrast infusion.

CT-Arteriography

Placing an angiographic catheter directly into the hepatic artery and then performing CT of the liver with contrast delivered through the hepatic artery catheter is a technique termed CT-arteriography. With infusion of contrast in this fashion, the liver enhances only minimally, because the portal vein delivers most of the blood flow to the liver as unenhanced blood, which dilutes the minimal

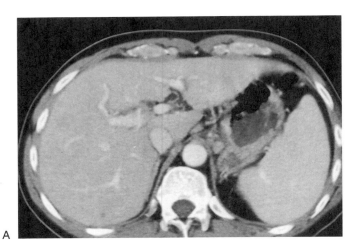
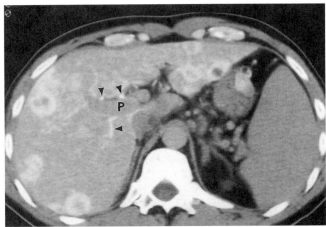

A

B

FIG. 16. Hepatocellular carcinoma (HCC) demonstrated at CT-arteriography. **A:** Portal venous-phase contrast-enhanced CT fails to demonstrate with confidence any liver tumor. **B:** CT at same level as **(A)** performed with contrast injected through a hepatic artery catheter shows only minimal enhancement of liver parenchyma. Dense enhancement of hepatic artery branches is seen *(arrowheads)*, and no enhancement is seen in the portal vein (P). Numerous foci of enhancing HCC are seen throughout the liver using this angiographic-assisted technique. (Reproduced with permission from Baron RL. Understanding and optimizing use of contrast material for CT of the liver. *AJR Am J Roentgenol* 1994; 163:323.)

contrast being delivered from the hepatic artery. Hypervascular tumors, however, such as hepatocellular carcinoma and hypervascular metastases, draw significant contrast-enhanced flow from the artery without any portal venous flow to dilute the contrast. This results in the tumor markedly enhancing against a background of minimally enhanced liver (Fig. 16). Although this approach can be helpful in certain circumstances, disadvantages of this technique make this an uncommonly used tool. Anomalous origins of branches of the hepatic artery are common arising from the superior mesenteric or gastric arteries, making evaluation of the entire liver impossible. In addition, heterogenous enhancement due to a variety of factors can make evaluation of liver parenchyma difficult (54,55). For practical purposes, this technique is limited to evaluation of patients with hepatocellular carcinoma in whom determination of the exact extent of tumor is essential, or a confusing clinical picture warrants further imaging clarification.

A variant of this procedure has been popularized predominantly in Japan, where infusion of an oil-based iodine contrast agent (lipiodol) into the hepatic artery is followed by subsequent CT imaging of the liver 7 to 10 days later (56,57). The normal liver densely traps the oil-based contrast and appears very dense if imaged shortly after such contrast infusion. However, by waiting approximately 1 week, most of the contrast is cleared from the normal parenchyma, leaving a background of unenhanced liver. Hepatocellular carcinoma, however, retains the lipiodol agent and appears as a dense nodule, allowing for easy detection and a target for biopsy, if necessary (Fig. 17). This can be particularly useful in patients with

cirrhosis, where the distorted liver architecture can make detection of hepatocellular carcinoma difficult. In addition, chemotherapeutic agents can be emulsified within the oil-based agent, which, when trapped within the tumor, can provide for a delayed-release, high-dose local treatment. Although this technique can certainly be helpful for diagnosis in some cases, its sensitivity is not as

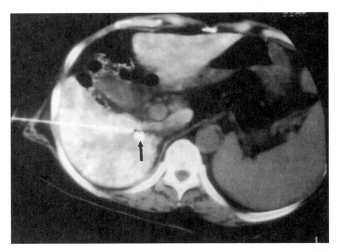

FIG. 17. Lipiodol CT detecting hepatocellular carcinoma. CT scan performed 7 days after hepatic artery infusion of lipiodol shows minimal retention of contrast diffusely throughout the liver. A small, dense focus of lipiodol retention is seen *(arrow)*, proven at biopsy to be hepatocellular carcinoma. The dense lipiodol makes a persistent target for percutaneous biopsy under CT guidance, as in this case, where the needle can be identified just before obtaining the biopsy specimen.

high as initially hoped, with recent studies showing only 50% to 80% of hepatocellular carcinoma foci retaining the contrast agent (57,58). It has not been shown to be helpful in evaluating metastatic liver disease.

CT-Arterial Portography

Placing a catheter into the superior mesenteric artery or splenic artery and performing the CT examination of the liver with contrast injected through the catheter provides contrast enhancement of the portal venous system and liver, bypassing the hepatic arterial supply. This technique is termed CT-arterial portography (CT-AP) and is generally considered the most sensitive nonoperative imaging technique for detecting liver neoplasms (6,7,9) (see Table 2). Such delivery of contrast markedly enhances liver parenchyma to degrees not possible with intravenous administration of contrast and, at the same time, prevents delivery of contrast to the tumor because the arterial system is bypassed. The resulting image is one of a markedly enhanced liver with hypodense tumors (Fig. 18). Studies with strong pathologic correlation (see Table 2) have shown that CT-AP detects between 81% and 94% of liver neoplasms of sufficient size to be seen at subsequent gross pathologic evaluation (5,6,9,11).

Because of the invasive nature of the test, as with CT-arteriography, it is usually reserved for patients who are potential candidates for resection of presumed isolated liver neoplasms (to ensure that the remainder of the liver is indeed tumor free), or to follow patients undergoing intra-arterial chemotherapy for whom the examination can be done while the catheter is in place for the therapy. In a large retrospective study, Small et al. (59) determined that CT-AP spared unnecessary surgery in 64% of patients referred for hepatic resection. It is important to realize, however, that although this technique is very sensitive, it is also nonspecific (60,61). Many lesions such as cysts and hemangiomas have no portal venous blood flow and appear as perfusion defects. Idiopathic intrahepatic portal obstruction and regions receiving collateral flow appear as defects and could be mistaken for tumor. Fortunately, most of these benign perfusion abnormalities have a characteristic appearance (wedge shaped and peripheral) or location (posterior aspect of segment 4; see Fig. 18) and can be differentiated from neoplasm. However, it is good advice to take a biopsy sample of any lesion seen at CT-AP before denying a patient potentially curative surgery for an otherwise isolated liver tumor. For small lesions, this may require proceeding with surgery but performing an intraoperative ultrasound-guided biopsy before commencing a liver resection. CT-AP can provide an excellent screen for the sonographer to locate the lesion for biopsy during surgery.

Magnetic Resonance Imaging

Magnetic resonance is an imaging tool based on differences of magnetic properties of atomic nuclei and the environment of those nuclei. Protons, abundant in the body's water and fat content, are used for conventional

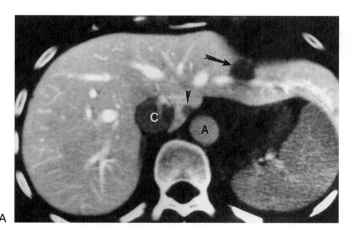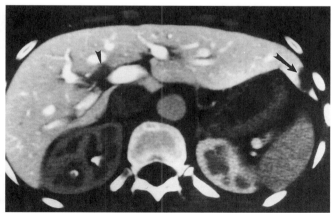

A
B

FIG. 18. CT-arterial portography (CT-AP) in patient with colon carcinoma metastasis to liver. **A:** Section near the superior aspect of the liver shows a colon carcinoma metastasis as a homogeneous, low-attenuation area *(arrow)* in the lateral segment. In the caudate lobe, a small hypodensity *(arrowhead)* was proven at surgery to be focal nodular hyperplasia. The dense liver enhancement is typical of CT-AP and is in marked contrast to the absent enhancement in the inferior vena cava (C) due to the lack of systemic contrast material. The minimal enhancement of the aorta (A) is due to slight reflux of contrast into the aorta during the injection. **B:** Scan in the same patient at a slightly inferior level shows an additional lesion in the lateral segment peripherally *(arrow)*, shown to be a hemangioma. A peripheral wedge-shaped lesion *(arrowhead)* is seen in the posterior aspect of segment 4, representing a benign perfusion abnormality commonly seen in this location because of aberrant gastric venous drainage to this region.

MRI. By applying an external, transient magnetic field gradient generated by a radiofrequency pulse, energy is absorbed by hydrogen nuclei. With the cessation of the external radiofrequency pulse, the nuclei release their energy, doing so by independent processes, termed T1 and T2. The relaxation times, or times to dissipate the energy, vary among different tissues, and it is these differences that are measured and transformed into gray-scale images. A discussion of the physics involved in creating images is beyond the scope of this chapter, and the reader is referred to basic MRI textbooks for more detail.

Technical parameters create different types of MR images, allowing for evaluation of different tissue characteristics by presenting tissues with varying signal intensity. Differences in signal intensity exist between normal liver and liver tumors and allow for detection of tumors, usually as a result of an increased water content in tumors. Common technical parameters include the TR (repetition time) and TE (echo time). By controlling these factors, images that are predominately T1 weighted (TR typically <300 and TE <20 mseconds) or T2 weighted (TR >1.5 seconds and TE >60 mseconds) can be produced. Spin echo images typically require lengthy imaging time (up to 14 minutes) to acquire, although multiple images of the entire liver are obtained. This results in motion artifact from breathing, vascular motion, and bowel peristalsis that can limit the spatial resolution of these images in some circumstances. Technical maneuvers of varying sorts can decrease the extent of the artifacts caused by such motion. Newer developments have resulted in fast spin echo sequences that can significantly

shorten the imaging time required to approximately 6 to 8 minutes. Breathholding imaging techniques using very short TR and TE create gradient echo images that can be obtained in a matter of seconds and allow use of dynamic contrast techniques very similar to those used for CT. Although these images are obtained rapidly, they usually have increased noise and poorer spatial resolution, so they most typically are used in conjunction with the higher–spatial-resolution images of spin echo imaging, or with contrast agents.

In practical clinical use, imaging the liver consists of several potential imaging sequences to display the liver anatomy and pathology. Spin echo images using both T1- and T2-weighted imaging parameters, gradient echo imaging with T1-weighted imaging parameters, and T2-weighted imaging with a fat-suppression technique (either spin echo imaging or inversion recovery imaging) are commonly used in evaluating the liver. Using a combination of these techniques, and including contrast agents with T1-weighted sequences, has resulted in detection of liver tumors with sensitivities that probably slightly exceed those of intravenous contrast CT in detecting specific numbers of neoplastic lesions (see Table 2) (3,6,7,62), although well controlled studies have been limited, and no comparative studies with pathologic correlation have been published using helical CT to optimize contrast use, as delineated in the section on CT.

Because of increased fluid content, most tumors have an appearance hypointense to liver on T1-weighted imaging and hyperintense to liver on T2-weighted imaging (Fig. 19). Exceptions to this are tumors containing a specific tissue content, such as blood or hemorrhage, fat,

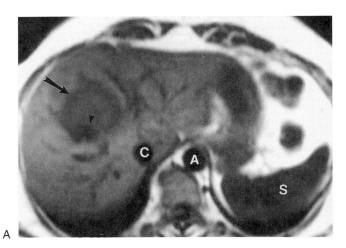

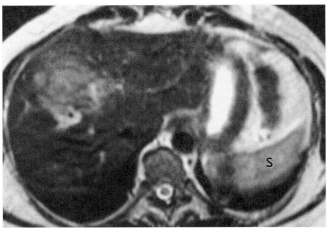

A

B

FIG. 19. Colon carcinoma metastasis to the liver. **A:** T1-weighted spin echo MR image shows the liver to be of higher signal intensity than the spleen (S), a normal relationship. A large colon carcinoma metastasis *(arrow)* appears of lesser intensity than surrounding liver. Vessels appear as a signal void on these images (note the inferior vena cava [C] and aorta [A] as well as the intrahepatic vessels). The colon metastasis can be seen encircling an intrahepatic vessel *(arrowhead)* appearing as a signal void at the periphery of the lesion. **B:** T2-weighted spin echo MR image at the same level as (A) shows the liver to be of lower signal intensity than the spleen (S), a normal relationship. The metastasis appears of higher signal intensity, approximating the intensity of the spleen.

melanin (Fig. 20), and others. These typically can be seen in certain tumors and help characterize such tumors because they result in high signal intensity changes on T1-weighted imaging (see discussion on characterization, later). These tumors typically still retain high signal intensity in T2-weighted images.

The availability of intravenous contrast agents has improved the ability of MRI to characterize tumors, and in some instances to detect tumors. Because of its inherent tissue contrast with unenhanced images, detection of most tumors is not improved with the use of the currently commercially available gadolinium chelates (63), which have pharmacokinetics similar to those of iodinated CT contrast agents. They do have an advantage in demonstrating hypervascular liver neoplasms, however, best demonstrated in hepatocellular carcinoma. Similar to CT, use of these agents combined with gradient echo fast imaging allows for arterial-phase contrast imaging and the detection of small hyperenhancing lesions that can be obscured during portal venous-phase imaging (64). These lesions are often well differentiated histologically and have unenhanced MR tissue characteristics and imaging appearances similar to those of normal liver, and therefore require contrast enhancement to overcome the lack of inherent tissue contrast differences.

Analogous to CT-AP, contrast material for MRI can be administered through an indwelling arterial catheter into the superior mesenteric artery or splenic artery, resulting in MR-arterial portography. Soyer et al. (10) reported detecting 94% of neoplastic lesions in subsequently resected liver specimens, compared with 87% for CT-AP.

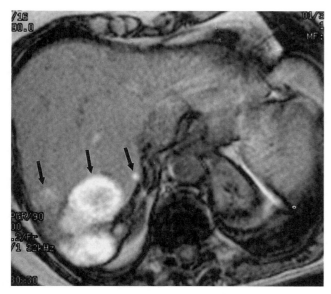

FIG. 20. Metastatic melanoma. T1-weighted gradient echo MR image shows several foci of melanoma *(arrows)* of high signal intensity compared with adjacent liver. Compare the appearance of these metastases with those of colon carcinoma shown in Fig. 19.

Because of the widespread use of CT as the predominant screening tool for abdominal neoplasms and the high sensitivity of CT-AP in detecting liver tumors, this technique has not achieved widespread use.

A distinct advantage in the past for MRI over CT has been its ability to characterize lesions. Although most neoplasms have a nonspecific appearance on T1- and T2-weighted imaging, certain benign lesions have very characteristic appearances. Specifically, lesions with very high fluid content such as cysts and hemangiomas typically have lesions with a very long T2, and therefore have a homogeneous, very–high-intensity appearance on T2-weighted images, termed the "light-bulb sign" (65,66). Particularly when using a long echo time (140 to 160 mseconds), these findings are indicative of such benign nonsolid lesions, because malignant lesions appear with a signal intensity only slightly greater than that of liver (Fig. 21). Although overlap of this appearance on T2-weighted images was reported for hypervascular neoplasms, these reports were based on using an echo time of 60 to 80 mseconds. By prolonging the echo time to 140 to 160 mseconds, such overlap is virtually eliminated (67). Use of intravenous gadolinium chelate contrast agents can also demonstrate dynamic enhancement characteristics (peripheral, nodular with centripetal enhancement) similar to those with CT, and can be used in confusing cases or for clarification (68).

Hepatocellular carcinoma can show other characteristic findings on MRI in a large percentage of cases, including high signal intensity on T1-weighted images and a peritumoral capsule of low signal intensity on T1-weighted images and high intensity on T2-weighted images (69,70).

Various MRI sequences can exquisitely demonstrate blood vessels and flow or lack thereof within the vessels. This can be extremely helpful in evaluating hepatocellular carcinoma and patients with cirrhosis. In particular, gradient echo imaging with technical parameters to accentuate flowing blood can give vessels an extremely high signal intensity, making them very conspicuous, and demonstrating thrombus as low-intensity regions (Fig. 22). Conversely, spin echo images that better demonstrate anatomic structures and neoplasms demonstrate vessels as a signal void. The presence of signal intensity within vascular structures on spin echo imaging is suggestive of thrombus, although slow flow and other technical phenomena can simulate this (71–73). In such cases, use of gradient echo imaging can confirm or exclude the presence of thrombus.

Newer contrast agents currently undergoing investigation are aimed at enhancing normal liver parenchyma for prolonged periods of time, allowing for static imaging. Such agents are typically incorporated into functioning hepatocytes or reticuloendothelial cells, and enhance the liver parenchyma but not tumors. Agents investigated to date in the United States include mangafodipir trisodium

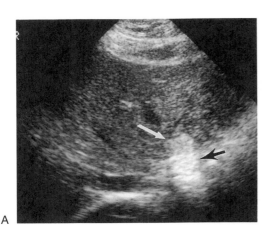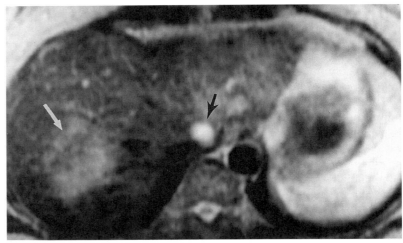

A

B

FIG. 21. Patient with colon carcinoma metastasis and cavernous hemangioma in the liver. **A:** Transverse ultrasound image shows the hemangioma *(white arrow)* as a homogeneous, hyperechoic, rounded lesion in a subcapsular position. Increased distal through-transmission of sound *(black arrow)* is seen. Note the lack of a surrounding hypoechoic halo, often seen with malignant liver lesions. **B:** T2-weighted MR image in a similar axial plane as (A) shows the hemangioma *(black arrow)* as homogeneously extremely bright, characteristic of hemangiomas. Note the difference between the signal intensity of the hemangioma and that of the large colon carcinoma metastasis *(white arrow)* in the right lobe. The metastasis is of slightly higher signal intensity than surrounding liver, but only mildly so, not approaching that of the hemangioma or the cerebrospinal fluid in the spinal canal.

(Mn-DPDP) (74,75) and ferrite oxide particles (76). The early results in tumor detection are promising, but their exact role in oncologic liver imaging awaits further investigations. Mn-DPDP produces excellent liver parenchymal enhancement, and metastatic tumors almost universally do not enhance. Well differentiated hepatocellular carcinoma with functioning hepatocytes, however, does

transfer the agent into the tumors, which can become isointense and not visualized with enhanced images. Although this is a potential problem, it can also be of benefit because some hepatocellular tumors can be visualized only because of their enhancement at MRI after Mn-DPDP administration. It may well be that, similar to CT, some tumors may require both enhanced and unenhanced MR images for optimal tumor detection (77).

Ultrasound

Ultrasonography uses sound waves generated by an electrical impulse. Sound waves reflected by tissues in the body are returned and transformed into electrical energy. Transducers used in medical imaging have a frequency of 3 to 15 MHz (million cycles per second, or the number of times the sound wave is generated per second). The higher the transducer's frequency, the superior the imaging resolution, although the poorer the tissue penetration. Thus, for superficial organs and thin patients, a higher-frequency transducer can be used (in the liver, this would be a 3.5- to 5-MHz transducer), whereas for deeper organs and large patients, a lower-frequency transducer would be used (for liver imaging, this would require a 2.25-MHz transducer). At the interface of tissues of different acoustic impedance, a reflective echo is generated. The greater the difference in density between the interfacing tissues, the higher the amplitude of the returning echo. The location of the echoes can be determined by the

FIG. 22. Hepatocellular carcinoma with portal venous tumor thrombus. Gradient echo MRI shows vessels such as the aorta (A) and the inferior vena cava (C) as of high signal intensity. Note the high intensity of the portal vein *(arrow)* is mostly replaced by lower signal intensity within the tumor thrombus. Such excellent vascular depiction is obtained without the use of contrast agents with these techniques.

differences in time required for echoes to travel to the interface and to return to the transducer—the shorter the time required, the closer the structure to the transducer.

The returning echoes are converted to imaging with use of a gray scale to differentiate the amplitude or strength of each returning echo. Most imaging units use a black background so that the echoes are shades of gray and white, with the brightest echoes representing the strongest-amplitude echoes from tissue interfaces of markedly different acoustic impedance (relating to tissue density and the speed of sound in the tissues). Sound may be absorbed, reflected, or scattered as it travels through the body and various tissue interfaces. Homogeneous regions with few or no tissue interfaces (such as through fluid) do not reflect echoes, resulting in anechoic regions. The lack of attenuation of the sound beam as it travels through such structures results in higher echo levels in structures distal to the fluid than other adjacent regions where the sound beam traveled through solid tissues to reach similar depths. Such acoustic enhancement can be used to characterize cystic lesions. Conversely, highly echogenic structures, with marked differences in acoustic impedance, such as at air–tissue or tissue–calcium interfaces, result in high-amplitude reflective echoes with little or no passage of the sound through to more distal regions of the body. This may create an anechoic distal "shadow" to the echogenic front, and allows for characterization of such abnormalities as due to one of these types of interfaces.

Current ultrasound scanners are capable of sending and receiving up to 30 images per second, with the resultant screen simulating a real-time environment rather than one of repeated image collections. This allows for evaluation of some structures over time (such as watching bowel peristalsis) and for further characterization of some structures. This has also allowed for the development of ultrasound contrast agents and the capability to watch blood flow with the use encapsulated microbubbles. With conventional gray-scale imaging, vessels are sonolucent and blood flow within lesions is not identified. With the use of encapsulated microbubble agents, vessels can be well delineated, as well as flow into some tumors (78). Early use of these agents has been for cardiac imaging, but the hope is that these may be helpful in the future for characterizing liver tumors.

Doppler ultrasound units are capable of measuring changes in the reflected echo frequency and determining the velocity of moving interfaces (such as blood flow). Color can be used to display the direction of flow and the relative magnitude of flow—usually the color is selected to display the direction of flow, and the shade of the color is used to display the relative magnitude of flow. An in-depth discussion of ultrasound physics is beyond the scope of this chapter, and the reader is referred to basic ultrasound textbooks for such a discussion.

The liver is a relatively easy organ to image with ultrasound because of its superficial location without overlying bowel gas. The anatomy can be well displayed, and there is the capability of displaying the liver in multiple planes, not limited to the axial plane as with CT. Unlike CT and MRI, ultrasound uses small fields of view with limited, "sector" scans of the regions viewed. It is portable, so that it can be used for intensive care unit patients. Its real-time capability makes it the instrument of choice for imaging directed biopsies of the liver (79) or for guiding intratumor injection of absolute ethanol for treating hepatocellular carcinoma (80). This very freedom to image also is one of ultrasound's drawbacks. There is a lack of methodical, rigid imaging to ensure production of images that cover the entire extent of the liver, as with CT and MRI. This, coupled with the limited sector visualization and lack of ultrasound's ability to demonstrate the entire cross-sectional anatomy, as well as the ability of CT to evaluate the chest, abdomen, and pelvis in one rapid examination, has resulted in CT becoming the standard imaging screening tool in the United States for the evaluation of the oncology patient. Recent comparative studies of ultrasound with other technologies in assessing its role in detecting liver neoplasia with good pathologic correlation are limited. One study by Lundstedt et al. (81) reported predicting specific lobe involvement with tumor in 71% of patients with ultrasound, compared with 48% for angiography and 82% for CT. Several studies have shown ultrasound not to fare as well as CT or MRI in predicting patients with neoplastic liver disease or in detecting specific numbers of liver lesions (see Tables 1 and 2). Leen et al. (8) reported a sensitivity of 48% for preoperative ultrasound in predicting the specific number of liver metastases from colon carcinoma, compared with 80% for CT. Such studies and general clinical experience have resulted in CT or MRI being the noninvasive screening and staging tools of choice for liver neoplastic disease. Nonetheless, when looking only at the liver or when attempting to characterize certain lesions, ultrasound excels in certain clinical situations, to be described later. As already mentioned, its value as a tool for guiding biopsies is unparalleled.

The one arena where ultrasound imaging for liver neoplasms is unsurpassed is that of intraoperative ultrasound, used before undertaking resection of liver neoplasms elsewhere in the liver. Intraoperative ultrasound has been shown to be equivalent to or slightly better than CT-AP (9), detecting up to 95% of liver tumors, and with very few false-positive results. Intraoperative ultrasound has the advantage of using high-frequency transducers (5 to 7.5 MHz) because of the closeness of the transducer to the organ. Lesions seen can be immediately sampled for biopsy under ultrasound guidance. Nonetheless, in my experience, the use of CT-AP can provide an excellent "roadmap" for intraoperative ultrasound, and it has not infrequently occurred that were it not for a preoperative CT portogram, the intraoperative ultrasound would have failed to detect a very small lesion that required

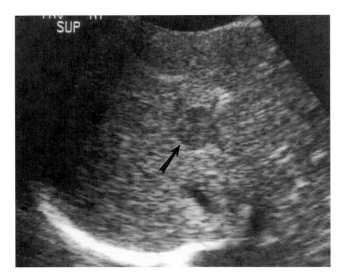

FIG. 23. Gallbladder carcinoma metastasis. The metastasis *(arrow)* appears as hypoechoic to the remaining liver parenchyma, which is increased in echogenicity because of diffuse fatty infiltration.

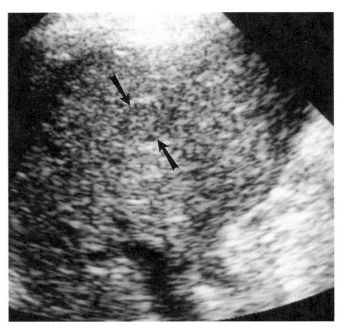

FIG. 24. Hepatocellular carcinoma. Ultrasound examination of the liver demonstrates diffuse heterogeneous liver parenchyma due to underlying cirrhosis. A small focus of hepatocellular carcinoma *(arrows)* is seen as predominantly isoechoic and identifiable because of a peripheral hypoechoic halo.

biopsy confirmation before undertaking an extensive liver resection.

The ultrasound appearance of most neoplastic lesions is nonspecific, demonstrating characteristics of a solid, space-occupying lesion different from surrounding liver parenchyma. The common appearances include hypoechoic lesions (Fig. 23), isoechoic with a hypoechoic halo (Fig. 24), hyperechoic lesions or foci of hyperechogenicity (usually indicative of calcification, such as with colon cancer or ovarian cancer metastases, although other lesions can rarely show this as well; Fig. 25), and focal or diffuse heterogeneity (Fig. 26). Rarely, malignant lesions appear homogeneously hyperechoic without a surrounding hypoechoic halo. Most tumors appear as well defined lesions, although infiltrative tumors such as lymphoma, breast carcinoma, and hepatocellular carcinoma can appear as ill-defined, heterogeneous disruption of the

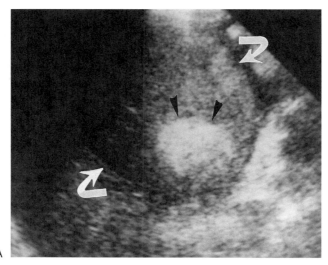

A

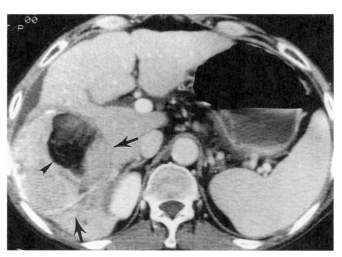

B

FIG. 25. Hepatocellular carcinoma. **A:** Transverse ultrasound image shows the tumor as a large, heterogeneous mass *(curved arrows)*. Portions of the tumor are markedly hyperechoic *(arrowheads)*. **B:** CT scan shows the large tumor *(arrows)* with characteristic foci of low attenuation *(arrowhead)* approximating the appearance of fat. Fatty material is typically echogenic at ultrasound and explains the findings in **(A)**.

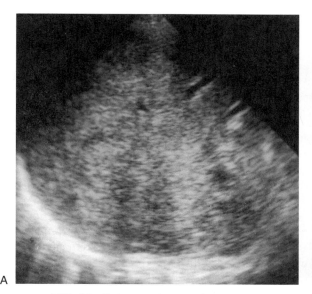
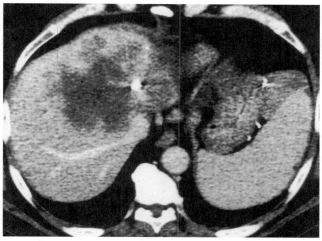

FIG. 26. Colon carcinoma. **A:** Transverse ultrasound image through the liver shows a diffusely heterogeneous appearance to the liver because of a large liver metastasis. **B:** CT image from approximately the same location as (**A**) shows the metastasis as appearing more homogeneous and hypodense to surrounding parenchyma.

normal liver parenchymal echo pattern. Particularly in cirrhosis, hepatocellular carcinoma can be ill defined and appreciated often only in retrospect, as a diffuse, heterogenous zone appearing slightly different from the distorted cirrhotic liver parenchyma (82).

Unfortunately, benign lesions such as focal nodular hyperplasia, liver cell adenoma, and regenerating nodules in cirrhosis can appear similar to all of the aforementioned ultrasound appearances of malignant lesions. Fortunately, the common benign lesions in the liver, cysts and cavernous hemangiomas, have relatively characteristic appearances at ultrasound and can be differentiated from underlying malignant lesions, depending on the clinical setting. Cysts, representing a homogeneous fluid medium, have an anechoic appearance with increased distal echogenicity (Fig. 27), a very different appearance from virtually all neoplastic lesions. Even necrotic or cystic tumors in the liver have some mural thickening or papillary projections that remove them from the benign cyst category (Fig. 28). The hemangioma has a series of characteristics at ultrasound that allow for its diagnosis in many clinical situations. It appears on ultrasound as a homogeneous, hyperechoic, usually small (<3 cm) mass without a surrounding hypoechoic halo in approximately 90% of cases (see Fig. 21). Increased through-echo transmission due to the liquid nature of these lesions is is another characteristic that aids in their characterization, particularly because this finding is not seen with echogenic solid masses that attenuate sound. Larger hemangiomas may more frequently demonstrate heterogenous appearances because of fibrosis and thrombosis, which may make it difficult

to differentiate them from malignant lesions, and occasionally small lesions can appear hypoechoic or heterogenous as well (see Fig. 9). Finally, the lack of change over time is a very helpful sign with any imaging modality, and ultrasound can be an inexpensive, easy method

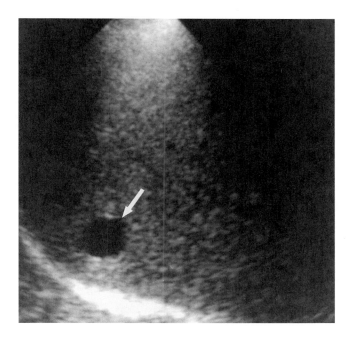

FIG. 27. Hepatic cyst. Sagittal ultrasound image shows the cyst *(arrow)* as homogeneously hypoechoic, with a sharp zone of transition without mural irregularity. Note the increased echogenicity passing distally through the lesion.

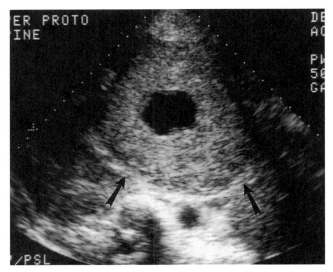

FIG. 28. Necrotic sarcoma metastasis. Transverse ultrasound image shows a large metastasis *(arrows)* with central necrosis appearing predominantly sonolucent. The margins of the necrosis show mural irregularity, which would not be seen with a simple cyst.

to perform such follow-up. It is important to recognize, however, that hemangiomas may change their size with follow-up imaging, as demonstrated in 18% of patients reported by Gibney et al. (83).

Hemodynamic characteristics of tumors as delineated by duplex and color Doppler ultrasound images may allow for differentiation of liver masses. Some investigators have shown that hepatocellular carcinoma shows a large Doppler shift, in contrast to hemangiomas and metastases, which show little or low shifts, respectively (84,85). Most investigations have been using this tool to differentiate hepatocellular carcinoma foci from benign lesions, but when investigators have included metastatic lesions, the findings are similar to those for hepatocellular carcinoma, limiting the specificity of Doppler ultrasound in differentiating among tumor types (85). The finding thought to be most representative of malignant tumors, that of a high peak systolic flow velocity, although most common in malignant lesions, can be seen in hemangiomas as well, although far less commonly (85). Most centers do not use Doppler characteristics to differentiate among liver masses.

Finally, recent studies have shown that duplex/color Doppler ultrasound measurement of hepatic perfusion ratios (ratio of hepatic arterial to total liver blood flow and the ratio of hepatic arterial to portal venous blood flow) can separate patients with overt liver metastases from those without (8,86). The role of such measurements is uncertain in the clinical treatment of patients and requires further studies for elucidation. The preliminary results suggest that abnormal flow characteristics may be helpful in identifying patients with small metastases not visualized at imaging.

EVALUATION OF PATIENTS WITH SUSPECTED LIVER NEOPLASIA

Computed tomography has become the screening and staging tool of choice for abdominal neoplastic disease based on its widespread availability, excellent anatomic depiction, and high sensitivity for liver tumor detection (see Table 1), as well as detection of neoplastic disease throughout the abdomen and chest. In most instances, this adequately stages the primary abdominal tumor and potential spread to the liver. Such easy, thorough staging is difficult with ultrasound. MRI equipment is not as widely available in the United States, and MRI is not currently thought to be as facile in staging disease throughout the abdomen (4,5), although its ability to detect liver neoplastic disease probably at least equals that of helical contrast CT, and may exceed it in the future with new contrast agent developments. In the clinical situation where it is necessary to characterize a liver mass suspected or known to be present, MRI is probably the tool of choice, although in many situations contrast-enhanced CT can be successful in this as well. The role of ultrasound is decreasing in screening for neoplastic disease, while it plays an increased role in guiding percutaneous biopsies and for intraoperative localization and detection of tumors.

Before the advent of helical CT scanning, it was generally acknowledged that patients being considered for surgical resection of liver neoplasms or selective intraarterial delivery of chemotherapeutic agents are inadequately staged by noninvasive imaging methods. Such patients have been thought to be best screened with CT-AP (6,87) to prevent unnecessary extensive surgery. Clearly, intraoperative ultrasound has the highest sensitivity of all the imaging methods (see Table 1), and should be undertaken in all cases before surgical resection. Whether helical CT and new MRI contrast agents can obviate the need for these invasive tests remains to be determined.

FUTURE DEVELOPMENTS IN LIVER IMAGING

Further improvement in imaging of neoplastic liver involvement is an ongoing challenge. Efforts at improvement are ongoing in many areas, centered on technological improvements and development of newer contrast agents.

The technological improvements the medical community can expect over the immediate few years will be for faster image acquisition, both with CT and MRI, which will allow for more optimal use of contrast agents as well as speedier individual examinations, lowering patient cost. The speed of image acquisition is becoming such that real-time imaging, similar to fluoroscopy, may soon be available, which would increase our ability to localize and sample or treat tumors with imaging guidance.

It is hoped that the ability to use imaging tools to go beyond the realm of displaying anatomy and anatomic distortions, to display altered metabolism, will become a reality in the coming years. Although the role of nuclear scintigraphy in imaging liver neoplasia has decreased dramatically, the advent of positron emission tomography (PET) scanning is bringing a resurgence of interest in liver scintigraphic imaging. The ability of PET scanning to demonstrate metabolic changes may help not only to detect liver tumors, but to follow therapy of patients and determine tumor viability after treatment. It is hoped that the anatomic display available with CT and MRI and the functional imaging of PET can be combined into functional anatomic displays of the liver.

Availability of new contrast agents for the liver is imminent. Recent interest has been solely aimed at MRI, although a resurgence of interest in developing similar agents for CT can be expected. Agents that are taken up by the reticuloendothelial system (large iron oxide particles) have undergone clinical trials and have demonstrated an increased ability to detect small tumors in preliminary reports (88). Agents that are taken up by hepatocytes (Mn-DPDP) are undergoing preliminary clinical investigations and have also been shown to increase detection of small tumors (75). Both of these types of agents (and others undergoing more basic investigation) are successful by enhancing normal liver, with tumors not taking up the agent and demonstrating an enhancement void. Obviously, in the further future, it would be desirable to develop agents that are tumor specific, analogous to or perhaps using monoclonal antibodies, that could be combined with active imaging agents that would display tumoral enhancement. Although no such agents have been developed for CT and MRI, the early development of monoclonal antibodies for imaging tumors with scintigraphy suggests this may be a possibility in the coming years. If scintigraphic evaluation of the liver becomes a reality, then we may expect such agents to be developed for CT or MRI that could combine both anatomic display with functional tumor imaging.

REFERENCES

1. Alderson PO, Adams DF, McNeil BJ, et al. Computed tomography, ultrasound and scintigraphy of the liver in patients with colon or breast carcinoma: a prospective comparison. *Radiology* 1983;149:225.
2. Knopf DR, Torres WE, Fajman WJ, et al. Liver lesions: comparative accuracy of scintigraphy and computed tomography. *AJR Am J Roentgenol* 1982;138:623.
3. Stark DD, Wittenberg J, Butch RJ, Ferrucci JT. Hepatic metastases: randomized, controlled comparison of detection with MR imaging and CT. *Radiology* 1987;165:399.
4. Chezmar JL, Rumancik WM, Megibow AJ, Hulnick DH, Nelson RC, Bernardino ME. Liver and abdominal screening in patients with cancer: CT versus MR imaging. *Radiology* 1988;168:43.
5. Vassiliades VG, Foley WD, Alarcon J, et al. Hepatic metastases: CT versus MR imaging at 1.5T. *Gastrointest Radiol* 1991;16:159.
6. Nelson RC, Chezmar JL, Sugarbaker PH, Bernardino ME. Hepatic tumors: comparison of CT during arterial portography, delayed CT, and MR imaging for preoperative evaluation. *Radiology* 1989;172:27.
7. Heiken JP, Weyman PJ, Lee JKT, et al. Detection of focal hepatic masses: prospective evaluation with CT, delayed CT, CT during arterial portography, and MR imaging. *Radiology* 1989;171:47.
8. Leen E, Angerson WJ, Wotherspoon H, Moule B, Cook TG, McArdle CS. Detection of colorectal liver metastases: comparison of laparotomy, CT, US, and Doppler perfusion index and evaluation of postoperative follow-up results. *Radiology* 1995;195:113.
9. Soyer P, Levesque M, Elias D, Zeitoun G, Roche A. Detection of liver metastases from colorectal cancer: comparison of intraoperative US and CT during arterial portography. *Radiology* 1992;183:541.
10. Soyer P, Laissy JP, Sibert A, et al. Focal hepatic masses: comparison of detection during arterial portography with MR imaging and CT. *Radiology* 1994;190:737.
11. Soyer P, Bluemke DA, Hruban RH, Sitzmann JV, Fishman EK. Hepatic metastases from colorectal cancer: detection and false-positive findings with helical CT during arterial portography. *Radiology* 1994;193:71.
12. Hagspiel KD, Neidl KF, Eichenberger AC, Weder W, Marincek B. Detection of liver metastases: comparison of superparamagnetic iron oxide-enhanced and unenhanced MR imaging at 1.5 T with dynamic CT, intraoperative US, and percutaneous US. *Radiology* 1995;196:471.
13. Kuszyk BS, Bluemke DA, Urban BA, et al. Portal-phase contrast-enhanced helical CT for the detection of malignant hepatic tumors: sensitivity based on comparison with intraoperative and pathologic findings. *AJR Am J Roentgenol* 1996;166:91.
14. Fink S, Chaudhuri K. Physiological considerations in imaging liver metastases from colorectal carcinoma. *Am J Physiol Imaging* 1991; 6:150.
15. Greenway CV, Stark RD. Hepatic vascular bed. *Physiol Rev* 1971; 51:23.
16. Baron RL. Understanding and optimizing use of contrast material for CT of the liver. *AJR Am J Roentgenol* 1994;163:323.
17. Foley WD. Dynamic hepatic CT. *Radiology* 1989;170:617.
18. Shuman WP, Adam JL, Schoenecker SA, et al. Use of a power injector during dynamic computed tomography. *J Comput Assist Tomogr* 1986; 10:1000.
19. Hollett MD, Jeffrey Jr RB, Nino-Murcia M, Jorgensen MJ, Harris DP. Dual-phase helical CT of the liver: value of arterial phase scans in the detection of small (≤ 1.5 cm) malignant hepatic neoplasms. *AJR Am J Roentgenol* 1995;164:879.
20. Ohashi I, Hanafusa K, Yoshida T. Small hepatocellular carcinomas: two-phase dynamic incremental CT in detection and evaluation. *Radiology* 1993;189:851.
21. Baron RL, Oliver JH, Dodd GD, Nalesnik M, Holbert BL, Carr BI. Hepatocellular carcinoma: evaluation with biphasic, contrast-enhanced helical CT. *Radiology* 1996;199:505.
22. Walkey MM. Dynamic hepatic CT: how many years will it take 'til we learn? *Radiology* 1991;181:17.
23. Chambers TP, Baron RL, Lush RM. Hepatic CT enhancement: Part II. Alterations in contrast material volume and rate of injection within the same patients. *Radiology* 1994;193:518.
24. Chambers TP, Baron RL, Lush RM. Hepatic CT enhancement: Part I. Alterations in the volume of contrast material within the same patients. *Radiology* 1994;193:513.
25. Heiken JP, Brink JA, McClennan BL, Sagel SS, Crowe TM, Gaines MV. Dynamic incremental CT: effect of volume and concentration of contrast material and patient weight on hepatic enhancement. *Radiology* 1995;195:353.
26. Freeny PC, Gardner JC, von Ingersleben G, Heyano S, Nghiem HV, Winter TC. Hepatic helical CT: effect of reduction of iodine dose of intravenous contrast material on hepatic contrast enhancement. *Radiology* 1995;197:89.
27. Brink JA, Heiken JP, Forman HP, Sagel SS, Molina PL, Brown PC. Hepatic spiral CT: reduction of dose of intravenous contrast material. *Radiology* 1995;197:83.
28. Heiken JP, Brink JA, McClennan BL, Sagel SS, Forman HP, DiCroce J. Dynamic contrast-enhanced CT of the liver: comparison of contrast

medium injection rates and uniphasic and biphasic injection protocols. *Radiology* 1993;187:327.

29. Paushter DM, Zeman RK, Scheibler ML, Choyke PL, Jaffe MH, Clark LR. CT evaluation of suspected hepatic metastases: comparison of techniques for IV contrast enhancement. *AJR Am J Roentgenol* 1989; 152:267.

30. Barnes PA, Thomas JL, Bernardino ME. Pitfalls in the diagnosis of hepatic cysts by computed tomography. *Radiology* 1981;141:129.

31. Wooten WB, Bernardino ME, Goldstein HM. Computed tomography of necrotic hepatic metastases. *AJR Am J Roentgenol* 1978;131:839.

32. Freeny PC, Marks WM. Hepatic hemangioma: dynamic bolus CT. *AJR Am J Roentgenol* 1986;147:711.

33. Freeny PC, Marks WM. Patterns of contrast enhancement of benign and malignant hepatic neoplasms during bolus dynamic and delayed CT. *Radiology* 1986;160:613.

34. Quinn SF, Benjamin GG. Hepatic cavernous hemangiomas: simple diagnostic sign with dynamic bolus CT. *Radiology* 1992;182:545.

35. Gaa J, Saini S, Ferrucci JT. Perfusion characteristics of hepatic cavernous hemangioma using intravenous CT angiography (IVCTA). *Eur J Radiol* 1991;12:228.

36. Jones EC, Chezmar JL, Nelson RC, Bernardino ME. The frequency and significance of small (less than or equal to 15 mm) hepatic lesions detected by CT. *AJR Am J Roentgenol* 1992;158:535.

37. Ottmar MD, Gonda RLJ, Leithauser KJ, Gutierrez OH. Liver function tests in patients with computed tomography demonstrated hepatic metastases. *Gastrointest Radiol* 1989;14:55.

38. Miller WJ, Baron RL, Dodd GD III, Federle MP. Malignancies in patients with cirrhosis: CT sensitivity and specificity in 200 consecutive transplant patients. *Radiology* 1994;193:645.

39. Freeny PC, Baron RL, Teefey SA. Hepatocellular carcinoma: reduced frequency of typical findings with dynamic contrast-enhanced CT in a non-Asian population. *Radiology* 1992;182:143.

40. Stevens WR, Johnson CD, Stephens DH, Batts KP. CT findings in hepatocellular carcinoma: correlation of tumor characteristics with causative factors, tumor size, and histologic tumor grade. *Radiology* 1994;191:531.

41. Teefey SA, Stephens DH, James EM, et al. Computed tomography and ultrasonography of hepatoma. *Clin Radiol* 1986;37:339.

42. Yoshikawa J, Matsui O, Takashima T, et al. Fatty metamorphosis in hepatocellular carcinoma: radiologic features in 10 cases. *AJR Am J Roentgenol* 1988;151:717.

43. Mathieu D, Grenier P, Larde D, Vasile N. Portal vein involvement in hepatocellular carcinoma: dynamic CT features. *Radiology* 1984;152: 127.

44. Schertz LD, Lee JKT, Heiken JP, Molina PL, Totty WG. Proton spectroscopic imaging (Dixon method) of the liver: clinical utility. *Radiology* 1989;173:401.

45. Ohtomo K, Baron RL, Dodd GD III, et al. Confluent hepatic fibrosis in advanced cirrhosis: appearance at CT. *Radiology* 1993;188:31.

46. Bernardino ME, Erwin BC, Steinberg HV, Baumgartner BR, Torres WE, Gedgaudas-McClees RK. Delayed hepatic CT scanning: increased confidence and improved detection of hepatic metastases. *Radiology* 1986;159:71.

47. Miller DL, Simmons JT, Chang R, et al. Hepatic metastasis detection: comparison of three CT contrast enhancement methods. *Radiology* 1987;165:785.

48. Phillips VM, Erwin BC, Bernardino ME. Delayed iodine scanning of the liver: promising CT technique. *J Comput Assist Tomogr* 1985;9:415.

49. Nelson RC. Techniques for computed tomography of the liver. *Radiol Clin North Am* 1991;29:1251.

50. Bressler EL, Alpern MB, Glazer GM, Francis IR, Ensminger WD. Hypervascular hepatic metastases: CT evaluation. *Radiology* 1987; 162:49.

51. DuBrow RA, David CL, Libshitz HI, et al. Detection of hepatic metastases in breast cancer: the role of nonenhanced and enhanced CT scanning. *J Comput Assist Tomogr* 1990;14:366.

52. Patten RM, Byun J-Y, Freeny PC. CT of hypervascular hepatic tumors: are unenhanced scans necessary for diagnosis. *AJR Am J Roentgenol* 1993;161:979.

53. Oliver JH, Baron RL, Federle MP, Rockette HP. Detecting hepatocellular carcinoma: the value of unenhanced or arterial phase CT imaging or both used in conjunction with conventional portal venous phase contrast-enhanced CT imaging. *AJR Am J Roentgenol* 1996;167:71.

54. Freeny PC, Marks WM. Computed tomographic arteriography of the liver. *Radiology* 1983;148:193.

55. Freeny PC, Marks WM. Hepatic perfusion abnormalities during CT angiography: detection and interpretation. *Radiology* 1986;159:685.

56. Nakakuma K, Tashiro S, Hiraoka T, Ogata K, Ootsuka K. Hepatocellular carcinoma and metastatic cancer detected by iodized oil. *Radiology* 1985;154:15.

57. Merine D, Takayasu K, Wakao F. Detection of hepatocellular carcinoma: comparison of CT during arterial portography with CT after intraarterial injection of iodized oil. *Radiology* 1990;175:707.

58. Taourel PG, Pageaux GP, Coste V, et al. Small hepatocellular carcinoma in patients undergoing liver transplantation: detection with CT after injection of iodized oil. *Radiology* 1995;197:377.

59. Small WC, Mehard WB, Langmo LS, et al. Preoperative determination of the resectability of hepatic tumors: efficacy of CT during arterial portography. *AJR Am J Roentgenol* 1993;161:319.

60. Fernandez MP, Bernardino ME. Hepatic pseudolesions: appearance of focal low attenuation in the medial segment of the left lobe at CT-arterial portography. *Radiology* 1991;181:809.

61. Peterson MS, Baron RL, Dodd GD III, et al. Hepatic parenchymal perfusion defects detected with CTAP: imaging–pathologic correlation. *Radiology* 1992;185:149.

62. Semelka RC, Shoenut JP, Kroeker M, et a. Focal liver disease: comparison of dynamic contrast-enhanced CT and T2-weighted fat-suppressed, FLASH, and dynamic gadolinium-enhanced MR imaging at 1.5T. *Radiology* 1992;184:687.

63. Carr D, Brown J, Bydder GM, et al. Gadolinium-DTPA as a contrast agent in MRI: initial clinical experience in 20 patients. *AJR Am J Roentgenol* 1984;143:215.

64. Peterson MS, Baron RL, Murakami T. Dynamic gadolinium-enhanced MR imaging of hepatic malignancies: utility of arterial and portal venous phase images (Abstract). *Radiology* 1995;197(P):176.

65. Stark DD, Felder RC, Wittenberg J, et al. Magnetic resonance imaging of cavernous hemangioma of the liver: tissue-specific characterization. *AJR Am J Roentgenol* 1985;145:213.

66. Wittenberg J, Stark DD, Forman BH, et al. Differentiation of hepatic metastases from hepatic hemangiomas and cysts by using MR imaging. *AJR Am J Roentgenol* 1988;151:79.

67. Bennett GL, Petersein A, Saini S, Hahn PF, Mayo-Smith WW, Gazelle GS. Liver lesion characterization: gadolinium chelates are not necessary for differentiating hemangiomas from metastases (Abstract). *Radiology* 1995;197(P):175.

68. Yoshida H, Itai Y, Ohtomo K, Kokubo T, Minami M, Yashiro N. Small hepatocellular carcinoma and cavernous hemangioma: differentiation with dynamic FLASH MR imaging with Gd-DTPA. *Radiology* 1989;171:339.

69. Itoh K, Nishimura K, Togashi K, et al. Hepatocellular carcinoma: MR imaging. *Radiology* 1987;164:21.

70. Kadoya M, Matsui O, Takashima T, et al. Hepatocellular carcinoma: correlation of MR imaging and histopathologic findings. *Radiology* 1992;183:819.

71. Zirinsky K, Markisz JA, Auh YH, et al. MR imaging of portal venous thrombosis: correlation with CT and sonography. *AJR Am J Roentgenol* 1988;150:283.

72. Levy HM, Newhouse JH. MR imaging of portal vein thrombosis. *AJR Am J Roentgenol* 1988;151:283.

73. Silverman PM, Patt RH, Garra BS, et al. MR imaging of the portal venous system: value of gradient-echo imaging as an adjunct to spin-echo imaging. *AJR Am J Roentgenol* 1991;157:297.

74. Rofsky NM, Weinreb JC, Bernardino ME, Young SW, Lee JK, Noz ME. Hepatocellular tumors: characterization with Mn-DPDP-enhanced MR imaging. *Radiology* 1993;188:53.

75. Hamm B, Vogl TJ, Branding G, et al. Focal liver lesions: MR imaging with Mn-DPDP—initial clinical results in 40 patients. *Radiology* 1992; 182:167.

76. Stark DD, Weissleder R, Elizondo G, et al. Superparamagnetic iron oxide: clinical application as a contrast agent for MR imaging of the liver. *Radiology* 1988;168:297.

77. Murakami T, Baron RL, Peterson MS, et al. Hepatocellular carcinoma: MR imaging with mangafodipir trisodium (Mn-DPDP). *Radiology* 1996;200:69.

78. Violante MR, Baggs RB, Tuthill T, et al. Particle-stabilized bubbles for enhanced organ ultrasound imaging. *Invest Radiol* 1991;26:S194.

79. Little A, Ferris J, Baron RL, Dodd GD. Image-guided percutaneous

hepatic biopsy: effect of ascites on the complication rate. *Radiology* 1996;199:79.

80. Livraghi T, Festi D, Monti F, Salmi A, Vettori C. US-guided percutaneous alcohol injection of small hepatic and abdominal tumors. *Radiology* 1986;161:309.

81. Lundstedt C, Ekberg H, Hederstrom E, Stridbeck H, Torfason B, Transberg KG. Radiologic diagnosis of liver metastases in colo-rectal carcinoma: prospective evaluation of the accuracy of angiography, ultrasonography, computed tomography and computed tomographic angiography. *Acta Radiol* 1987;28:431.

82. Dodd GD III, Miller WJ, Baron RL, Skolnick ML, Campbell WL. Detection of malignant tumors in end-stage cirrhotic livers: efficacy of sonography as a screening technique. *AJR Am J Roentgenol* 1992;159:727.

83. Gibney RG, Hendin AP, Cooperberg PL. Sonographically detected hepatic hemangiomas: absence of change over time. *AJR Am J Roentgenol* 1987;149:953.

84. Taylor KJ, Ramos I, Morse SS, Fortune KL, Hammers L, Taylor CR. Focal liver masses: differential diagnosis with pulsed Doppler US. *Radiology* 1987;164:643.

85. Numata K, Tanaka K, Mitsui K, Morimoto M, Inoue S, Yonezawa H. Flow characteristics of hepatic tumors at color Doppler sonography: correlation with arteriographic findings. *AJR Am J Roentgenol* 1993; 160:515.

86. Leen E, Goldberg JA, Robertson J, et al. Detection of hepatic metastases using duplex/color Doppler sonography. *Ann Surg* 1991;214: 599.

87. Sugarbaker PH, Nelson RC, Murray DR, Chezmar JL, Bernardino ME. A segmental approach to computerized tomographic portography for hepatic resection. *Surg Gynecol Obstet* 1990;171:189.

88. Ros PR, Freeny PC, Harms SE, et al. Hepatic MR imaging with ferumoxides: a multicenter clinical trial of the safety and efficacy in the detection of focal hepatic lesions. *Radiology* 1995;196:481.

CHAPTER 8

Surgical Treatment of Hepatic Metastases

Kelly M. McMasters and Mark S. Roh

The metastasis in the liver was removed by the transthoracic transdiaphragmatic approach. . . . A wedge removal of normal liver tissue varies from messy to alarming . . . The question was—how much blood? . . . The first incision into the liver outside the edge of the swelling produced an alarming gush of blood, which was soon seen to be coming from a divided vessel. In securing this vessel it was clear that the haemostat cut through the liver tissue like butter, but met with a resistance that could be appreciated when it reached the firmer tissue of Glisson's capsule in which the bleeding vessel lay. Thereupon the knife was laid aside.

—*Sir Heneage Ogilvie (1953)*

HISTORY OF HEPATIC RESECTION FOR METASTASES

Before the early 1900s, there were sporadic reports of liver resection, mainly for penetrating trauma. Most successful liver operations during this period were not major resections. L. McLane Tiffany of Baltimore has been credited with the first liver resection in the United States, in 1890. He debrided a walnut-sized mass of biliary calculi and debris from the left lobe of the liver, and it is unclear whether he resected any liver parenchyma. William Williams Keen of Jefferson Medical College in Philadelphia probably performed the first formal liver resection for tumor in the United States, in 1892. He performed three liver resections in the 1890s. Obvious concerns over hemorrhage and the technical challenge of performing major hepatic resections posed major obstacles to most surgeons. Results during this period were uniformly abysmal, with strikingly high mortality. Although Von Haberer in 1909, Wendell in 1910, Myer-May and Tung in 1939, Donovan and Santulli in 1945, Hershey in 1945, Honjo and Araki in

1949, and Lortat-Jacob and Robert in 1952 are all credited with early "anatomic" liver resections, it was the renewed interest in liver anatomy in the post-World War II period that led to rapid technical advances. With Couinaud's classification of the segmental anatomy of the liver in 1954, elective liver resection became more widespread. Brunschwig, Pack, and others in New York, Longmire and colleagues in Los Angeles, and McDermott and associates in Boston were early pioneers in the United States. Similar advances took place simultaneously in Asia. The first human liver transplantation by Starzl in 1963 signalled the beginning of a new era in liver surgery (1,2). A collective review of liver resections by Foster was presented before the James Ewing Society in 1970 (3). In this series, he reported 296 adult patients undergoing major hepatic resection for primary liver cancer with an operative mortality of 24%. Foster also reported 115 patients who underwent liver resection for metastatic lesions with an operative mortality rate of 17.3% and a 21% 5-year survival rate. This report provided support for performing liver resection for metastatic disease, which was very controversial at the time. Further support for liver resection for metastases was provided in the landmark monograph of Foster and Berman in 1977 (1). Other reports by Honjo and Mizumoto in 1974 (4), Lin in 1976 (5), Cady et al. in 1979 (6), Starzl et al. in 1980 (7), and Fortner et al. in 1981 (8) provided large series that established that major liver resection could be done safely, with operative mortality rates between 3% and 12%. Many other published series soon followed, but it was the pioneering work of Hughes and colleagues in establishing the Registry of Hepatic Metastases that defined the modern indications and results of liver resection for metastatic disease (9–11). Debate about the merits of surgical intervention in the face of liver metastases continues today, especially with the advent of new technology (cryosurgery, hepatic artery infusion chemotherapy, isolated liver perfusion therapy, and various interstitial therapies).

K. M. McMasters: University of Louisville-Brown Cancer Center, Louisville, Kentucky 40202.

M. S. Roh: Department of Surgical Oncology, University of Texas M. D. Anderson Cancer Center, Houston, Texas 77030.

COLORECTAL CANCER METASTATIC TO THE LIVER

Incidence and Natural History

Approximately 150,000 new cases of colorectal cancer are diagnosed each year in the United States (12). It is estimated that 15% to 25% of patients have liver metastases at the time of diagnosis of the primary tumor (13, 14). Metastatic disease develops in another 20% to 30% after resection of the primary tumor (15). Overall, synchronous or metachronous metastatic disease develops in at least 50% of patients with colorectal cancer (75,000 per year). Of these, about 60% (45,000) will have liver metastases (16), but only 20% (15,000) will have metastatic disease confined to the liver (17,18). Only about 25% of patients with liver-only metastases (3750) will have lesions that are amenable to resection (18–21). If all of these patients with resectable lesions were to undergo potentially curative surgical therapy, at most 30% (1125 patients) would be expected to survive more than 5 years (9,22–34). Although surgery offers the only chance for long-term survival in patients with liver metastases from colorectal cancer, it is apparent that only a small subset of patients with metastases can expect to benefit from surgical resection or ablation.

The diagnosis of liver metastases from colorectal cancer carries a poor prognosis. An analysis by Hughes et al. (10) of 1650 patients in the English literature with unresected colorectal metastases revealed only 11 5-year survivors. Only four of these patients had a histologically confirmed diagnosis of liver metastasis, and all of these patients died of their metastatic disease after 5 years. In a large series reported by Scheele and colleagues, there were no 5-year survivors among 983 patients with unresected colorectal liver metastases (27). Median survival was 14.2 months (N = 62) for patients with technically resectable metastases confined to the liver who did not undergo resection, and 6.9 months for patients with unresectable disease (N = 921) due to extensive hepatic disease, extrahepatic disease, or both. It seems reasonable to conclude that liver metastasis from colorectal cancer is almost uniformly fatal within 5 years of diagnosis. Although historical controls are never optimal, any treatment that achieves substantial 5-year survival in patients with liver metastases from colorectal cancer is believed to be meaningful.

Treatment Options

Systemic Chemotherapy

Because the detection of liver metastases heralds the development of systemic disease in most patients, systemic treatment is most appropriate. The ultimate demise of most patients with metastatic colorectal cancer, however, is often related to the tumor burden within the liver. In general, the response rate of hepatic metastases to chemotherapy correlates with the response rate of extrahepatic metastases from colorectal cancer. There are no good data, however, concerning the response rates and survival of patients with resectable liver metastases who receive systemic chemotherapy and do not undergo resection (35–37).

The most effective single agent against metastatic colorectal cancer is 5-fluorouracil (5-FU). Bolus administration of 5-FU alone results in variable response rates depending on the treatment schedule and the definition of response. In general, higher dose intensity correlates with better response rates, although toxicity is significant with more aggressive treatment regimens (38). Although a response rate of approximately 20% has been widely accepted in the literature (35–37), more recent studies using strict definitions of response suggest that the response rate of 5-FU bolus treatment is closer to 10% (38,39). Prolonged continuous infusion of 5-FU is more effective than bolus regimens and is associated with decreased toxicity. In one study using strict criteria for response, continuous infusion of 5-FU generated an overall response of 30%, compared with 7% for bolus treatment (39). However, there was no significant survival difference (median survival was 10 months for continuous infusion vs. 11 months for bolus 5-FU). Although survival may be prolonged among patients who respond to 5-FU, even the most effective 5-FU regimens have not improved overall survival reproducibly (35–37).

Various combination chemotherapy regimens based on 5-FU have been tested. Regimens consisting of 5-FU in combination with methylcyclohexylnitrosurea (methyl CCNU), vincristine, streptozotocin, methotrexate, mitomycin C, or cisplatin have been tested (35–37). The results of these trials may be summarized simply: variable response rates, increased toxicity, and no improvement in overall survival. Conventional combination chemotherapy has no proven benefit and is not recommended as standard treatment for metastatic colorectal cancer.

Modulation of 5-FU with leucovorin improves response rates in patients with metastatic colorectal cancer and may prolong survival. Of six prospective, randomized trials comparing intravenous 5-FU alone with 5-FU plus leucovorin in patients with metastatic colorectal cancer, five demonstrated higher response rates, and two demonstrated modest but statistically significant increases in overall survival for the combination regimen (40–45). The improvement in median survival was from 9.6 to 12.6 months (41) or from 7.7 to 12.2 months (44) for the groups receiving 5-FU or 5-FU plus leucovorin, respectively. Based on these results, the combination of 5-FU and leucovorin has become standard therapy for metastatic colorectal cancer.

It must be remembered, however, that regardless of the agents used, chemotherapy for colorectal liver metastases is only palliative, and confers no meaningful chance for long-term survival. Survival in most modern series is between 8 and 14 months for patients with metastatic colorectal cancer treated with chemotherapy. Although further trials are in progress, including agents such as alpha-interferon, it is doubtful that systemic chemotherapy with available agents will have a major impact on the course of colorectal metastases to the liver.

Regional Chemotherapy

Because the liver is the most frequent site of colorectal metastases, and metastatic disease within the liver is often the cause of death in these patients, regional treatments to prevent or treat liver metastases are theoretically attractive.

Portal Vein Infusion

Liver metastases that present soon after resection of the primary tumor (6 to 24 months) probably were present microscopically at the time of surgery. Several studies have investigated the adjuvant administration of chemotherapeutic agents (mainly 5-FU) through portal vein catheters placed at the time of resection of the primary tumor in an attempt to prevent or treat liver micrometastases. Taylor et al. (46) conducted the first randomized trial of adjuvant portal vein infusion of 5-FU, which demonstrated a decrease in subsequent development of liver metastases. Based on these results, several large, prospective, randomized trials comparing intraportal chemotherapy with surgery alone were initiated. In a follow-up study by Taylor and colleagues (47), a survival benefit was demonstrated in patients receiving adjuvant intraportal chemotherapy versus control subjects. However, a large randomized trial of 1158 patients with Dukes' A, B, and C colon cancers (NSABP C-02) did not demonstrate a decrease in the incidence of liver metastases in patients receiving intraportal chemotherapy. A significant disease-free survival advantage was apparent, although this was attributed to systemic effects of 5-FU (48). Additional trials have not demonstrated consistent benefit in terms of decreased incidence of liver metastases or increased overall survival (49–56).

Hepatic Artery Infusion

There has been much interest in hepatic artery infusion of chemotherapeutic agents for the treatment of colorectal liver metastases. The most effective drug for hepatic artery delivery is the 5-FU derivative, 5-FU deoxyribonucleoside (FUDR), because 90% of the drug is extracted in the first pass through the liver and less drug is delivered systemically (57,58). Early studies of chemotherapy delivered through the hepatic artery for colorectal liver metastases used external catheters and pumps and were associated with high complication rates, including hepatic artery thrombosis and catheter displacement (59–66). Subsequently, implantable pump and catheter systems were found to be associated with fewer complications (67–69) and were cost effective (70).

Several studies have investigated hepatic artery chemotherapy by implantable pumps using FUDR alone or in combination with other agents for the treatment of hepatic metastases from colorectal cancer. Response rates up to 88% have been reported for intra-arterial chemotherapy, and response to intra-arterial therapy has consistently exceeded that of systemic chemotherapy by two- to threefold (71–80). Although the response rates have been impressive, the effect on overall survival has been disappointing. Prospective, randomized trials conducted by the National Cancer Institute (80) and the Mayo Consortium (81) comparing systemic and intra-arterial chemotherapy failed to demonstrate a difference in overall survival, although subset analysis excluding patients with extra-hepatic (nodal) disease suggested a survival benefit to intra-arterial chemotherapy. The results of two other large studies from Memorial Sloan-Kettering Cancer Center (82) and the Northern California Oncology Group (83) comparing systemic FUDR to hepatic artery infusion of FUDR failed to demonstrate a survival difference. However, the results of these studies are confounded by a crossover provision: patients failing systemic therapy could subsequently receive intra-arterial therapy. If the crossover groups are excluded from analysis, prolonged survival is suggested for the groups receiving intra-arterial therapy. The only randomized study to demonstrate a statistically significant difference in overall survival was conducted in Paris and compared intravenous 5-FU to hepatic arterial infusion of FUDR in patients with colorectal liver metastases (84). The response rate among 82 patients receiving systemic 5-FU was 14% versus 49% in the intra-arterial group. Survival was significantly better for patients treated with intra-arterial FUDR (15 months) compared with those treated with intravenous 5-FU (11 months).

More recently, intra-arterial administration of FUDR plus leucovorin was evaluated in 66 patients with liver metastases from colorectal cancer (78). One- and 2-year survival rates were 86% and 62%, respectively, with a median survival of 28.8 months. The 5-year survival rate was only 7%, however. Biliary sclerosis occurred in 14% of patients. Although this was not a randomized, controlled trial, and is subject to all of the biases of an uncontrolled trial, the survival data are substantially better than other studies of systemic or intra-arterial chemotherapy. Therefore, the combination of intra-arterial FUDR and leucovorin deserves further study, and less toxic regimens are being tested.

After liver resection for metastases from colorectal cancer, recurrent metastatic disease develops in approximately 70% of patients, and half of these patients recur within the liver (10). Adjuvant hepatic arterial infusion chemotherapy of 5-FU after resection of liver metastases was studied in 20 patients in an attempt to reduce the rate of recurrent liver metastases (85). With a median follow-up of 33 months, 50% of patients experienced recurrence, 17% of which were in the liver only. Median survival was 39 months for patients without recurrence and 27 months for patients with recurrence. Others have investigated adjuvant hepatic artery chemotherapy after liver resection (86,87), but insufficient data are available to draw firm conclusions. A phase II, randomized, prospective trial of multiple metastasectomy combined with systemic and hepatic artery infusion chemotherapy for colorectal cancer metastatic to the liver conducted by the North Central Cancer Treatment Group is in progress.

Other agents are being investigated for intra-arterial chemotherapy. In a pilot study, hepatic artery infusion of interleukin-2 in combination with 5-FU and mitomycin C was performed in three patients with multiple liver metastases from colorectal cancer (88). Complete remission was obtained in all three patients as assessed by computed tomography (CT) scan and carcinoembryonic antigen (CEA) levels 2 to 3 months after treatment. One patient had a pelvic recurrence 14 months after starting treatment, whereas the other patients were still in remission at 25 and 22 months. Although preliminary, these results are impressive and will need to be confirmed. In an attempt to deliver higher doses of chemotherapy to the liver and minimize toxicity, a novel system that combines hepatic artery infusion chemotherapy with complete hepatic venous isolation and extracorporeal chemofiltration has been devised. Using this system, the total hepatic venous outflow was captured by a novel dual-balloon catheter placed in the inferior vena cava, filtered through an extracorporeal circuit containing carbon chemofilters to remove the chemotherapeutic agents from the circulation, and returned to the patient. A phase I trial suggests promise for this technology (89).

Overall, it is clear that chemotherapy delivered by hepatic arterial infusion results in considerable response rates that may confer a survival advantage in patients with metastatic disease confined to the liver. In an attempt to control the development of extrahepatic disease as well, combinations of systemic and intra-arterial chemotherapy have been tested in patients with colorectal liver metastases. One study comparing intra-arterial FUDR alone to the combination of intra-arterial and systemic FUDR demonstrated a decrease in the development of extrahepatic disease with combination therapy, but no survival difference (90). Other studies have demonstrated the feasibility of combination systemic and intra-arterial therapy (86,91–93), but the impact of this combination treatment on survival is not clear.

In summary, chemotherapy administered by hepatic arterial infusion results in higher response rates than systemic chemotherapy alone. The greater response has not been shown convincingly to translate into prolonged survival, probably because of the inability of this modality to control the spread of disease outside the liver. At best, intra-arterial chemotherapy is a palliative treatment for patients with unresectable liver metastases. At worst, it is an expensive, invasive, and potentially toxic therapy that provides no real benefit to the patient in terms of survival. Promising new regimens are being tested. Hepatic intra-arterial chemotherapy should not be considered standard therapy for patients with liver metastases from colorectal cancer, and should be performed only in the context of properly designed clinical trials.

Radiation Therapy

External-beam radiation therapy with and without systemic or hepatic artery infusion chemotherapy has been used for metastatic liver cancer. Radiation-induced toxicity is a major limitation, with radiation hepatitis, hepatic necrosis, and biliary fibrosis occurring at doses above 30 Gy (94–96). Unfortunately, this dose of radiation is tumoricidal in only a minority of patients, which explains the overall poor response to conventional external beam radiation therapy (97–99). Hepatic arterial infusion of 5-FU or FUDR as radiation sensitizers in combination with external beam radiation therapy resulted in responses ranging from 33% to 83%, although the duration of response was limited. Hepatic toxicity occurred in up to 30% of cases (100–105). The rationale for these regimens is that metastatic tumors derive most of their blood supply from branches of the hepatic artery, whereas the normal liver parenchyma receives most of its blood supply from the portal vein; intra-arterial chemotherapy with 5-FU or FUDR maximizes the exposure of the tumors to the radiosensitizers and minimizes the dose to the normal liver tissue (57,58). In an attempt to limit hepatic toxicity from radiation, Lawrence et al. (106) introduced the concept of dose–volume analysis for external-beam radiation to the liver. This is based on the fact that the tolerance of the liver to radiation depends both on the dose of radiation and the volume of liver treated. By combining boost treatment to gross tumor within the liver, concurrent use of intra-arterial FUDR, and hyperfractionation (1.5-Gy fractions given twice per day greater than 4 hours apart), up to 60 Gy was safely administered to the area of the tumor. In this study, a 48% objective response rate was observed, with an 8-month median duration of response. Although these techniques allow safe administration of doses of radiation that are potentially tumoricidal to the liver, more thorough investigation is necessary before external-beam radiation therapy is accepted as a safe and useful treatment modality for liver metastases.

Interstitial radiation therapy has been attempted to deliver higher doses or radiation directly to the tumor. In one study, 12 patients with inoperable liver metastases received iridium-192 implants at the time of exploratory laparotomy. The number of lesions treated varied from 1 to 11. In 10 patients with elevated CEA levels before treatment, 6 showed a decline in CEA within 2.5 months of treatment. Long-term follow-up is not yet available (107,108).

Percutaneous placement under ultrasound guidance of a high-intensity iridium-192 source directly into liver metastases from colorectal cancer has been performed in six patients (109). One-month follow-up revealed 25% regression in one patient and nonprogression in the remainder. Further investigation is warranted, but as yet there is no proven benefit for external beam or interstitial radiation therapy in the treatment of liver metastases.

Other Treatments

Various interstitial therapies have been designed to ablate liver tumors using freezing, hyperthermia, or chemical fixation (108).

Cryosurgery

Cryosurgery has been investigated for ablation of primary and metastatic liver tumors, and is discussed at length in Chapter 10. Initial results of cryosurgery for unresectable liver metastases have been comparable to those of surgical resection (110–116). This technique is appealing because it directs cryoablation to the tumors themselves, with minimal destruction of normal hepatic parenchyma. Previous experience with cryosurgery was limited to lesions deemed unresectable because of bilaterality, anatomic location, or comorbid disease. An expanded role for cryosurgery is being investigated as an adjunct to surgical resection. In patients with multiple liver metastases, cryoablation of deep central lesions or lesions close to major vascular structures can be used in combination with resection of more accessible lesions. This allows for an aggressive approach to multiple bilobar lesions combining cryoablation, segmental, and lobar resection. Because the fatal outcome of unresected liver metastases is certain, an aggressive approach to render the patient free of disease is worth studying and may improve the results of surgical treatment of liver metastases.

Hyperthermia

Hyperthermia can be induced by radiofrequency or microwave techniques, ultrasound, or laser technology. Of these, laser treatment appears the most promising (108). In an initial study, a neodymium–yttrium-aluminum garnet laser was used for ablation of hepatic tumors (117). At laparotomy, a quartz fiber tip was inserted into the tumor under intraoperative ultrasound guidance in two patients with hepatocellular carcinoma and eight patients with metastatic colorectal cancer. All patients had declines in alpha-fetoprotein or CEA levels, although survival was not mentioned. Another study examined the use of a similar laser in four patients with advanced liver malignancy. In one patient, an abscess developed within the area of necrosis, and one patient died from an air embolus when coaxial gas was used to cool the sapphire tip on the fiber (118).

Percutaneous placement of the laser fiber under ultrasound guidance was performed in 8 patients with 13 liver metastases and no extrahepatic disease (108). The average tumor diameter was 3 cm (range, 1.5 to 6 cm) in six patients with metastases from colorectal cancer and one each with gastric and breast cancer. No complications were observed. CT scans performed 6 to 8 weeks after treatment revealed that 6 of 13 metastases had greater then 50% necrosis, 2 metastases had less than 25% necrosis, and the remainder had no obvious necrosis or had increased in size. In general, the best responses were in the smaller metastases. Although still investigational, this technique has the advantages of being a minimally invasive technique targeted directly at the metastatic sites within the liver.

Alcohol Injection

Direct injection of ethanol into liver tumors is an effective method of providing palliation and occasionally cure of small (<3 cm) hepatocellular cancers. Several series have demonstrated that ethanol injection of small hepatocellular carcinomas results in survival rates that are comparable with or better than surgical resection (119–127). Mortality is rare, and major complications (intraperitoneal hemorrhage, shock, liver infarction, hemobilia) are infrequent, although pain and fever are common. Percutaneous injection of hot saline may be as effective as ethanol injection (128).

Little experience with percutaneous ethanol injection for metastatic liver tumors has been reported. Livraghi (129) treated a total of 30 patients with liver metastases, 29 of them with 51 focal lesions and 1 patient with 40% of the liver replaced by tumor. Primary tumors were colorectal in 19, gastric in 4, endocrine in 3, and 1 abdominal leiomyosarcoma. Response rates were related to size of the metastases, with complete response in 13 of 17 lesions <2 cm, 4 of 16 lesions 2 to 3 cm in size, 1 of 10 lesions 3 to 4 cm, and 0 of 8 lesions >4 cm. Survival data were not available. Hisa et al. (130) reported treatment of six patients with liver metastases by ethanol injection, and found that survival rates paralleled those of patients with hepatocellular carcinoma treated similarly. The site of the primary tumors was not mentioned, however.

Ethanol injection has been shown to be effective as a treatment for small hepatocellular carcinomas. Further study is necessary to determine if there is a role for this therapy for treatment of metastatic tumors to the liver. Ethanol injection may prove to be a useful modality for patients who are poor operative risks because of comorbid disease, or for patients with multiple small bilobar lesions that preclude resection.

Chemoembolization

Hepatic artery embolization or chemoembolization is a useful modality for palliation of hepatocellular carcinoma (131–133), as well as liver metastases from islet cell tumors (134), carcinoid tumors (135,136), and gastrointestinal leiomyosarcomas (137). The common denominator in determining response to chemoembolization is the hypervascularity of these types of liver tumors. No significant antitumor response has been demonstrated using embolization alone, chemoembolization with FUDR, or chemoembolization with cisplatin in patients with liver metastases from colorectal cancer, probably because of the relatively hypovascular nature of these tumors (70).

Hepatic Resection

Many excellent reviews and atlases are available that describe the technical aspects of hepatic resection. This section emphasizes the important technical aspects of liver resection used at M. D. Anderson (138,139).

Preoperative Evaluation

Because only a small fraction of patients with liver metastases have disease that is both confined to the liver and technically resectable, thorough preoperative staging is essential to prevent unnecessary abdominal exploration in patients with short life expectancy. Once liver metastases are diagnosed, it is imperative to search for contraindications to resection. Therefore, only lesions that can be resected with a negative margin should be considered. The presence of noncontiguous extrahepatic disease in lymph nodes or elsewhere (lung, peritoneum, adrenal, and other sites) should be considered a contraindication to resection. Only anecdotal 5-year survivors have been reported after liver resection in the face of extrahepatic disease. Although there is no consensus on the limits in terms of number of liver metastases that should be resected, survival is worse for patients with more than three or four liver metastases. Only patients with potentially resectable disease, no evidence of extrahepatic metastases, and acceptable operative risk should be explored.

Preoperative staging includes a history and physical examination focused on signs and symptoms of recurrent, metachronous, or metastatic disease, including rectal examination and stool guaiac testing. In addition, basic laboratory tests (complete blood count, liver function tests, coagulation profile, CEA level) and chest radiograph are obtained. Colonoscopy should be performed to check for metachronous lesions or recurrent disease if resection of the primary lesion was performed more than 3 months previously. Patients referred for surgical consultation usually have had an imaging study already performed (ultrasound, CT, or magnetic resonance imaging). The quality of this study may not be acceptable for accurate staging. A good-quality CT of the abdomen and pelvis with fine cuts through the liver is necessary to examine not only the liver, but to look for suspect lymphadenopathy (regional, retroperitoneal, and periportal). Occasionally, CT-guided fine-needle aspiration of enlarged lymph nodes can diagnose extrahepatic disease and prevent a nontherapeutic laparotomy. A properly performed CT scan can detect 80% to 90% of liver lesions. Despite careful preoperative staging, about 30% of patients have extrahepatic disease at operation.

A dynamic CT angiogram is obtained in all patients who are considered for resection. The purpose is twofold. It is more sensitive than routine CT scan and can detect small (1 to 2 cm) metastases, which can affect the treatment plan. A celiac and superior mesenteric artery arteriogram obtained at the same time provides valuable information because approximately 30% to 40% of patients have anomalous hepatic arterial anatomy.

Preoperative risk assessment takes into account the patient's overall medical condition, cardiac and pulmonary function, as well as evaluation of hepatic function. Advanced age is not a contraindication in otherwise healthy patients. Patients with cirrhosis have a much greater chance of fatal hepatic failure after major liver resection because of inadequate hepatic reserve. Despite careful preoperative evaluation, imaging, laboratory tests, and the judgment of experienced liver surgeons, it is not always possible to determine which patients will progress to liver failure.

Preparation

Patients are admitted on the day of surgery after an outpatient bowel cleansing regimen. Before the decision to proceed with resection, only a urinary catheter and minimal intravenous lines are placed. Once the decision to proceed with major resection is made, arterial and central venous catheters are placed. A Swan-Ganz catheter is occasionally necessary in patients with suboptimal cardiac function.

The patient is placed in the supine position on an operating table that can be flexed. The arms are extended and a roll is placed under the patient at the level of the 10th and 11th ribs. The operative field to be prepared includes the entire chest, abdomen, and both groins. Although most of this surface area is never needed for routine liver resection, this preparation allows for extension of the incision to a median sternotomy or thoracoabdominal incision for control of the suprahepatic inferior vena cava (IVC).

Exploration

The abdomen is explored through a right subcostal incision. The incision should be large enough to perform thorough exploration, but not so large as to cause undue discomfort or delay in recovery for those patients in whom contraindications to resection are found. All peritoneal surfaces are examined as well as the entire length of small and large bowel. The liver surface is inspected for miliary metastases or other obvious reasons to abort the planned procedure. Mesenteric and periaortic lymph nodes are examined and sampled for biopsy if abnormally enlarged, especially in the area of the base of the inferior mesenteric artery for patients with left colon or rectal primary tumors. The lesser sac is opened to evaluate the caudate lobe and the lymph nodes along the superior aspect of the pancreas, celiac axis, and superior mesenteric artery. The porta hepatis is carefully examined for lymphadenopathy, and any abnormal nodes are sampled for biopsy. It must be kept in mind that portal lymph nodes that feel soft and fleshy may contain tumor. It is important, therefore, to send frozen-section biopsy specimens of any enlarged nodes. Limited mobilization of the liver is then performed by incising the ligamentum teres and falciform ligament. The tumors are assessed by inspection and palpation, but the liver need not be completely mobilized at this stage unless it will affect the decision to proceed with the operation. This may be necessary for tumors located close to the IVC, porta hepatis, diaphragm, or other important structures. Intraoperative ultrasound (see Chap. 7) is then performed to search for nonpalpable tumors that were not visualized on preoperative imaging studies, define the vascular anatomy, and clarify the relationship of the tumors to major vascular structures. Intraoperative ultrasound has become an essential tool not only to determine resectability, but to define the tumor–vessel relationships necessary to plan segmental resections.

Mobilization of the Liver

If no contraindication to resection is identified, the incision is extended to a bilateral subcostal incision. The Goligher sternal lifting retractor is placed to provide optimal exposure of the liver and porta hepatis. The right lobe is mobilized by gently retracting the liver anteriorly and

to the left. A sterile linen glove placed on the retracting hand of the first assistant helps to maintain retraction without slipping of the liver.

The dissection begins at the right triangular ligament, proceeds to involve the anterior and posterior coronary ligaments, and extends medially to the IVC. In our hands, the best method of dissection to avoid troublesome hemorrhage from the short hepatic veins or damage to the major hepatic veins is to use the electrocautery to divide sequentially thin layers of tissue that are exposed with a long blunt-tipped clamp. By performing the dissection in this manner, the right adrenal gland and bare area of the liver are exposed, allowing the right lobe to be rotated into the wound. A right thoracic extension of the incision may be necessary if the liver cannot be mobilized safely because of the location of the tumor or a fibrotic liver. The left lobe is mobilized, if necessary, by completing the division of the falciform ligament until the IVC is exposed. The triangular and coronary ligaments are then incised, avoiding injury to the left phrenic vein and left hepatic vein as they course along the ventral border of these ligaments.

Hepatic Resection

When the decision has been made to proceed with liver resection, the type of resection must be considered carefully. Hepatic resections can be classified as either segmental or lobar, and are based on the segmental anatomy defined by Couinaud (Fig. 1). The liver comprises eight functional units (segments), each of which possesses a separate portal pedicle and draining hepatic vein. Precise knowledge of the anatomic organization of the liver and the distribution of the portal pedicles and hepatic veins is

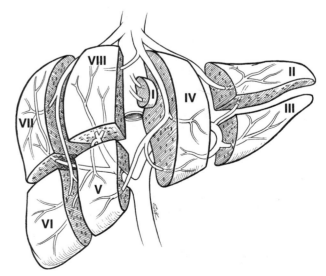

FIG. 1. Segmental anatomy of the liver as defined by Couinaud.

essential to perform liver resection safely, and especially important in planning segmental resection.

The goal of liver resection is to remove the tumor with at least a 1-cm margin of normal parenchyma. If this goal can be satisfied safely by segmental resection, there is no advantage to an anatomic lobectomy. Important factors to consider in deciding on the type of resection to perform are the size and location of the tumors. Large lesions (>4 cm) that are confined primarily to one anatomic lobe usually require a hepatic lobectomy. Tumors that are located adjacent to important intrahepatic vascular structures may require a lobectomy to be resected safely and with an adequate margin.

Lobar Resection

Right Hepatic Lobectomy

After the right lobe has been mobilized by dividing the coronary and triangular ligaments, the short hepatic veins are ligated and divided along the ventral surface of the IVC. The short hepatic veins are delicate and must be carefully ligated in continuity and divided. As the dissection proceeds cephalad, the right hepatic vein is identified. Although it is sometimes possible to encircle the right hepatic vein at this point, this maneuver is risky and can produce life-threatening hemorrhage. It should be attempted only if the ultrasound demonstrates a long (1 to 2 cm) trunk entering the IVC .

Dissection of the porta hepatis is performed next, beginning with a cholecystectomy and dissection of the common hepatic duct to expose the bifurcation. The right bile duct is dissected free, taking care to avoid troublesome bleeding from small periductal vessels. Before dividing the right duct, the left duct must be identified to avoid injury. In the event that the right duct cannot be dissected safely, it is identified and ligated during the parenchymal dissection.

The common hepatic artery is then identified and encircled with vessel loops. The right hepatic artery is identified and divided, taking care to identify and preserve the left hepatic artery. In 87% of cases, the right artery originates from the common hepatic artery to the left of the common hepatic duct and courses behind the hepatic duct. In 11% of cases, it passes in front of the duct.

With the common hepatic artery retracted to the left and the common hepatic duct retracted to the right, the portal vein is identified. The dissection is continued cephalad with both the right and left portal vein branches identified before the right portal vein is divided. Care must be taken to avoid stenosis of the left portal vein branch or thrombosis of the portal vein can result.

Division of the right portal vein and right hepatic artery provides a clear line of demarcation extending from the gallbladder bed toward the IVC. The proposed line of transection is marked on the liver surface with the electrocautery. The initial parenchymal dissection is performed with the electrocautery set to the highest intensity, cauterizing the small vascular and biliary structure near the liver surface. Once the transection has reached the 2-cm depth, large intrahepatic structures are encountered and the CUSA (Cavitron Ultrasonic Surgical Aspirator; Valley Lab, Boulder, CO) is used. When properly

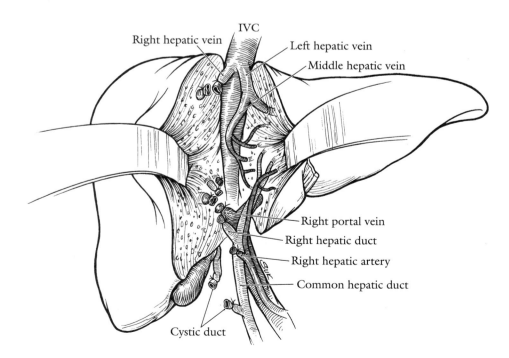

FIG. 2. Right hepatic lobectomy.

used, this device ultrasonically disrupts the hepatic parenchyma, exposing hidden arteries, ducts, and biliary radicals without dividing them. These structures can then be ligated or clipped and divided (Fig. 2).

Once the specimen has been removed, the tumor-free margins are assessed. The cut edge of the liver is treated with an argon beam coagulator, which reduces the incidence of bile leaks. If necessary, #2 chromic mattress sutures can be used to approximate the edges of the liver to further decrease the incidence of bile leak. If possible, a tongue of omentum is sutured to the cut edge of the liver. The transected falciform ligament is then reapproximated to prevent torsion and possible vascular compromise of the left lobe. Closed suction drains are are no longer routinely placed.

Left Hepatic Lobectomy

Left hepatic lobectomy is performed by dividing the falciform, triangular, and coronary ligaments to mobilize completely the left lobe. In cases in which tumor lies close to the hepatic venous drainage, mobilization of the right lobe may also be necessary. The left phrenic vein is identified, which empties into the left hepatic vein. The left and middle hepatic veins are very delicate structures and can receive multiple large side branches. The temptation to pass a right-angle clamp around the left hepatic vein must be resisted because this maneuver can produce damage to the hepatic vein branches or IVC that is extremely difficult to control. Only in rare cases is the left hepatic vein ligated before parenchymal transection.

Dissection of the porta hepatis is begun by identifying the common hepatic artery and tracing it to the bifurcation. The left hepatic artery is suture ligated and divided only after carefully identifying and preserving the right hepatic artery. Access to the common bile duct is facilitated by a cholecystectomy. The left bile duct, whose transverse part is extrahepatic, is identified, ligated, and divided after identifying and preserving the right hepatic duct.

Retraction of the common hepatic artery and the common hepatic duct exposes the portal vein. Dissection continues cephalad until the right and left branches are identified. The main trunk of the portal vein's left branch is separated into transverse and umbilical portions. The transverse part (pars transversa) is a 3.5-cm extrahepatic segment and usually gives off several small branches to adjacent liver tissue. These branches are ligated and divided. The umbilical part (pars umbilicus) curves forward as a continuation of the transverse part; it lies in the umbilical fissure and ends bluntly in an attachment to the ligamentum teres hepatis. The left portal vein branch is divided near the portal vein bifurcation and closed carefully to avoid compromising the lumen of the right portal vein.

Ligation of the left hepatic artery and portal vein produces a line of demarcation extending from the gallbladder bed to the IVC. The proposed line of transection is defined with the electrocautery, maintaining a 1-cm tumor-free margin. The parenchyma is transected as described earlier. The left hepatic vein is ligated at the end of the resection, with care taken to preserve the middle hepatic vein (Fig. 3).

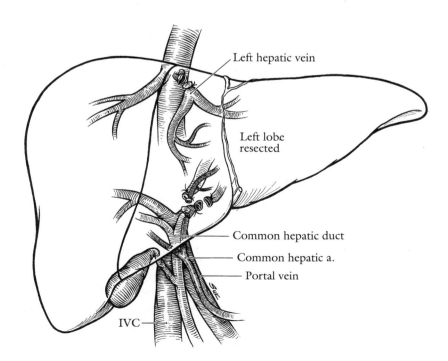

FIG. 3. Left hepatic lobectomy.

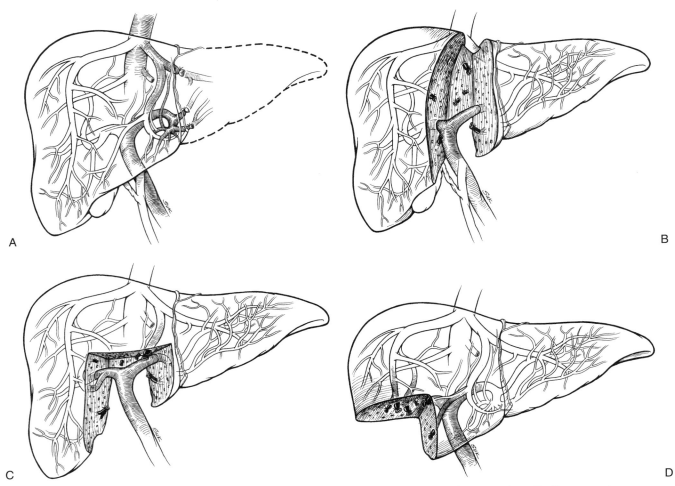

FIG. 4. A–D: Various types of segmental resection. **A:** Segment 2 and 3 resection. **B:** Segment 4 resection. **C:** Segment 4 and 5 resection. **D:** Segment 5 and 6 resection.

Trisegmentectomy

Right trisegmentectomy is a resection of the entire right lobe of the liver and the medial segment of the left lobe. The resection margin is marked by the falciform ligament. This resection removes 70% to 80% of the liver parenchyma and reduces portal venous flow by 75%. This procedure should be contemplated only in patients with normal liver function who are younger than 70 years of age. The usual indication for this procedure is a tumor located in the right anterior segment that involves the main anterior and posterior portal vein branches with extension into the medial segment of the left lobe.

Most of the steps in this procedure are identical to a formal right hepatic lobectomy. The right and left coronary and triangular ligaments are divided and the liver is mobilized to the IVC. The right bile duct, hepatic artery, and portal vein are ligated and divided, and the dissection is continued along the left hepatic artery up to its entrance at the umbilical fissure. After the hilar dissection has been completed, the entire retrohepatic vena cava and short hepatic veins are dissected away from the cau-

date lobe. Once the retrohepatic IVC has been separated from the liver, the middle and left hepatic veins are identified. The parenchyma is routinely transected using a Pringle maneuver. Care must be exercised to avoid injury to the blood supply of segments 2 and 3.

Left trisegmentectomy involves resection of the medial and lateral segments of the left lobe, the anterior segment of the right lobe, and occasionally parts of the caudate lobe. This is a difficult and potentially dangerous resection and is rarely indicated for metastatic disease (140).

Segmental Resection

Segmental resection significantly reduces blood loss, shortens operating time, lowers morbidity and mortality, and does not affect long-term survival compared with formal hepatic lobectomy. Segmental resection is particularly important to preserve liver parenchyma in patients with compromised liver function (eg, patients with cirrhosis) or if the volume of remaining liver after resection might be inadequate (eg, small left lobe). Segmentectomy

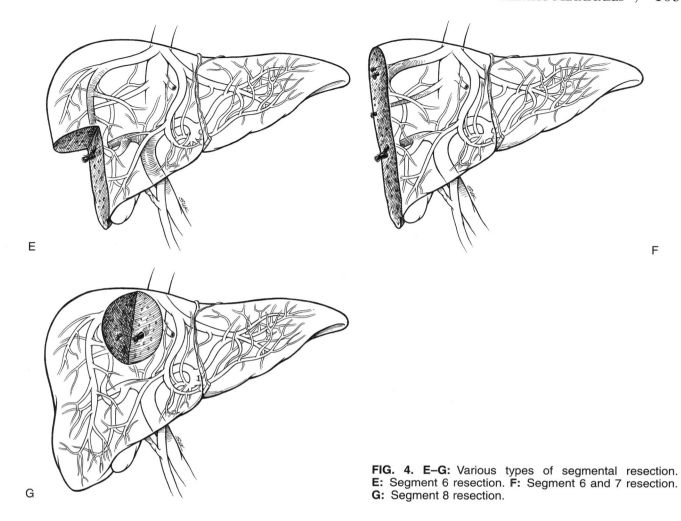

E

F

G

FIG. 4. E–G: Various types of segmental resection. **E:** Segment 6 resection. **F:** Segment 6 and 7 resection. **G:** Segment 8 resection.

also enables the surgeon to resect isolated bilobar metastases. This procedure can be performed safely in up to three isolated segments.

A segmentectomy is divided into three separate steps: 1) identification of the tumor and the involved portal pedicle and hepatic vein; 2) isolation and hemostatic control of the vascular structures; and 3) resection of the involved hepatic segments. Figure 4 illustrates various types of segmental resection.

Results of Liver Resection for Colorectal Metastases

Surgical resection of colorectal metastases to the liver in carefully selected patients improves both overall and disease-free survival, with 5-year survival rates ranging from 16% to 40% (Table 1). Operative mortality ranges from 0% to 14%, with less than 5% mortality in most modern series.

Much of our knowledge of prognostic factors in the surgical treatment of colorectal liver metastases is de-

rived from the Registry of Hepatic Metastases as reported by Hughes et al. (9–11).

The presence of extrahepatic metastases usually indicates incurable disease. Considering Registry data, the overall 5-year survival rate among 800 patients who underwent resection of metastases confined to the liver was 32%, and the 5-year disease-free survival rate was 24%. Twenty-five patients had concomitant resection of liver metastases and metastases in regional lymph nodes (celiac and hepatic). Despite resection of liver metastases and all gross nodal disease, the actuarial 5-year survival rate was only 4%, and there was only one actual 5-year survivor. Thirty-seven patients underwent resection of noncontiguous extrahepatic metastases (lung, peritoneum, adrenal, and other sites) at the time of resection of liver metastases. Despite being rendered clinically disease free by the surgical procedure, the 5-year survival rate was 20% and the 5-year disease-free survival rate was 4%. Some studies suggest that overall survival is no different among patients who undergo concomitant resection of liver and nonnodal (eg, lung) metastases compared with patients who undergo resection of metastases

TABLE 1. *Survival after hepatic resection for colorectal metastases*

Reference	No. of patients	Survival (%)			Operative Mortality (%)
		5 y	10 y	20 y	
Hughes et al., 1989 (9)	800	32			NA
Foster and Lundy, 1981 (31)	231	23			6
Scheele et al., 1991 (141)	219	39	28	18	5.5
Adson et al., 1984 (28)	141	25			4
van Ooijen et al., 1992 (142)	118	21			7.6
Savage and Malt, 1992 (143)	104	18			NA
Iwatsuki et al., 1989 (34)	86	38			0
Nordlinger et al., 1987 (144)	80	25			5
Ekberg et al., 1986 (145)	72	16			5.6
Fortner et al., 1984 (30)	65	40			7
Butler et al., 1986 (32)	62	34			10
Sesto et al., 1987 (146)	61	28	21		7
Lind et al., 1992 (147)	52	28			9
Wilson and Adson, 1976 (148)	54	28	19		1.7
Cobourn et al., 1987 (149)	41	25			0
Lise et al., 1990 (23)	39	32			5
Vogt et al., 1991 (150)	36	20			0
August et al., 1985 (24)	33	35			0
Coppa et al., 1985 (33)	25	25			4
Thompson et al., 1983 (151)	22	31			5
Cady and McDermott, 1985 (152)	20	30			0
Attiyeh and Wichern, 1988 (153)	20	35			0
Kortz et al., 1983 (154)	16	29			5
		Median Survival			
Steele et al., 1991 (22)	87	29 mo			2.7
Gennari et al., 1986 (25)	48	30 mo			2.1
Petrelli et al., 1985 (155)	36	22 mo			14
Bradpiece et al., 1987 (156)	24	30 mo			8

NA, not applicable.

confined to the liver. However, disease-free survival among patients with resected extrahepatic metastases is poor. Extrahepatic metastasis is a very poor prognostic sign, and resection of liver metastases in the face of extrahepatic disease, nodal or nonnodal, probably benefits very few patients (9,10,26–28,36,141–144,157–161).

The number of liver metastases affects outcome. The 5-year survival rate among patients with one, two, three, or four or more metastases resected was 37%, 34%, 9%, and 18%, respectively, in the Registry data. Although there was no difference in survival between patients with one or two resectable metastases, prognosis was clearly worse in patients with multiple metastases (9–11). This probably reflects a more aggressive tumor biology and the presence of undetectable hepatic or extrahepatic micrometastatic disease. High-quality preoperative imaging studies, careful intraoperative staging, and intraoperative ultrasonography may help identify patients with more extensive disease that is clinically unapparent. Other authors have also concluded that the number of metastases is an important prognostic factor, and most believe that resection of up to three or four metastases is warranted (24,28,31,36,145,157,158,162–165).

The distribution of resectable metastases (unilobar or bilobar) was not found to be a statistically significant factor in survival (9–11). There are conflicting data concerning the importance of size of metastatic lesions, and some studies have shown that lesions >5 cm in size have a worse prognosis (25,31,145,157,158,162,164,165). Size of the lesion alone should not dissuade the surgeon from resection, however, if technically feasible with negative margins.

It is important to resect liver metastases with an adequate surgical margin. In the Registry data, 5-year survival rates were 18%, 26%, and 44% for patients with positive margins, negative margins <1 cm, and negative margins >1 cm, respectively. Data from the University of Erlangen demonstrate the importance of negative surgical margins as well. Median survival was 26 months for patients with a margin <0.5 cm, 28 months for margins between 0.5 and 0.9 cm, and 44 months for patients with margins >1 cm. If dissection entered into the tumor during surgical resection, median survival was 18 months, even though the final surgical margins were negative (9–11). Although margins >1 cm are preferable, negative margins of <1 cm still confer survival advantage. The type of resection (anatomic, segmental, or wedge resection) is not crucial as long as adequate margins are obtained (24,36,145,152,157,158,164).

Stage of the primary tumor appears to have a marked effect on prognosis after resection of liver metastases. Five-year survival among Registry patients undergoing resection for liver metastases was 35% for patients with Dukes' stage B (negative mesenteric lymph nodes) primary tumors versus 28% for Dukes' C (positive mesenteric lymph nodes) tumors. Data from the University of Erlangen showed a more substantial difference in survival based on the stage of the primary lesion. The median survival for patients undergoing resection for hepatic colorectal metastases with Dukes' A and B tumors was 125 months, compared with a median survival of 28.6 months in those with Dukes' C lesions. Even more striking was the finding that, in patients with Dukes' A and B primary tumors, there was no difference in long-term survival between patients who had no liver metastases and those who underwent complete resection of liver metastases. Similarly, there was no significant difference in survival between patients with Dukes' C lesions without liver metastases versus those with resected liver metastases. These findings suggest that when hepatic metastases are curatively resected, they have little impact on survival (9–11). Other authors have emphasized the importance of stage of the primary tumor in determining prognosis after liver resection for metastatic colorectal cancer (28,30,36, 157–159,166).

Age, sex, and site of the primary tumor (colon vs. rectum) do not appear to be independent prognostic variables. A low preoperative CEA level may indicate improved survival, probably because an elevated CEA level indicates the presence of subclinical extrahepatic disease. A prolonged disease-free interval from the time of resection of the primary tumor (>1 year) may indicate a better prognosis, possibly indicating a more slowly growing tumor (9,10,28,31,36,157,158).

Although analysis of prognostic factors is a useful exercise, there remains no effective way to determine with certainty which patients will be alive 5 years after liver resection. In a frank and thoughtful review, Steele and Ravikumar (157) listed five rules to obtain the best outcome from liver resection for metastatic cancer:

1. Resect metastases only from colorectal cancer primary.
2. Resect only when no comorbid disease is present.
3. Resect only when there is no extrahepatic disease.
4. Resect three or fewer metastases (either unilobar or bilobar).
5. Resect all disease (ie, obtain tumor-free margins).

Adherence to these rules would select a subgroup of patients who would have the best 5-year survival statistics. However, most patients with technically resectable liver metastases do not fulfill all of these requirements.

Certainly patients with extrahepatic disease should not undergo resection, and tumor-free margins should always be obtained. The other rules should be considered relative. A quick review of the survival data reminds us that there is no effective systemic or regional treatment that can offer the hope of long-term survival. Given the certain fatal outcome in patients without resection versus a small chance of cure with resection, most patients choose the latter. In the absence of extrahepatic disease, technically resectable metastases should be resected regardless of the prognostic factors in patients with acceptable operative risk.

Complications

Operative mortality for resection of colorectal liver metastases ranges from 0% to 5% in most modern series. Although patients with cirrhosis can safely undergo liver resection, cirrhosis is associated with higher mortality rates, usually because of hepatic failure. Morbidity ranges from 15% to 45%. The most common complications include hemorrhage, coagulopathy, subphrenic abscess, bile leak (biloma and biliary fistula), hepatic failure, renal failure, wound infection and dehiscence, small bowel obstruction, gastrointestinal hemorrhage, atelectasis, pneumonia, and respiratory failure. Postoperative intra-abdominal fluid collections are usually adequately managed by percutaneous catheter drainage under CT or ultrasound guidance (36,158).

Patterns of Failure

Recurrent disease develops in about 60% to 75% of patients who undergo resection of hepatic metastases from colorectal cancer. The liver is the most common site of recurrent disease after resection of colorectal metastases. In most cases, however, recurrence in the liver after hepatic resection is accompanied by extrahepatic metastases or is too extensive to be resected again. In a large retrospective series from France (167), 1818 patients underwent resection of liver metastases from colorectal cancer with curative intent, and 1013 had documented recurrence. Of those patients with recurrent disease after liver resection, 638 (63%) had liver metastases, and 480 (47%) were thought to have disease confined to the liver. A total of 116 patients with liver-only metastases underwent repeat liver resection. Operative mortality was 0.9%. Two- and 3-year survival rates were 57% and 33% after the second liver resection, respectively. Twelve patients underwent a third hepatectomy with a mean survival of 15.2 months after the second resection.

These results and the observations of others (29, 168–176). support second (and even third) liver resection for recurrent colorectal metastases confined to the liver. The operative risk and potential survival benefit are similar with the first and second liver resection. Resection of pulmonary metastases, anastomotic recurrences, and other isolated metastases after liver resection may also improve survival. If careful preoperative staging demonstrates isolated recurrence after liver resection in the liver or lung, patients with acceptable operative risk should be offered the option of resection.

Liver Resection for Noncolorectal Metastases

Little information is available regarding results of liver resection for noncolorectal metastases. Table 2 summarizes the available literature on this topic. Patients with endocrine tumors metastatic to the liver have the best chance of long-term survival after liver resection (see Chap. 27). Liver resection for metastatic kidney tumors also appears to provide a significant proportion of 5-year survivors. Survival after liver resection for other types of tumors metastatic to the liver is associated with only anecdotal long-term survival. Even in colorectal cancer, only a small fraction of patients with metastatic disease (about 20%) have liver-only metastases, and of these only about 25% have lesions that are resectable. Most other types of cancer have even less propensity to metastasize exclusively to the liver; liver metastases in these patients almost uniformly signify the presence of systemic dis-

TABLE 2. *Survival after liver resection for metastases from noncolorectal primary sites*

Primary tumor	Operative survivors	Survival 2 y	Survival 5 y	Died of recurrence after 5 y
Nonendocrine				
Stomach	37	1/22	0/21	0
Breast	31	11/17	3/16	0
Testis	28	15/27	—	0
Wilms' tumor	21	10/18	6/14	0
Leiomyosarcoma	20	6/11	1/10	1
Melanoma	19	3/14	1/14	1
Kidney	15	6/9	4/8	0
Uterus and cervix	10	1/7	1/7	0
Pancreas	7	1/5	0/5	0
Ovary	7	0/3	0/3	0
Gallbladder	3	1/3	0/3	0
Others[a]	25	8/14	2/11	1
Endocrine				
Noncarcinoid[b]	16	6/7	5/7	2
Carcinoid	55	21/30	7/24	2

(Adapted from Table 4 in references 31 and 163. Additional data from references 149, 151, 154, 158, 164, 177–187.)

[a]Includes sarcomas (5), unknown primary (3), lung (3), hemangiopericytomatous meningioma (3), esophagus (2), duodenum (2), and 1 each: anus, teratoma, neuroblastoma, paraganglioma, pericytoma, seminoma, esophageal lymphoma.

[b]Includes adrenal (8), islet cell (4), medullary carcinoma of the thyroid (2), gastrinoma (2). Three adrenal, one islet cell, and one gastrinoma lived 5 years.

ease that is not amenable to surgical treatment. Patients with liver metastases from noncolorectal and nonendocrine tumors have a dismal chance at long-term survival. Nevertheless, patients with noncolorectal, nonendocrine tumors in whom an exhaustive metastatic workup fails to demonstrate extrahepatic disease may occasionally benefit from surgical treatment. It is our policy to consider liver resection for noncolorectal, nonendocrine metastatic tumors only if the tumor demonstrates a response to systemic chemotherapy.

Transplantation

Orthotopic liver transplantation (OLT) intuitively seems to be the ultimate means of obtaining surgical margins free of disease for patients with advanced liver tumors. However, experience with OLT for liver metastases from nonendocrine tumors has been dismal, with a 2-year survival rate of 14% (188). Similarly poor results have been reported for advanced cholangiocarcinoma. Many centers no longer perform OLT for malignant disease because of the relatively poor results compared with OLT for nonmalignant disorders, and the relative scarcity of donor organs. However, patients undergoing OLT for early stage (UICC stages I and II) hepatocellular cancer have been shown to have a 5-year survival of 60% or greater, although survival was poor for patients with more advanced disease (189,190). Furthermore, OLT results in 5-year survival rates of between 30% and 65% for fibrolamellar hepatocellular carcinoma, a variant of the disease that has a more favorable prognosis. In addition, OLT is thought to be an acceptable option for some patients with hepatoblastoma, hepatic epithelioid hemangioendothelioma, and neuroendocrine tumors metastatic to the liver. Development of adjuvant strategies to complement OLT for cancer may improve outcome (see review [191]).

CONCLUSIONS

Patients with untreated liver metastases have no reasonable chance for long-term survival. Systemic chemotherapy does not significantly alter the fatal course of patients with liver metastases. Radiation therapy has not been effective for control of liver metastases, although newer techniques may allow for more directed treatment and better results. Hepatic artery infusion of chemotherapeutic agents results in substantial improvement in response rates, but has not been shown convincingly to improve overall survival. Newer intra-arterial chemotherapeutic regimens, alone or in combination with systemic agents, may allow the impressive response rates to translate into prolonged survival. Chemoembolization is a noncurative technique that improves survival in patients with hypervascular hepatic tumors, but is not useful for colorectal metastases. Techniques to ablate liver metastases by alcohol injection, laser, ultrasound, microwave, and radiofrequency are under investigation and may prove to be useful therapeutic modalities. Cryoablation of colorectal metastases to the liver may be as effective as resection, and may play an important role as an adjunct to resection in patients with multiple metastases. Liver transplantation for advanced or metastatic cancer is indicated for only a few subsets of patients with more favorable tumors. Surgical resection of liver metastases remains the only proven therapy that has the potential for cure. Resection of liver metastases in selected patients with colorectal primaries results in approximately 30% 5-year survival. Surgical treatment of noncolorectal liver metastases has not been encouraging, with the exception of endocrine tumors, Wilms' tumor, and renal cancers. In most patients, however, the development of liver metastases signifies the presence of extrahepatic disease. Accordingly, survival of most patients with hepatic metastases is not improved by even the best strategies to resect, ablate, or otherwise control disease within the liver. The ultimate goal, therefore, is to develop effective systemic treatments in combination with locoregional therapy of hepatic metastases to benefit a larger proportion of patients.

PATIENT INFORMATION

Tumors that spread (or metastasize) to the liver usually have already spread elsewhere as well. Most of what we know about treating metastatic tumors in the liver comes from studies on patients with metastatic colon and rectal cancer. Other types of tumors that metastasize to the liver can occasionally be treated surgically as well.

Studies have shown that it is not generally beneficial to patients to resect liver tumors if there is metastatic tumor outside the liver, if the tumor cannot be completely removed, or if the liver contains tumors in many different areas. Some selected patients who do not show any evidence of spread of the tumor anywhere but the liver can undergo liver resection with the hope of cure. About 25% to 30% of patients who undergo liver resection for colorectal metastases live for 5 years or more. Although some of these patients die of their cancer after 5 years, many do not have recurrence of their cancer.

Therefore, only patients who have hope of a curative operation are taken to the operating room. At the operation, the surgeon examines the abdomen carefully for any sign of metastatic disease outside the liver. If any lymph nodes or nodules are found, they are sampled for biopsy and sent to the pathologist for immediate (frozen-section) analysis. If tumor is found, the surgeon would not proceed with liver resection. In such a case, systemic chemotherapy is the best option.

Occasionally, patients have liver tumors that are not easily resected or multiple tumors that do not allow for complete resection. Sometimes these patients can undergo cryosurgery instead of or in addition to resection. Cryosurgery consists of placing a probe into the center of the tumor and freezing it. The freezing and thawing kills the tumor cells, and from the available data, this appears to be as effective as removing the tumor in terms of survival.

Other treatments for liver metastases include hepatic artery infusion chemotherapy, radiation therapy, chemoembolization, and a variety of experimental procedures. None of these treatments has been shown definitely to improve survival of patients with liver metastases, and these procedures must be considered experimental. If you are not a candidate for standard therapy, your physician can give you information on experimental treatments for which you might be eligible.

The risks of liver resection or cryosurgery include death, which in the hands of most experienced liver surgeons is less than 5%. Other potential problems include, but are not limited to, bleeding that might require reoperation, infection or abscess, liver failure, kidney failure, bile leak, pneumonia or respiratory failure, small bowel obstruction, upper gastrointestinal bleeding, and problems with wound healing. The risk of having one or more of these problems ranges from 15% to 45%. Fortunately, most of the major complications are rare, and most patients who undergo liver resection or cryosurgery recover without difficulty. Finally, there is no guarantee that the tumor will not recur.

If you are a candidate for liver resection or cryosurgery, you must carefully consider the risks and benefits of the procedure in consultation with your surgeon. However, you must be aware that liver resection or cryosurgery are the only treatment options that offer any realistic hope of curing your cancer. All other options must currently be considered palliative; they are meant to prolong your life or make your life more comfortable. Be certain that you understand the goals, risks, and benefits of any treatment, medical or surgical, before you commit to it.

REFERENCES

1. Foster JH, Berman MM. Solid liver tumors. In: Ebert PA, ed. *Major problems in clinical surgery*. Philadelphia: WB Saunders; 1977.
2. Foster JH. History of liver surgery. *Arch Surg* 1991;126:381–387.
3. Foster JH. Survival after liver resection for cancer. *Cancer* 1970;26: 493–502.
4. Honjo I, Mizumoto R. Primary carcinoma of the liver. *Am J Surg* 128: 31–36,1974;
5. Lin T-Y. Recent advances in technique of hepatic lobectomy and results of surgical treatment for primary carcinoma of the liver. *Prog Liver Dis* 1976;5:668–682.
6. Cady B, Bonneral M, Fender HR Jr. Elective hepatic resection. *Am J Surg* 1979;137:514–521.
7. Starzl TE, Koep LJ, Weil R III, Lilly JR, Putnam CW. Right trisegmentectomy for hepatic neoplasms. *Surg Gynecol Obstet* 1980;150: 208–214.
8. Fortner JG, Maclean BJ, Kim DK, et al. The seventies evolution in liver surgery for cancer. *Cancer* 1981;47:2162–2166.

9. Hughes K, Scheele J, Sugarbaker PH. Surgery for colorectal cancer metastatic to the liver. *Surg Clin North Am* 1989;69:339–359.

10. Hughes KS, Simon R, Songhorabodi S, et al. Resection of the liver for colorectal carcinoma metastases: a multi-institutional study of indications for resection. *Surgery* 1988;103:278–288.

11. Hughes KS, Simon R, Songhorabodi S, et al. Resection of the liver for colorectal carcinoma metastases: a multi-institutional study of patterns of recurrence. *Surgery* 1986;100:278–284.

12. Wingo PA, Tong T, Bolden S. Cancer statistics 1995. *CA Cancer J Clin* 1995;45:8–30.

13. Bengmark S, Hafstrom L. The natural history of primary and secondary malignant tumors of the liver: I. the prognosis for patients with hepatic metastases from colonic and rectal carcinoma verified by laparotomy. *Cancer* 1969;23:198–202.

14. Morris MJ, Newland RC, Pheils MT, MacPherson JG. Hepatic metastases from colorectal carcinoma: an analysis of survival rates and histopathology. *Aust N Z J Surg* 1977;47:365–368.

15. Wood CB, Gillis CR, Blumgart LH. A retrospective study of the natural history of patients with liver metastases from colorectal cancer. *Clin Oncol* 1976;2:265–268.

16. Pestana C, Reitmayer RJ, Moertel CG, et al. The natural history of carcinoma of the colon and rectum. *Am J Surg* 1964;108:826–829.

17. Olsen RM, Perencevich NP, Molcolm AW, et al. Patterns of recurrences following curative resection of adenocarcinoma of the colon and rectum. *Cancer* 1980;45:2969–2974.

18. Welch JP, Donaldson GA. Detection and treatment of recurrent cancer of the colon and rectum. *Am J Surg* 1978;135:505–511.

19. Cady B. Natural history of primary and secondary tumors of the liver. *Semin Oncol* 1983;10:127–133.

20. Saenz NC, Cady B, McDermott WV Jr, Steele GD Jr. Experience with colorectal carcinoma metastatic to the liver. *Surg Clin North Am* 1989; 69:361–370.

21. Wilett CG, Tepper JE, Cohen AM, et al. Failure patterns following curative resection of colonic carcinoma. *Ann Surg* 1984;200:685–692.

22. Steele G Jr, Bleday T, Mayer RJ, et al. A prospective evaluation of hepatic resection for colorectal carcinoma metastases to the liver: Gastrointestinal Tumor Study Group Protocol, 6584. *J Clin Oncol* 1991;9:1105–1112.

23. Lise M, Dabian PP, Nitti D, et al. Colorectal metastases to the liver: present status of management. *Dis Colon Rectum* 1990;35:688–694.

24. August DA, Sugarbaker PH, Ottow RT. Hepatic resection of colorectal metastases. *Ann Surg* 1985;201:210–218.

25. Gennari L, Doi R, Bignami P, Bozetti F. Surgical treatment of hepatic metastases from colorectal cancer. *Ann Surg* 1986;203:49–54.

26. Cady B, Stone MD. The role of surgical resection of liver metastases in colorectal carcinoma. *Semin Oncol* 1991;18:399–406.

27. Scheele J, Stanfl R, Altendorf-Hofmann A. Hepatic metastases from colorectal carcinoma: impact of surgical resection on the natural history. *Br J Surg* 1990;77:1241–1246.

28. Adson MA, vanHeerden JA, Adson MH, Wagner JS, Ilstrup DM. Resection of hepatic metastases from colorectal cancer. *Arch Surg* 1984;119:647–651.

29. Asbun HJ, Hughes KS. Management of recurrent and metastatic colorectal carcinoma. *Surg Clin North Am* 1993;73:145–166.

30. Fortner JG, Silva JS, Golbey RB, Cox EB, Maclean BJ. Multi-variate analysis of a personal series of 257 consecutive patients with liver metastases from colorectal cancer. *Ann Surg* 1984;199:306–316.

31. Foster JH, Lundy J. Liver metastasis. *Curr Probl Surg* 1981;18: 157–202.

32. Butler J, Attiyeh FF, Daly JM. Hepatic resection for metastases of the colon and rectum. *Surg Gynecol Obstet* 1986;162:109–113.

33. Coppa GF, Eng K, Ranson JHC, Gouge TH, Localio SA. Hepatic resection for metastatic colon and rectal cancer. *Ann Surg* 1985;202: 203–208.

34. Iwatsuki S, Sheahan DG, Starzl TE. The changing face of hepatic resection. *Curr Probl Surg* 1989;26:283–379.

35. Hansen R. Systemic therapy in metastatic colorectal cancer. *Arch Intern Med* 1990;150:2265–2269.

36. Niederhuber JE, Ensminger WD. Treatment of metastatic cancer to the liver. In: DeVita VT Jr, Hellman S, Rosenberg S, eds. *Cancer: principles and practice of oncology.* 3rd ed. Philadelphia: JB Lippincott; 1993:2201–2224.

37. Cohen AM, Minsky BD, Schilsky RL. Colon cancer. In: DeVita VT Jr, Hellman S, Rosenberg S, eds. *Cancer: principles and practice of oncology.* 3rd ed. Philadelphia: JB Lippincott; 1993:929–977.

38. Lokich J, Ahlgren J, Gullo J, et al. A prospective randomized comparison of continuous infusion fluorouracil with a conventional bolus schedule in metastatic colorectal carcinoma: a Mid-Atlantic Oncology Program study. *J Clin Oncol* 1989;7:425–432.

39. Einhorn LH. Improvements in fluorouracil chemotherapy? *J Clin Oncol* 1989;7:1377–1379.

40. Petrelli N, Herrera L, Rustum Y, et al. A prospective randomized trial of 5-fluorouracil versus 5-fluorouracil and high-dose leucovorin versus 5-fluorouracil and methotrexate in previously untreated patients with advanced colorectal carcinoma. *J Clin Oncol* 1987;5: 1559–1565.

41. Erlichman C, Fine S, Wong A, Elhakim T. A randomized trial of fluorouracil and folinic acid in patients with metastatic colorectal carcinoma. *J Clin Oncol* 1988;6:469–475.

42. Valone FH, Friedman MA, Wittlinger PS, et al. Treatment of patients with advanced colorectal carcinomas with fluorouracil alone, high-dose leucovorin plus fluorouracil, or sequential methotrexate, fluorouracil, and leucovorin: a randomized trial of the Northern California Oncology Group. *J Clin Oncol* 1989;7:1427–1436.

43. Petrelli N, Douglass HO Jr, Herrera L, et al. The modulation of fluorouracil with leucovorin in metastatic colorectal carcinoma: a prospective randomized phase III trial. *J Clin Oncol* 1989;7: 1419–1426.

44. Poon MA, O'Connell MJ, Moertel CG, et al. Biochemical modulation of fluorouracil: evidence of significant improvement of survival and quality of life in patients with advanced colorectal carcinoma. *J Clin Oncol* 1989;7:1407–1418.

45. Doroshow JH, Multhauf P, Leong L, et al. Prospective randomized comparison of fluorouracil versus fluorouracil and high-dose continuous infusion of leucovorin calcium for the treatment of advanced measurable colorectal cancer in patients previously unexposed to chemotherapy. *J Clin Oncol* 1990;8:491–501.

46. Taylor I, Rowling JT, West C. Adjuvant cytotoxic liver perfusion for colorectal cancer. *Br J Surg* 1979;66:833–837.

47. Taylor I, Machin D, Mullee M, Trotter G, Cooke T, West C. A randomized controlled trial of adjuvant portal vein cytotoxic perfusion in colorectal cancer. *Br J Surg* 1985;72:359–363.

48. Wolmark N, Rockette H, Wickerham DL, Fisher B, Redmond C, other NSABP investigators. Adjuvant therapy of Dukes' A, B, and C adenocarcinoma of the colon with portal vein fluorouracil hepatic infusion: preliminary results of National Surgical Adjuvant Breast and Bowel Project Protocol C-02. *J Clin Oncol* 1990;8:1466–1475.

49. Metzger U, Mermillod B, Aeberhard P, et al. Intraportal chemotherapy in colorectal carcinoma as an adjuvant modality. *World J Surg* 1987; 11:452–458.

50. Ryan J, Heiden P, Crowley J, Bloch K. Adjuvant portal vein infusion for colorectal cancer: a 3-arm randomized trial. *Proceedings of the American Society of Clinical Oncology* 1988;7:361.

51. Metzger U, Laffer U, Castiglione M, Senn HJ. Adjuvant intraportal chemotherapy for colorectal cancer: four-year results of the randomized Swiss study (SAKK 40/81). *Proceedings of the American Society of Clinical Oncology* 1989;8:407.

52. Beart RW, Moertel CG, Wieland HS, et al. Adjuvant therapy of resectable colorectal carcinoma with 5-fluorouracil administered by portal infusion. *Arch Surg* 1990;125:897–901.

53. Wereldsma JCJ, Bruggink EDM, Meijer WS, Roukema JA, Van Putten WLJ. Adjuvant portal liver infusion in colorectal cancer with 5-fluorouracil/heparin versus urokinase versus control. *Cancer* 1990;65: 425–432.

54. Fielding PL, Hittinger R, Grace RH, Fry JS. Randomised controlled trial of adjuvant chemotherapy by portal-vein perfusion after curative resection for colorectal adenocarcinoma. *Lancet* 1992;340:502–506.

55. Schlag P. Regional chemotherapy: different operative techniques and clinical results. *Cancer Treat Rev* 1990;17:177–182.

56. Metzger U. Prevention of colorectal liver metastases. *European Clinics on Digestive Diseases Supplement Series (Vol. 1, Hepato-Gastroenterology)* 1992;39:31–38.

57. Ensminger W, Rosowsky A, Raso V, et al. A clinical–pharmacological evaluation of hepatic arterial infusions of 5-fluoro-2'-deoxyuridine and 5-fluorouracil. *Cancer Res* 1978;38:3784–3792.

58. Ensminger W, Gyves J. Clinical pharmacology of hepatic arterial chemotherapy. *Semin Oncol* 1983;100:736–743.

59. Grage TG, Vassilopoulos P, Shingleton WW, et al. Results of a prospective randomized study of hepatic artery infusion with 5-fluorouracil vs. intravenous 5-fluorouracil in patients with hepatic metas-

tases from colorectal cancer: a Central Oncology Group study. *Surgery* 1979;86:550–555.

60. Patt YZ, Mavligit GM, Chuang VP. Percutaneous hepatic arterial infusion (HAI) of mitomycin C and fluoxuridine (FUDR): an effective treatment for metastatic colorectal carcinoma in the liver. *Cancer* 1980;46:261–265.

61. Sullivan RD, Zurek WZ. Chemotherapy for liver cancer by protracted ambulatory infusion. *JAMA* 1965;194:481–486.

62. Watkins E, Khazei AM, Nahra KS. Surgical basis for arterial infusion chemotherapy of disseminated carcinoma of the liver. *Surg Gynecol Obstet* 1970;130:581–605.

63. Cady B, Oberfield RA. Regional infusion chemotherapy of hepatic metastases from carcinoma of the colon. *Am J Surg* 1974;127: 220–227.

64. Buroker T, Samson M, Correa J, et al. Hepatic artery infusion of 5-FUDR after prior systemic 5-fluorouracil. *Cancer Treat Rep* 1976;60: 1277–1279.

65. Oberfield RA, McCaffrey JA, Polio J, et al. Prolonged and continuous percutaneous intra-arterial hepatic infusion chemotherapy in advanced metastatic liver adenocarcinoma from colorectal primary. *Cancer* 1979;44:414–423.

66. Reed ML, Vaitkevicius VK, Al-Sarraf M, et al. The practicality of chronic hepatic artery infusion therapy of primary and metastatic hepatic malignancies: ten-year results of 124 patients in a prospective protocol. *Cancer* 1981;47:402–409.

67. Blackshear PJ, Dorman FD, Blackshear PL Jr, et al. The design and initial testing of an implantable infusion pump. *Surg Gynecol Obstet* 1972;134:51–56.

68. Buchwald H, Grage TB, Vassipoulos PP, et al. Intra-arterial infusion chemotherapy for hepatic carcinoma using a totally implantable infusion pump. *Cancer* 1980;45:866–869.

69. Ensminger WD, Niederhuber J, Dakhil S, et al. Totally implanted drug delivery system for hepatic arterial chemotherapy. *Cancer Treat Rep* 1981;65:393–400.

70. Patt YZ, Mavligit GM. Arterial chemotherapy in the management of colorectal cancer: an overview. *Semin Oncol* 1991;18:478–490.

71. Balch CM, Urist MM, Soong SJ, McGregor M. A prospective phase II clinical trial of continuous FUDR regional chemotherapy for colorectal metastases to the liver using a totally implantable drug infusion pump. *Ann Surg* 1983;198:567–573.

72. Niederhuber JE, Ensminger WD, Gyves J, et al. Regional chemotherapy of colorectal cancer metastatic to the liver. *Cancer* 1984;53: 1336–1343.

73. Shepard KV, Levin B, Karl RC, et al. Therapy for metastatic colorectal cancer with hepatic artery infusion chemotherapy using a subcutaneous implanted pump. *J Clin Oncol* 1985;3:161–169.

74. Kemeny MM, Goldberg DA, Browning S, et al. Experience with continuous regional chemotherapy and hepatic resection as treatment of hepatic metastases from colorectal primaries. *Cancer* 1985;55: 1265–1270.

75. Patt YZ, Boddie AW Jr, Charnsangavej C, et al. Hepatic arterial infusion with floxuridine and cisplatin: overriding importance of antitumor effect versus degree of tumor burden as determinants of survival among patients with colorectal cancer. *J Clin Oncol* 1986;4: 1356–1364.

76. Cohen AM, Schaeffer N, Higgins J. Treatment of metastatic colorectal cancer with hepatic artery combination chemotherapy. *Cancer* 1986;57:1115–1117.

77. Kemeny N, Daly J, Oderman P, et al. Hepatic artery pump infusion: toxicity and results in patients with metastatic colorectal carcinoma. *J Clin Oncol* 1984;2:595–600.

78. Kemeny N, Seiter K, Conti JA, et al. Hepatic arterial floxuridine and leucovorin for unresectable liver metastases from colorectal carcinoma. *Cancer* 1994;73:1134–1142.

79. Kemeny M. Regional chemotherapy for liver metastases from colorectal cancer. *European Clinics on Digestive Diseases Supplement Series (Vol. 1, Hepato-Gastroenterology)* 1992;39:18–23.

80. Chang A, Schneider PD, Sugarbaker PH, et al. A prospective randomized trial of regional versus systemic continuous 5-fluorodeoxyuridine chemotherapy in the treatment of colorectal liver metastases. *Ann Surg* 1987;206:685–693.

81. Martin JK, O'Connell MJ, Wieand HS, et al. Intra-arterial floxuridine vs. systemic fluorouracil for hepatic metastases from colorectal cancer. *Arch Surg* 1990;125:1022–1027.

82. Kemeny N, Daly J, Reichman B, et al. Intrahepatic or systemic infu-

83. Hohn DC, Stagg RJ, Friedman MA, et al. A randomized trial of continuous intravenous versus hepatic intraarterial floxuridine in patients with colorectal cancer metastatic to the liver: the Northern California Oncology Group Trial. *J Clin Oncol* 1989;7:1646–1654.

84. Rougier P, Laplanche A, Huguier M, et al. Hepatic arterial infusion of floxuridine in patients with liver metastases from colorectal carcinoma: long term results of a prospective randomized trial. *J Clin Oncol* 1992;10:1112–1118.

85. Curley SA, Roh MS, Chase JL, Hohn DC. Adjuvant hepatic arterial infusion chemotherapy after curative resection of colorectal liver metastases. *Am J Surg* 1993;166:743–748.

86. Wagman LD, Kemeny MM, Leong L, et al. A prospective, randomized evaluation of the treatment of colorectal cancer metastatic to the liver. *J Clin Oncol* 1990;8:1885.

87. Patt YZ, McBride CM, Ames FC, et al. Adjuvant perioperative hepatic arterial mitomycin C and floxuridine combined with surgical resection of metastatic colorectal cancer in the liver. *Cancer* 1987;59:867.

88. Okuno K, Ohnishi H, Nakajima I, et al. Complete remission of liver metastases from colorectal cancer by treatment with a hepatic artery infusion (HAI) of interleukin-2-based immunochemotherapy: reports of three cases. *Jpn J Surg* 1994;24:80–84.

89. Curley SA, Newman RA. From preclinical feasibility study to phase I clinical trial: pharmacologic evaluation during the development of a novel treatment system for liver tumors. *Cancer Bull* 1994;46:26–33.

90. Safi F, Bittner R, Roscher R, et al. Regional chemotherapy for hepatic metastases of colorectal carcinoma (continuous intraarterial versus continuous intraarterial/intravenous therapy). *Cancer* 1989;64: 379–387.

91. Seiter K, Kemeny N, Sigurdson E, et al. A phase I trial of hepatic artery fluorodeoxyuridine combined with systemic 5-fluorouracil for the treatment of metastases from colorectal cancer. *Regional Cancer Treatment* 1991;3:293–297.

92. Stagg RJ, Venook AP, Chase JL, et al. Alternating hepatic intra-arterial floxuridine and fluorouracil: a less toxic regimen for treatment of liver metastases from colorectal cancer. *J Natl Cancer Inst* 1991;83: 423–428.

93. Walther H, Kahle M, Filler RD. Hepatic artery infusion via an implantable catheter system using the 5-fluorouracil, leucovorin, mitomycin C regimen. *Regional Cancer Treatment* 1991;4:136–139.

94. Gunderson LL, Tepper JE, Biggs PJ, et al. Intraoperative plus or minus external beam irradiation. *Curr Probl Cancer* 1983;7:1–93.

95. Ingold JA, Reed GB, Kaplan HS, et al. Radiation hepatitis. *AJR Am J Roentgenol* 1965;93:200–208.

96. Wharton JT, Declos L, Gallager W, Smith JP. Radiation hepatitis induced by abdominal irradiation with cobalt 60 moving strip technique. *AJR Am J Roentgenol* 1973;117:73–80.

97. Borgelt BB, Gelger R, Brady LW. The palliation of hepatic metastases: results of the Radiation Therapy Oncology Group pilot study. *Int J Radiat Oncol Biol Phys* 1981;7:587–591.

98. Kinsella TJ. The role of radiation therapy alone and combined with infusion chemotherapy for treating liver metastases. *Semin Oncol* 1983;10:215–222.

99. Phillips R, Karnofsky DA, Hamilton LD, Nickson JJ. Roentgen therapy of hepatic metastases. *AJR Am J Roentgenol* 1954;71:826–834.

100. Barone RM, Byfield JE, Goldfarb PB, et al. Intra-arterial chemotherapy using an implantable infusion pump and liver irradiation for the treatment of hepatic metastases. *Cancer* 1982;50:850–862.

101. Herbsman H, Gardner B, Harshaw D, et al. Treatment of hepatic metastases with a combination of hepatic artery infusion chemotherapy and external radiotherapy. *Surg Gynecol Obstet* 1978;147:13–17.

102. Webber BM, Soderberg CH, Leone LA, et al. A combined treatment approach to management of hepatic metastases. *Cancer* 1978;42: 1087–1095.

103. Lokich JJ, Kinsella T, Perri J, et al. Concomitant hepatic radiation and intra-arterial fluorinated pyrimidine therapy: correlation of liver scan, liver function tests, and plasma CEA with tumor response. *Cancer* 1982;48:2569–2574.

104. Raju PI, Maruyama Y, DeSimone P, MacDonald J. Treatment of liver metastases with a combination of chemotherapy and hyperfractionated external radiation therapy. *Am J Clin Oncol* 1987;10:41–43.

105. Friedman M, Cassidy M, Levine M, et al. Combined modality therapy of hepatic metastases. *Cancer* 1979;44:906–913.

106. Lawrence TS, Dworzian LM, Walker-Andrews S, et al. Treatment of

cancers involving the liver and porta hepatis with external beam irradiation and intraarterial hepatic fluorodeoxyuridine. *Int J Radiat Oncol Biol Phys* 1991;20:555–561.

107. Natua RJ, Heres EK, Thomas DS, et al. Intraoperative single dose radiotherapy. *Arch Surg* 1987;122:1392–1395.

108. Masters A, Steger AC, Brown SG. Role of interstitial therapy in the treatment of liver cancer. *Br J Surg* 1991;78:518–523.

109. Dritschilo A, Grant EG, Harter KW, et al. Interstitial radiation therapy for hepatic metastases: sonographic guidance for applicator placement. *AJR American Journal of Roentgenology* 1986;146:275–278.

110. Ravikumar TS, Steele G Jr, Kane R, King V. Experimental and clinical observations on hepatic cryosurgery for colorectal metastases. *Cancer Res* 1991;51:6326–6327.

111. Ravikumar TS, Kane R, Cady B, et al. A 5-year study of cryosurgery in the treatment of liver tumors. *Arch Surg* 1991;126:1520–1524.

112. Onik G, Rubinsky B, Zemel R, et al. Ultrasound-guided hepatic cryosurgery in the treatment of metastatic colon carcinoma. *Cancer* 1991; 67:901–907.

113. Charnley RM, Thomas M, Morris DL. Effect of hepatic cryotherapy on serum CEA concentration in patients with multiple inoperable hepatic metastases from colorectal cancer. *Aust N Z J Surg* 1991;61: 55–58.

114. Steele G Jr, Ravikumar TS, Benotti PN. New surgical treatments for recurrent colorectal cancer. *Cancer* 1990;65:723–730.

115. Ravikumar TS, Steele GD Jr. Hepatic cryosurgery. *Surg Clin North Am* 1989;69:433–440.

116. Ravikumar TS, Kane R, Cady B, et al. Hepatic cryosurgery with intraoperative ultrasound monitoring for metastatic colon carcinoma. *Arch Surg* 1987;122:403–409.

117. Hashimoto D, Takami M, Ideezuki Y. In depth radiation therapy by Nd:YAG laser for malignant tumors of the liver under ultrasonic imaging. *Gastroenterology* 1985;88:A1663.

118. Schroder T, Hahl J. Laser induced hyperthermia in the treatment of liver tumors. *Lasers Surg Med Suppl* 1989;1:A53.

119. Livraghi T, Festi D, Monti F, et al. US-guided percutaneous alcohol injection of small hepatic and abdominal tumors. *Radiology* 1986;61: 309–312.

120. Livraghi T, Salmi A, Bolondi L. 3-year survival rate of small HCC treated by percutaneous ethanol injection: a study on 86 patients. *European Clinics on Digestive Diseases Supplement Series (Vol. 1, Hepato-Gastroenterology)* 1992;39:116–122.

121. Shina S, Yasuda H, Muto H, et al. Percutaneous ethanol injection in the treatment of liver neoplasms. *AJR Am J Roentgenol* 1987;149: 949–952.

122. Kotoh K, Sakai H, Sakamoto S, et al. The effect of percutaneous ethanol injection therapy on solitary hepatocellular carcinoma is comparable to that of hepatectomy. *Am J Gastroenterol* 1994;89:194–198.

123. Castells A, Bruix J, Bru C, et al. Treatment of small hepatocellular carcinoma in cirrhotic patients: a cohort study comparing surgical resection and percutaneous ethanol injection. *Hepatology* 1993;18: 1121–1126.

124. Ebara M, Ohto M, Sugiura N, et al. Percutaneous ethanol injection for the treatment of small hepatocellular carcinoma: study of 95 patients. *J Gastroenterol Hepatol* 1990;5:616–626.

125. Livraghi T, Bolondi L, Lazzaroni S, et al. Percutaneous ethanol injection in the treatment of hepatocellular carcinoma in cirrhotics: a study on 207 patients. *Cancer* 1992;69:925–929.

126. Vilana R, Bruix J, Bru C, et al. Tumor size determines the efficacy of percutaneous ethanol injection for the treatment of small hepatocellular carcinoma. *Hepatology* 1992;16:353–357.

127. Okuda K. Intratumor ethanol injection. *J Surg Oncol Suppl* 1993;3: 97–99.

128. Honda N, Guo Q, Uchida H, et al. Percutaneous hot saline injection therapy for hepatic tumors: an alternative to percutaneous ethanol injection therapy. *Radiology* 1994;190:53–57.

129. Livraghi T. Ultrasound guided percutaneous ethanol injection therapy of hepatic tumors and metastases. *Z Gastroenterol* 1993;31:260–264.

130. Hisa N, Ohkuma K, Fujikura Y, et al. Percutaneous ethanol injection therapy for hepatic tumors. *Seminars in Interventional Radiology* 1993;10:27–33.

131. Venook AP, Stagg RJ, Lewis BJ, et al. Chemoembolization for hepatocellular carcinoma. *J Clin Oncol* 1990;8:1108–1114.

132. Patt YZ, Chuang VP, Wallace S, et al. Hepatic arterial chemotherapy and occlusion for palliation of primary hepatocellular and unknown primary neoplasms in the liver. *Cancer* 1983;51:1359–1363.

133. Patt YZ, Charnsangavej C, Boddie A, et al. Treatment of hepatocellular carcinoma with hepatic arterial fluoxuridine, doxorubicin and mitomycin (FUDRAM) with or without hepatic artery embolization: factors associated with longer survival. *Regional Cancer Treatment* 1989; 2:98–104.

134. Ajani JA, Carrasco CH, Charnsangavej C, et al. Islet cell tumor metastatic to the liver: effective palliation by sequential hepatic artery embolization. *Ann Intern Med* 1988;108:340–344.

135. Wallace S, Carrasco C, Ajani J, et al. Embolization of neuroendocrine hepatic metastases. In: Levin B, ed. *Gastrointestinal cancer: current approaches to diagnosis and treatment.* Austin, TX: University of Texas Press; 1988:337–349.

136. Allison DJ, Modlin IM, Jenkins WJ. Treatment of carcinoid liver metastases by hepatic artery embolisation. *Lancet* 1977;2: 1323–1325.

137. Mavligit GM, Zukwiski AA, Salem P, et al. Durable regression of gastrointestinal leiomyosarcoma metastatic to the liver after hepatic arterial chemoembolization: infusion with cisplatinum, polyvinyl sponge and vinblastine. *Cancer* 1991;68:321–323.

138. Roh MS. Hepatic resection for colorectal liver metastases. *Hematol Oncol Clin North Am* 3:171–181.

139. Roh MS. Liver resection. In: Roh MS, Ames F, eds. *Advanced oncologic surgery.* 1984.

140. Hasegawa H, Yamasaki S, Makuuchi M, et al. Poor prognoses following left hepatic trisegmentectomies for cancer. *Jpn J Clin Oncol* 1989; 19:271–275.

141. Scheele J, Stangl R, Altendorf-Hofmann A, Gall FP. Indicators of prognosis after hepatic resection for colorectal secondaries. *Surgery* 1991;110:13–29.

142. van Ooijen B, Wiggers T, Meijer S, et al. Hepatic resections for colorectal metastases in the Netherlands. *Cancer* 1992;70:28–34.

143. Savage AP, Malt RA. Survival after hepatic resection for malignant tumors. *Br J Surg* 1992;79:1095–1101.

144. Nordlinger B, Parc R, Delva E, et al. Hepatic resection for colorectal metastases: influence on survival of preoperative factors and surgery for recurrences in 80 patients. *Ann Surg* 1987;205:256–263.

145. Ekberg H, Tranberg K-G, Andersson R, et al. Determinants of survival in liver resection for colorectal secondaries. *Br J Surg* 1986;73: 727–731.

146. Sesto ME, Vogt DP, Hermann RE. Hepatic resection in 128 patients: a 24-year experience. *Surgery* 1987;102:846–851.

147. Lind DS, Parker GA, Horsley JS III, et al. Formal hepatic resection of colorectal liver metastases. *Ann Surg* 1992;215:677–684.

148. Wilson SM, Adson MA. Surgical treatment of hepatic metastases from colorectal cancers. *Arch Surg* 1976;111:330–334.

149. Cobourn CS, Makowka L, Langer B, et al. Examination of patient selection and outcome for hepatic resection for metastatic disease. *Surg Gynecol Obstet* 1987;165:239–246.

150. Vogt P, Raab R, Ringe B, Pichlmayr R. Resection of synchronous liver metastases from colorectal cancer. *World J Surg* 1991;15:62–67.

151. Thompson HH, Tompkins RK, Longmire WP Jr. Major hepatic resection: 25-year experience. *Ann Surg* 1983;197:375–388.

152. Cady B, McDermott WV. Major hepatic resection for metachronous metastases from colon cancer. *Ann Surg* 1985;201:204–209.

153. Attiyeh FF, Wichern WA Jr. Hepatic resection for primary and metastatic tumors. *Am J Surg* 1988;156:368–373.

154. Kortz WJ, Meyers WC, Hanks JB, et al. Hepatic resection for metastatic cancer. *Ann Surg* 1984;199:182–186.

155. Petrelli NJ, Nambisan RN, Herrera L, Mittelman A. Hepatic resection for isolated metastasis from colorectal carcinoma. *Am J Surg* 1985; 149:205–209.

156. Bradpiece HA, Benjamin IS, Halevy A, Blumgart LH. Major hepatic resection for colorectal liver metastases. *Br J Surg* 1987;74:324–326.

157. Steele G Jr, Ravikumar TS. Resection of hepatic metastases from colorectal cancer: biological perspectives. *Ann Surg* 1989;210:127–138.

158. Hughes KS, Sugarbaker PH. Resection of the liver for metastatic solid tumors. In: Rosenberg SA, ed. *Surgical treatment of metastatic cancer.* Philadelphia: JB Lippincott; 1987:125–164.

159. Adson MA. Resection of liver metastases: when is it worthwhile? *World J Surg* 1987;11:511–520.

160. Murray KD. Excision of pulmonary metastasis of colorectal cancer. *Semin Surg Oncol* 1991;7:157–161.

161. Bozzetti F, Doci R, Bignami P, et al. Patterns of failure following surgical resection of colorectal cancer liver metastases. *Ann Surg* 1987; 205:264–270.

162. Foster JH. Survival after liver resection for secondary tumors. *Am J Surg* 1978;135:389–394.
163. Logan SE, Meier SJ, Ramming KP, et al. Hepatic resection of metastatic colo-rectal carcinoma: a ten year experience. *Arch Surg* 1982; 117:25–28.
164. Iwatsuki S, Byers WS Jr, Starzl TE. Experience with 150 liver resections. *Ann Surg* 1983;197:247–253.
165. Foster JH. Surgical treatment of metastatic liver tumors. *Hepatogastroenterology* 1990;37:182–187.
166. Wagner JS, Adson MA, van Heerden JA, et al. The natural history of hepatic metastases from colorectal cancer. *Ann Surg* 1984;199: 502–507.
167. Nordlinger B, Vaillant J-C, Guiget M, et al. Survival benefit of repeat liver resections for recurrent colorectal metastases: 143 cases. *J Clin Oncol* 1994;12:1491–1496.
168. Elias D, Lasser P, Hoang JM, et al. Repeat hepatectomy for cancer. *Br J Surg* 1993;80:1557–1562.
169. Stone MD, Cady B, Jenkins RL, et al. Surgical therapy for recurrent liver metastases from colorectal cancer. *Arch Surg* 1990;125:718–722.
170. Griffith KD, Sugarbaker PH, Chang AE. Repeat hepatic resections for colorectal metastases. *Surgery* 1990;107:101–104.
171. Vaillant J-C, Balladur P, Nordlinger B, et al. Repeat liver resections for recurrent colorectal liver metastases. *Br J Surg* 1993;80:340–344.
172. Bozzetti F, Bignami P, Montalto F, et al. Repeated hepatic resection for recurrent metastases from colorectal cancer. *Br J Surg* 1992;79: 146–148.
173. Dalton RR, Eisenberg BL. Surgical management of recurrent liver tumors. *Semin Oncol* 1993;20:493–505.
174. Huguet C, Bona S, Nordlinger B, et al. Repeat hepatic resection for primary and metastatic carcinoma of the liver. *Surg Gynecol Obstet* 1990;171:398–402.
175. Lange JF, Leese T, Castaing D, et al. Repeat hepatectomy for recurrent malignant tumors of the liver. *Surg Gynecol Obstet* 1989;169: 119–126.
176. Dagradi AD, Mangiante GL, Marchiori LA, et al. Repeated hepatic resection. *Int Surg* 1987;72:87–92.
177. Morrow CE, Grage TB, Sutherland DER, et al. Hepatic resection for secondary neoplasms. *Surgery* 1982;92:610–614.
178. Pommier RF, Woltering EA, Campbell JR, Fletcher WS. Hepatic resection for primary and secondary neoplasms of the liver. *Am J Surg* 1987;153:428–433.
179. Tomas-de la Vega JE, Donahue EJ, Doolas A, et al. A ten year experience with hepatic resection. *Surg Gynecol Obstet* 1984;159: 223–228.
180. Nims TA. Resection of the liver for metastatic cancer. *Surg Gynecol Obstet* 1984;158:46.
181. Stehlin JS, de Ipolyi PD, Greeff PJ, et al. Treatment of cancer of the liver: twenty years' experience with infusion and resection in 414 patients. *Ann Surg* 1988;208:23–35.
182. Kaneko T, Harada A, Isshiki K, et al. Hemangiopericytomatous meningioma metastasized to the liver: report of a case and review of the literature. *Jpn J Surg* 1993;23:644–648.
183. Gonzalez EM, Aguirre JI, Garcia JI, et al. Surgical treatment of hepatic metastases from malignant neoplasms of noncolorectal origin. *European Clinics on Digestive Diseases Supplement Series (Vol. 1, Hepato-Gastroenterology)* 1992;39:66–70.
184. Elias D, Lasser P, Spielmann M, et al. Surgical and chemotherapeutic treatment of hepatic metastases from carcinoma of the breast. *Surg Gynecol Obstet* 1991;172:461–464.
185. Yoshida K, Tamazaki S, Ota K, et al. A case report of meningioma with multiple liver metastases. *Kanzo (Acta Hepatica)* 1988;29: 1528–1534.
186. Hukill PB. Visceral metastasis from a meningioma: report of a case. *Ann Surg* 1960;152:804–808.
187. Goulet RJ Jr, Hardacre JM, Einhorn LH, et al. Hepatic resection for disseminated germ cell carcinoma. *Ann Surg* 1990;212:290–294.
188. Pichlmayr R. Is there a place for liver grafting for malignancy? *Transplant Proc* 1988;20:478.
189. Ringe B, Pichlmayr R, Wittekind C, et al. Surgical treatment of hepatocellular carcinoma: experience with liver resection and transplantation in 198 patients. *World J Surg* 1991;15:270–285.
190. Iwatsuki S, Starzl TE, Sheahan DG, et al. Hepatic resection versus transplantation for hepatocellular carcinoma. *Ann Surg* 1991; 214:221.
191. Gores GJ. Liver transplantation for malignant disease. *Gastroenterol Clin North Am* 1993;22:285–299.

CHAPTER 9

Infusional Chemotherapy of Hepatic-Metastatic Tumors

Joshua T. Rubin and Keith A. Dookeran

"...it is our impression that a better oncolytic effect is achieved more consistently with the higher local antimetabolite concentrations resulting from regional intra-arterial infusion than can be achieved by systemic administration. It remains uncertain, however, if regional infusion therapy with the available drugs will prove of practical clinical benefit."
—*Clarkson B, et al. Effects of continuous hepatic artery infusion of antimetabolites on primary and metastatic cancer of the liver. Cancer 1962;15:472–488.*

BACKGROUND

About 155,000 cases of colorectal cancer will be diagnosed in the United States this year (1). Hepatic metastases will develop in 35% to 40% of these patients (2,3), and almost one third of them will have little or no associated extrahepatic metastatic disease (3,4). The only curative therapy for patients with isolated hepatic-metastatic colorectal cancer is hepatic metastasectomy (5–12). Unfortunately, most patients with hepatic metastases are not appropriate candidates for this option.

Other treatment options appear to be of limited benefit. Systemic chemotherapy with 5-fluorouracil (5-FU)-based regimens has been associated with palliation and prolonged survival, but cure remains elusive (13–15). Our understanding of the mechanisms responsible for this lack of significant clinical efficacy remains inchoate. Resistance to the cytotoxic effects of chemotherapy has been thought to be mediated in any one of several ways. Tumor cells may develop resistance to chemotherapeutics through the expression of genes that encode the multiple drug resistance phenotype. This is acquired through the amplification or mutation of specific genes (16,17). The protein products of these genes are thought to mediate drug resistance in manifold ways that include altered transport of the drug across the plasma cell membrane, decreased drug metabolism to more active forms, increased drug detoxification, and alteration of the drug's protein target, rendering it less easily bound (18). Our understanding of the genetic events underlying these changes is incomplete. Efforts to target the few defined mechanisms of drug resistance have included the use of agents that bind to p-glycoprotein, like verapamil, and inhibitors of topoisomerase II. These interventions have met with little success, however.

Resistance to the direct toxic effects of chemotherapeutics may also be a manifestation of the low intratumoral concentrations associated with their intravenous administration. Increasing the dose intensity of chemotherapy has been identified as a strategy for overcoming resistance to many drugs. The concept of dose intensity identifies both the concentration of a drug to which a tumor is exposed and the duration of exposure as important variables determining efficacy (19–24). In vitro data suggest that the dose–response curve to most chemotherapeutics is steep. This steep dose–response curve obtains in animal models, as well (25). A relationship between dose intensity and response rate is also suggested by data accumulated in human trials (19,21,22,26). Dose intensification is generally proscribed by systemic toxicity.

Other impediments to drug delivery include the nonuniform blood supply within tumors that results in poor perfusion of the center of large tumors. Lack of well developed lymphatics and capillary leak contribute to elevated interstitial pressure seen within many tumors, as well (27–30).

Regional hepatic arterial chemotherapy was proposed as a rational approach to overcome drug resistance by

J. T. Rubin: Department of Surgery, University of Pittsburgh, Pittsburgh, Pennsylvania 15213.

K. A. Dookeran: The Mercy Cancer Institute, The Mercy Hospital of Pittsburgh, Pittsburgh, Pennsylvania 15219.

Sullivan et al. (31). They hypothesized that it would allow for the delivery of high concentrations of anticancer reagents selectively to tumors that far exceed the concentrations achieved through their systemic administration. The resulting high intratumoral concentrations of chemotherapeutics were anticipated to translate to greater tumor cell kill with less associated systemic toxicity.

The locoregional delivery of chemotherapeutics to hepatic-metastatic colorectal cancer as a means to dose-intensify therapy has a sound anatomic basis. Unlike normal liver parenchyma, which is supplied predominantly by the portal vein, liver metastases derive their blood supply mainly from the hepatic artery (32). Therefore, intrahepatic arterial infusion allows high concentrations of drugs to be delivered more selectively to hepatic tumors (33).

Hepatic arterial infusion has been shown to produce significantly higher tumor drug levels than those seen after intravenous or portal venous administration (32–34) and associated systemic toxicity is low for drugs that are sequestered in the liver like Floxuridine (FUDR) (35). Continuous infusion of FUDR for extended periods appears to be the optimal method of its delivery (36–38). This maintains drug levels for multiple cell cycles, producing a maximum antitumor effect (36).

Widespread use of hepatic arterial chemotherapy had been delayed by technical problems associated with vascular access. Percutaneous catheters and external pumps were associated with a significant risk of complications, including catheter migration, arterial thrombosis, infection, gastrointestinal hemorrhage, and bleeding (39–41). Development of implantable arterial catheters and ports overcame many of these problems (42–44).

There are two brands of implantable pump, both of which are similar in basic design (Table 1). The Infusaid Model 400 (Infusaid, Norwood, MA) and the Arrow Model 3000 (Arrow International, Walpole, MA) are constructed of titanium. Each is divided into two chambers by a metal bellows. The inner chamber is filled with drug or saline through a central silicone septum. The outer chamber surrounding the bellows contains Freon, which powers the pump. Filling the inner chamber expands the bellows and compresses the Freon gas in the outer chamber, turning it into liquid. The propellant, warmed by body temperature, is slowly converted to a gaseous state and exerts a constant pressure on the bellows surrounding the drug chamber. Compressing and collapsing the bellows forces infusate through an outlet flow mechanism and into the silicone catheter.

The Infusaid Model 400 has a side port for bolus injections. The Arrow Model 3000 uses a special needle for delivering boluses into a separate pathway within the main pump. The lifespan of each pump is limited only by the durability of the silicone septum, which should be accessed with nothing larger than a 22-gauge Huber needle. The septum is designed to tolerate as many as 1500 punctures with this needle.

An alternative to implantable pumps is the subcutaneous port. FUDR is delivered at a constant rate of infusion by an external pump, which the patient wears at all times. The port is continuously accessed with a butterfly Huber needle. We have found this to be more prone to catheter occlusion and less convenient for the patient.

SELECTION OF PATIENTS

Hepatic metastasectomy appears to be the most effective therapy for patients with isolated, hepatic-metastatic colorectal cancer who have fewer than four tumors (5–12). Patients with hepatocellular carcinoma limited to the liver and patients with solitary hepatic metastases from other primary tumors are also thought to be appropriate candidates for operative or ablative therapy. Most patients, however, have tumors that cannot be removed either as a result of their size, number, location, or propinquity to major vessels or ducts within the liver. Although these patients are usually treated with systemic chemotherapy, those whose tumors are isolated to the liver are potential candidates for regional chemotherapy.

Tumor burden should be considered in selecting patients for regional chemotherapy because it may affect operative morbidity and mortality. These may be prohibitively high among patients whose livers are significantly replaced with tumor. The impact of tumor burden on response to hepatic arterial chemotherapy is poorly understood. Allen-Mersh et al. reported that survival was not related to pretreatment tumor burden among patients who responded to hepatic arterial chemotherapy (45). However, Rougier et al. found that <30% hepatic replacement by tumor was associated with increased survival among all treated patients (46). Patients with concomitant extrahepatic metastatic disease are thought to be inappropriate candidates for hepatic artery chemotherapy (47).

Serum bilirubin above 2 g/dl, ascites, and portal vein obstruction have been associated with poor outcome after infusional chemotherapy. Poor performance status and significant comorbid medical illness defines patients whose quality of life may deteriorate as a result of treatment (48).

Because of the enhanced antitumor activity of regional chemotherapy, its use for the palliation of patients with symptomatic, hepatic-metastatic cancer is also thought to be appropriate. Finally, patients in whom dose-limiting

TABLE 1. *Comparison of intrahepatic arterial pumps*

Model	Weight	Height	Diameter	Volume	Septum diameter
Infusaid 400d	208 g	28 mm	89 mm[a]	50 ml	8 mm
Arrow 3000	137 g	34 mm	78 mm	30 ml	10.2 mm

[a]Diameter is exclusive of side port.

toxicity develops as a result of systemic chemotherapy may be more effectively treated by the intrahepatic arterial infusion of these drugs, provided there is a pharmacokinetic advantage to their intrahepatic arterial infusion, such as one sees with FUDR (35).

PRETREATMENT EVALUATION

Requisite preoperative screening varies according to the patient's health and comorbid diseases. Patients with hepatic-metastatic cancer require preoperative liver function tests and assessment of their prothrombin time. Patients who have been treated with systemic chemotherapy may have a variety of hematologic and renal abnormalities. These should be appropriately evaluated and corrected before surgery. Preoperative nutritional status is important because cachectic patients may find the presence of a sizable right lower quadrant, subcutaneous pump cumbersome.

Treatment conventionally requires placement of one or two hepatic artery catheters. Preoperative hepatic arteriography is requisite to determine whether this is technically feasible, because hepatic arterial anatomy varies significantly. Other preoperative radiographic studies should include abdominal and chest computed tomography scans, performed to detect extrahepatic metastatic disease. We have not found preoperative positron emission tomography scans or tagged monoclonal antibody scans useful, although their role continues to be investigated. Patients known to have manifested heparin-induced thrombocytopenia are probably not candidates for intrahepatic arterial chemotherapy because heparin must be used to maintain catheter patency.

METHODS

Hepatic arterial chemotherapy usually is administered through hepatic artery catheters connected to a subcutaneous port or pump. These devices have proven to be safer and less cumbersome than percutaneous catheters (42–44). Implanted pumps have been found to be less likely to become occluded than percutaneously placed ones (49). The experience of the surgeon is also closely associated with the incidence of technical complications (50).

Operative placement of hepatic arterial catheters is performed through a generous right subcostal incision. Preoperative antibiotics are routinely administered. The right upper quadrant should be meticulously explored for evidence of extrahepatic disease. Particular attention should be directed to the regional lymph nodes, which are sampled for biopsy to exclude occult nodal-metastatic disease. We usually defer extensive intraoperative evaluation of the liver, including ultrasound, because this information will not alter our operative plan. We do, however,

substantiate the radiographic findings suggesting that the hepatic-metastatic disease is unresectable.

Having excluded the presence of extrahepatic metastases, we ask that the pump be prepared for insertion. This requires that it be primed with heparinized saline, a procedure that is easily learned by a member of the surgical team. A detailed checklist is provided with the pump, which we have found to be helpful. Supplies necessary for pump preparation include a sterile thermometer, warm saline, and heparin.

Cholecystectomy is routinely performed to prevent drug-induced cholecystitis. The arterial supply to the liver is then exposed so that the common hepatic artery and the proper hepatic artery can be controlled with vessel loops. It is important to dissect out several centimeters of the common hepatic and proper hepatic arteries so that all branches to the proximal duodenum and the gastric antrum can be ligated and divided. This is requisite to prevent the development of chemotherapy-induced gastritis (51,52). For patients with conventional vascular anatomy, the gastroduodenal artery is exposed for a length of 2 to 3 cm and is ligated as far distally as possible. Care must be exercised in dissecting the gastroduodenal artery over the superior border of the pancreas because troublesome bleeding can occur at this point.

Before placing the catheter into the gastroduodenal artery, a subcutaneous pocket is created over the right lower quadrant of the abdomen into which the pump is placed and secured with proline sutures. The pump septum should be well-caudal to the transverse incision through which the pocket is fashioned. It should be covered with at least 1 cm of subcutaneous tissue but not so deep as to be difficult to palpate. The preattached catheter is passed into the abdominal cavity after being tunneled a short distance. Redundant catheter is looped and placed beneath the pump within its pocket. The intra-abdominal portion of the catheter should be lax to avoid tension at the level of the gastroduodenal artery.

A small arteriotomy is made in the gastroduodenal artery after the common hepatic artery and proper artery have been occluded with vessel loops or vascular clamps. The beaded catheter, having been cut flush with the most distal bead, is advanced through the arteriotomy to the junction of the gastroduodenal artery and the common hepatic artery. The catheter is secured in this position with silk ties placed around the gastroduodenal artery just proximal and distal to each bead. It is important to ensure that the catheter tip does not protrude beyond the gastroduodenal artery into the common hepatic artery lumen, because thrombosis of the proper hepatic artery is likely to develop. Once secured, the completeness of liver perfusion is determined by slowly injecting 5 ml of 10% fluorescein into the bolus port and evaluating the liver with a Wood's lamp.

Conventional hepatic arterial anatomy is present in only about 50% of humans and refers to a common hepatic artery that arises from the celiac trunk and that gives rise to the gastroduodenal artery and the proper hepatic artery. The proper hepatic artery then gives rise to a right and left hepatic artery several centimeters beyond the gastroduodenal artery origin. Common variations include "accessory" hepatic arteries, which usually arise from the left gastric artery or superior mesenteric artery and supply the left and right lobes of the liver, respectively. These accessory vessels can be ligated after placing the catheter in the usual fashion within the gastroduodenal artery. Another common variant is a "replaced" right hepatic artery arising from the superior mesenteric artery or a "replaced" left hepatic artery arising from the left gastric artery. In this case, only one artery arises from the proper hepatic artery. We ligate the smaller of the two arteries and cannulate the remaining vessel either through a side branch or by creating a side branch with Dacron. Before ligating a replaced right or left hepatic artery, the vessel should be clamped to ensure that any observed ischemia is transient.

Cannulation of the gastroduodenal artery in the setting of a marked common hepatic artery or celiac stenosis may result in significant hepatic ischemia by interruption of the reversed flow in the gastroduodenal artery, which, in effect, has become the source of arterial blood to the liver.

In this case, we cannulate the common hepatic artery and preserve the patency of the gastroduodenal artery.

If the gastroduodenal artery arises opposite the origin of the right and left hepatic artery, or if the proper hepatic artery is very short, misperfusion of the liver is likely. If this "trifurcation" variant of the common hepatic artery is encountered, we ligate one of the hepatic arteries and place a catheter in the gastroduodenal artery, as usual.

Some surgeons prefer to use two separate catheters when replaced hepatic arteries are encountered. In the absence of a proper hepatic artery, some surgeons recommend cannulation of the splenic artery and ligation of the left gastric and gastroduodenal arteries. They posit that perfusion of the lobe supplied by the ligated right or left hepatic artery is compromised and the delivery of chemotherapy is impaired. A recent randomized trial suggests that this concern may be justified (53).

CLINICAL RESULTS

Seven large prospective, randomized trials comparing intrahepatic arterial chemotherapy with systemic

TABLE 2. *Randomized trials of intrahepatic arterial FUDR*

Reference	Patients	Crossover	Dose[a]	Extrahepatic disease (portal LN/other site)	CR + PR (IA vs. IV)	Prior chemotherapy	Survival[b]
Allen-Mersh et al. (45)	100	N	FUDR 0. 2 IA[c]	Y/N[d]		N	405 vs. 226 d (P = 0.03)
Chang et al. (47)	64	N	FUDR 0. 3 IA[e] FUDR 0. 125 IV	Y/N[f]	62% vs. 17% (P < 0.003)	Y	2 y: 22% vs. 15% (P = 0.27)
Hohn et al. (56)	110	Y	FUDR 0.3 IA FUDR 0.075 IV[g]	Y/Y	42% vs. 10% (P = 0.0001)	Y[h]	
Kemeny et al. (55)	99	Y	FUDR 0.3 IA FUDR 0.15 IV	N/N	50% vs. 20% (P = 0.001)	N	
Martin et al. (57)	69	N	FUDR 0.3 IA 5-FU 500 mg/m² IV	Y/Y[i]	48% vs. 21% (P = 0.02)	N	13 m vs. 11 m (P = 0.53)
Rougier et al. (58)	163	N[g]	FUDR 0.3 IA 5-FU 500mg/m² IV[j,k]	?/N	43% vs. 9%		15 m vs. 11 m (P < 0.02)

[a]Starting dose. FUDR, in mg/kg/d, was administered by continuous IA or IV infusion for 14 days every 28 days. 5-FU, in mg/m²/d, was administered IV for 5 consecutive days every month.

[b]Survival is median survival unless stated otherwise.

[c]39 of 49 control patients did not receive systemic chemotherapy. The dose of 5-FU for the other 10 controls was not stated.

[d]It is not stated whether porta hepatis lymph nodes were closely evaluated for metastases. Although patients without evidence of extrahepatic disease on computed tomography scan were eligible, it is not stated whether patients with extrahepatic disease discovered at the time of surgery were eligible.

[e]Midway through the trial, the starting dose of FUDR was lowered to 0.2 mg/kg/d.

[f]Patients with extrahepatic metastases did not receive hepatic arterial chemotherapy, but were included in the survival analysis.

[g]The dose of FUDR was increased in 0.025-mg/kg/d increments each cycle until mild diarrhea was observed. The dose was then maintained at the previous dose level.

[h]Patients who received up to 10 g of 5-FU were eligible.

[i]Patients with extrahepatic metastases underwent tumor debulking.

[j]Patients receiving arterial FUDR could subsequently cross over to the systemic 5-FU arm.

[k]Half of the 82 control patients did not receive systemic chemotherapy.

LN, lymph node; CR, ; PR, ; IA, intrahepatic arterial; IV, intravenous; Y, yes; N, no; FUDR, 5-fluorouracil deoxyribonucleoside; 5-FU, 5-fluorouracil; CR, complete response; PR, partial response.

chemotherapy for the treatment of hepatic-metastatic colorectal cancer have been performed. The earliest was performed by Grage et al., who treated 74 patients with either one cycle of intrahepatic arterial 5-FU for 21 days or intravenous 5-FU for 8 days (54). Both groups were subsequently treated with intravenous 5-FU. Hepatic perfusion was performed by percutaneous catheters in 19 of the 31 treated patients. No patient had previously received chemotherapy. Neither clinical response nor survival differed between the treatment groups.

Table 2 compares the results of six large randomized trials that evaluated intrahepatic arterial FUDR. Kemeny et al. compared the intrahepatic arterial infusion of FUDR to its intravenous infusion in 99 patients, all of whom were free of nodal and extrahepatic disease as determined operatively (55). The response rate associated with intrahepatic arterial therapy was significantly greater than that seen with systemic FUDR (50% vs. 20%). The crossover design of this study precluded meaningful survival analysis.

Chang et al. also compared intrahepatic arterial with intravenous FUDR among patients with hepatic metastatic colorectal cancer (47). Patients found at operation to have extrahepatic disease (9 of 32 randomized to hepatic perfusion) were not treated with hepatic artery chemotherapy, although they were included in the survival analysis. Patients with regional nodal metastases discovered at celiotomy were included in this study. Although the response rate among patients treated with intrahepatic arterial FUDR exceeded that seen with its intravenous administration (62% vs. 17%), there was no difference in overall survival between these two groups. This lack of a survival advantage persisted even if the 11 patients who were randomized to but did not receive intrahepatic arterial therapy were excluded from the analysis.

Hohn et al. compared intrahepatic arterial FUDR to intravenous FUDR among 110 patients with hepatic-metastatic colorectal cancer (56). Patients found to have extrahepatic disease at the time of hepatic artery cannulation were not excluded. Patients who were noted to progress within the liver while being treated with systemic FUDR were crossed over to the intrahepatic arterial chemotherapy arm of this study. This precluded analysis for differences in survival. Clinical response and time to disease progression were both superior among patients treated with hepatic arterial FUDR, however.

Martin et al. randomized 69 patients to treatment with either intrahepatic arterial FUDR or intravenous 5-FU (57). Patients with extrahepatic disease discovered at the time of hepatic artery cannulation underwent tumor debulking and were included in this study. Intrahepatic arterial FUDR was associated with a higher response rate (48% vs. 21%) and prolonged interval to tumor progression. There was no apparent survival advantage, however.

The only two randomized trials that have demonstrated a survival advantage for intrahepatic arterial FUDR included untreated patients among the control subjects. Rougier et al. compared therapy with intrahepatic arterial FUDR to conventional therapy, which included either intravenous 5-FU or observation (58). The response rate among patients treated with hepatic arterial chemotherapy exceeded that seen among the 41 patients who were treated with systemic 5-FU (43% vs. 9%). Time to hepatic tumor progression was also superior (14.5 vs. 5.5 months). The median survival was significantly improved among patients treated with hepatic arterial FUDR (15 vs. 11 months). Allen-Mersh et al. conducted a similar study with 100 patients (45). In addition to improved median survival (405 vs. 226 days), they observed that intrahepatic arterial FUDR sustained quality of life more effectively than systemic 5-FU or expectant therapy.

These trials, with the exclusion of that conducted by Grage et al., formed the basis of a recent meta-analysis (59). For trials comparing intrahepatic arterial FUDR to intravenous therapy, a trend toward increased survival was observed for regional chemotherapy ($P = 0.14$). When all trials were considered in the survival analysis, there was a significant advantage associated with intrahepatic arterial therapy ($P = 0.0009$). The number of long-term survivors was also greater.

Any discussion of regional hepatic chemotherapy would be incomplete without considering its role as an adjuvant. Wagman et al. evaluated intrahepatic arterial chemotherapy after liver resection for hepatic metastases (60). Patients were randomized to regional chemotherapy or observation after being stratified based on the number of metastatic lesions. There was no apparent benefit associated with chemotherapy.

Morales et al. suggested that portal vein infusion of cytotoxic agents would inhibit the subsequent development of liver metastases after colon resection (61). The hypothesis that intraoperative manipulation may lead to portal venous dissemination of colon cancer was central to this approach. And mesenteric vein tumor emboli had been detected after colon resection for cancer (62). The salutary effects of adjuvant portal vein chemotherapy were demonstrated in a rat tumor model by Cruz et al. (63), and its safety in humans was demonstrated by Almersjo et al. (64).

These seminal observations served as the basis for six randomized, prospective trials (Table 3). Only two of these demonstrated a regional benefit for portal venous chemotherapy. Taylor et al. observed a decreased frequency in the development of liver metastases among all treated patients and increased survival among patients with Dukes' stage B colon cancer (65). Wereldsma et al. also observed a decreased frequency of liver metastases, but the subsequent development of metastases at other sites was also reduced, suggesting a systemic, not a regional, benefit of chemotherapy (66). Survival was not

TABLE 3. *Randomized trials of adjuvant portal vein chemotherapy*

Reference	Patients	Colon/rectum	Dukes' Stages	Recurrence	Survival
Taylor et al. (65)	244	Y/Y	A,B,C	Decreased in liver	Increased[a]
Metzger et al. (68)	378	Y/Y	A,B,C	No effect in liver / Decreased overall	Not evaluated
Wereldsma et al. (66)	304	Y/Y	A,B,C	Decreased in liver / Decreased systemic	No benefit
Wolmark et al. (69)	901	Y/N	A,B,C	No effect in liver	Increased at 4 y
Beart et al. (67)	219	Y/Y	B2,C	No effect in liver	No benefit
Fielding et al. (70)	398	Y/Y	A,B,C	No effect in liver	Increased after 3 y for stage C

[a]Increased survival among patients with Dukes' stage B colon cancer.
Y, yes; N, no.

prolonged in this study. Beart et al. demonstrated neither a regional nor systemic advantage to portal venous chemotherapy after resection of Dukes' stage B2 or C colorectal cancer (67). Metzger et al. observed a decrease in the overall recurrence risk without a concomitant regional benefit when patients were analyzed according to the intent to treat (68). Two trials, in addition to that of Taylor et al., have demonstrated a survival advantage among patients treated with portal vein infusion of 5-FU (69,70). A concomitant decrease in the development of liver metastases was not noted in these studies, suggesting that the salutary effects of chemotherapy were mediated systemically rather than regionally. One would have to conclude that the benefit of adjuvant portal vein chemotherapy is small at the dose intensity used in these studies, and the observed benefit is most likely mediated through a systemic rather than a regional antitumor effect.

MORBIDITY AND MORTALITY

The spectrum of toxicity associated with intrahepatic arterial infusion of FUDR differs from that seen with its intravenous administration (Table 4). Small numbers of patients have developed gastritis and duodenitis leading to bleeding. The risk of this toxicity has almost been eliminated by careful identification, ligation, and division of all vessels supplying the proximal duodenum and the gastric antrum (51). Management of this complication, often manifest by abdominal pain or gastrointestinal bleeding,

includes upper gastrointestinal endoscopy to evaluate the extent of gastritis, followed by the reinstitution of therapy at a reduced dose after sufficient time for healing. Hepatobiliary toxicity includes sclerosing cholangitis and hepatitis. Chemical cholecystitis is avoided by performing cholecystectomy routinely. Bile duct injury from FUDR occurs because the biliary blood supply is exclusively arterial. Although the addition of dexamethasone to the hepatic arterial infusion has reduced the risk of this sinister complication, very careful monitoring is required to prevent the development of multiple bile duct strictures and irreversible jaundice (71). Rising serum bilirubin, hepatic transaminases, or alkaline phosphatase should prompt dose modification or cessation of therapy and subsequent dose reduction. Endoscopic retrograde cholangiopancreatography may be necessary to evaluate patients whose jaundice does not improve.

Placement of the pump is well tolerated in carefully selected patients. Most patients are discharged from the hospital on the fourth or fifth postoperative day. Perioperative mortality varies from 0% to 4% in randomized trials. Morbidity related to the implant is infrequent and includes hematoma, seroma, infection, arterial thrombosis, and catheter dislodgement (see Table 4). Seromas almost always resolve with repeated aspiration. Great care should be taken to avoid injury to the catheter in the course of this procedure. Arterial thrombosis and catheter occlusion can be successfully managed in some patients with thrombolytic agents.

TABLE 4. *Toxicity of intrahepatic arterial chemotherapy*

	FUDR toxicity		Pump complications					
Reference	Sclerosing cholangitis	Gastritis/ gastric ulcer	Arterial thrombosis	Seroma	Hematoma	Infection	Dislodgment	Misperfusion
Allen-Mersh et al. (45)	0/51	0/51			2/51	3/51	5/51	
Chang et al. (47)	5/24	9/24						
Hohn et al. (56)	12/50	1/50		0	0	1/50	1/50	2/50
Kemeny et al. (55)	4/48	12/48						2/48
Martin et al. (57)	1/36	4/36	4/36	0	0	2/36	0	1/36
Rougier et al. (58)	19/81	19/81	8/81	4/81	8/81	0	0	1/81

FUDR, 5-fluorouracil deoxyribonucleoside.

PATIENT CARE CONSIDERATIONS

The preoperative and postoperative care of these patients is similar in most respects to that of any patient undergoing a major abdominal operation. With few exceptions, patients are admitted on the day of surgery through a same-day surgery unit. All of our patients receive preoperative doses of heparin subcutaneously and a broad-spectrum antibiotic intravenously. Heparin is discontinued when patients are fully ambulatory. Only one postoperative dose of antibiotic is administered. All patients are treated with antisecretory drugs to reduce further the risk for development of gastric mucosal toxicity.

We usually begin chemotherapy 2 weeks after surgery to avoid the pain associated with accessing a recently placed pump. Before this, we perform a ^{99}technetium-labeled macroaggregated albumin scan through the bolus port. This confirms both complete hepatic perfusion and the absence of gastric misperfusion. The latter, if detected, requires operative correction to avoid gastritis and gastric ulceration.

During chemotherapy, patients are closely monitored for evidence of hepatobiliary toxicity by checking their serum alkaline phosphatase, bilirubin, and aspartate aminotransferases (AST) every 2 weeks. The dose of FUDR is modified according to the results of these studies. For elevations of the aminotransferase (AST) greater than twice baseline, therapy is continued at 80% of the starting dose. The dose of FUDR is halved if the AST exceeds 3 times its baseline or if either the bilirubin or alkaline phosphatase exceed 1.5 times their baseline value. The dose of FUDR is held until hepatobiliary toxicity resolves if the AST reaches four times its baseline or the bilirubin or alkaline phosphatase reach two times their baseline (72). Patients in whom abdominal pain develops are not retreated until they are evaluated by endoscopy and found to be free of gastritis and gastric ulcer.

Estimated flow rates for each pump are established with the pump half full at normal body temperature and at sea level. However, the rate of drug delivery is not constant for reasons intrinsic to the design of the pump. The flow rate at full volume may be as much as 8% faster than the rate at low volume. At very low pump volume, the variation in flow rate may even be greater. For this reason, significant delay in refilling the pump is not recommended and the system should never be allowed to empty completely.

Changes in blood pressure, altitude, and body temperature also affect pump function and may necessitate modification of the drug concentration under certain conditions. Arterial hypertension reduces drug delivery by 3% for each 10 mmHg above a mean arterial pressure of 90 mmHg. Flow rate increases about 13% for every degree centigrade rise in body temperature. For this reason, patients should report persistent fever and the use of hot tubs and hot baths should be discouraged. For the same reason, heating pads should never be placed over the pump.

Every 1000-foot change in altitude may be associated with an 8% change in pump flow rate. Travel in a commercial airplane, although in a "pressurized" cabin, may increase drug delivery as much as 45%. Therefore, patients who fly frequently may require a change in drug concentration or a slower pump. Patients should also be advised to refrain from deep-sea diving.

Abdominal pain, fever, melena, and discomfort over the pump site should be reported immediately. Patients should be admonished to avoid contact sports. A product identification card should be carried at all times in the unlikely event the pump is detected by certain security systems.

Nothing larger than a 22-gauge Huber needle should be used to access the pump. Syringes smaller than a 10-ml capacity should not be used to flush or fill the pump because smaller syringes can generate excessive pressure. Bolus injections should not exceed 5 ml/minute. Finally, blood should never be aspirated through the pump or the bolus port. Use of the pump is straightforward and is well illustrated in product brochures. If prescribed guidelines are followed, pump malfunction is exceedingly rare.

ALTERNATIVE APPROACHES

Modification of hepatic blood flow by arterial embolization may allow for further dose intensification by either decreasing the washout of drugs from hypervascular tumors or by enhancing drug delivery to hypovascular ones. A variety of materials have been evaluated. Their effect on drug delivery depends, in part, on particle size and half-life once injected. More durable reagents such as polyvinyl sponge and gelatin may produce prolonged ischemia manifest by a debilitating postembolization syndrome consisting of fever, abdominal pain, and reversible hepatic dysfunction (73–79). This is exacerbated by the coadministration of chemotherapeutics. The recruitment of collateral circulation may decrease the efficacy of subsequent infusions (80–82).

Starch microspheres are cross-linked starch polymers with a mean diameter of 45 μm. Their half-life is short (about 30 minutes) as a result of degradation by serum amylase (83). They have been shown to decrease systemic levels of mitomycin C and 5-FU after hepatic arterial injection and increase blood flow to hypovascular tumors (84–89). Some evidence suggests that they may delay wash-out of drugs from hypervascular hepatic tumors after hepatic arterial injection (90). Their short half-life limits both morbidity and the development of hepatic arterial collaterals, but compromises their utility as vehicles to enhance the effects of FUDR, which requires prolonged cell exposure for maximum antitumor activity.

Vasoconstrictors have been shown to enhance drug delivery to hepatic tumors (91–94). This has been attributed to the insensitivity of aberrant tumor vasculature to the vasomotor effects of these reagents. The safety and efficacy of these drugs administered in combination with chemotherapy have not been extensively evaluated, and hemodynamic toxicity further limits their usefulness.

REFERENCES

1. Wingo PA, Tong T, Bolden S. Cancer statistics, 1995. *CA Cancer J Clin* 1995;45:8–31.
2. Nordinger B, Balludur P. Surgical management of hepatic metastases from large bowel cancer. In: Sugarbaker P, ed. *Hepatobiliary cancer.* Boston: Kluwer Academic Publishers; 1994:43–51.
3. Hughes KS, Sugarbaker RH. Resection of the liver for metastatic solid tumors. In: Rosenberg SA, ed. *Treatment of metastatic cancer.* Philadelphia: JB Lippincott; 1987:125–164.
4. Weiss I, Grundmann E, Torhorst J, et al. Haematogenous metastatic patterns in colonic carcinoma: an analysis of 1541 necropsies. *J Pathol* 1986;150:195–203.
5. Butler J, Attiyeh FF, Daly JM. Hepatic resection for metastases of the colon and rectum. *Surg Gynecol Obstet* 1986;162:109–113.
6. Nordinger B, Parc R, Delva E, et al. Hepatic resection for colorectal liver metastases. *Ann Surg* 1987;205:256–263.
7. Fortner JG, Silva JS, Golbey RB, Cox EB, Maclean BJ. Multivariate analysis of a personal series of 247 consecutive patients with liver metastases from colorectal cancer: I. treatment by hepatic resection. *Ann Surg* 1984;199:306–316.
8. Doci R, Gennari L, Bignami P, et al. One hundred patients with hepatic metastases from colorectal cancer treated by resection: analysis of prognostic determinants. *Br J Surg* 1991;78:797–801.
9. Adson MA, Van Heerden JA, Adson MH, Wagner JS, Ilstrup DM. Resection of hepatic metastases from colorectal. *Arch Surg* 1984;119:647–651.
10. Hughes KS, Simon R, Songhorabodi S, et al. Resection of the liver for colorectal carcinoma metastases: a multi-institutional study of patterns of recurrence. *Surgery* 1986;100:278–284.
11. Cobourn CS, Makowka L, Langer B, Taylor B, Falk R. Examination of patient selection and outcome for hepatic resection for metastatic disease. *Surg Gynecol Obstet* 1987;165:239–246.
12. Iwatsuki S, Esquivel CO, Gordon RD, Starzl TE. Liver resection for metastatic colorectal cancer. *Surgery* 1986;804–810.
13. Poon MA, O Connell MJ, Moertel CG, et al. Biochemical modulation of fluorouracil: evidence of significant improvement of survival and quality of life in patients with advanced colorectal carcinoma. *J Clin Oncol* 1989;7:1407–1418.
14. Nordic Gastrointestinal Tumor Adjuvant Therapy Group. Expectancy or primary chemotherapy in patients with advanced asymptomatic colorectal cancer: a randomized trial. *J Clin Oncol* 1992;10:904–911.
15. Scheithauer W, Rosen H, Kornek GV, Sebesta C, Depisch D. Randomized comparison of combination chemotherapy plus supportive care with supportive care alone in patients with metastatic colorectal cancer. *B Med J* 1993;306:752–755.
16. Biedler JL, Riehm H. Cellular resistance to actinomycin D in Chinese hamster cells in vitro: cross-resistance, radioautographic and cytogenic studies. *Cancer Res* 1970;30:1172–1184.
17. Scotto KW, Biedler JL, Melera PW. Amplification and expression of genes associated with multidrug resistance in mammalian cells. *Science* 1986;232:751–755.
18. Vickers PJ, Townsend AJ, Cowan KH. Mechanisms of resistance to antineoplastic drugs. *Critical Reviews in Dev Cancer Chemotherapy* (in press).
19. Hryniuk WM. The importance of dose intensity in the outcome of chemotherapy. In: DeVita VT, Hellman S, Rosenberg SA, eds. *Important advances in oncology 1988.* Philadelphia: JB Lippincott; 1988:121–142.
20. Hryniuk WM. Analysis of dose intensity for adjuvant chemotherapy trials in stage II breast cancer. *J Clin Oncol* 1986;4:1162–1170.
21. Hryniuk WM. Average relative dose intensity and the impact on design on clinical trials. *Semin Oncol* 1987;14:65–74.
22. Levin L, Hryniuk W. Dose intensity analysis of chemotherapy regimens in ovarian carcinoma. *J Clin Oncol* 1987;5:756–767.
23. Hryniuk W, Bush. The importance of dose intensity in chemotherapy of metastasis breast cancer. *J Clin Oncol* 1984;2:1281–1288.
24. Hryniuk W. Editorial: Is more better? *J Clin Oncol* 1986;4:621–622.
25. Skipper H. Data and analyses having to do with the influence of dose intensity and duration of treatment on lethal toxicity and the therapeutic response of experimental neoplasms. *Southern Research Institute Booklets,* 1986;13, and 1987;2–13.
26. DeVita VT, Hubbard SM, Longo DI. The chemotherapy of lymphomas: looking back, moving forward. The Richard and Hinda Rosenthal Foundation Award Lecture. *Cancer Res* 1987;47:5810–5824.
27. Jain RK. Transport of molecules across tumor vasculature. *Cancer Metastasis Rev* 1987;6:559–594.
28. Young JS, Lumsden CE, Stalker AL. The significance of the tissue pressure of normal testicular and of neoplastic tissue in the rabbit. *J Pathol Bacteriol* 1950;62:313–333.
29. Jain RK. Hemodynamic and transport barriers to the treatment of solid tumors. *Int J Radiat Biol* 1991;60:85–100.
30. Jain RK. Vascular and interstitial barriers to delivery of therapeutic agents in tumors. *Cancer Metastasis Rev* 1990;253–266.
31. Sullivan RD, Norcross JW, Watkins E. Chemotherapy of metastatic liver cancer by prolonged hepatic-artery infusion. *N Engl J Med* 1964;270:321–327.
32. Ridge JA, Bading JR, Gelbard AS, et al. Perfusion of colorectal hepatic metastases: relative distribution of flow from the hepatic artery and portal vein. *Cancer* 1987;59:1457–1553.
33. Sigurdson ER, Ridge JA, Kemeny N, Daly JM. Tumor and liver drug uptake following hepatic artery and portal vein infusion. *J Clin Oncol* 1987;5:1836–1840.
34. Daly MJ, Kemeny N, Sigurdson E, et al. Regional infusion of colorectal hepatic metastases. *Arch Surg* 1987;122:1273–1277.
35. Collins JM. Pharmacologic rationale for hepatic arterial therapy. *Recent Results Cancer Res* 1986;100:140–147.
36. Ensminger W. Hepatic arterial chemotherapy for primary and metastatic liver cancers. *Cancer Chemother Pharmacol* 1989;23(Suppl):S68–S73.
37. Speth PAJ, Kinsella TJ, Change AE, et al. Selective incorporation of iododeoxyuridine into DNA of hepatic metastases versus normal human liver. *Clin Pharmacol Ther* 1988;44:369–375.
38. Ensminger WD, Rosoksky A, Flaso V, et al. A clinical pharmacological evaluation of hepatic arterial infusion of 5-fluoro-2-deoxyuridine and 5-fluorouracil. *Cancer Res* 1978;38:3784–3792.
39. Cady B. Hepatic arterial patency and complications after catheterization for infusion chemotherapy. *Ann Surg* 1972;178:156–161.
40. Oberfield RA, McCaffrey JA, Polio J, et al. Prolonged and continuous percutaneous intra-arterial hepatic infusion chemotherapy in advanced metastatic liver adenocarcinoma from colorectal primary. *Cancer* 1979;44:414–423.
41. Reed ML, Vaitkevicius VK, Al-Sarraf M, et al. The practicality of chronic hepatic artery infusion therapy of primary and metastatic hepatic malignancies: ten year results of 124 patients in a prospective protocol. *Cancer* 1981;47:402–409.
42. Ensminger W, Niederhuber J, Dakil S, Wheeler R. Totally implantable drug delivery system for hepatic arterial chemotherapy. *Cancer Treat Rep* 1981;65:393–400.
43. Blackshear PJ, Dorman FD, Blackshear PL Jr, et al. The design and initial testing of an implantable infusion pump. *Surg Gynecol Obstet* 1972;134:51–56.
44. Buchwald H, Grage TB, Vassilopoulos PP, et al. Intra-arterial infusion chemotherapy for hepatic carcinoma using a totally implantable infusion pump. *Cancer* 1980;45:866–869.
45. Allen-Mersh TG, Earlam S, Fordy C. Quality of life and survival with continuous hepatic artery infusion for colorectal liver metastases. *Lancet* 1994;344:1255–1260.
46. Rougier P, Milan C, Lazorthes F, et al. Prospective study of prognostic factors in patients with unresected hepatic metastases from colorectal cancer. *Br J Surg* 1995;82:1397–1400.
47. Chang A, Schneider PD, Sigarbaker PH, et al. A prospective randomized trial of regional versus systemic continuous 5-fluorodeoxyuridine chemotherapy in the treatment of colorectal liver metastases. *Ann Surg* 1987;206:685–693.
48. Stagg RJ, Lewis BJ, Friedman MA, et al. Hepatic arterial chemotherapy for colorectal cancer metastatic to the liver. *Ann Intern Med* 1984;100:736–743.
49. Fordy C, Burke D, Earlam S, et al. Treatment interruptions and complications with two continuous hepatic artery floxuridine infusion systems in colorectal liver metastases. *Br J Cancer* 1995;72:1023–1025.

50. Kurtis A, Campbell R, Burns C, et al. Regional chemotherapy devices: effect of experience and anatomy on complications. *J Clin Oncol* 1993; 11:822–826.

51. Hohn DC, Stagg RJ, Price DC, Lewis BJ. Avoidance of gastroduodenal toxicity in patients receiving hepatic arterial 5-fluoro-2'-deoxyuridine. *J Clin Oncol* 1985;3:1257–1260.

52. Doria MI, Doria LK, Faintuch J, Levin B. Gastric mucosal injury after hepatic arterial infusion chemotherapy with floxuridine. *Cancer* 1994; 73:2042–2047.

53. Bruke D, Earlam S, Fordy C, Allen-Mersh TG. Effect of aberrant hepatic arterial anatomy of tumor response to hepatic artery infusion of floxuridine for colorectal liver metastases. *Br J Surg* 1995;82:1098–1100.

54. Grage TG, Vassilopoulos PP, Shingleton WW, et al. Results of a prospective randomised study of hepatic artery infusion with 5-fluorouracil vs intravenous 5-fluorouracil in patients with hepatic metastases from colorectal cancer: a Central Oncology Group study. *Surgery* 1979;86:550–555.

55. Kemeny N, Daly J, Reichman B, Geller N, Botet J, Oderman P. Intrahepatic or systemic infusion of fluorodeoxyuridine in patients with liver metastases from colorectal carcinoma. *Ann Intern Med* 1987;107: 459–465.

56. Hohn DC, Stagg RJ, Friedman MA, et al. A randomized trial of continuous intravenous versus hepatic intra-arterial floxuridine in patients with colorectal cancer metastatic to the liver: the Northern California Oncology Group Trial. *J Clin Oncol* 1989;7:1646–1654.

57. Martin J, O Connell M, Wieand H, et al. Intra-arterial floxuridine versus systemic fluorouracil for hepatic metastases from colorectal cancer: a randomized trial. *Arch Surg* 1990;125:1022–1027.

58. Rougier PH, Laplanche A, Huguier M, et al. Hepatic arterial infusion of floxuridine in patients with liver metastases from colorectal carcinoma: long term results of a prospective randomized trial. *J Clin Oncol* 1992;10:1112–1118.

59. Meta-Analysis Group in Cancer. Reappraisal of hepatic arterial infusion in the treatment of nonresectable liver metastases from colorectal cancer. *J Natl Cancer Inst* 1996;88:252–258.

60. Wagman LD, Kemeny MM, Leong L, et al. A prospective, randomized evaluation of the treatment of colorectal cancer metastatic to the liver. *J Clin Oncol* 1990;8:1885–1893.

61. Morales, F, Bell, M, McDonald, GO, et al. The prophylactic treatment of cancer at the time of operation. *Ann Surg* 1957;146:588–595.

62. Fisher ER, Turnbull RB Jr. The cytologic demonstration and significance of tumor cells in the mesenteric venous blood in patients with colorectal carcinoma. *Surg Gynecol Obstet* 1955;100:102–108.

63. Cruz EP, McDonald GO, Cole WH. Prophylactic treatment of cancer: the use of chemotherapeutic agents to prevent tumor metastases. *Surgery* 1956;40:291–296.

64. Almersjo O, Brandberg A, Gustavsson B. Concentration of biological active 5-fluorouracil in general circulation during continuous portal infusion in man. *Cancer Lett* 1975;1:113.

65. Taylor I, Machin D, Mullee M, Trotter G, Cooke T, West C. A randomized controlled trial of adjuvant portal vein cytotoxic perfusion in colorectal cancer. *Br J Surg* 1985;72:359–363.

66. Wereldsma JCJ, Bruggink EDM, Meijer WS, Roukema JA, van Putten WLJ. Adjuvant portal liver infusion in colorectal cancer with 5-fluorouracil/heparin versus urokinase versus control. *Cancer* 1990;65: 425–432.

67. Beart RW, Moertel CG, Wieand HS, et al. Adjuvant therapy for resectable colorectal carcinoma with fluorouracil administered by portal vein infusion. *Arch Surg* 1990;125:897–901.

68. Metzger U, Mermillod B, Aeberhard P, et al. Intraportal chemotherapy in colorectal carcinoma as an adjuvant modality. *World J Surg* 1987;11: 452–458.

69. Wolmark N, Rockette H, Wickerham DL, et al. Adjuvant therapy of Dukes A, B, C adenocarcinoma of the colon with portal-vein fluorouracil hepatic infusion: preliminary results of National Surgical Adjuvant Breast and Bowel Project C-02. *J Clin Oncol* 1990;8: 1466–1475.

70. Fielding LP, Hittinger R, Grance RH, Fry JS. Randomised controlled trial of adjuvant chemotherapy by portal-vein perfusion after curative resection for colorectal adenocarcinoma. *Lancet* 1992;340:502–506.

71. Kemeny N, Seiter K, Niedzwiecki D. A randomized trial of intrahepatic infusion of fluorodeoxyuridine with dexamethasone versus fluorodeoxyuridine alone in the treatment of metastatic colorectal cancer. *Cancer* 1992;69:327–334.

72. Kemeny N, Conti JA, Cohen A, et al. Phase II study of hepatic arterial floxuridine, leucovorin, and dexamethasone for unresectable liver metastases from colorectal carcinoma. *J Clin Oncol* 1994;12: 2288–2295.

73. Zou Y. Experimental canine hepatic artery embolization with polyvinyl alcohol microspheres. *Chung Hua Fang She Hsueh Tsa Chih* 1989;23: 330–332.

74. Goldberg JA, Willmott NS, Anderson JH, et al. The biodegradation of albumin microspheres used for regional chemotherapy in patients with colorectal liver metastases. *Nucl Med Commun* 1991;12:57–63.

75. Benita S, Fickat R, Benoit J, et al. Biodegradable cross-linked albumin microcapsules for embolization. *J Microencapsul* 1984;1: 317–327.

76. Anderson J, Angerson W, Willmott N, et al. Regional delivery of microspheres to liver metastases: the effects of particle size and concentration on hepatic distribution. *Br J Cancer* 1991;64:1031–1034.

77. Daniels J, Kerlan R, Dodds L, et al. Peripheral hepatic arterial embolization with crosslinked collagen fibers. *Invest Radiol* 1987;22: 126–131.

78. Cho KJ, Fanders B, Smid A, et al. Experimental hepatic artery embolization with a collagen embolic agent in rabbits: a microcirculatory study. *Invest Radiol* 1989;24:271–274.

79. Soulen MC. Chemoembolization of hepatic malignancies. *Oncology* 1994;8:77–93.

80. Plengvanit U, Chearanai O, Sindhvananda K, et al. Collateral arterial blood supply of the liver after hepatic artery ligation: angiographic study of 20 patients. *Ann Surg* 1972;175:105–110.

81. Nagasue N, Inokuchi K, Kobayashi M, et al. Hepatic de-arterialization for non-resectable primary and secondary tumors of the liver. *Cancer* 1976;38:2593–2603.

82. Wang LQ, Persson B, Bergqvist L, Bengmark S. Re-arterialization of liver tumors after various de-arterialization procedures. *J Surg Res* 1994;57:454–459.

83. Tuma, RF. The use of degradable starch microspheres for transient occlusion of blood flow and for drug targeting to selected tissues. In: Davis SS, et al, eds. *Microspheres and drug therapy: pharmaceutical, immunological, and medical aspects.* Amsterdam: Elsevier Science Publishers BV; 1984:189–203.

84. Johansson C-J, Teder H, Grönquist L, Gunnarsson P-O. Hepatic intraarterial administration of doxorubicin and degradable starch microspheres: a pharmacokinetic study in the rat. *Acta Oncol* 1994;33:39–42.

85. Wollner IS, Walker-Andrews SC, Smith JE. Phage II study of hepatic arterial degradable starch microspheres and mitomycin. *Cancer Drug Delivery* 1986;3:279–284.

86. Dahl EP, Fredlund PE, Tylen U, et al. Transient hepatic de-arterialization followed by regional intra-arterial 5-fluorouracil infusions as treatment for liver tumours. *Ann Surg* 1981;193:82–88.

87. Civalleri D, Scopinaro G, Balletto N, et al. Changes in the vascularity of liver tumors after hepatic arterial embolization with degradable starch microspheres. *Br J Surg* 1989;76:699–703.

88. Civalleri D, Scopinaro G, Gianantonio S, et al. Starch microsphere-induced arterial flow redistribution after occlusion of replaced hepatic arteries in patients with liver metastases. *Cancer* 1986; 58:2151–2155.

89. Civalleri D, Rollandi G, Simoni G, et al. Redistribution of arterial blood flow in metastases-bearing livers after infusion of degradable starch microspheres. *Acta Chir Scand* 1985;151:613–617.

90. Nott DM, Yates J, Grime SJ, et al. The effect of portal venous flow on the washout of a regionally injected marker substance ^{99m}Tc-methylene diphosphonate after hepatic arterial blockade with degradable starch microspheres. *Eur J Surg Oncol* 1992;18:347–352.

91. Ackerman N, Jacobs R, Bloom N, et al. Increased capillary flow in intrahepatic tumors due to α-adrenergic effects of catecholamines. *Cancer* 1988;61:1550–1554.

92. Bloom N, Kroop E, Sadjadi M, et al. Enhancement of tumor blood flow and tumoricidal effect of doxorubicin by intraportal epinephrine in experimental liver metastasis. *Arch Surg* 1987;122:1269–1272.

93. Vagianos C, Puntis M, Heppsson B, et al. Increased uptake of 5-FU in experimental liver tumours by simultaneous infusion of norepinephrine. *European Journal of Cancer Chemotherapy* 1991;64:212–214.

94. Hemingway D, Cooke T, Chang D, et al. The effects of intra-arterial vasoconstrictors on the distribution of a radiolabelled low molecular weight marker in an experimental model of liver tumour. *Br J Cancer* 1991;63:495–498.

CHAPTER 10

Cryoablation of Hepatic Metastases

Joshua T. Rubin

"We strongly believe that cryosurgical methods should be used only by surgeons familiar with liver anatomy and resection and experienced in liver surgery."
—*Blumgart and Fong, (76)*

BACKGROUND

The conventional treatment of metastatic cancer usually relies on systemic chemotherapy. The rationale for this approach is sound and is based on the observation that most of these patients usually have widespread disease. One exception to this pattern of dissemination is seen in patients with colorectal carcinoma, about 18,000 of whom develop isolated hepatic metastases every year. A significant subset of these patients appears to benefit from resection of their metastatic disease. More recently, hepatic cryosurgery as a substitute for or an adjunct to hepatic resection has become an increasingly important part of the surgical armamentarium.

The anodyne effects of refrigeration were purportedly appreciated by the Egyptians as early as 2500 B.C. (1). Among the earliest clinical reports in the Western scientific literature is a collection of anecdotes by Fay and Henny, which described cooling tumors using iced saline irrigation passed through hollow instruments (2). They observed tumor regression and palliation of patients suffering from readily accessible, locally advanced tumors such as those affecting the breast, skin, or cervix.

The need for more intense and localized hypothermia was recognized by Rowbotham et al. (3). They developed a cryoprobe that was cooled by 95% ethanol circulated at a temperature of $-110°C$. Patients with brain tumors were safely treated using this system.

The widespread availability of liquefied gases, particularly nitrogen, allowed for further refinements in cry-

otechnology. Cooper developed a cryogenic system that was a progenitor of those used today (4). It was cooled by liquid nitrogen circulated at $-196°C$ through a vacuum-insulated probe. He successfully treated 800 patients who had Parkinson's disease and other "disorders of involuntary movement" by ablating part of the basal ganglion. He suggested that this system was well suited to treating tumors in the liver, as well.

Growing interest in cyrosurgery for malignant tumors was accompanied by studies designed to elucidate the effects of controlled freezing on living tissues. Fraser and Gill studied the histologic changes that followed cryoablation of a serially transplanted carcinosarcoma in the liver of Sprague-Dawley rats (5). Eosinophilic necrosis developed in both the frozen liver and tumor within 24 hours. This was followed by increasing accumulation of granulocytes at the lesion's periphery and the formation of a well demarcated fibrous capsule within 5 days. Inward organization eventuated in near-complete resolution of the infarcted area, leaving a small residual scar. Cyst or abscess formation was rarely observed.

Fraser and Gill also demonstrated a steep temperature gradient extending radially from the $-190°C$ cryoprobe to the periphery of the ice ball. Their observation that the field of infarction extended peripherally to tissue cooled to only $-12°C$ suggested that mechanisms other than freezing were responsible for cell death. They hypothesized that cells close to the liquid nitrogen probe were destroyed as a result of rapid freezing and the formation of intracellular ice. Tissue farther from the probe was thought to experience slower cooling so that ice would form only in the extracellular fluid. The exclusion of solutes from this ice would lead to progressive hypertonicity of the yet-unfrozen extracellular fluid. Cells in this region would become dehydrated as water shifted into the extracellular space to maintain osmotic equilibrium. Fraser and Gill suggested that this shift of fluid to the extracellular compartment also led to dilatation of ves-

J. T. Rubin: Department of Surgery, University of Pittsburgh, Pittsburgh, Pennsylvania 15213-2582.

sels, vascular endothelial disruption, thrombosis, edema, and ischemia at the ice ball periphery.

These hypotheses concerning mechanisms of cell injury were subsequently reiterated by others. Whittaker studied the effects of freezing using electron microscopy and noted ice crystals only in cells close to the cryoprobe (6). Smith et al. (7) also applied electron microscopy to the study of tissue frozen with a liquid nitrogen probe. Normal rat livers treated for 3 minutes showed infarcts that extended well beyond the −160° probe. Vascular and sinusoidal dilatation and portal venous thrombosis were seen. These observations were consistent with Fraser and Gill's hypothesis that direct thermal injury was not responsible for all of the observed hepatic necrosis.

More recently, Rubinsky et al. evaluated the effects of rapid and slow freezing on normal rat liver using flat liquid nitrogen probes applied to the liver surface (8). They observed ice formation both intravascularly and intracellularly near the cryoprobe or when tissue was frozen rapidly. Tissue subjected to either slow freezing or tissue at a distance from the probe had ice only within the vessels, which were dilated. Surrounding cells were dehydrated. Vascular endothelial disruption was also seen. These findings corroborated Fraser and Gill's seminal observations and suggested that the mechanism of cell death within normal liver or hepatic tumors treated with liquid nitrogen probes is multifactorial.

Although cryoablation of normal liver and transplanted tumors in murine models was well tolerated, earlier observations by Ellis and Dragstedt using larger animals suggested that this would lead to infection of necrotic liver and the development of life-threatening hepatic abscesses (9). Healey et al. used a canine model to evaluate the consequences of leaving large volumes of frozen liver in situ (10). Liquid nitrogen-cooled probes were used to freeze as much as 20% of the liver. Multiple freeze–thaw cycles were used in some animals, and in others multiple hepatic lobes were treated. Although some dogs died after surgery secondary to acute bleeding, most survived and only one dog had an occult liver abscess. All dogs were treated with perioperative penicillin for 5 days. These findings, later confirmed in a similar model by Dutta et al., suggested that the risk of abscess formation after cryoablation of sizable hepatic tumors had probably been overstated (11).

Other technical aspects of hepatic cryosurgery were coincidentally addressed by several investigators using a variety of models. Gage et al. demonstrated the relative resistance of large arteries and veins to injury by liquid nitrogen (12). Although histologic changes within the vessel wall were apparent within 2 days of being frozen, these changes were transient and were never associated with the subsequent development of stenosis, rupture, or aneurysm formation. The common bile duct was not as resistant to freezing injury and often became acutely occluded because of edema. Fibrous stenosis of the common bile duct was often a late sequela of direct freezing of this structure.

The tendency of hepatic parenchyma to fracture and the protective effect of controlled, slow freezing and thawing were noted by Healey et al. (10) and Dutta et al. (11,13). They also evaluated the effect of hepatic cryosurgery on liver function, coagulation, and hematologic parameters. The hepatic transaminases aspartate aminotransferase (AST) and alanine aminotransferase (ALT), as well as alkaline phosphatase, were acutely elevated without associated abnormalities of bilirubin for a period of 1 to 3 weeks. A mild coagulopathy characterized by decreased fibrinogen, decreased platelet count, increased prothrombin time, and increased partial thromboplastin time was observed in a canine model. This was self-limited and was not associated with postoperative bleeding. Most dogs also manifested an increased white blood cell count. Neel et al. (14) and Fraser and Gill (5) described the potential benefits of multiple freeze–thaw cycles, larger probes, and close monitoring of the freezing zone.

Utsunomiya et al. may have been the first to apply liquid nitrogen-driven cryoprobes to the treatment of hepatic metastatic cancer in humans (15). Neither technical details nor the clinical course of their patients were provided in the abstract, however. Torigoshi et al. described four patients with hepatic metastatic colon cancer who were treated with cryosurgery and subsequently survived more than 1 year (16). Kuramoto and Kamegai used liquid nitrogen-driven cryoprobes to ablate large hepatic metastatic tumors in four patients (17). They described using three freeze–thaw cycles to effect complete destruction of the tumor. They also described using Avitene to achieve hemostasis in the cryoprobe tract. Their average blood loss was only 50 ml. Transient elevations of AST and ALT were noted but did not appear to be clinically significant.

The first large, published series of patients who underwent hepatic cryosurgery was reported by Zhou et al. in 1988 (18). They treated 60 patients with 3- or 5-cm liquid nitrogen-driven probes applied to the liver surface. Some patients were treated with concomitant or delayed resection of the frozen tumor, whereas others were treated with hepatic artery ligation or resection of synchronous liver metastases. They used multiple 15-minute freeze–thaw cycles or hepatic artery and portal vein occlusion to maximize tumor cell kill. Care was taken when freezing tumors near the hepatic hilum because the vulnerability of bile ducts to freezing had been previously described. They monitored the extent of freezing with thermocouples, which they perceived to be cumbersome and a limitation to the more widespread use of cryosurgery. They emphasized the need to protect surrounding organs from freezing, which they did with insulation. There was little apparent postoperative morbidity other than fever and reversible elevation of the ALT. Neither vascular injury nor bile leak were seen. There was no perioperative mortality reported. Resected tumors that had been previously frozen revealed histologic changes of coagulative necrosis circumscribed by a fibrous capsule.

Two subsequent innovations were central to the safe and effective application of hepatic cryosurgery as it is currently practiced. Inaccurate probe placement within deep-seated lesions and the cumbersome technique of monitoring freezing with thermocouples were obstacles to the consistent and complete destruction of hepatic parenchymal tumors. In 1984, Onik et al. described their experience using real-time ultrasound to guide probe placement and monitor tumor freezing (19). Using beef liver ex vivo, they observed a semicircular rim of high-amplitude echoes that slowly spread from the cryoprobe during freezing. This hyperechoic rim corresponded to the zero temperature front as it extended radially from the liquid nitrogen probe, and was thought to be due to changes in acoustic impedance associated with freezing. The ice ball had a hypoechoic center and showed acoustic shadowing posteriorly. During thawing, the hyperechoic rim was noted to recede until all that remained was a small hypoechoic area. These findings were subsequently duplicated in a canine liver model (20). Onik et al. had demonstrated that intraoperative ultrasound would allow for both the accurate placement of cryoprobes and accurate monitoring of the extent of tumor freezing.

The limited ability to freeze multiple lesions or to apply multiple freeze–thaw cycles to any individual lesion represented another obstacle to the more widespread application of hepatic cryosurgery. Most early clinical series used surface probes that could not adequately freeze deep-seated parenchymal metastases. Instruments that had been used in animal experiments were not well suited for use in humans because of the small probe diameters. In 1993, Dilley et al. developed a liquid nitrogen delivery system for Cryogenic Technology, Inc. (Ripley, UK) that allowed for the simultaneous use of two cryoprobes supplied by a 30-l tank (21). The maximum probe diameter was 9 mm. The hoses and hand pieces were sterilizable. Another system was developed by Chang et al. for Cryomedical Sciences (Rockville, MD) (22). This provided five independently controlled liquid nitrogen delivery systems that could be operated simultaneously. Both systems could circulate heated nitrogen gas to facilitate rewarming. The availability of multiple, independently operated probes of large diameter and with large liquid nitrogen reservoirs provided surgeons with great flexibility in attempting cryoablation of hepatic tumors.

SELECTION OF PATIENTS

The propensity of colorectal cancer metastases selectively to target the liver renders some patients curable by surgical means. Few selection criteria accurately predict patient outcome after hepatic metastasectomy, however.

Patients with more than three discrete hepatic metastases and patients with regional lymph node metastases are thought to be unsuitable candidates for curative resection (23–26). Patients who are thought to be medically unfit for general anesthesia and those with limited hepatic reserve are also poor candidates for hepatic metastasectomy. Relative contraindications to operative treatment of hepatic metastatic disease include advanced patient age and a carcinoembryonic antigen (CEA) value in excess of 200 ng/ml (24). Neither gender, primary tumor stage, primary tumor grade, tumor location, size of metastases, nor interval between removal of primary colon cancer and appearance of liver metastases have been consistently associated with patient outcome after surgery (23–26).

The indications for cryoablation are probably broader than those that are applied to the selection of patients for hepatic resection. Patients with multiple hepatic tumors distributed in such a way that hepatic resection would be technically impossible are candidates for cryoablation. Tumors situated centrally or straddling both the right and left lobes of the liver may be difficult to resect with adequate margins. These tumors may be treated with equal efficacy using cryoablation. Finally, patients with limited hepatic reserve are rarely candidates for resection because of the high risk of subsequent liver failure. Cryoablation represents a viable alternative for these patients because the amount of normal liver that is sacrificed with this technique is limited.

Between 15% and 40% of patients who undergo hepatic resection for metastatic disease eventually have recurrent disease within the liver without concomitant extrahepatic disease (26–31). The disease-free and overall survival of these patients seems to be extended by resection (32–37), but most of them are thought to be inoperable because previous hepatic surgery has left them with limited hepatic reserve. Cryoablation can be effectively applied in this subset of patients because its successful application is little affected by anatomic considerations such as previous hepatic surgery. Arguably, the more widespread use of hepatic cyrosurgery at the time of initial presentation might facilitate the subsequent management of recurrent, isolated hepatic-metastatic disease by obviating the need to sacrifice large amounts of normal liver tissue at the time of the first operation.

PRETREATMENT EVALUATION

Any operation of this magnitude requires careful patient selection to minimize the risk of perioperative cardiopulmonary complications. This has reduced the risk of myocardial mortality in most recent series to approximately 1% (23,31,38,39). For patients who are thought to be fit for surgery, the ultimate goal of pretreatment evaluation is to determine, as well as possible, that the metastatic disease is isolated to the liver and is limited in amount. Because a metachronous colon cancer subsequently develops in 3% to 5% of patients with colon cancer, colonoscopy should be selectively applied before hepatic resection. It is our practice to use chest, abdominal, and pelvic computed tomography (CT) scans to identify patients who have extrahepatic disease and are therefore inoperable. All patients are also evaluated by CT angioportography because the accuracy of conventional CT and magnetic resonance imaging (MRI) scans for defining the number of hepatic metastases is on the order of only 70% (40).

Recurrent disease develops in as many as 75% of patients after hepatic resection. This is undoubtedly present as undetectable micrometastatic disease at the time of resection. A cogent argument can be made that watchful waiting before instituting an aggressive preoperative evaluation will provide insight into the biology of a patient's metastatic disease. After a delay of several months, the absence of extrahepatic metastatic disease on preoperative CT scan may be a more reliable finding. For patients who have not received chemotherapy, its administration for several months before attempted resection may accomplish the same goal without the angst associated with expectant therapy. Understandably, issues other than tumor biology bear on the surgeon's decision concerning the timing of preoperative workup. For this reason, the approach to each patient may vary.

METHODS

Although we and others are developing laparoscopic techniques for hepatic cryosurgery, most patients require extensive celiotomy, abdominal exploration, and complete hepatic mobilization to apply cryosurgical techniques successfully to the treatment of hepatic-metastatic colorectal cancer. This allows for a complete assessment of the abdominal cavity and the porta hepatis. Complete mobilization of the liver is requisite for a detailed ultrasonographic assessment that best defines the extent of hepatic metastatic disease. A large abdominal incision and extensive mobilization of the liver are also necessary for the safe and accurate placement of cryoprobes. Finally, many of our patients require both hepatic resection and cryoablation (Table 1).

We have not routinely used extensive preoperative preparation for our patients. Nearly all of them are admitted through a same-day surgery unit. Everybody receives a preoperative dose of heparin subcutaneously and a preoperative dose of a broad-spectrum antibiotic intravenously. The operating room temperature is kept high and all intravenous solutions are warmed throughout the operation to maintain the patient's core body temperature.

After the satisfactory induction of general endotracheal anesthesia, a Foley catheter is placed and the patient is repositioned, supine, on the operating table so that an upper hand or Rochard retractor can be safely

TABLE 1. *Technical aspects of safe cryosurgery*

1. Generous abdominal incision
2. Complete mobilization of the liver
3. Cryoprobe placement through some normal liver
4. Avoid major ducts and vessels when placing cryoprobes
5. Do not freeze major bile ducts
6. Stabilize cryoprobe in relation to liver during freezing
7. Keep patient warm
8. Isolate cryoprobe from skin and viscera during freezing

placed at the head of the table. The temptation to place padding between the retractor bar and the patient's shoulder to protect the skin should be resisted because this may depress the shoulder and injure the brachial plexus. The retractor should be secured to the table well above the patient's shoulder so that if the patient is moved cephalad from retraction, the bar will not contact the shoulder. We routinely use upper and lower Bair Huggers (Augustine Medical, Inc., Eden Prairie, MN), which are placed at this time. Most patients are monitored with an arterial line and everybody has several large-bore intravenous catheters placed. Few patients are monitored with pulmonary artery catheters.

The patient's skin is prepared and draped from the pubis to the nipples. A generous bilateral subcostal incision is made, often with a cephalad extension to the left of the xiphoid process. The abdomen and the porta hepatis are carefully explored. Suspect lesions are sent for frozen-section evaluation. The operation is terminated at this point if extrahepatic metastatic disease is discovered.

The ligamentous attachments of the liver are divided in their entirety and ultrasound examination is performed. This may detect heretofore unrecognized hepatic metastases. If additional lesions are discovered, and if they number greater than four or five, we usually abort the operation. Ultrasound examination also allows us to begin to assess the technical difficulty of placing probes within the metastases.

A decision is made at this time regarding hepatic resection. For patients with small, superficial metastases, we perform nonanatomic wedge resections. For patients with lesions within segments two or three, we usually perform a left lateral segmentectomy. We usually resect lesions greater than 6 cm in diameter because they may be difficult to freeze in their entirety. The decision to resect or cryoablate individual hepatic metastases is a subjective one and, except for lesions that are too large to freeze, we believe that cryoablation and resection can be applied interchangeably.

Having decided to proceed with cryoablation, we first attend to several important details. The patient's core body temperature is checked because hypothermia significantly limits the duration of freezing. It is also prudent to assess the patient's volume status at this point. The tendency to administer large amounts of crystalloid or colloid in anticipation of hepatic resection may promote extensive or difficult-to-control bleeding and should be assiduously avoided. Hepatic resection or cryosurgery performed in a controlled manner is rarely associated with excessive blood loss. Dissection of the porta hepatis may facilitate the cryoablation of hepatic tumors by allowing for transient occlusion of hepatic blood flow, which has been found to be helpful when freezing larger lesions (21). Finally, complete mobilization of the liver, a generous incision, and adequate retraction provide greater latitude in the placement of cryoprobes.

Two widely used cryosurgical systems are the CMS Accuprobe (Cryomedical Sciences) and Cryotech (Candela Laser Corp., Wayland, MA). Both systems circulate liquid nitrogen through insulated probes. The CMS Accuprobes are available in 3- and 8-mm diameters. Candela cryoprobes are available in 3-, 5-, and 10-mm diameters. Cryotech also offers a variety of surface probes. Both systems allow for constant monitoring of probe temperature and rapid thawing of the probe tip. CMS Accuprobes are for single-patient use. Candela's probes are reusable, and may reduce operating expense. We use 8-mm Onik introducer sets (Cook Corporation, Bloomington, IN) or 3-mm Onik-Cohen percutaneous access sets (Cook Urological, Spencer, IN) for placement of the CMS Accuprobes. Liquid nitrogen tanks are required to drive the probes. It is useful to purchase carts on which these large tanks can be placed. The CMS Accuprobe system is large (52″ × 32″ × 54″) and weighs 600 lbs. It is powered by 208 volts. It may not easily fit into some operating rooms, and it may be difficult to transport. Its size should be taken into account when planning to establish a cryosurgical operative suite. The Candela system is smaller (52″ × 21.7″ × 23.6″) and weighs only 235 lbs. It is powered by conventional 110/120-volt lines.

Cryoprobes are placed using a modification of the Seldinger technique. An echogenic needle is placed through normal liver into a hepatic metastasis using ultrasound guidance. Onik et al. described using a linear-array transrectal ultrasound probe (41). We have not found use of this probe particularly advantageous and the 7.5-MHz convex-array probe has been adequate. We sterilize the ultrasound probes in Cidex before use. Others use sterile sleeves.

The needle is withdrawn from its sheath and a 0.038-inch, J-tipped guide wire is positioned with its tip at the farthest extent of the tumor (Fig. 1). The needle sheath is removed and a dilator and introducer sheath are then passed over the guide wire with ultrasound guidance. Once the tip of the dilator is at the farthest extent of the tumor, the wire and dilator are removed and the cryoprobe is passed through the introducer sheath with its tip positioned well within the tumor (Fig. 2). The introducer sheath is then withdrawn 1 cm beyond the proximal margin of the tumor so that it does not interfere with freezing. If multiple probes are to be used, they can be inserted at this time.

Positioning cryoprobes through some normal liver parenchyma minimizes the risk of liver fracture during freezing, facilitates hemostasis after freezing, and prevents postoperative bile leaks. The relationship between each metastasis and the surrounding vessels must be extensively evaluated ultrasonographically from all perspectives to avoid injuring major vessels and bile ducts. The shortest and most direct path to a tumor often is not the safest.

The selection of probe diameter is based on the size of the tumor to be frozen. We usually use the 8-mm probe unless we are freezing metastases less than 2 cm in diameter. Freezing is monitored ultrasonographically to ensure that the freezing zone, which appears as an echogenic rim, extends beyond the tumor margin about 1 cm (Fig. 3). We freeze each lesion for approximately 15 minutes. The circulation of liquid nitrogen is then stopped and the cryoprobe is allowed to thaw. When the tip of the cryoprobe reaches a temperature of 0°C, a second freeze–thaw cycle is performed. The application of a second freeze–thaw cycle is empiric and is based on data generated by Fraser and Gill (5) and Neel et al. (14) showing that tumor cell kill is more complete with multiple freeze–thaw cycles. During freezing, care must be taken to stabilize the cryoprobe in relation to the liver as the liver moves with diaphragmatic excursion. Too much torque on the cryoprobe can cause the frozen tumor to fracture at its junction with unfrozen liver. Hepatic parenchymal fracture has also been observed when

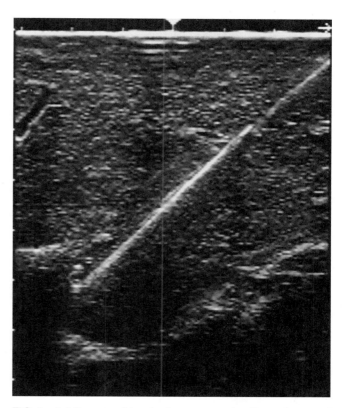

FIG. 1. A J-tipped guide wire is seen passing through normal liver parenchyma and with its tip lying at the distal border of a deep-seated hepatic-metastatic tumor.

freezing superficial lesions. After the last freeze–thaw cycle is completed, the cryoprobe and the introducer are removed and Surgicel (Johnson & Johnson, Arlington, TX) is packed into the probe tract using long forceps. Pressure is then applied to the tumor and the tract for about 10 minutes.

Tumors located close to vessels should be treated with special care. Larger vessels serve as heat sinks and tumors abutting them may be difficult to freeze completely. These tumors should be frozen by placing the probe adjacent to the blood vessel, which ensures that tumor lying on the vessel wall will be frozen. There appears to be little risk associated with freezing the blood vessel wall, provided that the probe is not withdrawn from the liver until the surrounding tissue has thawed and the probe is disengaged. Bile ducts are not as resilient and care should be taken to avoid placing the cryoprobe too close to the main biliary ducts. The more peripheral biliary radicals appear to be less of a concern. We routinely place closed suction drains around the liver to detect postoperative bile leaks. The abdominal incision is then closed and the patient is transferred to the recovery room or the intensive care unit for postoperative care.

CLINICAL RESULTS

The number of published series describing the clinical course of patients treated with hepatic cryosurgery is

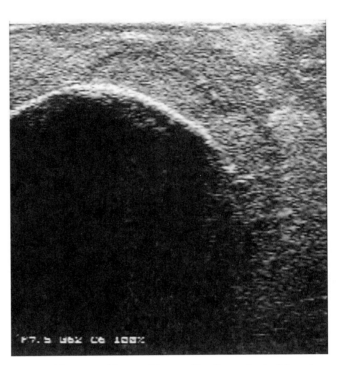

FIG. 3. Ultrasound is used to monitor the extent of freezing. The edge of the ice ball is seen as a hypoechoic arc.

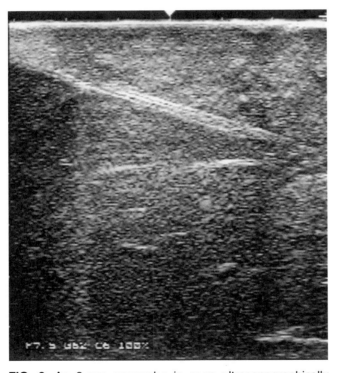

FIG. 2. An 8-mm cryoprobe is seen ultrasonographically with its tip at the distal margin of a hepatic-metastatic tumor. The introducer sheath has been pulled back and is seen casting a shadow posteriorly.

limited, both in number and in the detail with which the experience is reported (Table 2). The largest clinical series is that described by Zhou et al., who treated 113 patients, 107 of whom had hepatocellular carcinoma (42). There were no operative deaths, despite the observation that 86% of treated patients had cirrhosis. There was no mention of intraoperative patient temperature, estimated operative blood loss, transfusion requirement, or hospital stay. One patient had a hepatic abscess postoperatively. All patients had postoperative fevers.

Onik et al. described their experience treating 69 patients, 56 of whom had hepatic-metastatic colorectal cancer (41). The maximum number of metastases treated in any individual patient was 16. The range of tumor sizes was not described. Theirs is the only group that has reported any perioperative mortality. Three of their patients died: one as a result of a myocardial infarction and the other two as a result of liver failure. They also provided a detailed discussion of postoperative complications, which included hepatic fracture with significant intraoperative bleeding, a bile fistula, and a hepatic abscess. Pleural effusions were seen in all patients after surgery. All of their patients manifested myoglobinuria, which led to acute tubular necrosis on three occasions. The etiology of this complication remains an enigma.

Ravikumar et al. reported their experience treating 32 patients, 24 of whom had metastatic colorectal cancer (43). Few details of therapy were provided. There were no operative deaths and only two reported complications. One patient had a hepatic abscess, and a wound dehis-

TABLE 2. *Clinical series of hepatic cryosurgery*

Reference	Patient Numbers	Complications	Deaths	Survival
Zhou et al. (42)	*113—Total* 107—Hepatobiliary 4—Colon	Abscess—1/113	0	Cryo. only—15% Cryo. + resection—33% Resection of frozen tumor—60%
Onik et al. (41)	*69—Total* 56—Colon	Pleural effusion—69/69 Liver failure—1/69 Bile fistula—1/69 Liver abscess—1/69 Myoglobinuria—69/69 Renal failure—3/69	*3—Total* 2—Liver failure 1—MI	27% at 21 months
Charnley et al. (44)	*7—Total* 6—Colon 1—Carcinoid	0	0	Not provided
Ravikumar et al. (43)	*32—Total* 24—Colon 3—Hepatoma 2—Neuroendocrine 3—Miscellaneous	Subphrenic abscess—1/32 Wound dehiscence—1/32	0	78% of 18 patients with no residual tumor
Goodie et al. (45)	*26—Total* 24—Colon 1—Melanoma 1—Hepatoma	Liver failure—8/26 MI—1/26 Hypoglycemia—1/26	0	Not provided
Weaver et al. (46)	*47—Total* 47—Colon	Myoglobinuria—47/47 Reoperation for bleeding—6/47 Large effusion—7/47 Bile fistula—5/47	2—Coagulopathy	26 mo median

Cryo., cryosurgery; MI, myocardial infarction.

cence developed in another patient. All patients had postoperative fever. The median hospital stay was only 6 days.

Charnley et al. treated seven patients (44). Complications were not delineated, but there was no perioperative mortality. The maximum number of treated metastases in any individual patient was 12. The largest lesion treated was 6.5 cm. They reported an average hospital stay of only 7 to 10 days.

The most detailed clinical report is that of Goodie et al., who treated 26 patients (45). The maximum number of metastases in any particular patient was nine. The maximum tumor size was 12 cm. The lowest mean body temperature recorded was 35.2°C. The average blood loss per patient was 926 ml. Fourteen patients required red blood cell transfusions. There were no perioperative deaths. Nearly 30% of their patients experienced liver fracture in the process of freezing, five of whom required red blood cell transfusions. The average hospital stay was 6.8 days.

Most recently, Weaver et al. reported their experience treating 47 patients with hepatic cryosurgery with or without concomitant hepatic resection (46). Although not explicitly stated, many of their patients appear to have been included in their earlier series. As previously reported, myoglobinuria was observed in all treated patients, although renal toxicity did not develop in any of them. Postoperative bleeding requiring reoperation occurred in six patients. Seven patients required thoracentesis for clinically significant postoperative pleural effusions. Five patients had bile fistulas. There were two perioperative deaths due to coagulopathy.

It is difficult to glean meaningful survival data from these series. Zhou et al. reported a 5-year survival of 15% for all patients treated only with cryosurgery, 33% for patients treated with cryosurgery and concomitant hepatic resection, and 60% for patients treated with cryosurgery and resection of the frozen tumor (42). Ravikumar et al. reported that 78% of 18 patients who had no residual disease after cryosurgery survived 5 years (43). Onik et al. reported that 27% of 69 patients survived 21 months after cryosurgery (41). More recently, Weaver et al. reported a median survival of 26 months (46).

MORBIDITY AND MORTALITY

Complications uniquely associated with hepatic cryosurgery are usually easy to avoid (Table 3). The risk of hypothermia has received little detailed discussion in published clinical series of cryosurgery. The average low nasopharyngeal body temperature reported by Goodie et al. among a series of 26 patients was 35.2°C (45). Onik et al. reported that the surgical procedure had to be stopped frequently to rewarm patients, usually by lavaging the abdomen with warm saline (47). They reported that with the routine use of the Bair Hugger, the lowest mean body temperature was 35.3°C or about 1°C higher than that observed among patients in whom the Bair Hugger was not used. Use of the Bair Hugger in concert with other standard warming techniques obviated the need to rewarm patients with warm saline irrigations. We routinely use Bair Huggers and we warm all intravenous solutions. In addition, the ambient room temperature is kept high. The lowest mean body temperature among our patients after cryosurgery has been 38°C.

Onik et al. reported that acute tubular necrosis and renal failure developed in 3 patients among 69 undergoing cryosurgery (41). This was attributed to myoglobinuria, which they have invariably observed in all treated patients. Although myoglobinuria has not been reported by any other group, we still routinely administer prophylaxis to patients for this potential complication. All patients are placed on a 2 mcg/kg/minute dopamine infusion when freezing begins. We also routinely give patients a bolus of 50 mEq of sodium bicarbonate and begin a bicarbonate drip consisting of 50 mEq in 1 liter of D5½NS infused at 75 ml/hour. Finally, all patients receive a 25-g bolus of mannitol.

Freezing and thawing of the liver can cause fracture of the hepatic parenchyma. This is most likely to occur with rapid freezing and thawing of lesions situated close to the surface of the liver. We have noted that parenchymal fracture can also occur during freezing if torque is applied to the cryoprobe. Care must be exercised during freezing to ensure that the cryoprobe is moved with the liver as this organ migrates during ventilation. Although hepatic fracture can be associated with significant bleeding, this is usually not significant in amount and is easily controlled with pledgetted sutures.

In the course of cryoablation, care must be taken to isolate the liver from adjacent organs so that they are not injured by contact with frozen liver or the extrahepatic portion of the probe, which although insulated, still develops frost. This can be accomplished using insulated pads (Boundary, Columbus, MS) or dry laparotomy pads.

PATIENT CARE CONSIDERATIONS

The preoperative and postoperative care of these patients is similar in most respects to that of any patient undergoing a major abdominal operation. With few exceptions, patients are admitted on the day of surgery through a same-day surgery unit. All of our patients receive preoperative doses of heparin subcutaneously and a broad-spectrum antibiotic intravenously. These two medications are administered postoperatively, as well. Heparin is discontinued when patients are fully ambulatory. Only one postoperative dose of antibiotic is administered.

After surgery, patients are monitored for myoglobinuria every 12 hours. This is continued until two successive urine determinations are free of myoglobin. Until

TABLE 3. Morbidity unique to cryosurgery

1. Myoglobinuria
2. Hypothermia
3. Freeze injury to abdominal viscera
4. Hepatic parenchymal fracture
5. Hepatic abscess
6. Freeze injury to bile ducts

this time, all patients are treated with a dopamine infusion, 2 mcg/kg/minute, and a bicarbonate infusion titrated to keep the urinary pH close to 7.0. It is not unusual for patients to have nightly postoperative fever as high as 39°C. In the absence of evident infection, this is rarely evaluated. One or two closed suction drains are left in place until the patient resumes a regular diet. In the absence of bile drainage, the drains are removed before the patient's discharge from the hospital. Although thrombocytopenia and elevations of the prothrombin time have been described in these patients (46), we do not routinely follow these laboratory values.

ALTERNATIVE APPROACHES

Efficacious alternatives to ablation or resection for the treatment of hepatic-metastatic or primary hepatic tumors remain to be defined. Systemic chemotherapy with existing 5-fluorouracil (5-FU)-based regimens has been associated with response rates as high as 45% among patients with colorectal cancer (48–50). Prolonged survival has also been demonstrated (49,51,52). Response rates among patients with hepatocellular carcinoma treated with doxorubicin and cisplatin are similar (53). Nevertheless, cure remains elusive.

The locoregional infusion of chemotherapeutic agents represents another approach to the treatment of isolated hepatic tumors. The intrahepatic arterial delivery of chemotherapeutic agents as a means to dose-intensify therapy has a sound anatomic basis. Unlike normal liver parenchyma, which is supplied predominantly by the portal vein, liver tumors derive their blood supply from the hepatic artery (54). Therefore, intrahepatic arterial infusion allows high concentrations of drugs to be delivered more selectively to hepatic tumors (55). Associated systemic toxicity is low for drugs that are sequestered in the liver such as Floxuridine (FUDR) and 5-FU (56).

Intrahepatic arterial infusion of FUDR has been associated with response rates among patients with hepatic-metastatic colon cancer as high as 60% in phase III trials (57–60). However, because normal liver is also perfused by the hepatic artery, hepatic toxicity is marked, with as many 50% of treated patients requiring premature withdrawal from some reported protocols (57–60). An additional 25% of patients have required significant dose reductions. Most trials have used a relatively low dose of 0.25 mg/kg/day for 14 days to avoid drug-induced morbidity. Survival of patients treated with intrahepatic arterial chemotherapy has not been consistently shown to be prolonged compared with patients treated with systemic chemotherapy (57–63).

Attempts to improve the efficacy or decrease the toxicity of this approach have met with little success. Combining fluoropyrimidines with drugs known to biomodulate FUDR, such as leucovorin or cisplatin, has not been associated with a clinically significant increase in response rate (64–66). Associated toxicity appears to be enhanced, however. Although intrahepatic arterial infusions of dexamethasone have been associated with an amelioration of hepatic toxicity, their concurrent use with intrahepatic arterial FUDR does not appear to allow for meaningful dose intensification (67). The use of locoregional chemotherapy in the adjuvant setting, when tumor burden is minimal, has also been abortive (68).

Most recent published series suggest that hepatic resection applied to carefully selected patients with hepatic-metastatic colorectal cancer is associated with a 20% to 40% 5-year disease-free survival rate (25,27,28,31,38,39, 69–74). Perioperative mortality seems to be on the order of 2.5% to 5%, and is usually due to bleeding or liver failure (25,27,28,31,38,39,69–74). Hospital stay averages less than 2 weeks (75). Perioperative blood transfusion is required in about 50% of patients (76). Postoperative complications are common and include pleural effusions requiring drainage in 5% to 10% of patients (31), bile leak in 4% of patients (27,69), abscess in fewer than 10% of patients (27,31,38,39,69), and hepatic dysfunction in 3% to 8% of patients (27,39,69,75).

Less invasive ablative procedures for the treatment of hepatic-metastatic tumors have also been developed. It is difficult to compare the efficacy of these techniques with that of hepatic resection or cryoablation because of differences in patient selection, small patient numbers, varying definitions of response, and the preponderance of patients with hepatocellular carcinoma in reported clinical trials. The percutaneous injection of absolute alcohol or hot saline into hepatic tumors has been extensively evaluated (77–82). It is usually performed as an outpatient procedure and has been associated with very little morbidity and almost no mortality. It can be administered repeatedly and it has been well tolerated even by patients with limited hepatic reserve.

Giovannini and Seitz applied percutaneous alcohol injection to the treatment of 40 patients with hepatic-metastatic cancer, including 32 patients whose tumors were of colorectal origin (77). This series reviewed 352 treatment sessions for which no complications were observed. Complete response, as defined by complete necrosis on needle biopsy, was seen in only 31 of 55 treated tumors. Thirty-two percent of patients manifested normalization of their CEA value. Median survival of the 32 patients with hepatic-metastatic colorectal cancer was 28 months, with no patient surviving 4 years.

Shiina et al. treated 50 patients with alcohol injection but found that only 72% of treated hepatomas were completely destroyed (78). There was a 33% incidence of in-liver recurrence among the 98 patients treated with curative intent. Patients with multiple tumors tended to have higher recurrence rates.

At least three series have retrospectively compared percutaneous ethanol injection to hepatic resection among patients with hepatocellular carcinoma. Livraghi et al. observed better median survival (67% vs. 52%) among patients with solitary, small hepatocellular carci-

nomas treated with resection (79). The statistical significance of this difference was not evaluated, however. The survival of both treatment groups exceeded that of untreated control patients. Kotoh et al. observed equivalent survival between patients with small, solitary hepatomas treated with resection or ethanol injection (80). Castells et al. compared the results of surgical resection with those of percutaneous ethanol injection in the treatment of solitary hepatomas 4 cm or less in diameter (81). Only 23 of 30 ethanol-treated hepatomas were thought to be totally ablated, and there was a 60% in-liver recurrence rate among these patients. This did not compare favorably with 30 patients who underwent hepatic resection, 40% of whom manifested a subsequent hepatic recurrence. This difference was particularly significant for larger tumors. Of concern in this study was the observation that five patients who underwent resection were found to have additional tumors that had not been documented on preoperative evaluation. This suggests that minimally invasive ablative procedures leave unrecognized hepatic-metastatic or primary hepatic disease untreated and may compromise the chance to cure some of these patients.

Interstitial laser photocoagulation appears to offer the same advantages associated with percutaneous ethanol injection, yet at significantly greater cost. Most of the reported series have used the neodymium: yttrium-aluminum garnet laser (83–87). Hollow needles passed percutaneously into tumors, usually with ultrasound guidance, are used to guide placement of thin laser catheters. Photocoagulation is then monitored with ultrasound or nuclear MRI.

Amin et al. reported their experience treating 21 patients with metastatic liver tumors (83). All of the patients were either inoperable or too ill to undergo surgery. Patients with more than five metastases or tumors greater than 5 cm in diameter were excluded. This seems to be a follow-up of an earlier report by the same group. Forty-five of 55 treated tumors were thought to decrease in size by at least 50%. None of the patients manifested a significant decrease in CEA level. Six of 11 patients followed for at least 14 months manifested progression of the treated hepatic tumor.

Nolsœ et al. treated 16 metastases in 11 patients who had inoperable metastatic colorectal cancer (84). Only 12 of these lesions were thought to be completely destroyed as suggested by the results of ultrasound, fine-needle biopsy, or subsequent surgery. Vogl et al. treated 33 metastatic tumors in 20 patients using MRI to monitor photocoagulation (85). They observed only one partial response among 13 tumors smaller than 2 cm in diameter treated with interstitial laser therapy. At the end of 12 months of observation, an additional three tumors were thought to be stable in size. All of the other treated tumors manifested progression. Seventeen treated tumors measuring more than 2 cm were similarly resistant to photocoagulation. Only one of these tumors appeared to have regressed more than 50% 6 months after therapy. The remaining tumors were either larger or unchanged in size.

Amin et al. purportedly compared the efficacy of interstitial laser photocoagulation to percutaneous ethanol injection among patients with unresectable hepatic-metastatic colorectal carcinoma (88). Only 52% of the patients treated with laser photocoagulation manifested a complete response on CT scan, and some of these apparent responses were found to contain microscopic tumor when biopsy samples were examined. Results with ethanol injection appeared to be even less satisfactory, but the significance of this observation is unclear because the authors' experience with ethanol injection appears to have been limited at the time of this study. Survival data could not be interpreted because no patient was treated with ethanol injection alone.

Although percutaneous alcohol injection and laser photocoagulation are associated with little morbidity and little risk of mortality, their ability to treat tumors greater than 3 cm in diameter is limited and there is no clinical evidence that they are as effective as hepatic resection for curing or prolonging the survival of patients with hepatic-metastatic colorectal cancer. There are no data that either of these therapies is associated with significant palliation, either.

Cryoablation of hepatic tumors appears to be as effective as hepatic resection in controlling hepatic-metastatic or primary hepatic tumors. Both of these approaches appear to be more efficacious than ethanol injection or laser photocoagulation, neither of which can reliably ablate tumors completely if they measure more than 3 cm in diameter. Small tumors, though more susceptible to ablation, may elude detection by nonoperative evaluation and therefore may remain untreated.

There are several apparent advantages to hepatic cryoablation compared with resection. Available series suggest that hospital stay is shorter among patients who are treated with cryosurgery. Cryosurgery may render patients who have limited hepatic reserve or whose tumors are thought to be technically unresectable by virtue of their proximity to major vascular structures candidates for ablative therapy. The need for perioperative blood transfusion may be diminished when cryosurgery is used in lieu of hepatic resection. Several poorly controlled studies suggest that antitumor immune reactivity is enhanced in the course of cryosurgery (89–101). It remains to be defined whether this is due to fewer perioperative blood transfusions, sparing of normal liver, or the effects of freezing on tumor cells and their antigens. Other animal tumor models have actually demonstrated enhanced metastatic spread after cryosurgery (102,103).

Our experience at the University of Pittsburgh Medical Center suggests that most patients with operable hepatic-metastatic colorectal cancer are candidates for liver-conserving therapy with cryosurgery. The concomitant use of hepatic resection and cryoablation appears to be safe and uniformly effective in eradicating all detectable tumor. These techniques appear to be associated with prolonged survival and cure in a significant subset of patients.

REFERENCES

1. Tytus JS. *Cryosurgery: its history and development.* Springfield, IL: Charles C Thomas; 1968:3–18.
2. Fay T, Henny GC. Correlation of body segmental temperature and its relation to the location to carcinomatous metastases: clinical observations and response to methods of refrigeration. *Surg Gynecol Obstet* 1938;66:512–521.
3. Rowbotham GF, Haigh Al, Leslie WG. Cooling cannula for use in the treatment of cerebral neoplasms. *Lancet* 1959;1:12–15.
4. Cooper IS. Cryogenic surgery: a new method of destruction or extirpation of benign or malignant tissues. *N Engl J Med* 1963;268:743–749.
5. Fraser J, Gill W. Observations on ultra-frozen tissue. *Br J Surg* 1967;54:770–776.
6. Whittaker DK. Ice crystals formed in tissue during cryosurgery. *Cryobiology* 1974;11:202–217.
7. Smith JJ, Fraser J, MacIver AG. Ultrastructure after cryosurgery of rat liver. *Cryobiology* 1978;15:426–432.
8. Rubinsky B, Lee CY, Bastacky J, Onik G. The process of freezing and the mechanism of damage during hepatic cryosurgery. *Cryobiology* 1990;27:85–97.
9. Ellis JC, Dragstedt LR. Liver autolysis in vivo. *Arch Surg* 1930;20:8–16.
10. Healey WV, Priebe CJ, Farrer SM, Phillips LL. Hepatic cryosurgery. *Arch Surg* 1971;103:384–392.
11. Dutta P, Montes M, Gage AA. Experimental hepatic cryosurgery. *Cryobiology* 1977;14:598–608.
12. Gage AA, Fazekas G, Riley EE. Freezing injury to large blood vessels in dogs. *Surgery* 1967;61:748–754.
13. Dutta P, Montes M, Gage AA. Large volume freezing in experimental hepatic cryosurgery. *Cryobiology* 1979;16:50–55.
14. Neel HB, Riggle GC, Myers RS, Ketcham AS, Hammond WG. Apparatus modifications for experimental cryogenic surgery of cancer. *Cryobiology* 1971;8:501–505.
15. Utsunomiya J, Yaegashi K, Uehara K, et al. Clinical evaluations of cryosurgery of malignant lesions in general surgery. *Cryobiology* 1978;15:710.
16. Torigoshi Y, Ooke H, Kuramoto S, Yawagita K, Kamegai T. Hepatic metastasis of rectum and colon cancer. *Dig Dis Sci* 1986;31:125S.
17. Kuramoto S, Kamegai T. Cryosurgery for the liver tumor. *Cryobiology* 1978;15:710.
18. Zhou X-D, Tang Z-Y, Ma Z-C. Clinical evaluation of cryosurgery in the treatment of primary liver cancer: report of 60 cases. *Cancer* 1988;61:1889–1892.
19. Onik G, Cooper C, Goldberg HJ, Moss AA, Rubinsky B, Christianson M. Ultrasonic characteristics of frozen liver. *Cryobiology* 1984;21:321–328.
20. Onik G, Gilbert J, Hoddick W, et al. Sonographic monitoring of hepatic cryosurgery in an experimental animal model. *AJR Am J Roentgenol* 1985;144:1043–1047.
21. Dilley AV, Dy DY, Warlters A, et al. Laboratory and animal model evaluation of the Cryotech LCS 2000 in hepatic cryotherapy. *Cryobiology* 1993;30:74–85.
22. Chang Z, Finkelstein JJ, Ma H, Baust J. Development of a high-performance multiprobe cryosurgical device. *Biomed Instrum Technol* 1994;28:383–390.
23. Scheele J, Stangl R, Altendorf-Hoffman A, Gall FP. Indicators of prognosis after hepatic resection for colorectal secondaries. *Surgery* 1991;110:13–29.
24. Cady B, Stone MD, McDermott WV, et al. Technical and biological factors in disease-free survival after hepatic resection for colorectal cancer metastases. *Arch Surg* 1992;127:561–568.
25. Rosen CB, Nagorney DM, Taswell HF, et al. Perioperative blood transfusion and determinants of survival after liver resection for metastatic colorectal carcinoma. *Ann Surg* 1992;216:492–505.
26. Hughes KS, Simons R, Songhorabodi S, et al. Resection of the liver

for colorectal carcinoma metastases: a multi-institutional study of indications for resection. *Surgery* 1988;103:278–288.

27. Schalg P, Hohenberger P, Herfarth C. Resection of liver metastases in colorectal cancer: competitive analysis of treatment results in synchronous versus metachronous metastases. *Eur J Surg Oncol* 1990;16:360–365.

28. Butler J, Attiyeh FF, Daly JM. Hepatic resection for metastases of the colon and rectum. *Surg Gynecol Obstet* 1986;162:109–113.

29. Ekberg H, Tranberg KG, Andersson R, et al. Pattern of recurrence in liver resection for colorectal secondaries. *World J Surg* 1987;11:541–547.

30. Bozzetti F, Bignami P, Morabito A, Doci R, Gennari L. Patterns of failure following surgical resection of colorectal cancer liver metastases. *Ann Surg* 1987;205:264–270.

31. Nordinger B, Parc R, Delva E, et al. Hepatic resection for colorectal liver metastases. *Ann Surg* 1987;205:256–263.

32. Bozzetti F, Bignami P, Montalto F, Doci R, Gennari L. Repeated hepatic resection for recurrent metastases. *Br J Surg* 1992;79:146–148.

33. Griffith KD, Sugarbaker PH, Chang AE. Repeat hepatic resections for colorectal metastases. *Br J Surg* 1990;77:230–233.

34. Lange JF, Leese T, Castaing D, Bismuth H. Repeat hepatectomy for recurrent malignant tumors of the liver. *Surg Gynecol Obstet* 1989;169:119–126.

35. Valliant JC, Dalladur P, Nordlinger B, et al. Repeat liver resection for recurrent colorectal metastases. *Br J Surg* 1993;80:340–344.

36. Stone MD, Cady B, Jenkins RL, McDermott WV, Steele GD Jr. Surgical therapy for recurrent liver metastases from colorectal cancer. *Arch Surg* 1990;125:718–721.

37. Que FG, Nagorney DM. Resection of recurrent colorectal metastases to the liver. *Br J Surg* 1994;81:255–258.

38. Fortner JG, Silva JS, Golbey RB, Cox EB, Maclean BJ. Multivariate analysis of a personal series of 247 consecutive patients with liver metastases from colorectal cancer: I. treatment by hepatic resection. *Ann Surg* 1984;199:306–316.

39. Doci R, Gennari L, Bignami P, et al. One hundred patients with hepatic metastases from colorectal cancer treated by resection: analysis of prognostic determinants. *Br J Surg* 1991;78:797–801.

40. Heiken JP, Weyman PJ, Lee JKT. Detection of focal hepatic masses: prospective evaluation with CT, delayed CT, CT during arterial portography, and MR imaging. *Radiology* 1989;171:47–51.

41. Onik GM, Atkinson D, Zemel R, Weaver ML. Cryosurgery of liver cancer. *Semin Surg Oncol* 1993;9:309–317.

42. Zhou X-D, Tang Z-Y, Yu Y-Q, et al. The role of cryosurgery in the treatment of hepatic cancer: a report of 113 cases. *J Cancer Res Clin Oncol* 1993;120:100–102.

43. Ravikumar TS, Kane R, Cady B, Jenkins R, Clouse M, Steele G. A 5-year study of cryosurgery in the treatment of liver tumors. *Arch Surg* 1991;126:1520–1524.

44. Charnley RM, Doran J, Morris DL. Cryotherapy for liver metastases: a new approach. *Br J Surg* 1989;76:1040–1041.

45. Goodie DB, Horton MDA, Morris RW, Nagy LS, Morris DL. Anaesthetic experience with cryotherapy for treatment of hepatic malignancy. *Anaesth Intensive Care* 1992;20:491–496.

46. Weaver ML, Atkinson D, Zemel R. Hepatic cryosurgery in treating colorectal metastases. *Cancer* 1995;76:210–214.

47. Onik GM, Chambers N, Chernus SA, Zemel R, Atkinson D, Weaver ML. Hepatic cryosurgery with and without the Bair Hugger. *J Surg Oncol* 1993;52:185–187.

48. Petrelli N, Douglass H, Herrerra L, et al. The modulation of fluorouracil with leucovorin in metastatic colorectal carcinoma: a prospective randomized phase III trial. *J Clin Oncol* 1989;7:1419–1426.

49. Poon MA, O'Connell MJ, Moertel CG, et al. Biochemical modulation of fluorouracil: evidence of significant improvement of survival and quality of life in patients with advanced colorectal carcinoma. *J Clin Oncol* 1989;7:1407–1418.

50. Doroshow JH, Multhauf P, Leong L. Prospective, randomized comparison of FU versus FU and high-dose, continuous infusion leucovorin calcium for the treatment of advanced, measurable colorectal carcinoma in patients previously exposed to chemotherapy. *J Clin Oncol* 1990;8:491–501.

51. Nordic Gastrointestinal Tumor Adjuvant Therapy Group. Expectancy or primary chemotherapy in patients with advanced asymptomatic colorectal cancer: a randomized trial. 1992;10:904–911.

52. Scheithauer W, Rosen H, Kornek GV, Sebesta C, Depisch D. Randomized comparison of combination chemotherapy plus supportive care with supportive care alone in patients with metastatic colorectal cancer. *Br Med J* 1993;306:752–755.

53. Farmer DG, Rosove MH, Shaked A, Busuttil R. Current treatment modalities for hepatocellular carcinoma. *Ann Surg* 1994;219:236–247.

54. Ridge JA, Bading JR, Gelbard AS, et al. Perfusion of colorectal hepatic metastases: relative distribution of flow from the hepatic artery and portal vein. *Cancer* 1987;59:1547–1553.

55. Sigurdson ER, Ridge JA, Kemeny N, Daly JM. Tumor and liver drug uptake following hepatic artery and portal vein infusion. *J Clin Oncol* 1987;5:1836–1840.

56. Collins JM. Pharmacologic rationale for hepatic arterial therapy. *Recent Results Cancer Res* 1986;100:140–147.

57. Kemeny N, Daly J, Reichman B, et al. Intrahepatic or systemic infusion of fluorodeoxyuridine in patients with liver metastases from colorectal carcinoma. *Ann Intern Med* 1987;107:459–465.

58. Martin JK, O'Connell MJ, Wieand HS, et al. Intra-arterial floxuridine vs systemic fluorouracil for hepatic metastases from colorectal cancer. *Arch Surg* 1990;125:1022–1027.

59. Chang AE, Schneider PD, Sugarbaker PH, et al. A prospective randomized trial of regional versus systemic continuous 5-fluorodeoxyuridine chemotherapy in the treatment of colorectal liver metastases. *Ann Surg* 1987;206:685–693.

60. Hohn DS, Stagg RJ, Friedman MA, et al. A randomized trial of continuous intravenous versus hepatic intraarterial floxuridine in patients with colorectal cancer metastatic to the liver: the Northern California Oncology Group trial. *J Clin Oncol* 1989;7:1646–1654.

61. Buyse M. Reappraisal of hepatic arterial infusion in the treatment of nonresectable liver metastases from colorectal cancer: Meta-Analysis Group in Cancer. *J Natl Cancer Inst* 1996;88:252–258.

62. Allen-Mersh TG, Earlam S, Fordy C, Abrams K, Houghton J. Quality of life and survival with continuous hepatic-artery floxuridine infusion for colorectal liver metastases. *Lancet* 1994;344:1255–1260.

63. Rougier P, Laplanche A, Huguier M, et al. Hepatic arterial infusion of floxuridine in patients with liver metastases from colorectal carcinoma: long term results of a prospective randomized trial. *J Clin Oncol* 1992;10:1112–1118.

64. Kemeny N, Cohen A, Bertino JR, Sigurdson ER, Botet J, Oderman P. Continuous intrahepatic infusion of floxuridine and leucovorin through an implantable pump for the treatment of hepatic metastases from colorectal carcinoma. *Cancer* 1990;65:2446–2450.

65. Maeta M, Koga S, Shimizu N, et al. Intra-hepato-arterial chemotherapy with CDDP and 5-FU for metastases to the liver from colorectal and gastric cancers. *Eur J Cancer Clin Oncol* 1988;24:1199–1203.

66. Patt YZ, Boddie AW, Charnsangavej C, et al. Hepatic arterial infusion with floxuridine and cisplatin: overriding importance of antitumor effect versus degree of tumor burden as determinants of survival among patients with colorectal cancer. *J Clin Oncol* 1986;4:1356–1364.

67. Kemeny N, Seiter K, Niedzwiecki D, et al. A randomized trial of intrahepatic infusion of fluorodeoxyuridine with dexamethasone versus fluorodeoxyuridine alone in the treatment of metastatic colorectal cancer. *Cancer* 1992;69:327–334.

68. Wereldsma JCJ, Bruggink EDM, Meijer WS, Roukema JA, van Putten WLJ. Adjuvant portal liver infusion in colorectal cancer with 5-fluorouracil/heparin versus urokinase versus control: results of a prospective randomized clinical trial. *Cancer* 1990;65:425–432.

69. Scheele J, Stangl R, Altendorf-Hofmann A, Gall FP. Indicators of prognosis after hepatic resection for colorectal secondaries. *Surgery* 1991;110:13–29.

70. Adson MA, Van Heerden JA, Adson MH, Wagner JS, Ilstrup DM. Resection of hepatic metastases from colorectal. *Arch Surg* 1984;119:647–651.

71. Hughes KS, Simon R, Songhorabodi S, et al. Resection of the liver for colorectal carcinoma metastases: a multi-institutional study of patterns of recurrence. *Surgery* 1986;100:278–284.

72. Cobourn CS, Makowka L, Langer B, Taylor B, Falk R. Examination of patient selection and outcome for hepatic resection for metastatic disease. *Surg Gynecol Obstet* 1987;165:239–246.

73. Younes RN, Rogatko A, Brennan MF. The influence of intraoperative hypotension and perioperative blood transfusion on disease-free survival in patients with complete resection of colorectal liver metastases. *Ann Surg* 1991;214:107–113.

74. Iwatsuki S, Esquivel CO, Gordon RD, Starzl TE. Liver resection for metastatic colorectal cancer. *Surgery* 1986;100:804–810.

75. Cunningham JD, Fong Y, Schriver C. One hundred consecutive

hepatic resections: blood loss, transfusion, and operative technique. *Arch Surg* 1994;129:1050–1056.

76. Blumgart LH, Fong Y. Surgical options in the treatment of hepatic metastasis from colorectal cancer. *Curr Probl Surg* 1995;32:335–421.

77. Giovannini M, Seitz J-F. Ultrasound guided percutaneous alcohol injection of small liver metastases: results in 40 patients. *Cancer* 1994;73:294–297.

78. Shiina S, Tagawa K, Niwa Y, et al. Percutaneous ethanol injection therapy for hepatocellular carcinoma: results in 146 patients. *AJR Am J Roentgenol* 1993;160:1023–1028.

79. Livraghi T, Bolondi L, Buscarini L, et al, the Italian Cooperative HCC Study Group. No treatment, resection and ethanol injection in hepatocellular carcinoma: a retrospective analysis of survival in 391 patients with cirrhosis. *J Hepatol* 1995;22:522–526.

80. Kotoh K, Sakai H, Sakamoto S, et al. The effect of percutaneous ethanol injection therapy on small, solitary hepatocellular carcinoma is comparable to that of hepatectomy. *Am J Gastroenterol* 1994;89:194–198.

81. Castells A, Bruix J, Bru C, et al. Treatment of small hepatocellular carcinoma in cirrhotic patients: a cohort study comparing surgical resection and percutaneous ethanol injection. *Hepatology* 1993;18:1121–1126.

82. Honda N, Guo Q, Uchida H, Ohishi H, Hiasa Y. Percutaneous hot saline injection therapy for hepatic tumors: an alternative to percutaneous ethanol injection therapy. *Radiology* 1994;190:53–57.

83. Amin A, Donald JJ, Masters A, et al. Hepatic metastases: interstitial laser photocoagulation with real-time US monitoring and dynamic CT evaluation of treatment. *Radiology* 1993;187:339–347.

84. Nolsœ CP, Torp-Pedersen S, Burcharth F, et al. Interstitial hyperthermia of colorectal liver metastases with a US-guided Nd-YAG laser with a diffuser tip: a pilot clinical study. *Radiology* 1993;187:333–337.

85. Vogl TJ, Müller PK, Hammerstingl R, et al. Malignant liver tumors treated with MR imaging-guided laser-induced thermotherapy: technique and prospective results. *Radiology* 1995;196:257–265.

86. Masters A, Steger AC, Lees WR, Walmsley KM, Bown SG. Interstitial laser hyperthermia: a new approach for treating liver metastases. *Br J Cancer* 1992;66:518–522.

87. Dowlatshahi K, Bhattacharya AK, Silver B, Matalon T, Williams JW. Percutaneous interstitial laser therapy of a patient with recurrent hepatoma in a transplanted liver. *Surgery* 1992;112:603–606.

88. Amin Z, Brown SG, Lees WR. Local treatment of colorectal liver metastases: a comparison of interstitial laser photocoagulation and percutaneous alcohol injection. *Clin Radiol* 1993;48:166–171.

89. Tanaka S. Immunological aspects of cryosurgery in general surgery. *Cryobiology* 1982;19:247–262.

90. Ablin RJ. An appreciation: realization and application of cryoimmunotherapy. In: *Proceedings of the VI International Congress of Cryosurgery*. Casale Monferrato: Eurograf; 1988.

91. Ablin RJ, Guinan PD, Bruns GR, Al Sheik HI, Sadoughi N, Bush IM. Evaluation of cellular immunologic responsiveness in the clinical management of patients with prostatic cancer. *Urol Int* 1976;31:383–400.

92. Milleman LA, Weissman WD, Culp DA. Serum protein, enzyme and immunoglobulin responses following perineal cryosurgery for carcinoma of the prostate. *J Urol* 1979;123:710–712.

93. Ueda K, Ohtaguro K, Washida H, Jinno H, Fushimi N, Masegi T. Humoral immunity following double freezing of the prostate of patients with prostatic cancer. *Biomedical thermology* New York: Alan R. Liss: 1982;815–826.

94. Albin RJ, Fontana G, Cryoimmunotherapeutic Study Group. Cryoimmunotherapy: continuing studies toward determining a rational approach for assessing the candidacy of the prostatic cancer patient for cryoimmunotherapy and postoperative responsiveness—an interim report. *Eur Surg Res* 1979;11:223–233.

95. Bonney WW, Henstorf JE, Emaus SP, Lubaroff DM, Feldbush TL. Immunostimulation by cryosurgery: an orthotopic model of prostate and bladder cancer in the rat. *Monogr Natl Cancer Inst* 1978;49:375–381.

96. Ablin RJ, Bradley PF. Immunological aspects of cryosurgery. In: Bradley PF, ed. *Cryosurgery of the maxillofacial region*. Vol 1. Boca Raton, FL: CRC Press; 1986:78–99.

97. Bayjoo P, Rees RC, Goepel JR, Jacob G. Natural killer cell activity following cryosurgery of normal and tumour bearing liver in an animal model. *J Clin Lab Immunol* 1991;35:129–132.

98. Drylie DM, Jordan WP, Robbins JB. Immunologic consequences of cryosurgery. *Invest Urol* 1968;5:619–626.

99. Soanes WA, Gonder MJ, Ablin RJ. A possible immuno-cryothermic response in prostatic cancer. *Clin Radiol* 1970;21:253–255.

100. Soanes WA, Ablin RJ, Gonder MJ. Remission of metastatic lesions following cryosurgery in prostatic cancer: immunologic considerations. *J Urol* 1970;104:154–159.

101. Neel HB III, Ritts RE. Immunotherapeutic effect of tumor necrosis after cryosurgery, electrocoagulation, and ligation. *J Surg Oncol* 1979;11:45–52.

102. Zonnevylle JA, Zwaveling A. The influence of cryosurgery and electrocoagulation upon metastatic spread. *J Surg Oncol* 1984;27:131–134.

103. Yamashita T, Hayakawa K, Hosokawa M, et al. Enhanced tumor metastases in rats following cryosurgery of primary tumor. *Gann* 1982;73:222–228.

CHAPTER 11

Isolated Perfusion of the Liver

Douglas L. Fraker and H. Richard Alexander, Jr.

> Isolation is simple for the extremities . . . which have a single arterial inflow and a single venous outflow . . . [but] the technique for complete isolation of the liver is a relatively complicated procedure because of its anatomic peculiarity.
> —*Chung (2)*

BACKGROUND

Isolated perfusion is a surgical technique to selectively administer tumoricidal drugs intravascularly to specific organs or regions of the body, and was studied extensively in preclinical models in the late 1950s and early 1960s (2). Availability of perfusion equipment and techniques developed for cardiac surgery allowed investigators to perfuse oxygenated blood in a controlled recirculating system in terms of flow rates, perfusion pressures, oxygenation levels, and temperature. The theoretical advantage of isolation perfusion procedures is the ability functionally to separate the circulation to a particular area as a closed system from the rest of the native circulation to allow dose escalation of treatment drugs while limiting general systemic exposure. Drugs administered into the perfusate can be recirculated for a defined period of time and, at the conclusion of the treatment period, the perfusate with active agent is flushed out extensively such that when the native circulation is re-established, the overall systemic exposure is quite limited.

Experimental studies to perform isolation perfusion procedures of the extremities, the liver, the lung, the brain, and the pelvis were examined over 30 years ago (1–3). The clinical utility of an isolation perfusion procedure depends on the morbidity experienced by the patient because of the procedure; the degree of vascular isolation that can be achieved in the perfusion circuit, which par-

tially determines the ability to dose-escalate the antineoplastic agent; and the efficacy of the perfusate drug in terms of clinical outcome compared with alternative methods of treatment. For these reasons, isolated limb perfusion (ILP) for advanced extremity melanoma moved quickly to clinical applications (3,4) and has remained an accepted treatment modality for this particular clinical problem (see Chap. 25). While ILP was clinically used, isolated hepatic perfusion (IHP), although studied extensively in preclinical large animal models (5–7), did not immediately progress to clinical trials, with a single exception (8), for two reasons. First, the vascular anatomy of the liver is complex compared with an end organ or region such as an extremity. In terms of blood inflow, there is the dual system of the hepatic artery and the portal vein; there is extensive normal variability of the hepatic arterial anatomy; the hepatic venous drainage is through multiple short and variably sized hepatic veins into the retrohepatic inferior vena cava (IVC) over a long distance; and the relationship of the hepatic venous return to the short segment of the suprahepatic IVC, which also provides venous return from the kidneys and lower extremities, taken together make IHP a complicated procedure. A detailed discussion of the anatomic considerations and technical maneuvers of this procedure is presented in the Methodology section. The second major limitation of applying IHP clinically is the low expectations in terms of clinical response with available standard chemotherapeutic drugs. The potential morbidity for a surgical procedure as complex as IHP must be weighed against the potential benefit achieved for a given patient. The ability to achieve meaningful, durable responses against bulky hepatic metastases may be quite limited.

Despite continual reports of IHP in large animal models with variations in techniques, only a single clinical report was produced in over two decades (8). In the past 10 years, interest in the clinical application of IHP has been rekindled. Technical advances in terms of perfusion

D. L. Fraker: Department of Surgery, University of Pennsylvania, Philadelphia, Pennsylvania 19104.

H. R. Alexander, Jr.: Surgery Branch, National Cancer Institute, National Institutes of Health, Bethesda, Maryland 20854.

equipment and techniques, such as the use of venovenous bypass popularized by Starzl's group for liver transplantation procedures (9), were applied to improve the technique and safety of IHP. Also, recent reports that the addition of high-dose tumor necrosis factor (TNF) to the perfusate in ILP has improved outcome, with 90% complete response rates for extremity melanoma (10,11) even against bulky disease, has raised hopes that this treatment regimen may be applied with similar results in an IHP.

INDICATIONS

Isolated liver perfusion has the potential to treat primary and metastatic cancer confined to the liver. The overall utility of the approach depends on the natural history of the disease with regard to likelihood of recurrence and progression to extrahepatic sites. To alter outcome in terms of overall survival, a clinical condition in which disease remains confined to the liver and local hepatic progression is the predominant life-threatening problem is the ideal situation in which an effective regional treatment maximally benefits the patient.

Treatment of primary liver cancer by IHP is limited for the following reasons. First, a subgroup of patients have extrahepatic disease at the time of presentation and require systemic therapy. Also, the subgroup of patients presenting with focal lesions with no evidence of extrahepatic disease may be amenable to a hepatic resection for curative purposes (12). Finally, patients with hepatoma have a high likelihood of associated disease of the liver in the form of hepatitis or cirrhosis (12,13). Because IHP administers treatment agents to both the tumor as well as the liver parenchyma equally, pre-existing hepatic disease may increase the likelihood of hepatotoxicity and hepatic failure after treatment. Also, the presence of cirrhosis with the potential for elevated portal venous pressures would increase the technical difficulty of this vascular procedure. For the limited subgroup of patients with hepatoma with multifocal or otherwise unresectable disease with no evidence of extrahepatic spread and no significant underlying liver disease, IHP is a treatment option. For this small subgroup of patients, another aggressive surgical treatment option is hepatic transplantation (12).

Isolated hepatic perfusion has the greatest applicability for treatment of metastatic disease to the liver. The problems delineated previously for hepatoma do not exist for the most part for patients with metastatic disease. The most important feature for applying IHP for metastatic disease is the natural history of that particular histologic type. Metastatic colorectal cancer certainly represents the largest population of patients eligible for this procedure. Approximately half of patients with metastatic disease after the treatment of primary colorectal cancer present with evidence only of hepatic metastases (14). In one recent large autopsy series, almost a third of the patients who died with metastatic colorectal cancer had disease confined to the liver (15).

Two other unusual histologic types for which this technique may be applicable are gastrointestinal neuroendocrine tumors and ocular melanomas. Although these histologic types represent considerably fewer patients compared with colorectal cancer, the natural history of both is predominant recurrence in the liver, and there are limited alternative treatment options for those tumors. In over 75% of cases, gastrointestinal carcinoids and pancreatic endocrine tumors present with metastatic disease in the liver only (16). Systemic treatment with streptozotocin-based combination chemotherapy has limited response rates. Ocular melanoma when it metastasizes outside of the orbit presents with disease in the liver only in between 50% and 80% of patients in most series (17, 18). Combination chemotherapy and interleukin-2–based immunotherapy, which have efficacy against cutaneous melanoma, are much less effective for the treatment of metastatic ocular melanoma, giving these patients no effective systemic treatment alternatives (18). The success of ILP for cutaneous melanoma with the combination of melphalan plus TNF warrants trying to apply these same agents in IHP against metastatic ocular melanoma.

Other malignancies may in a minority of cases present with isolated liver metastases as a sole site of disease. Gastrointestinal visceral as well as retroperitoneal sarcomas are in this category, but are limited by further spread to the lungs as well as a high likelihood of extrahepatic intra-abdominal recurrence (14). However, for ocular melanoma, the lack of effective systemic chemotherapeutic agents and the activity reported against extremity sarcoma in ILP with currently available agents gives impetus to treatment of these patients with IHP if indicated. Other histologic types, such as renal cell carcinoma, adrenal carcinoma, breast cancer, cutaneous melanoma, and other gastrointestinal malignancies may occur in certain patients as liver-only metastatic disease. However, the natural history of these various histologies limits the appropriateness of aggressive regional therapy because these particular malignancies almost always spread or recur in extrahepatic sites.

METHODOLOGY

The primary technical challenges with IHP, as mentioned earlier, relate to the vascular anatomy of the liver. Any isolation perfusion procedure requires an inflow vessel or vessels and the placement of a catheter for venous return to create a closed circuit. Establishing both inflow to and outflow from the liver is complicated. Vascular inflow to the liver is provided by the smaller-caliber hepatic arterial system and the larger-caliber portal venous system. The portal vein anatomy is constant, with a single vessel of adequate length from where it exits under the head of the pancreas to its bifurcation in the hepatic hilum. Major advantages for using the portal vein to infuse perfusate drug into the liver are its large size and consistent anatomy. One potential disadvantage is that the blood supply of hepatic metastases is predominantly derived from the hepatic arterial vessels (19). Furthermore, infusional treatment studies in both preclinical and clinical models clearly show greater efficacy achieved through the hepatic arterial system compared with the portal vein (20).

The major disadvantage of using the hepatic arterial system for inflow during an IHP is its small caliber and the high incidence of normal anatomic variations (21). As a small-sized vessel, the ability to cannulate and generate flow rates that are high enough to perfuse and maintain liver viability through the hepatic artery is one consideration. Also, the technical challenge of cannulating and then re-establishing flow in the vessel at decannulation is potentially more difficult than with the portal venous system. The standard approach that alleviates many of these problems is to use the gastroduodenal artery (GDA) to place the hepatic arterial cannula (21). If the patient has standard arterial anatomy with an adequately sized GDA, then this vessel is dissected for a length 2 to 3 cm from its origin. The GDA is ligated distally and an arteriotomy is made well away from its origin from the common hepatic artery. A 2- or 3-mm arterial cannula is then placed through the arteriotomy in the GDA with the tip positioned in the common hepatic artery such that both the right and left hepatic arteries are perfused. If the GDA is small in caliber, it can be gently enlarged with coronary dilators to accommodate a 3-mm catheter in almost all cases. Decannulating with this approach is quite simple because when the cannula is removed, the GDA is simply ligated proximally, and the clamp is removed from the common hepatic artery such that blood flow to the liver is re-established quickly with no arterial suture line.

There are two major anatomic variations that complicate this technique to perfuse the liver through the hepatic arteries (21). First, the right hepatic artery may originate directly from the superior mesenteric artery. When this occurs, there usually are no side branches along the replaced right hepatic artery that can serve as a cannulation entry point, using a technique similar to the one described earlier for the GDA. In this case, the right hepatic artery is directly cannulated and then repaired using fine vascular sutures. The left hepatic artery is perfused through a separate cannula placed into the GDA, as described previously, and these two cannulas are linked to the inflow perfusion line by a Y-connector. A second common anatomic variation occurs when the left hepatic artery arises from the left gastric artery. In this case, there may be adequate gastric branches opposite the left hepatic artery such that one of these branches could be cannulated to feed into the left hepatic artery, similar to the technique used to cannulate the GDA. If not, a direct cannulation of the left hepatic artery can be achieved and, again, the right hepatic artery would be perfused in the

standard way through a GDA cannula and connected to the other arterial inflow with a Y-connector.

The venous return from the liver is primarily from two to three short, wide hepatic veins located superiorly near the suprahepatic IVC, as well as from small branches from the right lobe and the caudate lobe entering directly into the retrohepatic IVC. To capture all the hepatic venous return, direct cannulation of these multiple veins is clearly not possible. The only technique to achieve venous return during IHP is to cannulate the retrohepatic IVC directly, with control above and below the liver. Our approach to placement of this venous return cannula is to dissect a segment of infrahepatic IVC above the renal veins, including ligature of several caudate lobe venous branches to obtain more length. This segment of IVC is then clamped proximally and distally and the venous return cannula is placed directly into the retrohepatic IVC by a transverse venotomy. If the liver disease is bulky, such that hepatomegaly prevents dissection of a sufficient length of IVC, then an alternative cannulation approach is used. The IVC above and below the renal veins as well as both renal veins are dissected and clamped. A double pursestring stitch is placed in the IVC below the renal veins and the venous return cannula is passed through this pursestring and up into the retrohepatic IVC. Rumel tourniquets around this cannula above the renal vein isolate the hepatic venous return into this cannula when the renal vein clamps are removed.

These cannulation techniques to provide inflow to and outflow from the liver also block all venous return from below the diaphragm. Venous drainage from the gut, spleen, and pancreas returns to the heart by the portal vein and the liver circulation. Whether the portal vein or hepatic artery is used to provide perfusate inflow, the distal portal vein must be clamped. Similarly, to collect hepatic venous outflow, the IVC is clamped above the liver such that venous return from the kidney and lower extremities is also obstructed. Two different strategies have been used in both preclinical large animal studies and clinical trials to shunt venous return from below the diaphragm back to the heart. One approach is an internal shunt constructed with two concentric lumens—one to catch the venous return from the liver connected to the perfusion circuit, and a second, inner lumen to allow blood flow from the lower extremities and kidneys to continue back to the right atrium (22,23). The inner shunt tube has a sidearm that is placed in the distal portal vein to capture venous return from the gut and direct it back to the heart in a similar manner.

The second type of venous bypass shunt is an external system that establishes a pathway outside of the body to return blood to a large vein above the diaphragm. This external shunt is a Y-shaped circuit with inflow from both the portal vein and the distal IVC. The outflow from the shunt is directed into a catheter in the internal jugular vein (in most preclinical models) or to the axillary/subclavian vein (clinical trials). The most practical version of this external venovenous bypass shunt was developed by Starzl and coworkers for hepatic transplantation procedures and cannulates the distal IVC through a cutdown on the saphenous vein (9). The inflow is provided by a small axillary incision, with the direct cannulation of this vein positioning the tip of the cannula into the innominate vein.

The biggest problem with the internal shunt is that, because of the way that it is constructed, the inner lumen in quite small and resistance to flow may be high (22). Also, because it is a contained system, there is no way actively to pump or assist flow through the shunt. Therefore, a significant gradient builds up over this shunt, with decreased venous return and venous engorgement of the gut, kidneys, and lower extremities. On the other hand, the external shunt can be actively pumped (24). Most commonly, a centrifugal pump is used with no reservoir in the circuit such that all venous return collected is pumped into the axillary vein. Furthermore, by accessing the distal IVC through the saphenous vein instead of through direct cannulation, this arm of the shunt can be maintained during clamping and manipulation of the IVC such that minimal hemodynamic shifts occur during cannulation and decannulation.

An additional advantage of the external shunt with a centrifugal pump is that it establishes a constant reservoir of systemic blood that can be used to monitor perfusate leak continuously during the IHP (25). An analogous system using ^{131}I-albumin was developed to monitor perfusate leak during TNF limb perfusion (10). The equipment required for this leak detection system includes a gamma counter, which in an ILP is placed over the precordium with output adapted to a continuous strip chart or digital recorder. Once surgical isolation is achieved, a calibration dose of 20 μCi of ^{131}I-albumin is injected into the circuit, and after this distributes throughout the systemic circulation, it establishes an incremental count from the relatively constant systemic blood maintained in the heart and great vessels. A 10-fold higher dose (200 μCi ^{131}I-albumin) is then injected into the perfusate and any increase in counts from the precordial gamma counter represents a "leak" of the perfusate to the systemic circulation. This system used for ILP cannot be adapted to monitor perfusate leak during IHP because of the proximity of the liver to the precordial probe detection device. When the perfusate dose of radionuclide would be injected into the liver perfusion circuit, scatter to the probe over the heart would make data from this system uninterpretable. Another site of a constant systemic blood line distant from the liver is needed to provide continuous monitoring. Attempts were made to place a gamma counter over the skull based on central nervous system/sagittal sinus blood volume, but the amount of counts from this site was not sufficient (unpublished observations, D. L. Fraker and H. R. Alexander, National Cancer Institute, Bethesda, MD). The centrifugal pump

provides a constant volume reservoir of approximately 75 ml, and the gamma counter can then be positioned directly over this reservoir. Compared with the ILP system described previously using a precordial monitor, a leak of the perfusate would not be detected as quickly as with the monitor placed over the venous bypass circuit; however, it does provide a system that can reliably assess leak of perfusate drug during an IHP.

The sequential steps to perform an IHP at the National Cancer Institute (NCI) are shown in Tables 1 to 3. Initially, a small subcostal incision is made to evaluate for carcinomatosis. If no evidence of obvious extrahepatic spread is noted, the incision is extended to a bilateral subcostal, with a midline extension to the xiphoid process if needed. The goal of the dissection before perfusion is to isolate the liver such that it is attached only by the IVC superiorly and inferiorly and by the three portal structures—hepatic artery, portal vein, and common bile duct (Table 1). With this dissection, the only source of perfusate leak short of a clamp becoming dislodged is col-

TABLE 1. *Steps to perform an isolated liver perfusion: initial dissection*

1. Limited incision to evaluate for extrahepatic disease
2. Bilateral subcostal incision ± midline extension to xiphoid
3. Complete mobilization of all attachments of liver including
   Suprahepatic IVC, tying phrenic branches
   Retrohepatic IVC, tying right adrenal vein
   Infrahepatic IVC, tying caudate lobe branches
   Porta hepatis dissection, skeletonizing hepatic artery, bile duct, and portal vein
4. Cholecystectomy
5. Dissection of right saphenous vein and left axillary vein

IVC, inferior vena cava.

TABLE 2. *Steps to perform an isolated liver perfusion: cannulation, perfusion, and flush*

1. Heparinize systemically with 200 U/kg
2. Place 16–20-Fr cannula into saphenous vein and pass into distal IVC
3. Place 18–22-Fr cannula into axillary vein
4. Clamp IVC above renal veins and start shunt flow at 800–1200 ml/min
5. Place venous return cannula (24 Fr) in retrohepatic IVC
6. Cannulate distal portal vein (18–20 Fr) and shunt portal flow increasing flow rate to 1500–2000 ml/min
7. Place temperature probe into proximal portal vein for core liver temperatures
8. Ligate gastroduodenal artery distally, clamp hepatic artery, and cannulate to perfuse proper common hepatic artery
9. Clamp suprahepatic IVC and begin perfusion
10. Flow rates set at 500–750 ml/min
11. At conclusion of treatment, flush liver with 2500 ml crystalloid/colloid through hepatic artery and gravity-flush proximal portal vein with 1 liter

IVC, inferior vena cava.

TABLE 3. *Steps to perform an isolated liver perfusion: decannulation*

1. Unclamp suprahepatic IVC
2. Remove arterial cannula from GDA; ligate proximal GDA and unclamp common hepatic artery
3. Remove retrohepatic IVC venous return cannula and repair IVC
4. Unclamp IVC and remove saphenous vein shunt cannula; decrease shunt flow
5. Turn off venous shunt, clamp portal vein shunt line, decannulate, and repair portal vein
6. Gravity-drain blood in shunt tubing into left axillary vein
7. Decannulate and repair left axillary vein
8. Obtain hemostasis and close abdominal incision

IVC, inferior vena cava; GDA, gastroduodenal artery.

laterals in and around the common bile duct. The gallbladder is removed to prevent chemical cholecystitis and to eliminate a possible source of perfusate leakage.

The steps required to establish the circuit and the shunt to perform an isolated limb perfusion are shown in Table 2. The only possible time of hemodynamic compromise, when venous return is limited significantly, is when the portal vein is clamped before positioning the shunt cannula in this vessel.

Similarly, during decannulation (Table 3), the only time in which venous return to the heart is obstructed is when the portal vein is clamped and the venotomy is being repaired. The steps for decannulation shown in Table 3 are ordered as shown because we have found that decannulating the IVC and repairing it to establish native flow through this large vessel makes the patient more stable during the clamping and repair of the portal vein.

SPECIAL INSTRUMENTATION

The equipment needed for performing IHP, apart from standard vascular surgical equipment, relates to the perfusion pump, the venous bypass pump, and the equipment used to monitor leakage of perfusate by radioactive tracer technique (Fig. 1). The equipment for a perfusion circuit consists of a pump, a heater–cooler unit to warm the perfusate, a pressure monitor, and temperature probes. We use a standard roller pump to perfuse the liver, and the perfusion flow rate is controlled with this pump and the mean arterial (inflow line pressure) is monitored. The disposable equipment used in each IHP includes tubing, filters, an oxygenator, and a heat exchanger. A custom-made pack for pediatric cardiac surgery in which the prime volume of the circuit is limited is most appropriate.

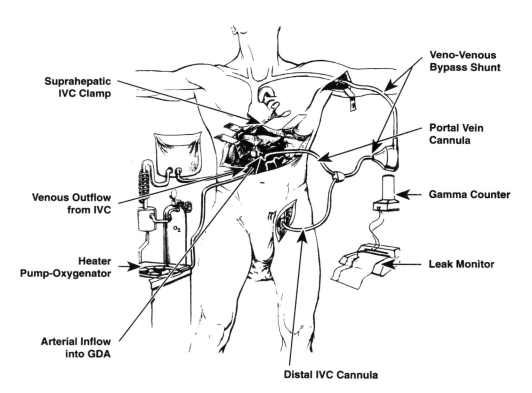

FIG. 1. The operative setup used at the National Cancer Institute to perform an isolated hepatic perfusion. The circuit shown on the patient's right circulates the perfusate with drug to the liver only. The veno-venous bypass circuit with the gamma counter used as a leak-monitoring device is shown on the patient's left.

Our system requires a 900- to 1000-ml prime consisting of one unit of packed red blood cells, saline, and heparin (25). The circuit has a reservoir into which the venous return drains by gravity. The reservoir is useful because it also provides a visual assessment of perfusate leakage to systemic circulation (decreasing reservoir volume) or a systemic-to-perfusate communication (increasing reservoir volume). Limited changes in reservoir volume during IHP may represent redistribution of blood between the perfusion circuit and the liver, with no real leak.

The venovenous bypass circuit requires a Bio-Medicus (Minneapolis, Minnesota) centrifugal pump (9). A perfusion pack designed as a liver transplantation circuit, including the Y-shaped tubing and the Bio-Medicus reservoir attachment, is commercially available. The cannulas used in both circuits are standard disposable straight venous cannulas ranging between 14 and 22 Fr in diameter. We use a small, olive-tipped, 2- to 3-mm arteriotomy cannula for placement in the GDA for arterial inflow to the liver.

The equipment used to monitor perfusate leakage includes a gamma counter attached to a movable arm such that it can be positioned at various angles. A mobile thyroid counter unit is optimal because it can be used for both IHP and ILP. The detector on these units is well shielded, which is necessary for this application. The signals from the gamma counter are electronically adapted such that for every 10- to 30-second period, it generates an average number of counts detected, which is then read out on a strip chart recorder or a digital meter.

SPECIAL PRECAUTIONS

Patient selection for an aggressive regional surgical approach such as IHP is crucial, and patients must be screened for extrahepatic disease, amount and distribution of hepatic metastases, and other systemic medical conditions. The tests used to screen for extrahepatic disease depend on the histologic status of that particular patient's disease, but at minimum a complete chest, abdominal, and pelvic computed tomography (CT) scan is required. In ocular melanoma and other conditions, a head CT or magnetic resonance imaging (MRI) scan may also be indicated.

In terms of the bulk of the liver disease, patients with over 50% of their hepatic parenchyma replaced may have problems with IHP for two reasons. First, all of the normal liver is treated in an identical manner to the tumor within the liver, such that the likelihood of morbidity from liver failure is greater with bulky tumor and limited normal reserve. Eligibility requirements from the NCI IHP protocol include a bilirubin less than 2.0 mg/dl with normal coagulation panels as a measure of hepatic function. A second problem with bulky disease is that it may not be possible technically to dissect, isolate, and perfuse the liver in that circumstance. Large lesions that are sclerotic, particularly in the right lobe, prevent upward and medial deflection of the liver to expose the retrohepatic IVC. Similarly, large surface metastases that are soft and necrotic may rupture on mobilization and present a problem with bleeding during treatment with heparinization. A final situation in which disease can prevent performing this procedure is bulky and invasive tumor near the suprahepatic IVC at the junction with the hepatic veins. This region of the IVC must be circumferentially dissected, tying off any phrenic branches to allow a suprahepatic clamp to be placed that does not obstruct venous return. Large tumor nodules in this area invading the diaphragm may prohibit safe dissections to accomplish these goals.

Isolated hepatic perfusion may result in some hemodynamic fluctuations during cannulation and decannulation, and use of high-dose TNF in IHP causes a cascade of secondary mediators that results in a hyperdynamic state for 24 to 48 hours. For this reason, we perform IHP with a Swann-Ganz pulmonary artery catheter in place. Patients are left intubated overnight the day of the procedure to control ventilation. Pre-existing cardiopulmonary disease places the patient at significant risk for complications, and this experimental approach should not be offered to patients who do not have normal or near-normal performance status.

CLINICAL TRIALS

The clinical application of IHP, as noted earlier, has been infrequent. The initial application was over 30 years ago by Ausman, who treated five patients with nitrogen mustard and saw no responses, but acceptable toxicity (8). Two teams of investigators have applied IHP in the 1980s in clinical trials (Table 4). Skibba and coworkers in Wisconsin treated eight patients in a protocol in which no chemotherapy drug was administered, but the liver was heated to 42°C for 4 hours (26,27). Five patients with metastatic colon cancer, two with melanoma, and one with cholangiocarcinoma were treated. Two patients died after surgery, but of the six survivors, five were reported to be responders. However, these investigators defined response as changes seen on CT scans consistent with central tumor necrosis, tumor necrosis by biopsy, or stable disease with extrahepatic progression. No response data in terms of decrease in size of the treated lesions using standard criteria were reported (26,27).

Aigner et al., working in Germany, treated over 30 patients primarily with colorectal metastases with high-dose 5-fluorouracil (mean dose, 1000 mg) and mild hyperthermia (28,29). Unfortunately, most of these patients were treated with IHP in conjunction with other therapeutic modalities, including postoperative intra-arterial infusional therapy, such that the impact from IHP alone cannot be clearly delineated. Aigner et al. did report and publish CT changes in which tumors had central

TABLE 4. *Results of published trials using isolated hepatic perfusion to treat solid tumors of the liver*

Reference	N	Drugs	Temperature	Time	Clinical outcome
		Treatment Regimen			
Ausman, 1961 (8)	5	Nitrogen mustard 0.2–0.4 mg/kg	37°	NA	One postoperative death; no response data
Aigner et al., 1984 (29)	32	5-Fluorouracil 1000 mg	40°	60 min	No standard response data; 12 patients IHP only; median survival 8 months; 20 patients IHP plus intra-arterial chemotherapy, median survival 12 months
Skibba and Quebbeman, 1986 (27)	8	None	40–42.5°	4 h	No standard response data; five patients evidence of tumor necrosis, two postoperative deaths due to liver failure
van Zuidewign et al., 1993 (31)	9	Mitomycin C 30 mg/m^2	NA	80 min	One complete response; seven other undefined responses; three hepatic vein occlusions with one death
van Zuidewign et al., 1993 (31)	6	Melphalan 0.75–1.25 mg/kg	NA	80 min	Two objective partial responses

NA, information not available; IHP, isolated hepatic perfusion.

hypoperfusion or what they termed "target lesions" similar to the changes seen by Skibba and Quebbeman with hyperthermia alone (27,29). Clearly, IHP can produce an effect against large metastatic adenocarcinoma deposits, specifically causing central necrosis.

Recently, groups in The Netherlands, Sweden, and the United States have been performing IHP in clinical protocols evaluating the addition of TNF into the perfusate (30). Van Zuidewign and colleagues in Leiden recently reported IHP with mitomycin C or melphalan (31). Nine patients received an 80-minute IHP with mitomycin C at 30 mg/m^2. Seven patients had "clear response" by CT scans, with one complete response. Mitomycin C in IHP is limited by the toxicity of hepatic vein obstruction, and one postoperative death occurred because of this complication, with two other patients needing peritoneovenous shunt (31).

Because of this toxicity, the investigators switched to melphalan at 1 mg/kg, with two of six patients treated having an objective response. There were no problems reported with hepatic venous obstruction in the melphalan subgroup. This trial has subsequently been extended to add TNF to melphalan, which reproduces the ILP regimen.

Fraker et al. at the NCI have completed an IHP protocol with low-dose interferon-gamma and escalating-dose TNF (30). The NCI trial differs from all previous clinical IHP studies in that only the hepatic artery is cannulated for perfusate inflow, and the external venovenous shunt is used to maintain venous return as well as to provide a source for perfusate leak monitoring. Finally, Holmberg and colleagues in Sweden are developing a similar approach, combining TNF and melphalan but at doses considerably lower than those used by Fraker's and van Zuidewign's groups (32). The reported TNF dose is only 0.7 µg/kg, which is 5% to 10% of the amount of agent currently used at the NCI. The melphalan dose in this study is also considerably lower, at 0.5 mg/kg. The current trial at the NCI combining melphalan with TNF and hyperthermia has demonstrated an apparent improvement in response rates compared with TNF alone for both colorectal metastases and ocular melanoma, but it is too early to assess the duration of response (unpublished observations, D. L. Fraker and H. R. Alexander, NCI). The various techniques and clinical questions being asked from ongoing trials of IHP are shown in Table 5.

TABLE 5. *Ongoing clinical trials incorporating high-dose TNF in isolated hepatic perfusion*

Location	NCI, United States (30)	Netherlands[a]	Sweden (32)
Infusion vessels	Hepatic artery alone	Hepatic artery and portal vein	Hepatic artery and portal vein
Venous shunt	External	Internal initially, now external	Internal
Treatment regimen			
Initial	Escalating-dose TNF 0.3, 0.6, and 1.0 mg, 2.0 + 0.2 mg interferon	Escalating-dose melphalan 1.0, 2.0, 3.0 ml, 4.0 mg/kg	TNF 0.7 µg/kg, melphalan 0.5 mg/kg
Current	Alternative escalating-dose TNF 1.0, 1.5, 2.0, 2.5, 3.0 mg with melphalan 1.0, 1.5, 2.0, 2.5, 3.0 mg/kg	Melphalan 1.0 mg/kg plus escalating-dose TNF 0.4, 0.8, 1.2, 1.6, 2.0 mg	
TNF Source	Knoll	Boehringer	Knoll

[a] A. M. M. Eggermont, personal communication (Rotterdam Cancer Institute, Rotterdam, Netherlands).
TNF, tumor necrosis factor.

MORBIDITY AND MORTALITY

One consistent effect of IHP is the transient elevation in liver function chemistries after this procedure. Skibba and Quebbeman reported the time course and degree of these changes after IHP with hyperthermia (27). Fraker et al. had seen similar changes of greater magnitude after IHP with TNF or TNF plus melphalan (unpublished results, NCI). These changes in serum transaminases peak on the second postoperative day and then return to baseline levels in all patients, and are most likely indicative of a centrolobular necrosis due to ischemia from performing the cannulation and decannulation, and from the hyperthermic IHP treatment. Irreversible liver toxicity has not been seen in the NCI trial, but did occur in two patients in Skibba and Quebbeman's series in whom liver necrosis and hepatic failure developed, which resulted in postoperative death (27). These patients were treated for a longer time (4 hours) with more significant hyperthermia (42°C). Holmberg et al. commented on postoperative hepatic and renal toxicity after perfusion with low-dose TNF and melphalan (32). As mentioned earlier, mitomycin C causes a specific problem with hepatic vein occlusion, creating a Budd-Chiari syndrome with hepatic vein obstruction, resulting in this series in one death in nine patients (31).

In summary, IHP may be technically performed safely using the shunt approach described previously. The degree of direct cytotoxicity using mild hyperthermia plus melphalan-based chemotherapy perfusions is acceptable. It remains to be determined whether further dose escalation of melphalan in conjunction with high-dose TNF in the perfusate can result in durable, meaningful clinical responses, as seen in ILP (10). Also, whether the dose of TNF can be escalated to levels that are currently used in ILP while maintaining an acceptable level of systemic toxicity is under investigation.

ALTERNATIVE TREATMENT STRATEGIES

Regional therapy directed against primary or metastatic disease in the liver can be divided into two broad categories. One approach is a direct destruction of tumor by physical or chemical means. A second approach is a regional vascular-based therapy that allows treatment of the entire liver by infusion/perfusion of the blood vessels. Direct destruction of tumor is disadvantageous in that even if all disease can be effectively eliminated, the patients are at risk for development of recurrent disease in other areas of the liver that remain untreated (33). The vascular therapy has the disadvantage that currently available agents that have been used in the various systems have limited durable response rates, such that the survival benefits over systemic therapy have been difficult to demonstrate.

Current direct therapeutic strategies include the use of cold with cryosurgery to freeze tumor (34); the use of heat with percutaneously placed electrodes to destroy tumor (35); and percutaneous injection of ethanol into tumor (36). These treatments are limited by the size and location of lesions that can be treated because the tumor and liver or other adjacent structures are destroyed indiscriminately. Metastatic lesions close to essential vascular or biliary structures as well as those of large size are not amenable to local therapy. Vascular-based therapies, in addition to IHP, include placement of a pump or port to provide continuous infusional hepatic arterial therapy (37–39); chemoembolization, which recently has been shown not to increase survival significantly in patients with hepatoma (40); and percutaneous hepatic perfusion with hemofiltration (41). The variety of treatment strategies attests to the magnitude of the clinical problem presented by solid tumors of the liver, as well as to the fact that no single therapeutic approach has shown dramatic success.

PATIENT ASSESSMENT

Isolated hepatic perfusion delivers a single treatment at a defined point in time during the perfusion operation. Assessment of response and toxicity in this situation is simplified by this single treatment course. That is, preoperative scans taken shortly before IHP document the size and amount of disease. In our experience, MRI scans give a better delineation between tumor mass and normal liver and allow more precise objective measurement of lesions to be taken to assess response (Fig. 2). Objective responses are defined as decrease in tumor size in a standard manner using sequential measurements over time. In addition to size changes, contrast-enhanced CT scans or gadolinium-enhanced MRI scans can show a change in tumor vascularity reflecting antitumor effects, but this cannot be quantitated into a definition of response. Furthermore, for patients with colorectal carcinoma in whom carcinoembryonic antigen (CEA) is elevated before surgery, sequential determination of CEA levels at postoperative time points is another indication of response.

Toxicity is similarly assessed by standard criteria in the postoperative period. Because the physical manipulations required to perform IHP result in biochemical toxicity to the liver, hepatic toxicity that returns to baseline should not be considered a dose-limiting feature in evaluating different regimens in phase I trials. Similarly, the magnitude of a surgical procedure such as an IHP, with a prolonged period of anesthesia, results in systemic toxicities, and separation of effects due to the surgery versus the drug administered may be difficult.

PATIENT INFORMATION

Isolated liver perfusion is a major surgical procedure during which the blood vessels to and from the liver are

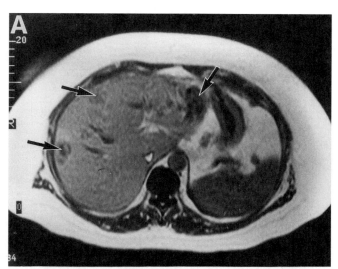

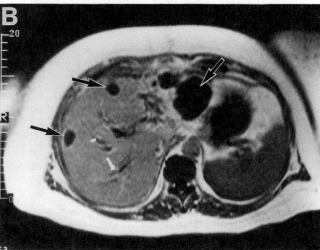

FIG. 2. Preoperative **(A)** and postoperative **(B)** magnetic resonance imaging scans (gadolinium-enhanced, T1-weighted images) from a patient with metastatic colon cancer treated with isolated hepatic perfusion using 0.6 mg tumor necrosis factor and 0.2 mg interferon-gamma with mild hyperthermia at the Surgery Branch, National Cancer Institute. Note the dramatic change in the degree of perfusion in the postoperative scans, in which the lesions appear uniformly dark (arrows) with no perfusion on this contrast-enhanced image.

controlled so that very high concentrations of chemotherapy drugs can be administered to the area where the tumor is located. By isolating the blood flow to the liver from the rest of the body, large amounts of drug that would be toxic if given by arm vein can be used. Isolated liver perfusion is recommended for patients who have tumor located exclusively within the liver but have failed to respond to conventional forms of treatment. Radiologic studies to show that there is no spread to other parts of the body such as the brain, lungs, or elsewhere in the abdomen are important before recommending this type of treatment. Also, before undergoing isolated liver perfusion, patients need to have a radiographic study called an angiogram to show the anatomy of the blood vessels to the liver.

The operation to perform an isolated liver perfusion is a lengthy procedure done under general anesthesia. It requires an abdominal incision to isolate collateral branches of blood flow to the liver. Small incisions also are made in the groin and armpit to shunt the blood from the lower body around the liver into a large vein draining directly back into the heart. A machine like the one used in open heart surgery circulates blood and medications through tubes such that the treatment is delivered only into the liver during the operation.

Complications of the surgical procedure include, like any major operation, bleeding, infection, and the risk of anesthesia. Other complications specific to isolated liver perfusion include potential damage to the normal liver tissue because it is also receives the same treatment agents directed toward the tumor. This complication could result in abnormal blood clotting, jaundice, ascites, or potentially complete liver failure. Other complications not related to the liver include problems in other organ systems due to side effects from the drugs acting on the liver. These side effects can include cardiac failure, pulmonary edema, and renal failure.

Isolated liver perfusion is a highly experimental and aggressive form of treatment. It has been used in a fairly limited number of patients in the United States and Europe. However, a similar operation called isolated limb perfusion for patients who have disease extensively spread throughout the arm and leg has been used in a much larger number of patients. The current treatment drugs used in the limb perfusion trials have given excellent results, and attempts are being made to reproduce these results in a liver perfusion setting.

REFERENCES

1. Chung WB, Moore JR, Mersereau W. A technique of isolated perfusion of the liver. *Surgery* 1962;51:508–511.
2. Shingleton WW, Parker RT, Mahaley, S. Abdominal perfusion for cancer chemotherapy. *Ann Surg* 1069;152:583–593.
3. Creech O, Krementz ET, Ryan RF, Winblad JN. Chemotherapy of cancer: regional perfusion utilizing an extracorporeal circuit. *Ann Surg* 1958;148:616–632.
4. Stehlin JS. Hyperthermic perfusion with chemotherapy for cancers of the extremities. *Surg Gynecol Obstet* 1969;129:305–308.
5. Mulcare RJ, Solis A, Fortner JG. Isolation and perfusion of the liver for cancer chemotherapy. *J Surg Res* 1973;15:87–95.
6. Boddie AW Jr, Booker L, Mullins JD, Buckley CJ, McBride CM. Hepatic hyperthermia by total isolation and regional perfusion in vivo. *J Surg Res* 1979;26:447–457.
7. Sindelar WF. Method of isolation-perfusion of the liver in the pig. *Am Surg* 1984;50:557–563.
8. Ausman RK. Development of a technic for isolated perfusion of the liver. *N Y State J Med* 1961;61:3393–3397.
9. Shaw BW, Martin DJ, Marquez JM, et al. Venous bypass in clinical liver transplantation. *Ann Surg* 1984;200:524–533.
10. Lienard D, Ewalenko P, Delmotti JJ, Renard N, Lejeune FJ. High-dose recombinant tumor necrosis factor alpha in combination with interferon gamma and melphalan in isolation perfusion of the limbs for melanoma and sarcoma. *J Clin Oncol* 1992;10:52–60.

11. Lienard D, Lejeune F, Ewalenko I. In transit metastases of malignant melanoma treated by high dose rTNFα in combination with interferon-gamma and melphalan in isolation perfusion. *World J Surg* 1992;16: 234–240.

12. Farmer DG, Rosove MH, Shaked A, Busuttil RW. Current treatment modalities for hepatocellular carcinoma. *Ann Surg* 1994;219: 236–247.

13. Tsukuma H, Hiyama T, Tanaka S, et al. Risk factors for hepatocellular carcinoma among patients with chronic liver disease. *N Engl J Med* 1993;328:1797–1801.

14. Niederhuber JE, Ensminger WD. Treatment of metastatic cancer to the liver. In: DeVita VT, Hellman S, Rosenberg SA, eds. *Cancer: principles and practice of oncology.* Philadelphia: JB Lippincott; 1993: 2201–2224.

15. Weiss L, Grundman E, Torhurst J, et al. Hematogenous metastatic patterns in colonic carcinoma: an analysis of 1541 necropsies. *J Pathol* 1986;150:195–203.

16. Norton JA, Levin B, Jensen RT. Cancer of the endocrine system. In: DeVita VT, Hellman S, Rosenberg SA, eds. *Cancer: principles and practice of oncology.* Philadelphia: JB Lippincott; 1993:1333–1435.

17. Lorigan JG, Wallace S, Mavligit GM. The prevalence and location of metastases from ocular melanoma: imaging study in 110 patients. *AJR Am J Roentgenol* 1991;157:1279–1281.

18. Rajpal S, Moore R, Karakousis CP. Survival in metastatic ocular melanoma. *Cancer* 1983;52:334–336.

19. Lin G, Lunderquist A, Hägerstrand I, Boijsen E. Postmortem examination of the blood supply and vascular pattern of small liver metastases in man. *Surgery* 1984;96:517–526.

20. Sigurdson ER, Ridge JA, Kemeny N, Daly JM. Tumor and liver drug uptake following hepatic artery and portal vein infusion in man. *J Clin Oncol* 1987;5:1836–1840.

21. Campbell KA, Burns RC, Sitzmann JV, Lipsett PA, Grochow LB, Niederhuber JE. Regional chemotherapy devices: effect of experience and anatomy on complications. *J Clin Oncol* 1993;11:822–826.

22. Van de Velde D, Kothuis BJL, Barenbrug HWM, et al. A successful technique of *in vivo* isolated liver perfusion in pigs. *J Surg Res* 1986; 41:593–599.

23. Aigner K, Walther H, Tonn J, et al. First experimental and clinical results of isolated liver perfusion with cytotoxics in metastases from colorectal primary. *Recent Results Cancer Res* 1983;86:99–102.

24. Diebel LN, Wilson RF, Bender J, Paules B. A comparison of passive and active shunting for bypass of the retrohepatic IVC. *J Trauma* 1991; 31:987–990.

25. Fraker DL, Alexander HR, Thom AK, et al. Technique of isolated hepatic perfusion for the treatment of metastatic cancer using tumor necrosis factor. *Surgery* 1997 (submitted for publication).

26. Skibba JL, Quebbeman EJ, Komorowski RA, Thorsen KM. Clinical results of hyperthermic liver perfusion for cancer in the liver. In: Aigner KR, Patt YZ, Link KH, Kreidler J, eds. *Regional cancer treatment.* Basel: Karger; 1988:222–228.

27. Skibba JL, Quebbeman EJ. Tumoricidal effects and patient survival after hyperthermic liver perfusion. *Arch Surg* 1986;121:1266–1271.

28. Aigner KR, Walther H, Link KH. Isolated liver perfusion with MMC/5-FU: surgical technique, pharmacokinetics, clinical results. In: Aigner KR, Patt YZ, Link KH, Kreidler J, eds. *Regional cancer treatment.* Basel: Karger; 1988:229–246.

29. Aigner KR, Walther H, Tonn JC, Link KH, Schoch P, Schwemmle K. Die isolierte Leberperfusion bei fortgeschrittenen Metastasen kolorektaler Karzinome. *Onkologie* 1984;7:13–21.

30. Fraker DL, Alexander HR, Thom AK. Use of tumor necrosis factor in isolated hepatic perfusion. *Circ Shock* 1994;44:45–50.

31. van Zuidewign DBW, de Brauw LM, Marinelli A, Keijzer HJ, van Bockel JH, Van de Velde CJH. Isolated liver perfusion with mitomycin-C or melphalan in patients with hepatic metastases (Abstract). *Proceedings of the Society of Surgical Oncology* 1993;46:198.

32. Holmberg SB, Hafström L, Lindner P, et al. Hyperthermic liver perfusion with tumor necrosis factor and chemotherapy (Abstract). *Eur J Surg Oncol* 1994;20:317.

33. Ebara M, Ohto M, Shinagawa T, et al. Natural history of minute hepatocellular carcinoma smaller than three centimeters complicating cirrhosis: a study of 22 patients. *Gastroenterology* 1986;90:289–298.

34. Ravikumar TS, Kane R, Cady B, Jenkins R, Clouse M, Steele G Jr. A 5-year study of cryosurgery in the treatment of liver tumors. *Arch Surg* 1991;126:1520–1524.

35. Rossi S, di Stasi M, Buscarini E, et al. Percutaneous radiofrequency interstitial thermal ablation in the treatment of small hepatocellular carcinoma: report of 24 patients. *The Cancer Journal of Scientific American* 1995;1:72–79.

36. Sironi S, Livraghi T, Angeli E, et al. Small hepatocellular carcinoma: MR follow-up of treatment with percutaneous ethanol injection. *Radiology* 1993;187:119–123.

37. Patt YZ. Regional hepatic arterial chemotherapy for colorectal cancer metastatic to the liver: the controversy continues. *J Clin Oncol* 1993; 11:815–819.

38. Martinelli DJ, Wadler S, Bakal CW, et al. Utility of embolization or chemoembolization as second-line treatment in patients with advanced or recurrent colorectal carcinoma. *Cancer* 1994;74:1706–1712.

39. Higuchi T, Kikuchi M, Okazaki M. Hepatocellular carcinoma after transcatheter hepatic arterial embolization. *Cancer* 1994;73:2259–2267.

40. Groupe d'Etude et de Traitment du Carcinome Hepatocellulaire. A comparison of lipiodol chemoembolization and conservative treatment for unresectable hepatocellular carcinoma. *N Engl J Med* 1995;332: 1256–1261.

41. Ravikumar TS, Pizzorno G, Bodden W, et al. Percutaneous hepatic vein isolation and high-dose hepatic arterial infusion chemotherapy for unresectable liver tumors. *J Clin Oncol* 1994;12:2723–2736.

Diagnosis of Central Nervous System Metastases

Nicholas J. Patronas and Myles B. Koby

... Life is short, the Art long, Opportunity fleeting, Experience treacherous, Judgment difficult ...
—*Hippocrates (460–357 B.C.)*

This chapter discusses the imaging methods currently used in clinical practice for the diagnosis of metastatic lesions to the central nervous system (CNS). The parameters that influence the sensitivity and specificity of these methods are examined, and indications to solve specific diagnostic problems are addressed. Understanding the strengths and weaknesses of each modality provides the foundation for uses and limitations in the evaluation of metastatic disease. The variety of diagnostic methods available to study the metabolic activity and the biologic behavior of brain tumors are reviewed. Some of these studies shed light on the chemical environment of brain tumors, and others show changes that occur under the influence of various therapeutic regimens.

The presence of brain metastases in patients with primary malignancies dramatically changes the prognosis as well as the management of these patients. Successful treatment of a solitary brain metastasis can substantially improve longevity and quality of life for cancer patients. This in turn has renewed interest in the diagnosis of metastatic disease. If any of the therapeutic approaches are to be maximally successful, it is of paramount importance to define precisely the extent of involvement. The number, size, and location of brain metastases must be accurately demonstrated, and metastases must be distinguished from lesions with similar characteristics. In addition, brain imaging is required to assess the response to therapy and plays an important role in the diagnosis of complications that may occur during the course of disease.

N. J. Patronas: Department of Radiology, National Institutes of Health, Clinical Center, Bethesda, Maryland 20892.

M. B. Koby: Department of Diagnostic Radiology, Michigan State University, Lansing, Michigan 48910.

BACKGROUND

An important question often raised when dealing with malignant tumors is how often these tumors give rise to CNS metastases. The incidence of CNS metastasis during the course of systemic malignancies varies widely in published reports. These discrepancies are best explained by the different biases that influence the results of these studies. Differences in demographic composition are major factors in biased conclusions. The method of diagnosis used, including autopsy, surgery, or imaging, also influences the results of these studies (1). Thus, older reports based mainly on autopsy data indicate that brain metastasis occurred in 6.3% to 15% of cancer patients who died as a result of their disease (2–4). More recent reports indicate that this complication occurs in 25% to 30% of patients with cancer (5,6).

The proportion of cerebral metastasis among all tumors found in the intracranial cavity has been reported to range from 13.5% to 41% (7,8). These results are also influenced by demographic and institutional biases, but it is currently believed that brain metastases comprise 20% to 25% of all clinically detected tumors (1,9).

Studies evaluating the variable propensity of primary tumors to metastasize to the CNS have shown that lung cancer is the most common. In most cases of lung cancer, metastatic deposits occur early in the course of the disease and are often multiple. Breast cancer is the second most common primary tumor metastasizing to the CNS. This is usually a late event, taking place after failure of different therapies (1). Melanoma, cancers of the genitourinary tract, leukemia, and lymphoma are next in frequency, followed by carcinomas of the gastrointestinal tract, head and neck carcinomas, and sarcomas. In a large series, it is reported that 63% of all metastatic brain tumors have their origin from carcinoma of the lung, breast, and genitourinary tract, and melanoma (4). These malignancies, with the addition of leukemia and lymphoma, are also responsible for most meningeal metastases.

The distribution of these tumors in the compartments of the CNS is useful in both the diagnosis and the management of patients with intracranial metastatic tumors. Thus, it has been estimated that 80% to 85% of brain metastases are located in the cerebrum and 15% to 20% in the structures below the tentorium (4,10). The frontal and parietal lobes of the cerebral hemispheres are most commonly affected, in direct proportion to the larger volume of these lobes (11,12). Metastatic brain tumors are commonly encountered at the corticomedullary junction and in the border zones of cerebral vascular territories. Finally, certain primary malignant tumors have a predilection to metastasize to certain sites of the CNS. Thus, pelvic tumors, such as carcinomas of the prostate and uterus, and tumors of the gastrointestinal tract metastasize to the posterior fossa with increased frequency (4, 10,11). Although not proven, it has been suggested that local environmental factors are responsible for this preferred site of metastasis.

The intracranial epidural space, the meninges, and the spinal canal are also affected by metastases, producing symptoms identical to those of primary lesions in these areas. The incidence of metastatic tumors to the intracranial epidural space is not well documented. It is known that tumors in this location usually spread as a result of direct extension from metastatic deposits in the bony calvarium. Tumors with a high propensity to metastasize to bone, such as breast, prostate, lung, thyroid, and renal carcinomas, commonly present with intracranial epidural lesions (13).

In autopsy studies, the intracranial meninges were involved in 4% of patients who died from malignant tumors (14). This incidence is probably increasing as a result of longer survival in treated cancer patients.

The incidence of metastatic tumors in the spinal canal is also difficult to ascertain. The vertebrae represent a common site of secondary tumor deposits, often accompanied by tumor growth into the epidural space of the spinal canal. Metastases to the spinal column may not always produce symptoms because patients not infrequently succumb to their primary disease before cord compression. It has been reported that up to 5% of patients with metastatic tumors develop symptoms from spinal canal involvement, and that 97% of them are caused by extradural cord compression. Intramedullary metastases are rare. In most cases, the involvement of the spinal meninges occurs as an extension of intracranial meningeal carcinomatosis (14–16).

PATHOGENESIS

The departure of tumor cells from the primary tumor site, the implantation of these cells in a remote organ, and the development of a metastatic colony follows a specific pattern and occurs in stages. The first barrier that neoplastic cells cross at the site of their origin is the basement membrane. An impermeable basement membrane that demarcates a mass and clearly separates it from its surroundings is a constant feature of benign tumors. On the other hand, the basement membrane is poorly formed or absent in malignant tumors, and when identifiable, is always breached by neoplastic cells. The degree of maturation of the basement membrane and the extent to which it is permeated by the neoplastic cells represents an index of the malignant potential of a neoplasm.

The invasion of the basement membrane by tumor cells follows a three-step process. Initially, special receptors on the surface of these cells recognize a glycoprotein (laminin) of the basement membrane to which they attach. This attachment is followed by proteolysis of type IV collagen of the basement membrane by a specific collagenase found in tumor cells. Once an area of the membrane is dissolved, the final step of locomotion follows, during which neoplastic cells exhibit increased mobility, allowing them to cross through the defective membrane and to move between other cells into the interstitial space, where they may start replicating. Using similar mechanisms of invasion, tumor cells may penetrate the basal membrane of the capillaries and enter the lumen of the vessels. Once within the intravascular compartment, neoplastic cells can escape the primary tumor site and may establish colonies in different organs (17,18).

As a rule, these free tumor cells are arrested in the first capillary or lymphatic bed encountered. Thus, the first organ of metastasis to a large degree can be predicted from the anatomic routes that tumor cells are obliged to follow. At the new site, by further invading the capillaries or the small venules, tumor cells may again enter the systemic circulation and gain access to wider spread.

Most of the circulating tumor cells are destroyed by the defense mechanisms of the immune system. Perhaps more important, the mechanical shearing-stress forces that these tumor cells are exposed to during the journey from the site of origin to the site of their destination can cause them to die (19). Cells that do manage to survive may be implanted and produce metastatic colonies in different organs at a rate that is roughly proportional to the blood flow of these organs. Once a neoplastic cell is attached to the wall of a capillary, the endothelial cells retract, allowing direct contact of the tumor cells with the basal membrane. At this point, the same mechanisms used by the tumor cells to penetrate the basement membrane at the primary site are repeated so that tumor cells eventually enter the interstitial space of the host organ.

Some primary tumors metastasize preferentially to certain organs, which suggests that factors other than those dictated by anatomic or circulatory considerations play a significant role. It is believed that the development of metastatic colonies is regulated by the target organs. The regulatory mechanisms of this process are the topic of active research. It has been suggested that the target organ either uses chemical signals to attract neoplastic cells or that the endothelial cells of the vasculature of these organs possess a special affinity for certain types of tumor cells. Finally, it is recognized that the presence of neoplastic cells in the interstitial space of an organ is not always synonymous with the development of a new tumor colony, because other autocrine growth mechanisms or factors from the local tissues must be mobilized to promote the development of a tumor (20).

In the case of CNS metastasis, tumor cells arrive in the intracranial cavity by the arterial route. Because 15% to 20% of the cardiac output enters the cerebral circulation, it is not surprising that the brain is a common site of metastatic deposits. Tumor cells of any primary neoplasm can enter the arterial circulation after passing through the pulmonary capillary bed. The proximity of lung carcinoma to the pulmonary vascular bed provides a rationale for the high incidence of brain metastases from this primary. Clusters of tumor cells are found lodged in small arteries at the gray–white matter junction, where the luminal diameter changes abruptly from 100 to 200 mm to 50 to 150 mm. This mechanism is thought to provide a plausible explanation for the high frequency of small tumor nodules commonly found at the gray–white matter interfaces (1). The venous route has also been implicated as a possible mode of access to the posterior fossa. The venous system of the posterior fossa is in direct communication with the venous plexus of the spinal canal (Batson's plexus). It has been theorized that tumor cells from metastatic deposits in the spinal column enter this plexus and are then taken into the intracranial circulation by retrograde flow (21). This route of intracranial metastasis is not unequivocally proven (3). On rare occasions, tumor cells may pass from the venous circulation to the arterial through an atrial septal defect that remains patent in a small percentage of individuals, potentially permitting bidirectional flow (22).

Tumor seeding to the leptomeninges takes place primarily by the arterial route, although an alternative mode of involvement may result from neoplastic cells that escape the ependymal surface or the choroid plexuses and circulate in the cerebrospinal fluid (CSF). In contrast, the dura may be seeded by neoplastic cells of the arterial circulation, or be invaded by metastatic calvarial lesions either directly or from circulating cells in the small venules shared by both (23–26).

The involvement of the epidural space in the intracranial cavity or in the spinal canal usually occurs as a result of direct extension of metastatic tumor in the bone. Hematogenous seeding of tumor into the epidural space in the absence of bony abnormality has been documented in only a few exceptional cases. Finally, tumors of the head and neck may invade the intracranial space through direct extension, using the foramina of the skull base. Rarely, these tumors may extend intracranially by perineural spread (13,27).

PATHOLOGY

Macroscopically metastatic tumors may be discolored, allowing them to be differentiated from normal tissues. This is a result of alteration in tumor circulation, microscopic hemorrhagic elements, and, in melanoma, the presence of melanin. Metastatic tumors are often round, firm, and well demarcated from the adjacent brain parenchyma, which has a softer texture in the presence of edema. When small (<1.5 cm), these tumors are usually solid, but as they become larger, they frequently outgrow their blood supply and central necrosis develops. Some tumors, such as melanomas and choriocarcinomas, have a propensity to bleed and may present as a hematoma. Hemorrhagic brain metastases have also been reported in a variety of other neoplasms, including renal cell and thyroid carcinomas. In exceptional cases, calcifications are detected in metastatic brain lesions.

A variable amount of edema is nearly always present surrounding a metastatic tumor. This edema is vasogenic, produced by extravasation of fluid and proteins from the intravascular compartment into the interstitial spaces. The defective walls of the tumoral capillary bed and the ischemic abnormalities that occur in the brain near the tumor are responsible for the exit of fluid.

Microscopically, metastatic tumors resemble the primary tumor of their origin. The margins of these tumors insinuate into the normal brain by forming projections that first alter the normal architecture and eventually destroy neuronal elements. Tumor often extends along the perivascular Virchow-Robin spaces in a sheath-like fashion, and can be traced to the surface of the brain. Neovascularity is evident within the tumor parenchyma, characterized by immature vessels with endothelial cells containing abundant vesicles and defective tight junctions. Astrocytic reaction is also present in the surrounding brain, and the adjacent myelin is pale due to edema.

Involvement of the leptomeninges presents as plaques of meningeal thickening spread over a variable area on the surface of the brain. Occasionally, a nodular tumor formation develops from the meninges and invaginates into the brain, giving the appearance of an intraparenchymal lesion. In other instances, meningeal tumor masses form within the intracranial subarachnoid cisterns, and rarely in the internal auditory canals. Involvement of the ependymal ventricular walls occurs either as an extension of metastatic brain disease or concomitantly with meningeal carcinomatosis. The infiltrated ependyma is thickened or forms nodular projections into the ventricles.

The ventricular system may have compression deformities from adjacent tumor masses or may be abnormally dilated. Dilatation is caused by obstruction at the foramina of Monro, the aqueduct of Sylvius, or the outlet foramina of the fourth ventricle. Ventricular enlargement can also occur when the flow of CSF in the subarachnoid spaces is disturbed or when the absorption of CSF by the arachnoid villi is impaired. Both of these complications may occur with meningeal carcinomatosis (1,13).

CLINICAL SYMPTOMS

Because of the availability of diagnostic imaging modalities, more asymptomatic patients with metastases to the CNS are being diagnosed on screening and follow-up examinations. The detected lesions are often small with minimal or no edema; therefore, the mass effect associated with these lesions is insufficient to produce symptoms. Typically, however, the time from the development of the first symptom to the discovery of CNS lesion ranges from 3 to 6 months (28).

The appearance of symptoms is usually insidious and progressive, but occasionally an abrupt onset of neurologic deficit mimicking stroke is the first indication of intracranial metastasis. Acute symptoms are the result of hemorrhage, seizure, or frank tumor emboli (29,30).

In older reports, headaches were the most common presenting symptom in patients with intracranial metastases, occurring in 53% to 88% of cases. This is due to increased intracranial pressure, commonly occurring in the morning and spontaneously resolving, only to return each following day, becoming progressively worse.

When headache is accompanied by ataxia, the possibility of cerebellar/posterior fossa metastases must be considered. This can rapidly advance to cause obstruction of the fourth ventricular exit foramina with acute hydrocephalus. Progressive headache and somnolence signify imminent herniation. Papilledema is another nonspecific finding indicative of increased intracranial pressure, but is usually a late event, often found after the diagnosis of intracranial metastases has been made.

Most of the remaining symptoms are specific to the location of the metastatic lesion. Focal motor weakness is a common presenting symptom found with lesions directly or indirectly affecting the motor pathways. Motor deficit can be elicited in as many as 66% of patients by careful neurologic examination. Confusion or behavioral changes have been reported to occur in 31% to 36% of patients, but appropriate neuropsychological testing may yield up to twice this incidence of cognitive impairment. Seizures occur in 15% to 29% of patients with intracerebral metastasis, and are more frequent with leptomeningeal disease. Vision disturbances (27%), vertigo (24%), and aphasia (10%) are also common symptoms. Lesions of the hypothalamus and pituitary gland, although less common, produce specific endocrine dysfunction, including panhypopituitarism, diabetes insipidus, and hyperprolactinemia. Masses in the parasellar region may result in cranial neuropathies presenting as visual impairment (optic nerve or chiasmatic compression), diplopia (cavernous sinus involvement, III, IV, and VI cranial nerve compromise), and motor-sensory alteration (trigeminal ganglion/V cranial nerve) (3,14,28,31–33).

IMAGING MODALITIES

Computed Tomography

Soon after its invention, computed tomography (CT) was applied to the diagnostic problem of metastases. It was a breakthrough in the diagnosis of this disease, demonstrating hitherto unseen lesions.

Computed tomography uses a fan beam of photons or x-rays, emitted from different directions. These x-rays, by virtue of their short wavelength, penetrate the brain. In passing through the brain, the beam is partially absorbed by a quantity dependent on the electron density and effective atomic number of the tissues it encounters. Brain images are presented on a two-dimensional matrix composed of small picture elements (pixels), each depicting a small volume of tissue in a given location (voxel). The radiographic density in each pixel is proportional to the absorption of x-rays that took place in the corresponding voxel, and is measured in Hounsfield units (HU) (34–36).

In most living tissues, the differences in x-ray absorption (contrast) are relatively small, limiting the diagnostic value of CT. To overcome this problem, the use of contrast material is necessary. The compounds used are salts of iodinated acids, whose large molecules diffuse into the interstitial space only when the blood–brain barrier is a disrupted. The presence of iodine in tissues such as a brain tumor dramatically increases the absorption of x-rays in those areas, providing contrast that distinguishes lesions from normal brain (37).

The radiographic features of metastatic brain tumors are evaluated on both precontrast and contrast-enhanced examinations. On noncontrast studies, these tumors may be isodense, hypodense, or hyperdense with respect to normal brain. When isodense, small metastatic brain tumors are usually not seen, whereas large tumors are evident by the mass effect they produce. The signs of mass effect include effacement of cortical sulci, deformity or obliteration of a cistern or a fissure, deformity of a ventricular wall, shift of midline structures, or transtentorial herniation. When cerebral edema has developed or when the tumor has become necrotic, the density decreases and the tumor is more apparent (38–42).

Occasionally, metastatic brain tumors exhibit increased density compared with normal brain on the noncontrast examinations. This is a feature of highly cellular tumors with relatively small interstitial spaces and a high nuclear–cytoplasmic ratio. A few solid tumors, including small cell carcinoma of the lung, lymphoma, and melanoma, demonstrate this hyperdensity. Hyperdensity is also observed in hemorrhagic metastatic tumors such as melanoma, choriocarcinoma, and, less frequently, in other neoplasms (Fig. 1). The density of these hyperdense tumors (75 to 100 HU), is greater than normal brain (35 and 50 HU). Abnormal increased density, even greater than that observed in hemorrhagic masses, is present in metastatic tumors with calcifications. This is a finding often noted in osteogenic sarcomas, but also observed infrequently in a variety of other tumors, including small cell carcinomas of the lung, adenocarcinomas of the gastrointestinal tract, and carcinomas of the breast (43,44) (Fig. 2).

On contrast-enhanced studies, metastatic brain tumors nearly always enhance; their radiographic density increases so that lesions as small as 5 mm in diameter become detectable. Contrast material significantly improves the diagnostic yield of CT, not only by showing metastatic lesions that are unsuspected on the noncontrast examination but by demonstrating multiple lesions (37, 45). To improve the diagnostic accuracy of the enhanced study, various investigators have increased the amount of injected iodine from 37 to 80 g. In one report, examinations performed with a higher dose of iodine revealed additional metastatic lesions in 50% of cases and improved lesion conspicuousness (46). Another group of investigators combined double dose with delayed scanning 90 minutes after injection and showed that the diagnostic yield improved by 11.5% (47,48). Metastatic tumors, when small, are usually solid, nodular lesions that enhance homogeneously. As the tumor increases in size and becomes necrotic, ring-like enhancement ensues (Fig. 3). The thickness of the enhancing ring is not uniform and its inner border is irregular. Infrequently, necrotic tumors

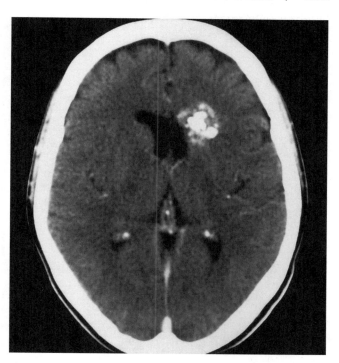

FIG. 2. Metastatic adenocarcinoma to the left frontal lobe. Postcontrast computed tomography shows a calcified mass adjacent to the left frontal horn, which is compressed. Abnormal enhancement is present in the noncalcified tumor parenchyma.

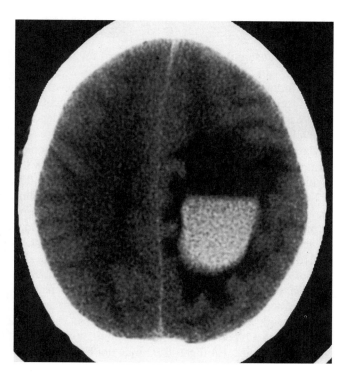

FIG. 1. Hemorrhagic metastatic melanoma. Unenhanced brain computed tomography shows a hyperdense lesion in the left cerebral hemisphere representing hemorrhage in a pre-existing cavitary metastasis. Its horizontal superior border represents a fluid level characteristic of recent hemorrhage.

loose their round shape and assume an irregular configuration. Unfortunately, these imaging features cannot be used to identify the site of origin of these neoplasms. In addition, there is considerable overlap between features of primary and metastatic tumors.

The infiltrated leptomeninges of meningeal carcinomatosis demonstrate linear enhancement within the cortical sulci on the medial aspect or on the convexities of the cerebral hemispheres (Fig. 4). The leptomeninges in the basal cisterns are commonly involved by carcinomatosis and demonstrate abnormal enhancement and increased thickness. Similar findings are also present when there is involvement of the falx or the tentorium (49–51).

The clinical experience of the past 20 years has revealed a number of disadvantages of CT scanning in the diagnosis of metastatic brain tumors. CT studies often cannot identify tumors smaller than 5 mm in diameter in spite of the improved sensitivity achieved with the use of iodinated contrast material. Artifacts, caused by hardening of the x-ray beam as it passes through the skull, usually obscure small lesions located on the brain surface and may even obscure larger lesions in the posterior fossa, where these artifacts are more prominent. Furthermore, the normal density of the calvarial bones does not permit visualization of the underlying dura, and therefore meningeal carcinomatosis of the dura cannot be appreciated. The diagnostic yield for meningeal carcinomatosis

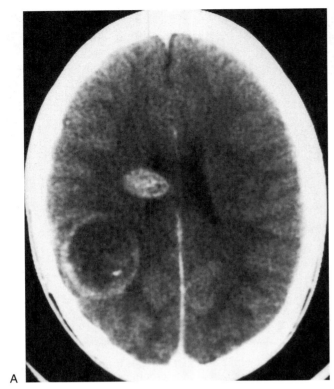 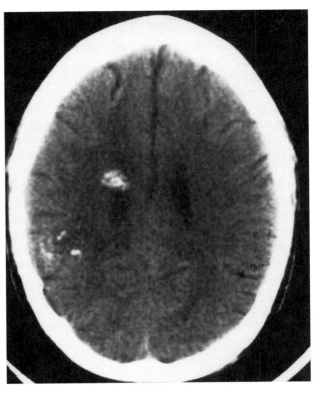

A   B

FIG. 3. Metastatic Ewing's sarcoma to the right cerebral hemisphere in an 18-year-old man. **A:** Post-contrast computed tomography shows solid and cavitary masses, demonstrating homogeneous and ring-like enhancement, respectively. **B:** After irradiation, dystrophic calcifications are noted in the tumor sites. Enhancement is no longer present, indicating absence of residual tumor.

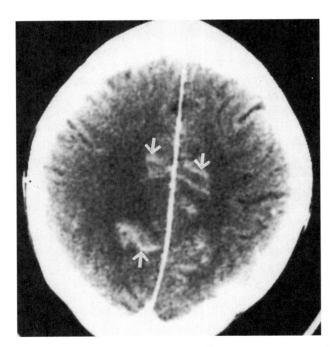

FIG. 4. Leptomeningeal metastasis. Postcontrast computed tomography demonstrates typical abnormal enhancement in the leptomeninges (arrows) on the medial aspect of both cerebral hemispheres.

is low, because only advanced meningeal involvement is detected with this method.

The iodinated contrast materials used in CT have a myriad of problems related to their use. These agents are known to produce a variety of side effects, the incidence of which is reported to be as high as 5% to 12%. Severe anaphylactic reactions associated with acute cardiopulmonary failure occur in 1 in 1000 injected patients, whereas the incidence of death is between 1:12,000 to 1:75,000 (52–54). Patients with a prior history of allergy to iodine may not be eligible for contrast-enhanced CT examination or may require premedication. In most cases, the development of a major reaction is unpredictable and cannot be excluded by prior testing. Iodinated contrast agents are also known for their nephrotoxicity. Contrast-induced acute renal failure has been reported in 15% to 42% of patients with azotemia, and this incidence is even greater in patients with azotemia and diabetes mellitus. Therefore, patients with a blood urea nitrogen >20 mg/100 ml or with serum creatinine >1.4 mg/100 ml may not be safely studied with iodinated contrast agents. Other risk factors include cardiovascular diseases, severe pulmonary decompensation, bronchial asthma, pheochromocytoma, sickle cell disease, multiple myeloma, diabetes mellitus, dehydration, advanced age, and severe debilitation (55–58).

More recently, a new group of iodinated contrast agents has been introduced. These newer contrast agents are nonionic and have low osmolarity, producing fewer undesirable side effects. Although these contrast agents do not entirely eliminate iodine-related complications, having similar nephrotoxic profiles, they produce far fewer allergic and idiosyncratic reactions. Overall, they are much safer, but unfortunately are considerably more expensive, making their routine use problematic (59–61).

Computed tomography has largely been displaced by magnetic resonance imaging (MRI) in the evaluation of brain metastases. It is currently used primarily for claustrophobic patients, or in patients with known contraindications to MRI examinations. CT continues to have a role in the assessment of tumors that involve the bony calvarium or the spine. Fine bone detail is shown very well by CT, which is helpful in distinguishing early destructive metastatic bone lesions from benign changes, such as venous lakes in the diploic space, which occasionally mimic metastasis on MRI studies. Finally, CT may be preferred for its low cost and greater speed.

Magnetic Resonance Imaging

Magnetic resonance imaging of the brain has become the diagnostic modality of choice in the evaluation of patients with suspected CNS metastases. Superior soft tissue contrast and multiplanar orientation are strengths of MRI. These allow better appreciation of the anatomy and internal architecture of various organs, particularly the brain.

Magnetic resonance imaging images hydrogen nuclei in molecules, which are abundant in most body tissues. The image contrast of MRI depends on four parameters: the concentration of protons, the blood flow, and the relaxation times, T1 and T2. Relaxation times are specific properties of protons in the various tissues measured when placed in a homogeneous magnetic field and exposed to radiofrequency pulses.

The concentration of protons in the tissues is proportional to their water content, whereas the relaxation times are influenced by the molecular structure in which hydrogen is incorporated. Liquids with hydrogen in molecular water have long T1 and T2 values, whereas body tissues with hydrogen incorporated in larger molecules have short T1 and T2 values (62–64). Similarly, cancer cells and edematous body tissues have longer T1 and T2 values than normal tissues, a fundamental observation made by Damadian in 1971 that established the rationale for the diagnosis of cancer by MRI (65).

By appropriate choice of pulse sequences, images are produced in which the signal intensity (high signal intensity is bright; low signal intensity is dark) depends on differences in T1, T2, or a combination of both. In clinical MRI, the terms "T1-weighted" or "T2-weighted" have emerged and are useful in the choice of scanning techniques and interpretation of images. T1-weighted images provide anatomic detail because the brain parenchyma and CSF differ on T1. Most pathologic entities affect T2, and therefore the T2-weighted pulse sequences produce images most sensitive to pathologic processes.

Magnetic resonance imaging studies are performed before and after intravenous administration of contrast material when intracranial spread of neoplasm is suspected. Gadolinium (Gd) is an element of the lanthanide series, which, by virtue of its seven unpaired electrons, alters the local magnetic environment of the hydrogen nuclei. This shortens the T1 value of the tissues in which gadolinium concentrates and increases their signal intensity. Gadolinium, bound to different chelating agents, is commercially available in ionic and nonionic formulations and has been found to be safe and stable for intravenous injection. The safety factor of these compounds is 10-fold greater than that of the iodinated contrast agents used in CT (66–72).

Most small, solid metastatic tumors without peritumoral edema exhibit signal characteristics similar to normal brain parenchyma and may not be detectable on nonenhanced T1-weighted sequences. Tumors with significant necrosis or adjacent parenchymal edema demonstrate a low T1 value and can be visualized in these studies.

Metastatic tumors are often hyperintense compared with normal brain on T2-weighted studies because of the increased intrinsic T2 value of the neoplastic tissues (73, 74). The T2-weighted technique is sensitive in demonstrating peritumoral edema, which is also hyperintense (Fig. 5). Because both tumor and surrounding edema have high signal, the tumor margins may not be discernible on T2-weighted images (75,76). The additive effect of hyperintensity of tumor to that of edema is helpful in demonstrating otherwise unapparent small metastases. In other instances, small tumors located near the brain surface or a sulcus are easily obscured by the hyperintensity of the adjacent CSF (77,78). Some metastatic tumors, especially adenocarcinomas, retain the signal characteristics of the primary tumor, which is of lower signal intensity on T2-weighted sequences than normal brain, and are hypointense compared to white and gray matter (79,80) (Fig. 6).

Metastatic brain tumors enhance on postcontrast T1-weighted examinations and demonstrate the same morphologic characteristics seen on CT studies: homogeneous enhancement of the solid tumors and ring-like enhancement of tumors with central necrosis (Fig. 7). Administration of 0.1 mmol/l Gd-DTPA/kg body weight significantly increases the signal intensity of the tumor within 8.5 minutes. Tumor enhancement is maintained for 30 to 40 minutes, followed by a gradual decrease in signal intensity. Tumors with necrotic cavities exhibit delayed uptake of the contrast agent in the cavitary component, with a maximum signal intensity at between 48 and 68 minutes (81).

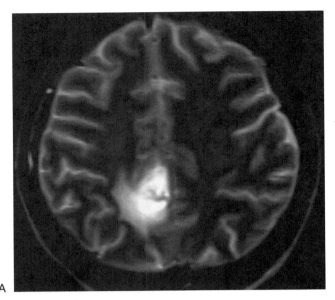
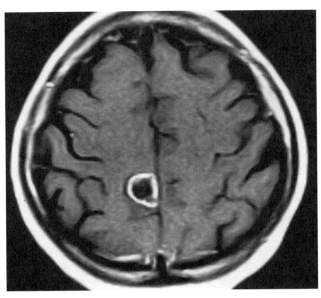

A

B

FIG. 5. Metastatic ovarian carcinoma. **A:** Axial T2-weighted magnetic resonance image (MRI) shows the lesion in the right parietal lobe. The neoplastic tissue cannot be separated from its cavitary component or from the surrounding edema because all three elements of this tumor have similar T2 values. **B:** Postcontrast T1-weighted MRI demonstrates enhancement in the viable part of the tumor, forming a ring around the necrotic center.

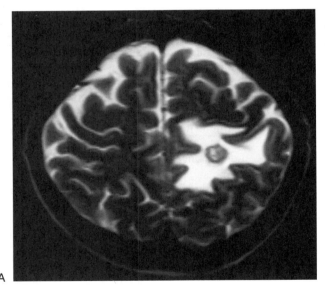
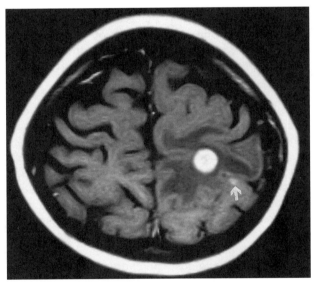

A

B

FIG. 6. Relatively hypointense metastatic adenocarcinoma to the left parietal lobe. **A:** Axial T2-weighted magnetic resonance image (MRI) shows the tumor to be relatively hypointense with respect to the surrounding edema, which is markedly hyperintense. An ill-defined hyperintensity is identified in the center of this lesion, representing early necrosis. **B:** Postcontrast T1-weighted MRI shows intense and homogeneous enhancement of the tumor, creating the false impression of a solid rather than cavitary tumor. A smaller enhancing tumor nodule (arrow) is also present in the left parietal lobe, which was not visible on the T2-weighted study.

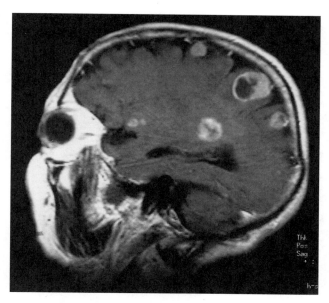

FIG. 7. Metastatic breast carcinoma in a 74-year-old woman. Sagittal postcontrast T1-weighted magnetic resonance image of the the brain reveals multiple brain tumors with and without central necrosis. The irregular inner border of the cavitary lesions is considered to be one of the features of metastatic tumors, which in many instances distinguishes them from abscesses.

Improvement in the sensitivity of MRI has been sought by increasing the dose of injected contrast. Various investigators have used triple doses of a contrast agent and observed an increase in the number of detected metastatic lesions as well as greater enhancement of the lesions (82–86). Other investigators have used magnetization transfer, a newer MRI pulse sequence, and shown that the number and conspicuousness of the lesions detected were greater compared with conventional techniques (87–90).

The MRI findings described for precontrast and postcontrast studies are not specific for tumor metastases, because other brain lesions can present with similar findings. The signal intensity measurements of individual lesions in various MRI techniques, the morphology of tumor as seen on enhanced studies, and the multiplicity of lesions do not significantly contribute to tissue characterization. Furthermore, these signs are not useful in predicting the site of tumor origin (91).

Magnetic resonance imaging is sensitive in demonstrating even small amounts of hemorrhagic elements within certain metastatic lesions, but because many different tumors may hemorrhage, the diagnostic value of this finding is limited. The signal abnormalities of blood products in the parenchyma of a metastatic tumor are useful in dating the age of hemorrhage. If the hemorrhagic event occurred within 48 hours of the examination, there is an abundance of deoxyhemoglobin, which is hypointense on T2-weighted and gradient echo sequences. At this stage, the T1-weighted sequence of the lesion is isointense to normal brain. As the hematoma ages over several days to several weeks, deoxyhemoglobin is converted to methemoglobin from the periphery of the mass to its center. Methemoglobin increases the signal intensity of hemorrhagic lesions on both T1- and T2-weighted techniques. Finally, in weeks to months, blood products in the form of hemosiderin are trapped within macrophages as well as in the interstitial spaces of the tumor, producing low signal intensity on T2-weighted and gradient echo sequences that persists throughout life (92). Because a certain amount of healing time is necessary for phagocytosis to take place in the tumor bed, hemosiderin deposition is usually encountered in hemorrhagic tumors that have been successfully treated by either radiation or surgery. In metastatic melanotic melanomas, the presence of melanin increases lesion signal intensity, having paramagnetic properties that shorten the T1 value of the tumor. Melanomas are also known for their tendency to bleed; therefore, it is not possible to determine whether this hyperintensity is due to presence of melanin or to hemorrhage, particularly in the acute and subacute phases (93,94).

In the case of meningeal carcinomatosis, there are two typical patterns. The first is leptomeningeal involvement, with enhancement in a gyral pattern, extending into the sulci or other subarachnoid spaces. The second pattern is dural infiltration, with curvilinear enhancement following the contours of the inner table of the skull. Unlike CT, cortical bone is hypointense on MRI and provides the appropriate contrast necessary to discern dural meningeal involvement (95–98) (Fig. 8).

Contrast-enhanced MRI reveals abnormalities in 36% to 66% of patients with positive CSF cytology (99). This compares unfavorably with the 80% to 85% yield achievable with multiple spinal taps. In a study comparing MRI contrast-enhanced images with CSF sampling, a high yield of CSF cytology (80%) is achieved only in patients with leptomeningeal carcinomatosis, whereas in those with dural involvement, CSF is positive in 21% of cases (100).

Currently, contrast-enhanced, T1-weighted studies provide the best method for the diagnosis of metastatic brain tumors. The intensity of enhancement is superior to that achieved with contrast-enhanced CT, whereby lesions as small as 2 mm in diameter can routinely be detected. The presence of edema, other associated abnormalities in the tumor bed such as hemorrhage, and other unrelated brain lesions, are best demonstrated by MRI. Finally, the bone artifacts on CT that obscure brain tumors and meningeal lesions are not encountered with MRI.

Single-Photon Emission Computed Tomography (SPECT) and Positron Emission Tomography (PET)

Brain tumors have been studied using a number of radiotracers. The bulk of this research has been with primary intracranial neoplasms, but the same methods have also been applied to metastatic brain tumors. Two basic

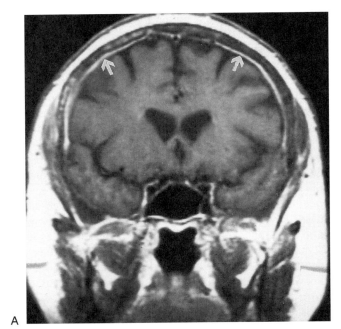 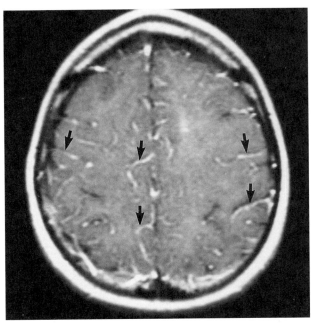

FIG. 8. Meningeal carcinomatosis on postcontrast magnetic resonance imaging. **A:** Prostate carcinoma metastatic to the dura matter. There is increased thickness and abnormal enhancement of the dura, showing high signal intensity (arrows) along the hypointense inner table of the skull. **B:** Metastatic lymphoma to leptomeninges. The linear hyperintensities noted within the cortical sulci (arrows) represent abnormal enhancement of the involved leptomeninges.

techniques have been explored for tumor imaging. The first uses isotopes that decay by emission of single photons. The second approach is to use isotopes that decay by positron emission. With either technique, a radioactive species is coupled to an organic compound to improve specificity.

Technetium-99m tagged to hexamethylpropylene amine oxime (HMPAO) and iodine-123 iodoamphetamine (IMP) are perfusion agents that have been used to study regional cerebral blood flow. Intravenous injection with dynamic data acquisition has shown increased tracer concentration in vascular primary and metastatic tumors. Static delayed images have revealed persistent abnormal uptake in tumors as well as a definite correlation between abnormal tumor vascularity and tumor grade. Therefore, SPECT imaging with perfusion agents is a relatively noninvasive predictor of tumor aggressiveness (101–105). Tracer uptake is not always specific for malignancy, however, because other factors, including amine receptors or the glutathione content of various cells, can also influence tracer concentration. Thus, nonmalignant lesions, including meningiomas and angiomas, may demonstrate increased activity. Conversely, cavitary metastatic lesions with a thin rim of viable peripheral tumor suffer from the limited spatial resolution of the SPECT instrument and may be photopenic (106).

Thallium-201 is another single-photon emitter that, having chemical properties similar to potassium, can pass through the cellular membrane (107,108). The accumula-

tion of this tracer into the tumor depends on various factors that include blood flow, degree of disruption of the blood–brain barrier, cellular membrane permeability, and tumor histologic type (109–111). SPECT studies with Tl-201 have shown abnormal increased concentration in most high-grade tumors that is not influenced by glucocorticoid administration (112). Low-grade gliomas show less prominent tracer concentration, whereas there is no appreciable uptake in gliotic scars. Dierckx et al performed SPECT scans with Tl-201 in 14 patients with metastatic brain tumors, and in 1 of them the tumor was entirely missed, whereas in 2 others additional masses measuring less than 1.5 cm in diameter were undetected (105). Because most of the tumors in the study were large, it could be concluded that this method should not be used for tumor detection.

Technetium-99m–labeled methoxyisobutylisonitrilen (hexamibi) has been used and has shown increased uptake in brain tumors, but its concentration is less than that achieved by Tl-201. An additional problem with this tracer is that it accumulates in normal choroid plexus and can obscure nearby tumors (113).

Positron emission tomography is the other method of radionuclide imaging, using short-lived isotopes that decay by positron emission. Three positron emitters are commonly used in PET. The first, fluorine-18 attached to deoxyglucose, an analogue of glucose (fluorodeoxyglucose; FDG), is used to measure the rate of glucose utilization in brain lesions (114). The second, carbon-11 attached to the amino acids methionine and tyrosine or thymidine, provides markers of protein and DNA synthesis (115). The third, oxygen-15 administered either by continuous inhalation or intravenous injection of radioactive water ($H_2^{15}O$), is used to measure cerebral blood flow, oxygen extraction fraction, and oxygen metabolic rate in tumors and other tissues (116–119).

Positron emission tomography studies with FDG have shown that uptake is influenced by the histologic grade of the tumor. Tumors of high grade have an increased rate of glucose use (Fig. 9), whereas in tumors of low grade the glucose consumption is diminished (120,121). Furthermore, in gliomas, PET studies with FDG have shown that the rate of glucose use accurately depicts tumor biologic behavior, and its predictive value for survival is better than histologic grade (122,123).

The use of PET-FDG in the evaluation of metastatic brain tumors was explored by Griffeth et al (124). They found that 21 of 31 lesions (68%) had increased activity and could be easily identified, whereas 10 other tumors with metabolic activity lower than or equal to normal brain were not visible. It was also noted that the metabolic activity in metastatic tumors of different histologic types is highly variable, and thus the method is not useful for determining tumor origin.

Positron emission tomography studies with carbon-11 methionine performed in patients with brain tumors showed abnormally increased tracer accumulation in tumor parenchyma. This method was proven to be superior to CT or MRI in defining tumor margins, which invariably extend beyond the areas of disrupted blood–brain barrier. PET studies with carbon-11 methionine do not discriminate between high- and low-grade tumors, because both have abnormal increased activity. Carbon-11 methionine PET is therefore a good method for defining tumor extension, but a poor indicator of tumor aggressiveness (125–128).

Besides methionine, thymidine and tyrosine labeled with carbon-11 have been used in PET studies to assess DNA and protein synthesis, and, indirectly, cellular proliferation. Such studies, performed mainly in patients with primary brain tumors, have shown abnormal increased activity in the tumor parenchyma, with only minimal tracer concentration in normal brain. Thus, the contrast between normal and pathologic tissues was proved to be superior to achieved with the PET-FDG method, providing a sensitivity of tumor detection in the range of 80% to 92% of cases. Because metastases are usually smaller than primary tumors, this high diagnostic yield is not expected in these type of tumors. Furthermore, similar to observations made with carbon-11 methionine studies, the tracer concentration did not sufficiently differ between the various intracranial tumors; therefore, the method is not useful in evaluating tumor aggressiveness (129–131).

Oxygen-15–labeled water PET studies are used to evaluate the vascularity of various tumors during the first pass through the cerebral circulation. The oxygen-15 inhalation method is also applied in primary and metastatic tumors, showing decreased oxygen extraction frac-

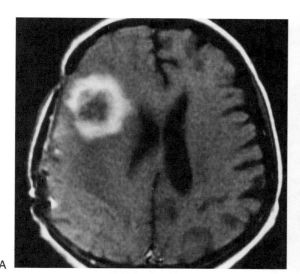
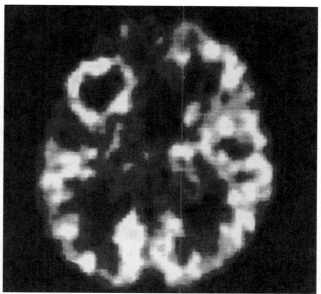

FIG. 9. Metastatic brain tumor studied with magnetic resonance imaging (MRI) and positron emission tomography with fluorodeoxyglucose (PET-FDG). **A:** Postcontrast T1-weighted MRI demonstrates a ring-like enhancing mass in the right frontal lobe. **B:** PET-FDG study shows increased glucose consumption in the periphery of the lesion, representing viable tumor. The is no activity in the necrotic center. (Courtesy of Dr. Ramesh Raman.) (See also Color Plate 2.)

tion and decreased oxygen use, which has been attributed to the increase in anaerobic glycolysis known to occur in these tumors (118,132,133).

The experience of the past several years has revealed that neither SPECT nor PET examinations are appropriate for the diagnosis of metastatic brain tumors because of poor spatial resolution compared with CT or MRI. As a result of this shortcoming, small or largely cavitary metastatic tumors are often missed. PET and SPECT studies can, however, be useful to select an appropriate biopsy site in heterogeneous tumors, thus avoiding sampling errors (134). They are important in assessing response to therapy and are also useful in the evaluation of experimental drugs (105,135–137). Finally, PET studies are invaluable in solving diagnostic problems that arise when ring-like enhancing lesions are found in CT or MRI studies in patients with metastatic malignancies. In neoplastic processes, the metabolic activity of the lesion is increased, whereas in abscesses or postradiation necrosis there is low activity (138,139).

Functional Imaging of the Central Nervous System

A number of imaging methods have been developed that demonstrate brain function superimposed on anatomy. Focal functional brain activity is provoked by different motor or sensory paradigms performed during a PET or MRI examination. With these methods, a functional map of the brain can be generated in patients with intracerebral lesions, which provides important information in treatment planning approaches.

Because neurons use glucose almost exclusively for their metabolic needs, functional activity is associated with an increased rate of glucose metabolism. This was confirmed in PET studies performed with FDG that showed increased concentration of the radioactive compound in functionally stimulated areas of the brain (140–143).

Neuronal activity is closely linked to regional cerebral blood flow and blood volume. PET studies using ^{15}O-labeled water during various provocative paradigms have shown augmented local cerebral blood flow associated with a minimal increase in oxygen consumption (144–146).

Local circulatory changes at the capillary and postcapillary level that occur during functional stimulation can also be appreciated with MRI techniques. Functional MRI is performed using gradient echo or echo planar sequences. Alteration in the local cerebral circulation has been studied during intravenous administration of gadolinium and rapid scanning techniques permitting evaluation of signal changes during the first pass of this contrast agent through the brain vessels (147–149). Similar observations have also been made using deoxyhemoglobin formed during oxygen exchange at the capillary bed (150). This technique is known as the blood oxygen level-dependent (BOLD) method, and has proven more practical because it eliminates the need for exogenous injection of contrast agent and can be repeated multiple times.

Both gadolinium and deoxyhemoglobin alter the local magnetic environment of the circulating protons and the protons in the immediate vicinity of the capillaries. This is known as susceptibility effect, which reduces the T2 value of the tissues, suppressing their signal intensity when a gradient echo or a T2-weighted sequence is used. The protons outside the capillary lumen are subjected to the altered magnetic field by these paramagnetic agents, and therefore the circulatory changes observed have qualitative rather than quantitative values.

In functional MRI, the various task paradigms, such as repetitive movement of the fingers, produce an increase in the local circulation of the functionally activated cortex. This causes a more rapid washout of gadolinium, with resultant increased signal in the stimulated region. When the BOLD technique is used, the increase in the

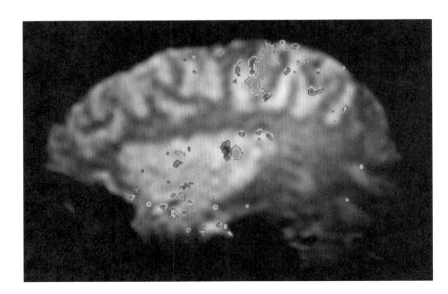

FIG. 10. Functional magnetic resonance imaging using the blood oxygen level-dependent technique. Parasagittal image of the left cerebral hemisphere obtained during repetitive movements of the right hand. The activated motor cortex demonstrates increased signal. (Courtesy of Dr. Lucie Pannier.) (See also Color Plate 3.)

local circulation is not accompanied by an increase in oxygen extraction; thus, the concentration of deoxyhemoglobin is proportionally decreased. In both cases, the suppressive effect of the paramagnetic agents is minimized by the accentuated local circulation, which results in increased signal intensity of the activated region (151) (Fig. 10). Functional MRI has been used not only to produce functional maps that are useful in treatment planning of patients with primary or metastatic brain tumors, but to assess recovery of function in the post-treatment period after cerebral injury and adaptation to altered anatomy (152–154).

Local circulatory changes that occur in brain tumors can also be appreciated in MRI studies that are performed with intravenous administration of contrast material and rapid acquisition of images during the first pass of the contrast material through the vascular bed of these lesions. The susceptibility effect of gadolinium decreases the signal intensity in brain tumors proportional to their blood volume. Similar to the observations made in SPECT imaging with diffusion agents, these studies were able to demonstrate the differences in the vascular architecture of brain tumors, which often correlates with their biologic behavior (155–157).

Magnetic Resonance Spectroscopy

Magnetic resonance spectroscopy (MRS) is a technique that can provide metabolic information in living tissues. Unlike MRI, which produces images representative of T1 and T2 values of tissue, MRS presents frequency spectra with peaks reflecting concentrations of metabolites. Protons and phosphorus-31 are the nuclei primarily studied by MRS in proton and phosphorus spectroscopy. The position of each peak depends on the chemical environment of the various substances and its relation to water, in the case of proton spectroscopy, or to phosphocreatine (PCr) in phosphorus-31 spectroscopy (158).

Proton spectroscopy detects metabolites such as lactate, total creatine (PCr/Cr), choline, N-acetyl aspartate (NAA), lipids, and some amino acids. These substances are found in the millimolar concentration range, producing weak signals requiring suppression of the water signal for their detection. Each molecule has a specific chemical shift, which is expressed in parts per million on a frequency plot.

Magnetic resonance spectroscopic imaging or chemical shift imaging has emerged as a new method able to display metabolites in an image format. High-speed, three-dimensional techniques have also been developed for spectroscopic imaging that provide superior spatial resolution. Metabolic maps of NAA, choline, lactate, and Cr can thereby be produced that depict the relative concentration of these molecules in tumors and brain tissues (159–161).

In phosphorus spectroscopy, high-energy compounds such as PCr and adenosine triphosphate as well as phosphomonoesters (PME), phosphodiesters (PDE), and inorganic phosphate are studied. Intracellular pH can also be determined by the chemical shift of the inorganic phosphate peak (162,163).

Magnetic resonance spectroscopy has the potential of showing metabolic changes before the development of structural abnormality. In brain tumors, this method has been applied to evaluate the chemical alterations that take place during their development and to appreciate better their biology. Most of the observations made thus far relate to primary brain tumors, but can also be applied to the metastatic tumors. Choline, a product of phospholipid metabolism, is elevated in brain tumors, reflecting increased membrane turnover. Lactate is also increased in brain tumors because of anaerobic glycolysis, the level of which correlates with tumor grade. NAA, a neuronal cell marker, and total Cr are decreased in brain tumors (164–170). Phosphorus-31 spectroscopy has revealed increased PME and PDE in neoplasms. These changes are considered to be due to alterations of membrane turnover in rapidly proliferating tissues (163). Furthermore, phosphorus-31 spectroscopic studies revealed intracellular alkaline pH in tumors formally believed to be acidic (165,171).

Bruhn et al (172) studied metastatic breast tumors with proton spectroscopy and found that the tumor spectra do not contain signal from Cr/PCr and NAA resonances, but exhibit strong contributions from choline and lipids. Abnormal increased lipids were also found by Kugel et al (166) in three metastatic tumors. In addition, a number of investigators have reported increased lactate in these tumors (165,167). In a recent study, Sijens et al evaluated a large variety of metastatic brain tumors by localized proton MRS (173). Abnormal increased choline and reduced NAA were detected in the tumor parenchyma. In addition, the metabolic ratios of NAA/choline, Cr/choline, and NAA/Cr were similar in all tumors but distinctly different from normal brain tissue. The abnormal metabolic ratios found in these tumors were similar to those reported in primary brain tumors. The authors concluded that proton MRS is a valuable method to exclude metastatic tumor as the cause of a focal brain disorder, but cannot be used to discriminate between metastases and primary tumors or to identify the origin of metastases.

An extensive research effort is underway to identify metabolic alterations by MRS that could accurately reflect the tumor grade. This is an important goal, given the heterogeneous nature of these tumors, with important implications in the management of these patients. Current research efforts also focus on parameters that may be predictive of the therapeutic value of certain drugs. Furthermore, considerable effort is being made to assess the value of MRS in documenting response to therapy in the post-treatment period. To date, MRS plays an auxiliary role in the evaluation of brain tumors, and is not considered an appropriate technique for the initial diagnosis (159,167,170,174,175).

DIFFERENTIAL DIAGNOSIS

A number of non-neoplastic diseases may occur with a systemic malignancy. These diseases can present with neurologic symptoms related to the CNS that mimic the typical presentation of metastasis. Similarly, these non-neoplastic processes can take place in individuals without any systemic neoplasm, causing symptoms indistinguishable from CNS metastases. When this occurs, establishing the correct diagnosis becomes a critical issue in patient management. Although clinical and laboratory data are indispensable in the evaluation of these patients, imaging studies often elucidate these diagnostic problems. The following are the disease categories that are considered: primary intracranial tumors, infections, granulomatous disease, ischemic events and hemorrhage, vascular malformations and aneurysms, and multiple sclerosis (MS).

Primary Intracranial Tumors

Primary intracranial neoplasms can originate from the calvarium, the meninges, or the brain parenchyma. Primary calvarial neoplasms are solitary, unlike metastatic tumors, which are often multiple. Multiplicity of lesions is the first distinguishing feature between these two entities. Most primary calvarial tumors are benign, with smooth, well defined, and occasionally sclerotic margins. Conversely, tumors metastatic to the calvarium demonstrate a destructive, permeative pattern with irregular borders and a poorly defined transitional zone from tumor to adjacent normal bone. Malignant primary calvarial neoplasms also present with this type of bone destruction, which is typical of their aggressive behavior. The differences in the type of bone destruction are best demonstrated on plain radiographs or CT images. Furthermore, both primary malignant and metastatic brain tumors are often accompanied by a soft tissue component projecting intracranially or extracranially. The soft tissue portion of the tumor enhances on postcontrast studies and often contains calcifications, ossified densities, or bone fragments. The common primary malignant tumors of the skull are chondrosarcoma, osteosarcoma, and chordoma. Other mesenchymal tumors (sarcomas) occur less frequently. Most of these tumors arise from the skull base, whereas most metastatic tumors are found in the cranial vault because of its larger bony surface (176).

Neoplasms originating from the meninges and intracranial nerves, and other, less common lesions found in the subarachnoid space, can also be mistaken for metastatic tumors. Analysis of the imaging features in each of these entities may provide the information needed to establish the correct diagnosis.

Meningiomas are the most common extra-axial tumors. The configuration of these tumors is characteristic, having a flat surface with meningeal attachment and a convex surface abutting or compressing the adjacent brain. Meningiomas may have psammomatous calcifications within their parenchyma. This type of calcification is unique in meningiomas, producing a uniform increased density that is best imaged on noncontrast CT examinations. On MRI, most meningiomas are isointense to gray matter on both T1- and T2-weighted images, with homogeneous enhancement after contrast administration (177). Metastatic tumors to the meninges can occasionally present as nodular formations that compress the underlying brain. These lesions develop in the advanced stages of meningeal carcinomatosis, and should not be mistaken for meningiomas because they are usually multiple and are accompanied by generalized enhancement of the meninges.

Occasionally, aggressive meningiomas invade the skull and produce bony abnormalities indistinguishable from primary or metastatic calvarial malignant neoplasms. These unusual tumors have a sizable soft tissue component with the epicenter inside the cranial cavity. Although associated masses are also found in primary or metastatic calvarial tumors, in most instances masses confined within the epidural space are flat, their shape being influenced by the thick underlying dura.

Metastatic tumors involving the pituitary stalk and the pineal body may pose difficult diagnostic problems. These sites lack a blood–brain barrier and normally enhance on postcontrast studies. Metastatic tumors to these areas extrinsically compress or infiltrate the adjacent brain and produce symptoms and imaging abnormalities similar to those associated with the other lesions that occur in these two locations (178).

Involvement of the suprasellar meninges and pituitary stalk is common in neurosarcoidosis and Langerhans cell histiocytosis, both of which present as mass lesions that may invaginate into the hypothalamus. The CT and MRI findings of these entities are often indistinguishable from metastasis. The clinical and laboratory data as well as a search for other involved organs are crucial in establishing a diagnosis. A favorable response to a therapeutic trial with glucocorticoids is characteristic of sarcoidosis (179,180).

Primary neoplasms that occur in the suprasellar region include pituitary adenomas, craniopharyngiomas, germ cell tumors, meningiomas, and dermoid and epidermoid tumors. Pituitary adenoma is the most common suprasellar tumor. Because these tumors originate within the pituitary gland, the epicenter is always located within the sella turcica. Large adenomas with suprasellar extension are often associated with erosion of the sellar floor. Metastasis can occur within a normal pituitary gland or within a pituitary adenoma. There are no reliable imaging features to differentiate pituitary metastasis from nonfunctioning adenomas, because both present with enlargement and abnormal enhancement of the gland.

Craniopharyngiomas usually have cysts as well as calcification in their solid component, best shown with CT.

Both of these findings are uncommon with metastatic tumors. On MRI studies, craniopharyngiomas present as enhancing masses attached to the pituitary stalk, with good demonstration of the cystic portions, but calcified elements are rarely identifiable. Meningiomas may occur in this region and present as a mass with meningeal attachment on the planum sphenoidale or the diaphragm sellae. Dermoid and epidermoid tumors commonly contain fat, which can be detected by MRI or CT. The presence of fat in these well marginated tumors is virtually diagnostic. Germ cell tumors in this location are indistinguishable from metastasis unless they are calcified. These tumors are in direct contact with the pituitary stalk and enhance intensely, similar to metastases. Germ cell tumors typically occur in the pediatric age group, almost exclusively in boys, producing hormonal disturbances that may be a guide for diagnosis (181,182).

Tumors in the region of the pineal body include primary pineal tumors, gliomas of the quadrigeminal plate, and meningiomas of the incisura. Each of them can mimic metastasis both clinically and radiographically. A distinguishing feature of pineal body tumors is the presence of calcification in the tumor mass, which is best shown on CT. Meningiomas in this location have features already described, including a flat surface of meningeal attachment, homogeneous enhancement, and isointensity to normal brain on both T1- and T2-weighted MRI. A cerebral arteriogram demonstrates meningeal arterial feeders, a characteristic feature of meningiomas. Gliomas of the quadrigeminal plate may be indistinguishable from metastatic tumors, and may require a stereotactic biopsy to establish a diagnosis (183).

Neuromas arising from the cranial nerves present as enhancing masses, often producing erosions in the adjacent bone that can simulate metastases. These tumors are found along the known paths of the intracranial nerves in the cerebellopontine angle cisterns, the parasellar regions, and the jugular foramen. Similar to metastases, neuromas have a radiographic density equal to or lower than that of normal brain on CT. On MRI studies, their signal intensity is decreased on T1- and increased on T2-weighted images. Unlike metastases, which cause irregular bone destruction, neuromas produce smooth, well marginated bony erosions at the base of the skull owing to chronic compression (184).

Because most intracranial metastatic tumors are found within the brain parenchyma, distinguishing these tumors from primary cerebral neoplasms is critical but often difficult. Most primary intra-axial tumors are of glial origin with variable malignant potential. Low-grade gliomas often present as focal mass lesions within the brain displacing adjacent structures. Infiltrative low-grade gliomas are intermingled with normal brain, from which they cannot be separated. The mass effect of these tumors is very subtle, manifest only as effacement of cortical sulci. Except on rare occasions, particularly in the pediatric age group, the blood–brain barrier in low-grade gliomas is not disrupted, and therefore there is no abnormal contrast enhancement. Although the unenhanced CT or MRI images demonstrate density or signal intensity changes similar to those seen with metastatic tumors, the absence of enhancement because of the intact blood–brain barrier separates low-grade gliomas from metastases. In those low-grade gliomas that enhance, other parameters such as the age of the patient, tumoral calcifications, or the presence of fluid-filled cysts adjacent to but not within the enhancing mass are signs favoring glioma.

High-grade glial tumors are the most common intra-axial tumors in adults; as a rule, they enhance intensely and present as solid masses or with a central cavity similar to that of metastases. They are surrounded by edema, and the combined presence of tumor and edema produces profound mass effect. Separation of high-grade gliomas from metastases often cannot be made by imaging studies, and operative or stereotactic biopsy is needed. High-grade gliomas are infiltrative, forming irregular projections within the adjacent brain. The necrotic cavity and the tumor projections at their periphery produce a garland-like pattern of enhancement common to these tumors. This pattern may be a distinguishing feature, because it is unusual in metastatic tumors (185,186).

Infections

Infectious processes often produce diagnostic dilemmas. Bacterial, fungal, protozoan, parasitic, and viral infections involving the brain present with imaging abnormalities that may be similar to those seen with brain tumors. Mass effect is a constant feature in all brain lesions of infectious etiology, where a ring-like or a nodular enhancing focus is often encountered. Like metastases, they are often found at the gray–white matter interface, surrounded by edema.

Several authors have described helpful imaging features for distinguishing infectious brain abnormalities from tumor metastasis. It has been observed that the enhancing wall in most abscesses is of uniform thickness and usually is thin. Cavitary tumors, however, have ragged, irregular walls of variable thickness. On T2-weighted MRI, the walls of some brain abscesses are hypointense, a finding attributed to paramagnetic species such as free radicals present in the adjacent inflamed tissues. This feature is not specific for abscesses, however, because metastatic cavitary adenocarcinomas may exhibit signal intensity that is lower than the necrotic center or that of the adjacent brain tissue on T2-weighted images. Multiplicity is a feature that may be present in some infections, such as toxoplasmosis, candidiasis, or cysticercosis, but is more frequent in brain metastases. In addition, the coexistence of multiple ring-enhancing lesions accompanied by solid, nodular-enhancing lesion also favors metastatic disease.

Temporal changes frequently are more important than morphologic signs in distinguishing inflammatory from neoplastic lesions. Brain abscesses are preceded by cerebritis, which presents with low density on CT, hypointensity on T1-, and hyperintensity on T2-weighted MRI sequences. Early in its evolution, the inflammatory process is poorly defined, with mass effect largely due to edema. On postcontrast studies, there is either no enhancement or mild, heterogeneous enhancement. As the inflammatory processes continues to evolve, there is tissue destruction, breakdown of the blood–brain barrier, and cavity formation, which can be indistinguishable from cavitary metastasis (Fig. 11). Metastatic disease begins with a solid, nodular, homogeneously enhancing lesion that eventually cavitates and presents with ring-like enhancement. Conversely, infectious processes evolve from an ill-defined abnormality, cerebritis, to a cavitary lesion, an abscess (187–189).

Involvement of the choroid plexus by an infectious process is a rare complication occurring with increased frequency in immunocompromised patients. The causative agents are either bacterial, fungal, or parasitic, producing intraventricular abnormalities identical to metastases. In both infectious and neoplastic processes, the volume of the choroid plexus is increased, causing obstruction to the flow of CSF and ventricular distention, which may be generalized or may only affect a horn of the lateral ventricle. Furthermore, both disease entities increase the normally observed enhancement in the choroid plexus. Finally, tumors as well as infections can spread to the ventricular wall, a complication that becomes apparent by the presence of linear enhancement along its ependymal layer.

The imaging feature that can be used to distinguish neoplasms from infections is that in the latter, the involvement is more diffuse, often extending in both lateral ventricles, whereas in neoplasms, a solitary mass is usually found in one area of the choroid plexus (190).

When the meninges are involved by a neoplastic or infectious process, the distinction between the two becomes problematic. In both instances the meninges are abnormally thickened and enhance intensely. It has been suggested that leptomeningeal involvement is more common in infectious processes, whereas dural involvement is more often associated with neoplastic processes (191). Although this may be a valid observation, there is considerable overlap between the two, which limits the value of this finding. For this reason, CSF analysis is indispensable in establishing the correct diagnosis, whereas enhanced MRI images continue to play an important role in assessing response to treatment.

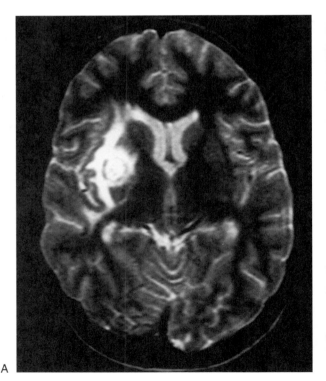
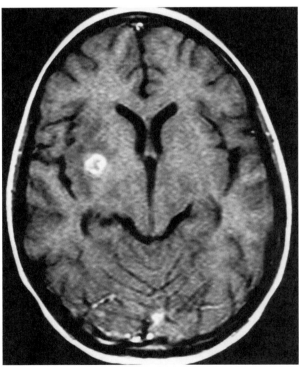

FIG. 11. Toxoplasmosis abscess mimicking tumor. **A:** Axial T2-weighted brain magnetic resonance image shows an irregular, hyperintense lesion in the basal ganglia caused by the abscess and edema in the surrounding brain. Within the lesion, a faint hypointense rim is identified. This finding has been attributed to paramagnetic species such as free radicals. **B:** Postcontrast T1-weighted image demonstrates abnormal enhancement in the wall of the abscess cavity, whereas the edema is not seen as well with this technique.

Granulomatous Disease

Granulomata are brain lesions that develop during the course of a granulomatous disease. Tuberculosis, sarcoidosis, and fungal infections are among the most common causes. The target organ in these entities is the meninges, from which the inflammation extends into the brain parenchyma. The granulomatous process in the brain is often accompanied by tissue necrosis with cavity formation, although on other occasions a solid inflammatory mass develops. Perilesional edema nearly always accompanies these abnormalities, which, in addition, invariably demonstrate disruption of the blood–brain barrier, presenting either as a nodular or as a ring-like area of enhancement on CT or MRI. At this stage, distinction of neoplastic from granulomatous disease is quite difficult. Careful observation of the enhancing peripheral margins of such a lesion may reveal irregularities that favor the diagnosis of a granuloma, whereas well demarcated margins are more often seen in metastatic tumors.

As the granulomatous process matures, the size of the lesion decreases, the edema is partially or completely resolved, and calcium is deposited in its parenchyma. Partially calcified granulomata have diminished enhancement, usually at the periphery of the lesion. In heavily calcified granulomata, abnormal enhancement cannot be appreciated on CT. Identification of calcifications in a partially enhancing brain lesion strongly favors the diagnosis of a granulomatous disease because calcification in metastatic tumors is rare (189,192–194).

Ischemic Events and Hemorrhage

Ischemic infarctions can mimic metastatic tumors, having similar clinical and imaging features. The findings on noncontrast CT or MRI studies are those of mass effect and edema, which are not specific for either entity. On contrast-enhanced studies, infarctions often have a curvilinear or a gyral pattern of enhancement, which is different from the nodular or cavitary lesions typical of metastatic disease. The temporal evolution also is different in the two entities, with infarction gradually diminishing in size. As gliotic scar develops in the infarcted area, the enhancement resolves. Metastases, however, relentlessly continue to grow, producing more mass effect and enhancement (195).

Spontaneous cerebral hematomas and hemorrhagic metastatic tumors share similar density changes on CT and signal abnormalities on MRI examinations. Enhanced studies may provide the information for a diagnosis of tumor if there is pathologic enhancement beyond the margins of the hemorrhagic lesion. This usually represents a nonhemorrhagic area of the neoplasm. Peripheral enhancement is also found in hematomas, but is observed days to weeks later during the stage of resolution. This is due to the granulation tissue that develops around the subsiding hemorrhagic mass (196).

Vascular Malformations and Aneurysms

Cavernous hemangiomas are congenital vascular anomalies that can be mistaken for metastatic tumors because both lesions have a rounded configuration and intense enhancement on contrast studies. Cavernous hemangiomas exhibit no mass effect and there is no edema in the adjacent brain parenchyma, unlike brain metastases. In addition, on noncontrast CT studies, cavernous hemangiomas demonstrate increased density because of the blood pool they contain, whereas neoplasms are usually hypodense. Cavernous hemangiomas frequently have calcifications, a rare finding in metastatic tumors. On T1- and T2-weighted MRI sequences, cavernous hemangiomas demonstrate a heterogeneous pattern of increased and decreased signal intensity because of the presence of methemoglobin and hemosiderin, which are secondary to microscopic hemorrhagic and endovascular thrombotic events. The differences observed on CT and MRI examinations are sufficient to distinguish cavernous hemangiomas from metastatic tumors (197).

Venous angiomas are another type of congenital vascular malformation, usually found incidentally in normal individuals. These lesions consist of small venules converging into a larger vein that empties into a dural sinus. Venous angiomas occasionally hemorrhage, producing symptoms due to the local effects of the hematoma. They invariably enhance on contrast studies, and can be confused with metastatic tumors. The internal architecture of these lesions, however, differs from that of tumors because the individual venules are easily discernible, demonstrating a linear enhancing pattern, whereas the larger draining vein shows flow void on T2-weighted MRI sequences (198).

The nidus of an arteriovenous malformation presents on CT or MRI as a space-occupying lesion that enhances with contrast. This congenital vascular anomaly is nearly always solitary. In the classic presentation, enhancing, tortuous arteries and veins are seen around the lesion on contrast-enhanced studies. On noncontrast CT studies, the lesion is hyperdense compared to normal brain, with occasional calcifications. Both these findings are uncommon in metastatic tumors. Finally, MRI examinations invariably demonstrate flow void, further documenting the vascular nature of the lesion. The thrombosis and hemorrhage that frequently occur within the lesion also show characteristic signal changes (199).

Giant cerebral aneurysms typically originate from a proximal segment of the cerebral arteries or from the vessels of the circle of Willis and invaginate into the brain, presenting as parenchymal masses. Partially thrombosed giant aneurysms commonly develop curvilinear calcifications in the thrombus lining the wall of the aneurysm that are evident on nonenhanced CT studies. The multiplanar capability of MRI is helpful in establishing the anatomic relationship of an aneurysm to its parent vessel. The flow void of the circulating blood in the sac of the aneurysm is best appreciated on T2-weighted sequences. Thrombus formation within an aneurysm is recognized by the characteristic appearance of the various stages of blood degradation products on MRI. On postcontrast studies, the patent portion of an aneurysm enhances on CT or MRI in a fashion identical to any other blood pool or vascular structure inside the cranial cavity (200,201).

Multiple Sclerosis

The diagnosis of MS is based on clinical criteria. Careful consideration of the neurologic complications and their evolution in combination with a variety of laboratory data usually establishes the diagnosis. Diagnostic problems arise in MS patients with atypical presentation who, in the course of their investigation, are examined by CT or MRI. Active demyelinating lesions in patients with MS enhance in a nodular or ring-like fashion, with an appearance identical to metastatic tumors. Most of these lesions are located in the white matter adjacent to the lateral ventricles, the corpus callosum, or in the white matter cephalad to the lateral ventricles, rather than at the corticomedullary junction, as is typical of metastatic lesions. Another feature is that there are usually multiple nonenhancing lesions present on T2-weighted MRI sequences, a finding characteristic of MS (Fig. 12). These nonenhancing plaques are present in greater numbers than enhancing lesions (202,203).

PROBLEMS EVALUATING POST-THERAPEUTIC CHANGES

In the post-treatment period, the focus of attention is centered on the tumor and imaging plays an important role in evaluating the results of therapy. Measurement of tumor diameters on pretreatment CT or MRI studies and comparison with those on the post-treatment examinations provides an objective assessment of any change in tumor size. In patients with cavitary tumors, changes in the thickness of the enhancing rim can be used as an indication of therapeutic response. However, an increase in the diameter of the cavity, even if the thickness of the enhancing rim diminishes, represents an ominous sign of progression. Linear measurements of tumor size often can be mislead-

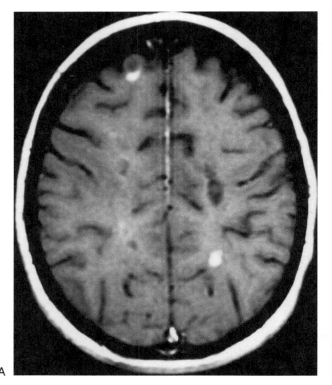
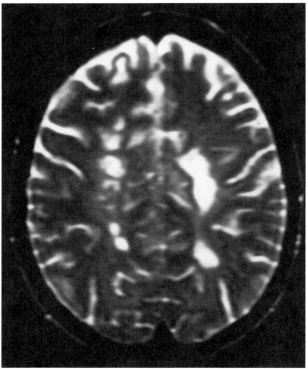

A B

FIG. 12. Multiple sclerosis presenting with findings similar to brain metastasis. **A:** Postcontrast magnetic resonance image (MRI) shows one solid lesion in the left parietal lobe and a second cavitary lesion in the right frontal lobe. Both abnormalities enhance in a fashion similar to tumors. **B:** A T2-weighted MRI shows multiple additional lesions in the periventricular white matter that did not enhance. The combination of findings is characteristic for multiple sclerosis.

ing because of a variety of technical factors, such as positioning of the patient's head, slice thickness, or intensity of enhancement related to exposure parameters of the film. These problems need to be considered, particularly when marginal changes in tumor size are observed. To minimize such errors inherent to linear measurements, newer techniques have recently become available that enable the observer to calculate the volume of the enhancing tumor expressed in cubic centimeters. A postcontrast MRI study is performed using three-dimensional data acquisition and a T1-weighted gradient echo pulse sequence for volume measurement. A method of data analysis known as segmentation techniques, using computer programs that rely upon thresholding, sums all voxels containing enhancing tumor tissues. Segmentation techniques currently represent the most accurate method for measuring initial tumor burden and changes after treatment (204).

In clinical practice, an MRI or a CT examination must be obtained in the immediate post-therapy period to serve as a baseline. An imaging study at this time is also useful in interpreting the patient's symptoms, because increasing edema, hemorrhage, and shift of the midline structures can develop, particularly in the postsurgical period, all of which significantly contribute to symptomatology. Furthermore, the demonstration of abnormal enhancement at the tumor bed in the immediate post-therapy period documents the presence of residual tumor. In surgically treated patients, abnormal enhancement develops days to weeks after surgery, and in such cases two possibilities are considered. The first is granulation tissue formation and the other is recurrent tumor. During this period, distinction of granulation tissue formation around the postoperative cavity from recurrent tumor is not possible by either MRI or CT. This information is often desirable, however, because adjuvant chemotherapy or radiation therapy may be considered in these patients. Experience has shown that the enhancement due to granulation tissue can persist for months but eventually involutes. Recurrent tumors, however, continue to demonstrate new growth manifest by increasing enhancement.

The only imaging modality available to address these diagnostic problems is the PET-FDG examination, which shows increased metabolic activity in recurrent or residual tumors and hypometabolism in patients with enhancement of non-neoplastic etiology. PET-FDG is useful in evaluating brain tumors not only after surgery but, more importantly, after radiation or chemotherapy (137). Furthermore, it can also be used to assess the effectiveness of experimental therapies administered to patients with brain tumors. Regardless of the type of treatment, a favorable response is accompanied by a decrease in the rate of glucose consumption. It should be noted that measurements of glucose use by PET have relative values, requiring normalization by comparison with unaffected normal brain. This is important for results to be meaningful, particularly in serial studies. Another limitation of PET is its poor spatial resolution, which ranges from 6 to 10 mm. Therefore, the rate of glucose use is underestimated in cavitary tumors. This occurs because the measured value of the viable tumor rim is contaminated by the necrotic portion of the tumor, which has no metabolic activity, and by the peritumoral edematous brain, which also has diminished activity.

Positron emission tomography with FDG is the method of choice for the differentiation of tumor recurrence from postradiation necrosis (138,139). On a PET-FDG study, abnormal increased activity at the tumor site indicates recurrent neoplasm. If the tumor site is hypometabolic, however, either radiation necrosis or combined tissue necrosis with quiescent tumor is present. The absence of increased metabolic activity on these studies does not entirely exclude some residual tumor.

Magnetic resonance spectroscopy studies have also been performed in patients with brain tumors treated with both chemotherapy and radiation therapy. Investigators have reported increased PCr and PDE, as well as decreased PME, after radiation therapy of intracranial lymphoma (205). Increased inorganic phosphorus, PME, and PCr have also been reported in gliomas treated with irradiation. The findings in these studies suggest that MRS can potentially provide a deeper understanding of the biochemical alterations occurring during and after the treatment of brain tumors. The results obtained to date are not sufficiently conclusive for MRS to be used for the assessment of tumoral response to therapy (162,206).

Brain images obtained after treatment of intracranial tumors often demonstrate changes in the brain parenchyma distant to the tumor bed. These abnormalities can produce symptoms identical to recurrent tumor and, if incorrectly interpreted, can result in diagnostic errors. During the induction period, patients treated with systemic chemotherapy pass through a hypercoagulable stage and occasionally develop intravascular thrombosis that affects primarily the venous side of the circulation. Thrombosis of one or more small cortical cerebral veins results in obstruction of blood flow and development of focal edema. Clinically, this complication presents with seizures, visual disturbances, or motor deficits, any of which then raise the question of metastatic neoplasm. MRI is superior to CT in demonstrating the changes, showing characteristic T2 and proton density hyperintensity in the cortical gray matter, with variable extension into the adjacent white matter. There is usually no significant mass effect or abnormal enhancement. As a rule, thrombosis of small cortical veins does not result in cerebral infarctions. Instead, both the clinical symptoms and MRI hyperintensities are usually transient, requiring no specific treatment (207). If a large cortical vein develops thrombosis, this may result in a hemorrhagic infarct with or without hematoma that, depending on its size and location, may require surgical evacuation.

Patients receiving systemic or intrathecal chemotherapy, like methotrexate, cytarabine, or BCNU, are at risk

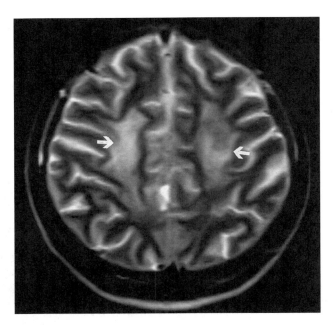

FIG. 13. Postradiation leukomalacia in a patient with ovarian carcinoma. Axial T2-weighted magnetic resonance image shows a broad zone of abnormal increased signal intensity in the white matter of the cerebral hemispheres, characteristic of leukomalacia (arrows). A smaller focus of hyperintensity is present at the tumor site.

for development of abnormalities in the white matter and may present with symptoms of CNS dysfunction. These lesions are hyperintense on T2-weighted MRI images, are not apparent on the T1-weighted sequences, and usually do not enhance. Such white matter abnormalities, if they develop during treatment or in the immediate post-treatment period, represent acute demyelination or edema that may be transient and often disappears after cessation of chemotherapy. In more severe cases, chemotherapy-related white matter abnormalities progress to myelomalacia with permanent and irreversible lesions and clinical deficits (208–210).

Delayed effects on the brain occur particularly in patients who have received whole-brain irradiation. These patients are at high risk of incurring diffuse cerebral atrophy, leukomalacia, or a combination of both (Fig. 13). Brain atrophy diagnosed on CT and MRI presents with enlargement of the cortical sulci and ventricles. Segmentation techniques may also be used to quantitate the degree of parenchymal loss, particularly in older patients. Leukomalacia may developed independently or concomitantly with atrophy and presents with scattered focal or confluent hyperintensities on T2- and proton density-weighted MRI sequences. Similar to leukomalacia after chemotherapy, these lesions are permanent and often progressive, representing irreversible white matter damage. Rarely, such an injury progresses to the formation of cystic cavities, but because they have no mass effect or enhancement, they

should not be confused with recurrent tumors. Children and aged individuals are more vulnerable to the development of leukomalacia—children because of the injury to immature white matter, and the elderly because of preexisting arteriosclerotic vessels, representing an additional burden of treatment. It is well recognized that chemotherapeutic agents act synergistically with radiation to produce leukomalacia. It is also known that both the atrophic brain changes and leukomalacia are associated with mental decline, which may be revealed only in psychometric testing (211).

Vasculopathy is another complication of radiation therapy with distinct imaging features on CT and MRI studies. Vascular damage caused by radiation primarily affects small vessels, the endothelial cells of which are most vulnerable. During the reparative process of a microvascular injury, calcium is deposited in the wall of the damaged vessels. This calcific vasculopathy is best demonstrated in CT studies as areas of abnormal density, and is usually not seen on MRI studies. Radiation-related calcified lesions are characteristically found at the corticomedullary junction and in the basal ganglia, and are often accompanied by cerebral atrophy. Postirradiation vasculopathy is also appreciated in MRI studies, which are particularly sensitive to microscopic hemorrhagic events occurring about the injured walls of small vessels. Gradient echo or T2-weighted sequences best show the scattered hypointense lesions in the brain parenchyma that are due to hemosiderin deposits, and are characteristic for this condition. On rare occasions, the damaged wall of these vessels may actually rupture and produce a frank hematoma, easily diagnosed by MRI or CT.

In conclusion, a number of imaging modalities are available to evaluate intracranial tumors. These methods are indispensable for the diagnosis and assessment of therapeutic results. MRI is the most sensitive method for tumor detection and follow-up. Functional MRI, demonstrating physiology superimposed over anatomy, is still evolving, and has already found applications in surgical planning. MRS is a method with great potential, able to portray chemical and metabolic changes in different brain lesions. The usefulness of this modality in the management of metastatic brain tumors is at this time uncertain. PET methods have been applied in a variety of primary brain tumors and in tumors metastatic to the brain. PET imaging is a potentially powerful tool to assess response to therapy, but with less sensitivity and spatial resolution than MRI. In spite of this, PET-FDG is to date the method of choice for diagnosing postradiation necrosis and differentiating this complication from recurrent brain tumor.

REFERENCES

1. Henson RA, Urich H. Cancer and the nervous system. *The neurological manifestation of systematic malignant disease.* Oxford: Blackwell Scientific Publications; 1982:7–58.

2. Willis RA. *The spread of tumors of the human body* (3rd ed). London: Butterworths; 1973:251–258.
3. Cairncross G, Posner J. The management of brain metastases. In: Walker MD, ed. *Oncology of the nervous system.* Boston: Martinus Nijhoff Publishers; 1983:341–377.
4. Posner JB, Chernik NL. Intracranial metastases from systemic cancer. *Adv Neurol* 1978;19:579–592.
5. Patchell RA. Brain metastases. *Neurol Clin* 1991;9:817–824.
6. Black PM. Brain tumors. *N Engl J Med* 1991;324:1555–1564
7. Globus JH, Meltzer T. Metastatic tumors of the brain. *Archives of Neurology and Psychiatry* 1942;48:163–226.
8. Percy AK, Elveback LR, Okazaki H, Kurland LT. Neoplasms of the central nervous system: epidemiologic consideration. *Neurology* 1972; 22:40–48.
9. Courville CB. *Pathology of the central nervous system* (3rd ed). Mountain View, CA: Pacific Press Publishing Association; 1950:368–375.
10. Takakura K, Sano k, Hojo S, Hirano A. *Metastatic tumors of the central nervous system.* Tokyo: Igaku-Shoin, 1982.
11. Delattre JY, Krol G, Thaler HT, Posner JB. Distribution of brain metastases. *Arch Neurol* 1988;45:741–744.
12. Vieth RG, Odorn GL. Intracranial metastases and their neurosurgical treatment. *J Neurosurg* 1965;23:375–383.
13. Russell DS, Rubistein LJ. *Pathology of tumors of the nervous system.* 5th ed. Baltimore: Williams & Wilkins; 1989:825–842.
14. Posner JB. Management of central nervous system metastases. *Semin Oncol* 1977;4:81–91.
15. Baron KD, Hirano A, Araki S, et al. Experiences with metastatic neoplasms involving the spinal cord. *Neurology* 1959;9:91–106.
16. Edelson RN, Deck MDF, Posner JB. Intramedullary spinal cord metastases: clinical and radiographic findings in 9 cases. *Neurology* 1972;22:1222–1231.
17. Liotta LA, Rao NC, Terranova VP, Barsky S, Thorgeirsson U. Tumor cell attachment and degradation of basement membranes. In: Nicolson GL, Milas L, eds. *Cancer invasion and metastasis: biologic and therapeutic aspects.* New York: Raven Press; 1984:169–176.
18. Katz DA, Liotta LA. Tumor invasion and metastasis in the central nervous system. *Progress in Neuropathology* 1986;6:119–131.
19. Nicolson GL, Irimura T, Nakajima M, Estrada J. Metastatic cell attachment to and invasion of vascular endothelium and its underlying basal lamina using endothelial cell monolayers. In: Nicolson GL, Milas L, eds. *Cancer invasion and metastasis: biologic and therapeutic aspects.* New York: Raven Press; 1984:145–167.
20. Liotta LA, Kohn E. Cancer invasion and metastasis. *JAMA* 1990;263: 1123–1126.
21. Batson CV. Function of vertebrae veins and their role in spread of metastasis. *Ann Surg* 1940;112:138–149.
22. Thompson T, Evans W. Paradoxical embolism. *Q J Med* 1929;23: 135–150.
23. Olson ME, Chernick NL, Posner JB. Infiltration of the leptomeninges by systemic cancer: a clinical and pathological study. *Arch Neurol* 1974;30:122–137.
24. Gonzalez-Vitale JC, Garcia-Benuel R. Meningeal carcinomatosis. *Cancer* 1976;37:2906–2911.
25. Wasserstrom WR, Glass P, Posner JB. Diagnosis and treatment of leptomeningeal metastases from solid tumors: experience with 90 patients. *Cancer* 1982;49:759–772.
26. Del Regato JA. Pathways of metastatic spread of malignant tumors. *Semin Oncol* 1977;4:33–38.
27. Kokkoris PC. Leptomeningeal carcinomatosis: how does cancer reach the pia-arachnoid? *Cancer* 1983;51:154–160.
28. Mahaley MS Jr. Commentary on diagnosis and surgical management of metastatic brain tumors. *J Neurooncol* 1987;4:191–193.
29. O'Neil BP, Dinapoli RP, Okazaki H. Cerebral Infarction as a result of tumor embolisms. *Cancer* 1987;60:90–95.
30. Rogers LR. Cerebrovascular complications in cancer patients. *Oncology* 1994;8:23–30.
31. O'Neil BP, Buckner JC, Coffey RJ, Dinapoli RP, Shaw EG. Brain metastatic lesions. *Mayo Clin Proc* 1994;69:1062–1068.
32. Eapen L, Vachet M, Catton G, et al. Brain metastases with an unknown primary: a clinical perspective. *J Neurooncol* 1988;6:31–35.
33. Trillet V, Catajar JF, Croisile B, et al. Cerebral metastasis as first symptom of bronchogenic carcinoma. *Cancer* 1991;67:2935–2940.
34. Hounsfield GN. Computerized transverse axial scanning tomography: Part I. description of the system. *Br J Radiol* 1973;46:1016–1022.
35. Boyd DP, Parker DL. Basic principles of computed tomography. In:

Moss AA, Gamsu GE, Genant HK, eds. *Computed tomography of the body.* Philadelphia: WB Saunders; 1983:1–21
36. Brooks RA, DiChiro G. Principles of computed assisted tomography (CAT) in radiographic and radioisotopic imaging. *Phys Med Biol* 1976; 21:689–732.
37. Kramer RA, Janetos GP, Perlstein G. An approach to contrast enhancement in computed tomography of the brain. *Radiology* 1975; 116:641–647.
38. Deck MDF, Messima AV, Sackett JF. Computed tomography in metastatic disease of the brain. *Radiology* 1976;119:115–120.
39. Kane RC. Brain scans for metastasis. *JAMA* 1978;239:2115–2116.
40. Potts DG, Abbott GF, von Sneidern JV. National cancer institute study: evaluation of computed tomography in the diagnosis of intracranial neoplasms: III. metastatic tumors. *Radiology* 1980; 136:657–664.
41. Dublin AB, Norman D. Fluid–fluid level in cystic cerebral metastatic melanoma. *J Comput Assist Tomogr* 1979;3:650–652.
42. Dupont MG, Baleriaux-Waha D, Kuhn G, Bollaert A, Jeanmart L. Computerized axial tomography in the diagnosis of cerebral metastasis. *Comput Tomogr* 1981;5:103–113.
43. Enzmann DR, Kramer R, Norman D, Pollock J. Malignant melanoma metastatic to the central nervous system. *Radiology* 1978;127:177–180.
44. Handa J, Nakasu Y, Kamijyo Y. Calcified metastatic carcinoma of the brain. *Surg Neurol* 1980;14:67–70.
45. Latchaw RE, Gold LHA, Tourje EJ. A protocol for the use of contrast enhancement in cranial computed tomography. *Radiology* 1978;126: 681–687.
46. Davis JH, Davis KR, Newhouse J, Pfister RC. Expanded high iodine dose in computed cranial tomography: a preliminary report. *Radiology* 1979;131:373–380.
47. Hayman LA, Evans RA, Hinck VC. Delayed high iodine dose contrast computed tomography cranial neoplasms. *Radiology* 1980;136: 677–684.
48. Shalen PR, Hayman LA, Wallace S, Handel SF. Protocol for delayed contrast enhancement in computed tomography of cerebral neoplasia. *Radiology* 1981;139:397–402.
49. Enzmann DR, Krikorian J, Yorke C, et al. Computed tomography of leptomeningeal spread of tumor. *J Comput Assist Tomogr* 1978;2:448–455.
50. Ascherl GF, Hilal SK, Brisman R. Computed tomography of disseminated meningeal and ependymal malignant neoplasms. *Neurology* 1981;31:567–574.
51. Lee YY, Glass JP, Geoffray A, Wallace S. Cranial computed tomographic abnormalities in leptomeningeal metastasis. *AJNR Am J Neuroradiol* 1984;5:559–563.
52. Ansell G, Tweedie MCK, West CR, Evans P, Couch L. The current status of reaction to intravenous contrast media. *Invest Radiol* 1980;15 (Suppl):S32–S39.
53. Hartman GW, Hattery RR, Witten DM, Williamson B Jr. Mortality during excretory urography: Mayo Clinic experience. *AJR Am J Roentgenol* 1982;139:919–922.
54. Shehadi WH. Contrast media adverse reactions: occurrence, recurrence and distribution patterns. *Radiology* 1982;143:11–17.
55. Lalli AF. Urography shock reaction and repeated urography. *AJR Am J Roentgenol* 1975;125:264–268.
56. Stormorken H, Skalpe IO, Testart MC. Effect of various contrast media on coagulation fibrinolysis and platelet function: an in vitro and in vivo study. *Invest Radiol* 1986;21:348–354.
57. Lasser EC, Berry CC, Talner LB, et al. Pretreatment with corticosteroids to alleviate reactions to intravenous contrast material. *N Engl J Med* 1987;317:845–849.
58. Greenberger PA, Patterson R, Tapio CM. Prophylaxis against repeated radiocontrast media reaction in 857 cases: adverse experience with cimetidine and safety of β-adrenergic antagonists. *Arch Intern Med* 1985;145:2197–2200.
59. Peck WW, Slutsky Ra, Hackney DB, Mancini GBJ, Higgins CB. Effects of contrast media on pulmonary hemodynamics: comparison of ionic and non-ionic agents. *Radiology* 1983;149:371–374.
60. Katayama H, Yamaguchi K, Kozuka T, Takashima T. Adverse reactions to ionic and nonionic contrast media: a report from the Japanese Committee of Safety of Contrast Media. *Radiology* 1990;175:621–628.
61. McClennan BL. Ionic and nonionic iodinated contrast media: evolution and strategies for use. *AJR Am J Roentgenol* 1990;155:255–233.
62. Lauterbur PC. Image formation by induced local interaction: examples employing NMR. *Nature* 1973;242:190–191.
63. Jones JP, Partain CL, Mitchell MR, et al. Principles of magnetic reso-

nance. In: Kressel HY, ed. *Magnetic resonance annual.* New York: Raven Press; 1985:71–111.

64. Pykett IL, Newhouse JH, Buonanno FS, et al. Principles of nuclear magnetic resonance imaging. *Radiology* 1982;143:157–168.

65. Damadian R. Tumor detection by nuclear magnetic resonance. *Science* 1971;171:1151–1153.

66. Weinmann HJ, Grier H. Paramagnetic contrast media in MNR tomography: basic properties and experimental studies in animals. *Magn Reson Med* 1984;1:271.

67. Gadian DG, Payne JA, Bryant DJ, Young IR, Carr DH, Bydder GM. Gadolinium-TPA as a contrast agent in MR imaging: theoretical projections and practical observations. *J Comput Assist Tomogr* 1985;9: 242–251.

68. Wolf GL. Current status of MR imaging contrast agents: special report. *Radiology* 1989;172:709–710.

69. Brasch RC, Bennet HF. Considerations in the choice of contrast media for MR imaging. *Radiology* 1988;166:897–899.

70. Oskendal AN, Hals P. Biodistribution and toxicity of MR imaging contrast media. *J Magn Reson Imaging* 1993;3:157–165.

71. Hendrick RE, Haacke EM. Basic physics of MR contrast agents and maximization of image contrast. *J Magn Reson Imaging* 1993;3: 137–148.

72. Sobol WT. Magnetic resonance contrast agents: physical basis of relaxation. *Neuroimaging Clin N Am* 1994;4:27–42.

73. Bottomley CJ, Hardy RE, Argersinger RE, Allen-Moore G. A review of ¹H nuclear magnetic resonance relaxation in pathology: are T1 and T2 diagnostic? *Med Phys* 1987;14:1–37.

74. Fullerton GD. Physiologic basis of magnetic relaxation. In: Stark DD, Bradley WG, eds. *Magnetic resonance imaging.* St Louis: Mosby; 1988:36–55.

75. Tice HM, Jones KM, Mulkern RV, et al. Fast spin-echo imaging of intracranial neoplasms. *J Comput Assist Tomogr* 1993;17:425–431.

76. Russel EJ, Geremia GK, Johnson CE, et al. Multiple cerebral metastases: detectability with Gd-DTPA-enhanced MR Imaging. *Radiology* 1987;165:609–617.

77. Healy ME, Hesselink JR, Press GA, Middleton MS. Increased detection of intracranial metastases with intravenous Gd-DTPA. *Radiology* 1987;165:619–624.

78. Davis PC, Hudgins PA, Peterman SB, Hoffman JC Jr. Diagnosis of cerebral metastases: double-dose delayed CT vs contrast enhanced MR imaging. *AJNR Am J Neuroradiol* 191;12:293–300.

79. Carrier DA, Mawad ME, Kirkpatrick JB, Schmid MF. Metastatic adenocarcinoma to the brain: MR with pathologic correlation. *AJNR Am J Neuroradiol* 1994;15:155–159.

80. Egelhoff JC, Ross JS, Modic MT, Masaryk TJ, Estes M. MR imaging of metastatic GI adenocarcinoma in brain. *AJNR Am J Neuroradiol* 1992;13:1221–1224.

81. Schorner W, Laniado M, Niendorf Hp, Schuber C, Felix R. Time-dependent changes in image contrast in brain tumors after gadolinium-DTPA. *AJNR Am J Neuroradiol* 1986;7:1013–1020.

82. Runge VM, Wells JW, Nelson KL, Linville PM. MR imaging detection of cerebral metastases with a single Injection of high-dose gadoteridol. *J Magn Reson Imaging* 1994;4:669–673.

83. Niendorf HP, Laniado M, Semmler W, Schorner W, Felix R. Dose administration of gadolinium-DTPA in MR imaging of intracranial tumors. *AJNR Am J Neuroradiol* 1987;8:803–815.

84. Yuh WTC, Engelken JD, Muhonen MG, Mayr NA, Fisher DJ, Ehrhardt JC. Experience with high-dose gadolinium MR imaging in the evaluation of brain metastases. *AJNR Am J Neuroradiol* 1992;13: 335–345.

85. Yuh WTC, Fisher DJ, Runge VM, et al. Phase III multicenter trial of high-dose gadoteridol in MR evaluation of brain metastases. *AJNR Am J Neuroradiol* 1994;15:1037–1051.

86. Kuhn MJ, Hammer GM, Swenson LC, Youssef HT, Gleason TJ. MRI evaluation of "solitary" brain metastases with triple-dose gadoteridol: comparison with contrast-enhanced CT and conventional-dose gadopentetate dimeglumine MRI studies in the same patients. *Comput Med Imaging Graph* 1994;18:391–399.

87. Grossman RI, Gomori JM, Ramer KN, Lexa FJ, Schnall MD. Magnetization transfer: theory and clinical applications in neuroradiology. *Radiographics* 1994;14:279–290

88. Boorstein JM, Wong KT, Grossman RI, Bolinger L, McGowan JC. Metastatic lesions of the brain imaging with magnetization transfer. *Radiology* 1994;191:799–803.

89. Kurki TLI, Niemi PT, Lundbom N. Gadolinium-enhanced magnetization transfer contrast imaging of intracranial tumors. *J Magn Reson Imaging* 1992;2:401–406.

90. Finelli DA, Hurst GC, Gullapali RP, Bellon EM. Improved contrast of enhancing brain lesions on postgadolinium, T1-weighted spin-echo images with use of magnetization transfer. *Radiology* 1994;190: 553–559.

91. Asari S, Makabe T, Katayama S, Itoh T, Tsuchida S, Ohmoto T. Configurational MR characteristics of metastatic brain tumors. *Comput Med Imaging Graph* 1992;16:389–395.

92. Gomori JM, Grossman RI, Goldberg HI, Zimmerman RA, Bilanuik LT. Intracranial hematomas: imaging by high field MR. *Radiology* 1985;157:87–93.

93. Amer MH, Al-Sarraf M, Baker L, Vaitkevicius VK. Malignant melanoma and central nervous system metastases. *Cancer* 1978;42: 660–668.

94. Atlas SW, Grossman RI, Gomori JM, et al. Imaging of intracranial metastatic melanoma. *J Comput Assist Tomogr* 1987;11:577–582.

95. Davis PC, Friedman NC, Fry SM, Maldo JA, Hoffman JC, Braun IF. Leptomeningeal metastasis: MR imaging. *Radiology* 1987;163: 449–454.

96. Cordoliani YS, Christian D, Pharaboz C, Jeanbourquin D, Schill H, Cosnard G. Primary cerebral lymphoma in patients with AIDS: MR findings in 17 cases. *AJR Am J Roentgenol* 1992;159:841–847.

97. Yousem DM, Patrone PM, Grossman RI. Leptomeningeal metastasis: MR evaluation. *J Comput Assist Tomogr* 1990;14:255–261.

98. Sze G. Diseases of the intracranial meninges: MR imaging features. *AJR Am J Roentgenol* 1993;160:727.

99. Olson ME, Chemik NL, Posner JB. Infiltration of the leptomeninges by systematic cancer: a clinical and pathological study. *Arch Neurol* 1974;30:122–137.

100. Paakko E, Patronas NJ, Schellinger D. Meningeal Gd-DTPA enhancement in patients with malignancies. *J Comput Assist Tomogr* 1990;14: 542.

101. Biersack HJ, Grunwald F, Kropp J. Single photon emission computed tomograph imaging of brain tumors. *Semin Nucl Med* 1991;21:2–10.

102. Winchell HS, Horst WD, Braun WH, Oldendorf WH, Hattner R, Parker H. N-Isopropyl-(I¹²³)p-iodoamphetamine: single-pass brain uptake and wash-out; binding to brain synaptosomes and localization in dog and monkey brain. *J Nucl Med* 1980;21:947–952.

103. Reba RC, Holman BL. Brain perfusion radiotracers. In: Diksic M, Reba RC, eds. *Radiopharmaceuticals and brain pathology studied with PET and SPECT.* Boston: CRC Press; 1991:35–65.

104. Neirinckx RD, Canning LR, Piper IM, et al. Technetium-99m d,l-HM-PAO: a new radiopharmaceutical for SPECT imaging of regional cerebral blood perfusion. *J Nucl Med* 1987;28:191–202.

105. Dierckx RA, Martin JJ, Dobbeleir A, Crols R, Neetens I, De Deyn PP. Sensitivity and specificity of thallium-201 single-photon emission tomography in the functional detection and differential diagnosis of brain tumors. *Eur J Nucl Med* 1994;21:621–633.

106. Suess E, Malessa S, Ungersbock K, et al. Technetium-99m-d,l-hexamethylpropyleneamine oxime (HMPAO) uptake and glutathione content in the brain tumors. *J Nucl Med* 1991;32:1675–1681.

107. Elgazzar Ah, Fernandez-Ulloa M, Silberstein EB. Thallium-201 as a tumour-localizing agent: current status and future considerations. *Nucl Med Commun* 1993;14:96–103.

108. Sehweil AM, KcKillop JH, Milroy R, Wilson R, Abdel-Dayem HM, Omar YT. Mechanism of thallium-201 uptake in tumours. *Eur J Nucl Med* 1989;15:376–379.

109. Kim KT, Black KL, Marciano D, et al. Thalium-201 SPECT imaging of brain tumors: methods and results. *J Nucl Med* 1990;31:965–969.

110. Carvalho PA, Schwartz RB, Alexander E, et al. Detection of recurrent gliomas with quantitative thallium-201/technetium-99m HMPAO single-photon emission computerized tomography. *J Neurosurg* 1992;77: 565–570.

111. Yoshii Y, Satou M, Yamamoto T, et al. The role of thallium-201 single photon emission tomography in the investigation and characterization of brain tumors in man and their response to treatment. *Eur J Nucl Med* 1993;20:39–45.

112. Borggreve F, Dierckx RA, Crols R, et al. Repeat thalium-201 in cerebral lymphoma. *Funct Neurol* 1993;8:95–101.

113. Macapinlac HA, Scott A, Caluser C, et al. Comparison of thalium-201 and Tc-99m methoxy isobutylisontrile (MIBI) with MRI in the evaluation of recurrent brain tumors (Abstract). *J Nucl Med* 1992;31:867.

114. Sokoloff L, Reivich M, Kennedy C, et al. The (¹⁴C) deoxyglucose method for the measurement of local cerebral glucose utilization: the-

ory, procedure, and normal values in the conscious and anesthetized albino rat. *J Neurochem* 1977;28:897–916.

115. Oldendorf WH. Brain uptake of radiolebeled aminoacids, amines and hexoses after arterial injection. *Am J Physiol* 1971;221:1629–1639.

116. Jones T, Chesler DA, Ter-Pogossian MM. The continuous inhalation of oxygen-15 for assessing regional oxygen extraction in the brain of man. *Br J Radiol* 1976;49:339–343.

117. Frackowiak R, Lenzi G, Jones T, et al. Quantitative measurement of regionalcerebral blood flow and oxygen metabolism in man using ^{15}O and positron emission tomography: theory, procedure and normal values. *J Comput Assist Tomogr* 1980;4:727–736.

118. Ito M, Lammertsma AA, Wise RJ, et al. Measurement of regional cerebral blood flow and oxygen utilization in patients with cerebral tumors using ^{15}O and positron emission tomography: analytical techniques and preliminary results. *Neuroradiology* 1982;23:63–74.

119. Mazziotta JC, Phelps ME. Positron emission tomography studies of the brain. In: Phelps M, Mazziotta J, Schelbert H, eds. *Positron emission tomography and autoradiography: principles and applications for the brain and heart.* New York: Raven Press; 1986:493–579.

120. Di Chiro G, De LaPaz RL, Brooks RA, et al. Glucose utilization of cerebral gliomas measured by (^{18}F) fluorodeoxyglucose and positron emission tomography. *Neurology* 1982;32:1323–1329.

121. Davis WK, Boyko OB, Hoffman JM, et al. (^{18}F)2-fluoro-2-deoxyglucose-positron emission tomography corelation of gadolinium-enhanced MR imaging of central nervous system neoplasia. *AJNR Am J Neuroradiol* 1993;14:515–523.

122. Patronas NJ, Di Chiro G, Kufta C, et al. Prediction of survival in glioma patients by means of positron emission tomography. *J Neurosurg* 1985;62:816–822.

123. Alavi JB, Alavi A, Ahawluk J, et al. Positron emission tomography in patients with glioma: a predictor of prognosis. *Cancer* 1988;62:1074–1078.

124. Griffeth LK, Rich KM, Dehdashti F, et al. Brain metastasis from non-central nervous system tumors: evaluation with PET. *Radiology* 1993;186:37–44.

125. Bergstrom M, Collins JP, Ehrin E, et al. Discrepancies in brain tumor extent as shown by computed tomography and positron emission tomography using (^{68}Ga) EDTA, (^{11}C) glucose and (^{11}C) methionine. *J Comput Assist Tomogr* 1983;7:1062–1066.

126. Ericson K, Lilja A, Bergstrom M, et al. Positron emission tomography with (^{11}C methyl)-L-methionine, (^{11}C)D-glucose, (^{68}Ga)-EDTA in supratentorial tumors. *J Comput Assist Tomogr* 1985;9:683–689.

127. Bergstrom M, Ericson K, Hagenfeldt L, et al. PET study of methionine accumulation in glioma and normal brain tissue: competition with branched chain amino acids. *J Comput Assist Tomogr* 1987;11:208–213.

128. Ogawa T, Shishido F, Kanno I, et al. Cerebral glioma: evaluation with methionine PET. *Radiology* 1993;186:45–53.

129. Mosskin M, Ericson K, Hindmarsh H, et al. Positron emission tomography compared with magnetic resonance imaging and computed tomography in supratentorial gliomas using multiple stereotactic biopsies as reference. *Acta Radiol* 1989;30:225–232.

130. Borght TV, Pauwels S, Lambotte L, et al. Brain tumor imaging with PET and 2-(carbon-11) thymidine. *J Nucl Med* 1994;35:974–982.

131. Pruim J, Willemsen ATM, Molenaar WM, et al. Brain tumors: L-(1-C-11) tyrosine PET for visualization and quantification of protein synthesis rate. *Radiology* 1995;197:221–226.

132. Rhodes CG, Wise RJ, Gibbs JM, et al. In vivo disturbance of the oxidative metabolism of glucose in human cerebral gliomas. *Ann Neurol* 1983;14:614–626.

133. Lammertsma AA, Ito M, McKenzie CG, et al. Quantitative tomographic measurements of regional cerebral flow and oxygen utilization in patients with brain tumors using oxygen-15 and positron emission tomography. *J Cereb Blood Flow Metab* 1981;1(Suppl 1):S567–S568.

134. Hanson MW, Glantz MJ, Hoffman JM, et al. FDG-PET in the selection of brain lesions for biopsy. *J Comput Assist Tomogr* 1991;15:796–801.

135. Coleman RE, Hoffman JM, Hanson MW, Sostman HD, Schold SC. Clinical application of PET for the evaluation of brain tumors. *J Nucl Med* 1991;32:616–622.

136. Kim EE, Chung SK, Haynie TP, et al. Differentiation of residual or recurrent tumors from post treatment changes with F-18 FDG PET. *Radiographics* 1992;12:269–279.

137. Di Chiro G, Oldfield E, Wright DC, et al. Cerebral necrosis after radiotherapy and/or intra-arterial hemotherapy of brain tumors: PET and neuropathological studies. *AJNR Am J Neuroradiol* 1987;8:1083–1091.

138. Patronas NJ, Di Chiro G, Brooks RA, et al. (^{18}F) Fluorodeoxyglucose and positron emission tomography in the evaluation of radiation necrosis of the brain. *Radiology* 1982;144:885–889.

139. Doyle WK, Budinger TF, Valk PE, Levin VA, Gutin PH. Differentiation of cerebral radiation necrosis from tumor recurrence by (^{18}F)FDG and ^{82}Rb positron emission tomography. *J Comput Assist Tomogr* 1987;11:563–570.

140. Mazziotta JC. Physiological anatomy: functional brain imaging presents a new problem to an old discipline. *J Cereb Blood Flow Metab* 1984;4:481–483.

141. Mazziotta JC, Phelps ME. Human sensory stimulation and deprivation: PET results and strategies. *Ann Neurol* 1984;15(Suppl 1):S50–S60.

142. Reivich M, Gur R, Alavi A. Positron emission tomographic studies of sensory stimuli, cognitive process and anxiety. *Hum Neurobiol* 1983;2:25–33.

143. Chadwick DJ, Whelan J, eds. Exploring brain functional anatomy with positron tomography. *Ciba Found Symp* 1991;163:1–287.

144. Raichle ME. Circulatory and metabolic correlates of brain function in normal humans. In: Plum F, ed. *The nervous system: higher functions of the brain.* Bethesda, MD: American Physiological Society; 1987:643–674.

145. Fox PT, Raichle ME. Focal physiological uncoupling of cerebral blood flow and oxidative metabolism during somatosensory stimulation in human subjects. *Proc Natl Acad Sci USA* 1986;83:1140–1144.

146. Fox PT, Raichle ME, Mintum MA, Dence C. Nonoxidative glucose consumption during focal physiologic neural activity. *Science* 1988;241:462–464.

147. Rosen BR, Belliveau JW, Vevea JM, Brady TJ. Perfusion imaging with NMR contrast agents. *Magn Reson Med* 1990;14:249–265.

148. Belliveau JW, Kennedy DN, McKinstry RC, et al. Functional mapping of the human visual cortex by magnetic resonance imaging. *Science* 1991;254:716–719.

149. Le Bihan D. Theoretical principles of perfusion imaging: application to magnetic resonance imaging. *Invest Radiol* 1992;27(Suppl. 2):S6–S11.

150. Ogawa S, Lee TM, Nayak AS, Glynn P. Oxygenation-sensitive contrast in magnetic resonance image of rodent brain at high magnetic fields. *Magn Reson Med* 1990;14:68–78.

151. Menon RS, Ogawa S, Kim SG, et al. Functional brain mapping using magnetic resonance imaging: signal changes accompanying visual stimulation. *Invest Radiol* 1992;27:S47–S53.

152. Kwong KK, Belliveau JW, Chesler DA, et al. Dynamic magnetic resonance imaging of the human brain activity during primary sensory stimulation. *Proc Natl Acad Sci USA* 1992;89:5675–5679.

153. Connelly A, Jackson GD, Frackowiak RJ, et al. Functional mapping of activated human primary cortex with a clinical MR imaging system. *Radiology* 1993;188:125–130.

154. Jack CR, Thompson RM, Butts RK, et al. Sensory motor cortex: correlation of presurgical mapping with functional MR imaging and invasive cortical mapping. *Radiology* 1994;190:85–92.

155. Patronas NJ, Turner R, Le Bihan D, Fulham M, Schellinger D, Di Chiro G. Echo planar imaging with contrast agent in studying brain perfusion. *Neuroradiology* 1991;33:267–268.

156. Gowland P, Mansfield P, Bullock P, Stehlink M, Worthington B, Firth J. Dynamic studies of gadolinium uptake in brain tumors using inversion-recovery echo-planar imaging. *Magn Reson Med* 1992;29:241–258.

157. Nagele T, Petersen D, Klose U, et al. Dynamic contrast enhancement of intercranial tumors with snapshot-FLASH MR imaging. *AJNR Am J Neuroradiol* 1993;14:89–98.

158. Jackson EF. In vivo magnetic resonance spectroscopy in humans: a brief review. *Am J Physiol Imaging* 1994;314:146–154.

159. Meyerhoff DJ, MacKay S, Baker A, Schaefer S, Weiner MW. Magnetic resonance spectroscopy. In: Higgins CB, Hricak H, Helms CA, eds. *Magnetic resonance imaging of the body.* 2nd ed. New York: Raven Press; 1992:287–302.

160. Luyten PR, Marien AJH, Heindel W, et al. Metabolic imaging of patients with intracranial tumors: H-1 MR spectroscopic imaging and PET. *Radiology* 1990;176:791–799.

161. Posse S, DeCarli C, Le Bihan D. Three-dimensional echo-planar MR spectroscopic imaging at short echo times in the human brain. *Radiology* 1994;192:733–738.

162. Negendank W. Studies of human tumors by MRS: a review. *NMR Biomed* 1992;5:303–324.

163. de Cartaines D, Larsen VA, Podo F, Carpinelli G, Briot O, Henriksen O.

In vivo ^{31}P MRS of experimental tumours. *NMR Biomed* 1993;6: 345–365.

164. Ross B, Michaelis T. Clinical applications of magnetic resonance spectroscopy. *Magn Reson Q* 1994;10:191–247.

165. Howe FA, Maxwell RJ, Saunders DE, Brown MM, Griffiths JR. Proton spectroscopy in vivo. *Magn Reson Q* 1993;9:31–59.

166. Kugel H, Heindel W, Ernestus RI, Bunke J, du Mesnil R, Friedmann G. Human brain tumors: spectral patterns detected with localized H-1 MR spectroscopy. *Radiology* 1992;183:701–709.

167. Fulham MJ, Bizzi A, Dietz MJ, et al. Mapping of brain tumor metabolites with proton MR spectroscopic imaging: clinical relevance. *Radiology* 1992;185:675–686.

168. Alger JR, Frank JA, Bizzi A, et al. Metabolism of human gliomas: assessment with H-1 MR spectroscopy and F-18 fluorodeoxyglucose PET. *Radiology* 1990;177:633–641.

169. Herholz K, Heindel W, Luyten PR, et al. In vivo imaging of glucose consumption and lactate concentration in human gliomas. *Ann Neurol* 1992;31:319–327.

170. Segebarth CM, Baleriaux DF, Luyten PR, den Hollander JA. Detection of metabolic heterogeneity of human intracranial tumors in vivo by 1-H NMR spectroscopic imaging. *Magn Reson Med* 1990;19:62–76.

171. Oberhaensli RD, Hilton-Jones D, Bore PJ, Hands LJ, Rampling RP, Radda GK. Biochemical investigation of human tumors in vivo with phosphorus-31 magnetic resonance spectroscopy. *Lancet* 1986;2:8–11.

172. Bruhn H, Frahm J, Gyngell ML, et al. Noninvasive differentiation of tumors with use of localized H-1 MR spectroscopy in vivo: initial experience in patients with cerebral tumors. *Radiology* 1989;172:541–548.

173. Sijens PE, Knopp MV, Brunetti A, et al. ^{1}H MR Spectroscopy in patients with metastatic brain tumors: a multicenter study. *Magn Reson Med* 1995;33:818–826.

174. Peeling JS, Sutherland G. High-resolution ^{1}H NMR spectroscopy studies of extracts of human cerebral neoplasms. *Magn Reson Med* 1992;24:123–136.

175. Ott D, Henning J, Ernst T. Human brain tumors: assessment with in vivo proton MR spectroscopy. *Radiology* 1993;186:745–752.

176. Smirniotopoulos JG, Olmsted WW. Primary and secondary neoplasms of the skull. In: Putman CE, Ravin CE, eds. *Textbook of diagnostic imaging*. Philadelphia: WB Saunders; 1994:106–125.

177. Siegelman ES, Mishkin MM, Taveras JT. Past, present and future of radiology of meningioma. *Radiographics* 1991;11:899–910.

178. Johnsen DE, Woodruff WW, Alen IS, et al. MR imaging of the sellar and juxtasellar regions. *Radiographics* 1991;11:727–758.

179. Miller DH, Kendall BE, Barter S, et al. MRI in central nervous system sarcoidosis. *Neurology* 1988;38:378–383.

180. Seltzer S, Mark AS, Atlas SW. CNS sarcoidosis: evaluating with contrast-enhanced MR imaging. *AJNR Am J Neuroradiol* 1991;12:1227–1233.

181. Sherman JL, Stern BJ. Sarcoidosis of the CNS: comparison of unenhanced and enhanced MR images. *AJNR Am J Neuroradiol* 1990;11:915–923.

182. Chong BW, Newton TH. Hypothalamic and pituitary pathology. *Radiol Clin North Am* 1993;31:1147–1183.

183. Smirniotopoulos JG, Rushing EJ, Mena H. Pineal region masses: differential diagnosis. *Radiographics* 1992;12:577–596.

184. Osborn AG. Miscellaneous tumors, cysts and metastases. In: Osborn AG, ed. *Diagnostic neuroradiology*. St Louis: Mosby; 1994:626–670.

185. Watanabe M, Tanaka R, Takeda N. Magnetic resonance imaging and histology of cerebral gliomas. *Neuroradiology* 1992;35:463–469.

186. Atlas SW. Adult supratentorial tumors. *Semin Roentgenol* 1990;25:130–154.

187. Enzmann DR, Britt RH, Placone R. Staging of human brain abscess by computed tomography. *Radiology* 1983;146:703–708.

191. Zimmerman RD, Weingarten K. Neuroimaging of cerebral abscesses. *Neuroimaging Clin N Am* 1991;1:1–16.

188. Berkovich AJ. Infections of the nervous system. In: Barkovich AJ, ed. *Pediatric neuroimaging*. New York: Raven Press; 1992:293–325.

190. Patronas NJ, Makariou E. MRI of choroidal plexus involvement in intracranial cryptococcosis. *J Comput Assist Tomogr* 1993;17:547–550.

191. Phillips ME, Ryals TJ, Kambhu SA, Yuh WTC. Neoplastic vs inflammatory meningeal enhancement with Gd-DTPA. *J Comput Assist Tomogr* 1990;14:536–541.

192. Enzmann DR. Central nervous system infections. In: Putman CE, Ravin CE, eds. *Textbook of diagnostic imaging*. Philadelphia: WB Saunders; 1994:225–242.

193. de Castro CC, Hesselink JR. Tuberculosis. *Neuroimaging Clin N Am* 1991;1:119–139.

194. Bazan C III, Rinaldi MG, Rauch RR, Jinkins JR. Fungal infections of the brain. *Neuroimaging Clin N Am* 1991;1:57–88.

195. Bryan RN, Levy NM, Whitlow WD, Killian JM, Preziosi TJ, Rosario JA. Diagnosis of acute cerebral infarction: comparison of CT and MR imaging. *AJNR Am J Neuroradiol* 1991;12:611–620.

196. Gomori JM, Grossman RI, Hackney DB, Goldberg HI, Zimmerman RA, Bilaniuk LT. Variable appearances of subacute intracranial hematomas on high-field spin-echo MR. *AJNR Am J Neuroradiol* 1987;8:1019–1026.

197. Savoiardo M, Strada L, Passerini A. Intracranial cavernous hemangioma: neuroradiologic review of 36 operated cases. *AJNR Am J Neuroradiol* 1983;4:945–950.

198. Lasjaunias P, Burrows P, Planet C. Developmental venous anomalies (DVA): the so-called venous angioma. *Neurosurg Rev* 1986;9:100–105.

199. Smith HJ, Strother CM, Kikuchi Y, et al. MR imaging in the management of supratentorial intracranial AVMs. *AJNR Am J Neuroradiol* 1988;9:225–235.

200. Pinto RS, Kircheff II, Butler AR, Murali R. Correlation of computed tomographic, angiographic, and neuroradiological changes in giant cerebral aneurysms. *Radiology* 1979;132:85–92.

201. Alvarez O, Hyman RA. Even echo MR rephasing in the diagnosis of giant intracranial aneurysm. *J Comput Assist Tomogr* 1986;10:699–701.

202. Offenbacher H, Fazekas F, Schmidt R, et al. Assessment of MRI criteria for a diagnosis of MS. *Neurology* 1993;43:905–909.

203. Giang DW, Poduri KR, Eskin TA, et al. Multiple sclerosis masquerading as a mass lesion. *Neuroradiology* 1992;34:150–154.

204. Clarke LP, Velthuizen RP, Camacho MA, et al. MRI segmentation: methods and applications. *Magn Reson Imaging* 1995;13:343–368.

205. Smith SR, Martin PA, Davies JM, Edwards RHT, Stevens AN. The assessment of treatment response in non-Hodgkin's lymphoma by image guided 31P magnetic resonance spectroscopy. *Br J Cancer* 1990;61:485–490.

206. Sijens PE, van Dijk P, Oudkerk M. Correlation between choline level and Gd-DTPA enhancement in patients with brain metastases of brain carcinoma. *Magn Reson Med* 1994;32:549–555.

207. Patronas NJ, Argyroloulou M. Intravascular thrombosis as a possible cause of transient cortical brain lesions: CT and MRI. *J Comput Assist Tomogr* 1992;16:849–855.

208. Ball WS, Prenger EC, Ballard ET. Neurotoxicity of radio/chemotherapy in children: pathologic and MR correlation. *AJNR Am J Neuroradiol* 1992;13:761–776.

209. Baker WJ, Royer GL, Weiss RB Jr. Cytarabine and neurologic toxicity. *J Clin Oncol* 1991;9:679–693.

210. Paako E, Vainionpaa L, Lanning M et al. White mater changes in children treated for acute lymphoblastic leukemia. *Cancer* 1992;70:2727–2733.

211. Johnson BE, Patronas N, Hayes W, et al. Neurologic, computed tomographic and magnetic resonance imaging abnormalities in patients with small-cell lung cancer: further follow-up of 6- to 13-year survivors. *J Clin Oncol* 1990;8:48–56.

CHAPTER 13

Surgical Treatment of Brain Metastases

Jeffrey W. Campbell, Ian F. Pollack, and Donald C. Wright

. . . the surgical removal of single brain metastases followed by radiotherapy results in substantially longer survival and a better quality of life than treatment with radiotherapy alone.
—*R.A. Patchell et al., 1990*

BACKGROUND

It is estimated that over 1.3 million Americans will be diagnosed with cancer in 1996. Over 550,000 people will die from cancer, making it second only to heart disease as a cause of death in the United States (1). Between 8% and 26% of patients who die with cancer will have metastases to the central nervous system (CNS) at autopsy (2–5), resulting in approximately 50,000 to 140,000 people who will die with CNS metastases in 1996. It is estimated that symptoms will develop in two thirds to three quarters of these patients before death (6). In contrast, approximately 18,000 Americans will be diagnosed with primary CNS tumors in 1996 (1). Although it would appear that the incidence of symptomatic CNS metastases is several times the incidence of primary CNS tumors, review of hospital records reveals that primary and metastatic CNS tumors are diagnosed in equal numbers (7), possibly reflective of underreporting of CNS metastases in patients with progression of systemic disease.

History

The treatment of patients with CNS metastases has changed substantially over the last 35 years. In the 1950s,

J. W. Campbell: Department of Neurosurgery, University of Pittsburgh, Presbyterian-University Hospital, Pittsburgh, Pennsylvania 15213.

I. F. Pollack: Department of Neurosurgery, University of Pittsburgh, Children's Hospital, Pittsburgh, Pennsylvania 15213.

D. C. Wright: Department of Neurosurgery, George Washington University Medical Center, Washington, DC 20037.

steroids were found to temporarily improve symptoms of patients suffering from intraparenchymal brain metastases (8). A small improvement in survival was noted, extending the median survival from approximately 1 month to 2 months (9,10). In the 1970s, whole-brain radiation became the standard therapy for CNS metastases, again increasing median survival to approximately 4 months while improving the functional status of the patient (9,11).

In the 1980s, surgical resection of solitary metastatic disease in select patients was found to double survival compared to treating with radiation alone (12). In the 1990s, improved surgical techniques and the popularization of radiosurgery have extended the indications for surgical intervention to patients with multiple or deep metastases (13–15). Despite the improvements in surgical interventions, brain metastases are four times less likely to be resected than are primary CNS tumors, a bias that may result in part from a misunderstanding by referring clinicians of the efficacy and safety of surgery for metastatic disease (16).

Rationale

When choosing an appropriate therapy for cancer, it is important to distinguish between the goal of a cure and the need for palliation of symptoms (17). In that context, therapies designed to cure systemic cancer often result in temporary morbidity to the patient, with the belief that long-term benefit will result. Because approximately 55% of patients with systemic cancer survive for more than 5 years (1), aggressive therapy aimed at curing the primary disease may be justified in most patients.

In contrast, the likelihood of a cure is much lower for patients with distant metastases, decreasing the long-term benefits of some aggressive therapies and making their short-term morbidity unacceptable. For example, less than 10% of patients with metastases to the CNS survive for 5 years despite current medical or surgical intervention (18,19). In such patients, therapies that reduce symptoms and improve the quality of the patient's remaining life may be more clinically relevant than "curative" therapies. Because CNS metastases are often associated with neurologic deficits that can be devastating to the patient, palliative therapy must be directed at reducing neurologic symptoms and controlling intracranial disease while minimizing treatment-induced morbidity.

INDICATIONS FOR SURGICAL RESECTION

Parenchymal Metastases

Two recent, prospective, randomized trials have established surgical resection with postoperative radiation as superior to radiation alone for certain patients with solitary parenchymal brain metastases (20–22) (Fig. 1). Eligible patients for these trials were at least 18 years of age with a documented systemic cancer and moderate level of function (Karnofsky ≥70 [21] or World Health Organization scale ≥2 [20,22]). Patients who were excluded had radiosensitive primary tumors

(eg, small cell lung cancer, lymphoma [20–22], germ cell tumor, multiple myeloma, and leukemia [21]), leptomeningeal disease, tumors inaccessible to surgery (20–22), or life expectancy less than 6 months (20,22). Both studies documented a survival advantage as well as an improved functional status of patients with surgical resection and postoperative radiation compared with radiation alone. This survival advantage was lost in the presence of progressive extracranial disease (20,22). Therefore, surgical resection with postoperative radiation is the traditional gold standard for patients with solitary metastases of relatively radioresistant tumors (Table 1) and stable extracranial disease. This group comprises roughly 25% of all patients with intracranial metastases (19,23,24).

The treatment of solitary metastases with active extracranial disease is controversial. Some studies have demonstrated an improved outcome for patients with active extracranial disease who underwent surgical resection with postoperative radiation versus radiation alone, with a survival advantage of approximately 5 months (23). In addition, several studies demonstrate similar outcomes for patients with solitary metastases in the presence or absence of extracranial disease (25,26). In contrast, one of the aforementioned prospective, randomized trials for solitary metastatic disease found no

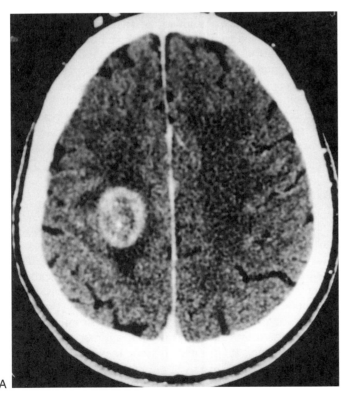
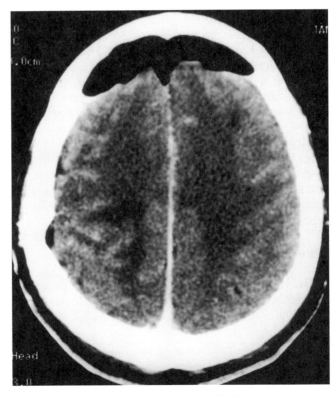

FIG. 1. A: A 49-year-old woman with lung cancer with a contrasted computed tomography (CT) scan revealing a solitary parietal metastasis. **B:** A contrasted CT scan on the first postoperative day reveals mild pneumocephaly and complete resection of the tumor.

TABLE 1. *Radiosensitivity of selected brain metastases (6,17,21)*

Radiosensitivity	Primary tumor
High	Small cell lung cancer, lymphoma, leukemia, germ cell tumor, neuroblastoma, Wilms' tumor
Medium	Adenocarcinoma (breast, lung), squamous cell cancers (lung, cervical, bladder), Ewing's sarcoma
Low	Colon adenocarcinoma, melanoma, renal cell carcinoma, sarcomas

improvement in survival or functional status for patients undergoing surgical resection and postoperative radiation in the presence of extracranial disease (20,22). In addition, one retrospective series found a decrease in median survival with the presence of extracranial disease from 22 to 6 months ($P < 0.001$) (27), similar to the median survival reported for radiation alone (11, 20–22). The poor survival for patients with extracranial disease is primarily due to progression of systemic disease, because surgical resection does decrease the incidence of local CNS recurrences (21). Therefore, surgical intervention may benefit patients whose solitary parenchymal brain metastasis is likely to cause significant morbidity before the patient succumbs to systemic disease, particularly with tumors that are not highly radiosensitive (see Table 1). In addition, because up to 11% of solitary CNS lesions that radiographically resemble metastatic disease in patients with systemic cancer are not metastases (21), stereotactic biopsy may be indicated to guide nonsurgical treatment, even if surgical resection of a solitary CNS lesion is not deemed appropriate (28).

Until recently, most investigators concluded that surgical resection did not benefit the 50% of patients with multiple CNS metastases (6,29–31). Several recent studies seem to support this contention, demonstrating no survival advantage for patients who undergo incomplete resection of multiple CNS metastases (32,33). However, when complete resection of all intracranial tumors is accomplished, survival rates and functional status equal those of patients with resections of solitary metastases (32). In addition, results from radiosurgical treatment of multiple metastases imply that treatment of all intracranial lesions results in improved survival over radiation therapy alone (14,15,34). Even when resection of all intracranial metastases is not feasible, patients may still benefit from resection of selected lesions, especially with tumors that are resistant to radiation. In particular, metastases that are imminently life threatening or causing significant neurologic dysfunction that may improve with debulking of the mass should be resected if the patient is likely to survive for a reasonable period of time (35–37) (Fig. 2).

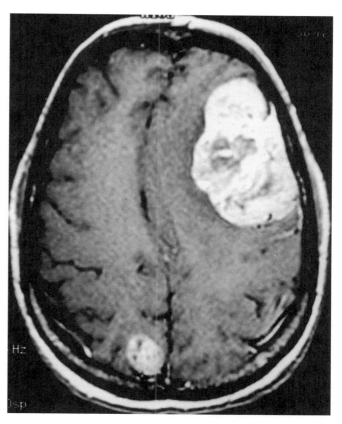

FIG. 2. A 55-year-old man with renal cancer. Magnetic resonance imaging with a short TR and contrast reveals a large left frontal metastasis and smaller right occipital metastasis. The patient underwent surgical resection of the frontal tumor because of its mass effect, followed 2 weeks later by radiosurgery for the occipital lesion.

Recurrent metastases are often difficult to treat because previous whole-brain radiation may preclude further radiation. Even in patients with radiographically complete surgical resections, 20% will have recurrent tumor at the site of resection, and an additional 10% to 20% will have CNS metastases distant to the initial site (21). The same criteria used to select patients for initial surgical resection are applicable to those with recurrent metastases. In appropriately selected patients, reoperation may yield significant improvements in survival and functional status (38,39). In rare cases, multiple operations may be beneficial in extending the duration of high-quality survival, particularly if alternate therapeutic approaches have been exhausted (38).

Leptomeningeal Metastases

Ten to 40% of patients with CNS metastases have leptomeningeal involvement at autopsy. Of these, roughly 70% have evidence of other CNS involvement (4,5). The signs and symptoms of leptomeningeal metastases typically involve diffuse cerebral dysfunction (headache, change in mental status, nausea, vomiting) and cranial nerve palsies (especially III, IV, VI, VII, and VIII) (40–42). These metastases are diffuse and unresectable, resulting in a median survival similar to that for patients who receive radiation therapy without surgical resection for parenchymal metastases (42). Patients with concomitant parenchymal metastases are unlikely to benefit from surgical resection, with the possible exception of intraparenchymal lesions that are imminently life threatening or causing significant neurologic dysfunction from mass effect (35,37).

Standard therapy for leptomeningeal metastases includes radiation and intrathecal chemotherapy (42). Intraventricular instillation of the chemotherapeutic agents through an Ommaya reservoir may improve their efficacy against intracranial disease (42,43).

Skull and Dural Metastases

Forty percent of patients with intracranial metastases have involvement of the skull or dura at autopsy (4,5). Of these, 50% have no other intracranial involvement (4). These lesions rarely cause significant neurologic deterioration unless they compress a venous sinus or reach considerable size and impinge on the underlying brain. In these cases, most patients benefit from surgical resection of the lesion (30). It appears that resection of asymptomatic dural metastases does not significantly improve survival or functional status.

SPECIAL INSTRUMENTATION AND AGENTS

Preoperative Imaging

As noted earlier, the number and location of intracranial metastases are critical factors in determining which surgical or nonsurgical therapies will provide the greatest benefit to the patient. The most sensitive means for detecting small intracranial metastases is magnetic resonance imaging (MRI) with high-dose contrast (44–46). Nearly twice as many metastases are identified on an MRI with high-dose contrast than with normal-dose contrast or computed tomography (CT) scanning (44).

Metastases that arise near eloquent brain, such as the motor strip or speech centers, are of particular concern for operative morbidity. Various strategies to identify the proximity of the lesion to eloquent areas are used, the simplest of which is MRI multiplanar imaging with or without three-dimensional reconstruction. Careful inspection of a high-quality MRI is vital to determine the safest surgical approach. At times, the metastatic lesion distorts the natural anatomy so that identification of eloquent areas is difficult on conventional MRI. In such cases, functional MRI can provide accurate physiologic data as to the precise location of the motor strip and speech centers. If the metastasis occurs in a presumed speech center, a Wada test, where Amytal is sequentially injected into each carotid territory to produce temporary dysfunction of one hemisphere, may be useful to determine hemispheric dominance.

Preoperative Medications

Since the 1950s, glucocorticoid therapy has been the mainstay of acute treatment for peritumoral edema from CNS metastases (8). Prompt clinical improvement is seen in over 70% of patients with neurologic deficits. Dexamethasone is the preferred steroid because of its low mineralocorticoid activity and low rate of inducing steroid psychosis (6). The standard initial dose is 10 mg followed by 16 mg/day in four divided doses. Patients with stable intracranial disease may benefit from several days of steroid therapy before surgical resection. This allows reduction in peritumoral edema, potentially lowering the morbidity from perioperative brain swelling (17,30,47).

The use of perioperative anticonvulsant therapy is controversial. Nearly all investigators support their use in the 15% of patients with CNS metastases who suffer from seizures at presentation (12,37,48). Although seizures will develop in an additional 10% of patients after initial presentation, prophylactic anticonvulsant therapy does not appear to be beneficial. In addition, interactions between anticonvulsants and steroids can adversely affect the patient's medical management (48). Two possible exceptions are patients with metastatic melanoma, who have a 50% incidence of seizures, and patients with marked mass effect, where the acute rise in intracranial pressure associated with a seizure could be fatal (35).

Intraoperative Imaging

Most intraparenchymal brain metastases do not extend to the pial surface, so intraoperative visualization may be difficult (30,49). When the pia over the tumor is normal, gentle palpation of the cortical surface may detect a subcortical firmness (49). If this approach also fails to localize the tumor, several intraoperative imaging techniques can guide the surgeon to the tumor, obviating the need for unnecessary cortical exploration. Two-dimensional, realtime ultrasonography is an efficient technique for localizing subcortical lesions after a craniotomy has been performed (17,30). However, small lesions may not be well visualized with this technique (49). Although ultrasound cannot be used to guide the location or size of the craniotomy performed, this modality is indispensable when intraoperative visualization does not reveal the location of the lesion.

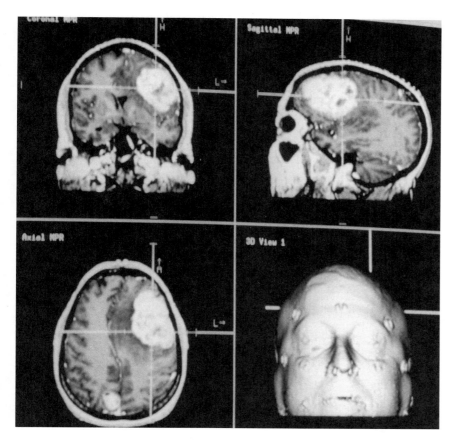

FIG. 3. The left frontal craniotomy for the patient from Fig. 2 is aided with frameless stereotaxy using the ISG/Wand (Elekta, Stockholm, Sweden). A sterile wand attached to a mechanical arm is pointed to a site of interest in the surgical field, resulting in precise localization of that point on three-dimensional imaging obtained before surgery. This provides precise placement of the craniotomy and aids in identifying the borders of the tumor.

Traditional and frameless stereotaxy provide for more precise localization of the tumor and surgical planning and minimize the size of the craniotomy performed. Traditional stereotactic surgery involves the preoperative fixation of a frame to the skull followed by imaging with either CT or MRI. This rigid framework is able to direct the surgeon to within 1 mm of a desired target (49), and even deep parenchymal metastases can be removed with minimal morbidity (13). Frameless stereotaxy involves correlation of cutaneous fiducial points on the patient with those on preoperative imaging. After proper registration of surface fiducial points, placement of a mechanical wand to a site of interest within the operative field leads to a three-dimensional display of the location on the imaging study, accurate to within approximately 3 mm (30) (Fig. 3). Stereotactic techniques require additional preoperative preparation, but remove much of the uncertainty as to the location of even the deepest parenchymal lesions, and allow the surgeon to plot a trajectory to the tumor that minimizes injury to functionally significant cortex.

Intraoperative Instrumentation

To minimize morbidity associated with resection of metastatic tumors near areas of eloquent brain, several intraoperative techniques can be used to define accurately the motor strip or speech centers. One technique uses somatosensory evoked potentials with direct cortical measurements. The central gyrus is identified by where the phase of the cortical response reverses from negative to positive, leading to accurate identification of the motor strip. Another technique uses direct cortical stimulation, which can be used at low voltage to produce a response (ie, movement or sensation) or at higher voltage to suppress a normal function (ie, speech arrest). Testing for sensation or speech requires an awake patient and can be performed only with a patient who is cooperative and able to communicate appropriately.

Removal of tumors that are firm and fibrotic is often difficult using standard operative instruments. The ultrasonic aspirator, which morselizes tissue with high-frequency ultrasound and removes the pieces through suction, can be of great assistance in these cases (17). The central portion of larger tumors can be easily removed with the ultrasonic aspirator, facilitating the resection of the tumor capsule.

SPECIAL PRECAUTIONS

Both spontaneous and iatrogenic intracranial hemorrhage may complicate CNS metastases. The rate of spontaneous intratumoral hemorrhage from CNS metastases is approximately 3%, with a particularly high incidence associated with choriocarcinoma, malignant melanoma, and renal cell carcinoma, although the most common histologic type associated with peritumoral hemorrhage is bronchogenic carcinoma because of its higher metastatic prevalence (50). In addition, systemic cancer is often associated with abnormalities in coagulation that can lead to spontaneous intracranial hemorrhage distant from the site of metastasis, most often seen in patients with lymphoma or leukemia (51). Chemotherapy induced thrombocytopenia may increase the risk of intratumoral bleeding and elective surgery for tumor removal is best deferred until platelet counts have recovered (30).

All patients must be carefully screened for evidence of coagulopathy before surgical intervention. Ideally, the platelet count should be above 100,000 with normal coagulation (prothrombin time, partial thromboplastin time) and bleeding times. Even if the patient needs urgent surgical intervention for impending herniation, significant alterations in coagulation that cannot be sufficiently corrected often result in postoperative hemorrhages that are themselves life threatening. Even with normal coagulation, many metastases are highly vascular and can result in significant intraoperative blood loss or postoperative hemorrhage unless meticulous hemostasis is achieved throughout the operation. To this end, it is important that the surgeon use all the standard instruments of intraoperative hemostasis, including irrigation, bipolar cautery, oxidized cellulose, and considerable patience (50).

METHODS

Surgical resection of intracranial metastases uses techniques of microneurosurgery common to most intraparenchymal tumor operations. Preoperative planning is perhaps the most important component of the operation, with determination of a surgical trajectory that provides adequate access to the tumor with the lowest likely morbidity to the patient. Tumors that are deep or small should be approached using stereotactic techniques to minimize unnecessary manipulation of the cortex (13,49). Many surgeons prefer to use traditional or frameless stereotaxy for even relatively superficial metastases to provide exact guidance to the tumor location and minimize the size of the craniotomy needed (47).

Because most patients receive postoperative radiation, linear scalp incisions are used when feasible to improve healing of the wound (52). Safe tumor resection requires sufficient illumination, often with the aid of a headlight, and magnification of vision using loupes or a microscope (17). Superficial lesions are approached with a cortical incision made longitudinally in an overlying gyrus, with an effort to preserve as much of the pial vasculature as possible. In general, this incision should provide the shortest possible route to the tumor while minimizing cortical injury and need only be long enough to provide adequate access to the entire tumor. Deeper lesions can be approached through an overlying sulcus with the aid of stereotactic techniques to minimize cortical manipulation (13,52).

Most metastatic tumors appear encapsulated and are easily dissected from the surrounding brain (49). With large or fibrous tumors, the ultrasonic aspirator facilitates rapid removal of the tumor with minimal disturbance of normal cortex. To minimize brain manipulation, the tumor capsule should be progressively rolled away from the surrounding cortex, with the use of self-retaining retractors when necessary (49,52). Even after gross total resection of a well encapsulated tumor, biopsy of the surrounding brain may reveal microscopic deposits of tumor cells that should be removed to provide the patient with the best possible outcome (49).

TABLE 2. *Surgical resection with postoperative radiation versus radiation alone for solitary metastatic disease*

		Survival (No. Patients)[a]		FIS[b]	
Author	Histology	Surgery	RTx	Surgery	RTx
Vecht et al. (22)[c]	All	10 (32)	6 (31) $P = 0.04$	7.5	3.5 $P = 0.06$
	Stable extracranial disease	12 (22)	7 (21) $P = 0.02$	9	4 $P = 0.01$
Patchell et al. (21)[c]	All	9 (25)	3.5 (23) $P < 0.01$	8.8	2 $P < 0.005$
Patchell et al. (23)	All	19 (43)	9 (43) $P = 0.00002$		
Mandell et al. (53)	Non-small cell lung	16 (35)	4 (69) $P < 0.0001$		
Stevens et al. (54)	Melanoma	11 (24)	8.5 (4)		
Rosenstein et al. (55)	Bladder	19 (7)	8 (20) $P = 0.13$		
DiStefano et al. (56)	Breast	14 (7)	4 (87)		

[a]Median survival in months. Number of patients in each group is within parentheses.
[b]Functionally independent survival (FIS) in months.
[c]Randomized, prospective studies.
RTx, radiation therapy.

TABLE 3. *Complete versus incomplete resections of CNS metastases*

Author	Histology	Survival (no. patients)[a]	
		GTR	Subtotal
Stevens et al. (54)	Melanoma	12 (21)	5 mo (3)
Sundaresan and Galicich (57)	Non-small cell lung	28 (28)	10 (15)
			P < 0.001
White et al. (58)	All	8 (87)	5 (35)
Hazuka et al. (33)	All	15 (9)	11 (19)
			P = 0.05

[a]Median survival in months. Number of patients in each group is within parentheses.
GTR, gross total resection.

CLINICAL RESULTS

Solitary Metastases

Most patients with solitary brain metastases benefit from surgical resection in addition to radiation, especially with stable extracranial disease (21–23,53–56) (Table 2). Patients randomized to surgical resection with postoperative radiation compared with those who received only radiation demonstrate improved median survival (9 to 12 vs. 3.5 to 7 months) and prolonged functionally independent survival (7.5 to 9 vs. 2 to 4 months) (21,22). The acute palliation of symptoms is similar for patients undergoing surgical resection with postoperative radiation (76% to 89%) compared with those who receive only radiation (72% to 84%) (23,27, 32,53). Factors that increase median survival for patients undergoing surgical resection include gross total resec-

TABLE 4. *Extracranial disease with surgical resections of CNS metastases*

Author Progressive[c]	Histology	Survival (no. patients)[a]	
		Stable[b]	
Vecht et al. (22)[d]	All	12 (22)	5 (10)
			P = 0.06
Galicich et al. (25)	All	6 (26)	6 (41)
Sundaresan and Galicich (27)	All	22 (63)	6 (62)
			P < 0.001
Sundaresan and Galicich (57)	Non-small cell lung	24 (31)	6 (19)
			P < 0.001
Hagen et al. (60)	Melanoma	19.2 (17)	3.7 (18)
			P < 0.001

[a]Median survival in months. Number of patients in each group is within parentheses.
[b]Stable extracranial disease.
[c]Evidence of progressive extracranial disease.
[d]Prospective, randomized trial.

TABLE 5. *Duration between initial diagnosis of primary tumor and development of CNS metastases with surgical resection*

Author	Histology	Survival (no. patients)[a]	
		<12 months	>12 months
Galicich et al. (25)	All	7 (41)	4 (24)
Yardeni et al. (26)	All	14 (26)	66 (24)
			P < 0.05

[a]Median survival in months. Number of patients in each group is within parentheses.

tion of the CNS metastasis (54,57,58) (Table 3), lack of active systemic disease (22,25,27,57) (Table 4), prolonged latency between diagnosis of primary tumor and CNS metastasis (25,26) (Table 5), supratentorial location of metastasis (22,26,27,58) (Table 6), and age younger than 60 years (20,59).

Multiple Metastases

The efficacy of surgical intervention for multiple CNS metastases remains unclear, but seems to depend heavily on whether a gross total resection of all CNS disease can be achieved (Fig. 4). Hazuka et al. (33) reported that patients who underwent surgical resection of multiple metastases had diminished median survival compared with patients with solitary metastases (5 vs. 12 months, *P* = 0.05). However, only 1 of the 18 patients with multiple metastases underwent a complete resection of all intracranial tumors. Bindal et al. (32) reported similar results for 30 patients with multiple metastases who underwent incomplete resections, with a median survival of 6 months. In contrast, an additional 26 patients with multiple metastases who underwent complete resections of all intracranial tumors had a median survival (14 months) and palliation of symptoms (83%) similar to those of a matched cohort of patients with solitary metastases and complete resections (median survival, 14 months; palliation, 84%).

Recurrent Metastases

Patients with recurrences after resection of CNS metastases are considered for reoperation if the recurrent tumor is surgically accessible and the patient's functional status and systemic disease warrant aggressive therapy (38,39). Median survival after the second operation is 9 to 11.5 months, similar to that reported for initial resection of CNS metastases. Over 50% of these patients may require an additional resection for a second recurrence, with a median survival of 8.6 months from the third operation (38). Factors that predict a longer survival

TABLE 6. *Location of tumor with surgical resections*

Author	Histology	Survival (no. patients)[a]	
		Supratentorial	Infratentorial
Vecht et al. (22)[b]	All	11 (26)	5 (5) $P = 0.08$
Yardeni et al. (26)	All	7.5 (56)	2 (14) $P < 0.0001$
Sundaresan and Galicich (27)	All	12 (106)	7 (19) $P < 0.05$
White et al. (58)	All	11 (85)	6 (37)

[a]Median survival in months. Number of patients in each group is within parentheses.
[b]Prospective, randomized study.

after reoperation include absence of systemic disease, Karnofsky performance scale ≥70, age <40 years, and time to recurrence >4 months. Breast cancer and melanoma are associated with poorer survival (38).

Postoperative Radiation

The use of postoperative radiation is controversial, especially in patients with complete resection of their intracranial tumor. Most studies show a survival advantage and a decreased incidence of significant CNS recurrences when postoperative radiation is used (60–63) (Table 7). Smalley et al. (62) stratified their 229 patients into eight categories by total versus subtotal resection, progressive versus stable extracranial disease, and postoperative radiation. In patients with progressive extracranial disease, postoperative radiation does not significantly prolong median survival, which was approximately 6 months for all four categories (total or subtotal resection with or without postoperative radiation). In contrast, patients with either total or subtotal resections and stable extracranial disease had significant prolongation of median survival with irradiation (see Table 7).

MORBIDITY AND MORTALITY

Advances in surgical technique and instrumentation have made intracranial surgery for resection of metas-

tases progressively safer for the patient. Most recent series have reported 30-day mortality under 5%, with many of these deaths resulting from progression of systemic disease (13,21,23,32,53,57,59) (Table 8). Operative morbidity ranges from 8% to 31%, with the lower percentages often not including medical complications (13, 21–23,32,53,57,59). Patients who receive radiation without surgical intervention have 30-day morbidity and mortality similar to those who undergo surgical resection (21, 22), suggesting that the natural course of the systemic disease may contribute significantly to the morbidity and mortality reported for surgical resections. The most common complications reported after surgical resection are postoperative neurologic worsening (2% to 9%) (13,53, 57,59), hemorrhage into the surgical bed (1.5% to 7%) (22,32,53,57), infection (0.9% to 7%) (22,32,53,59), and respiratory dysfunction (2% to 6%) (22,53,57).

ALTERNATIVE APPROACHES

Radiosurgery

The indications and efficacy of radiosurgery are discussed in detail in Chapter 14. This technique is quickly becoming the treatment of choice for patients with deep, multiple, or recurrent metastases because of its low morbidity and high efficacy in even radioresistant tumors (28,66,67). In addition, radiosurgery may be more cost effective than open surgical resection (68) and may ulti-

TABLE 7. *Influence of postoperative radiation on median survival and central nervous system recurrences*

Author	Histology	Survival (no. patients)[a]		Brain failure[b]	
		RTx[c]	No RTx[d]	RTx	No RTx
DeAngelis et al. (61)	All	20.6 (79)	14.4 (19)	22%	46% $P = 0.034$
Smalley et al. (62)[e]	All	15.6 (46)	8.4 (75) $P < 0.001$		
Smalley et al. (62)[f]		13.2 (20)	3 (8) $P < 0.001$		
Smalley et al. (63)	All	21 (34)	11.5 (51) $P < 0.001$	21%	85% $P = 0.0001$
Hagen et al. (60)	Melanoma	8.4 (19)	8.3 (16)	24%	85% $P < 0.05$
Armstrong et al. (64)	Non-small cell lung	10 (32)	14 (32)	47%	38%

[a]Median survival in months. Number of patients in each group is within parentheses.
[b]Central nervous system recurrence resulting in symptoms or death.
[c]Postoperative radiation.
[d]No postoperative radiation.
[e]Patients with complete resection of intracranial disease and no evidence of extracranial progression.
[f]Patients with incomplete resection of intracranial disease but no evidence of extracranial progression.

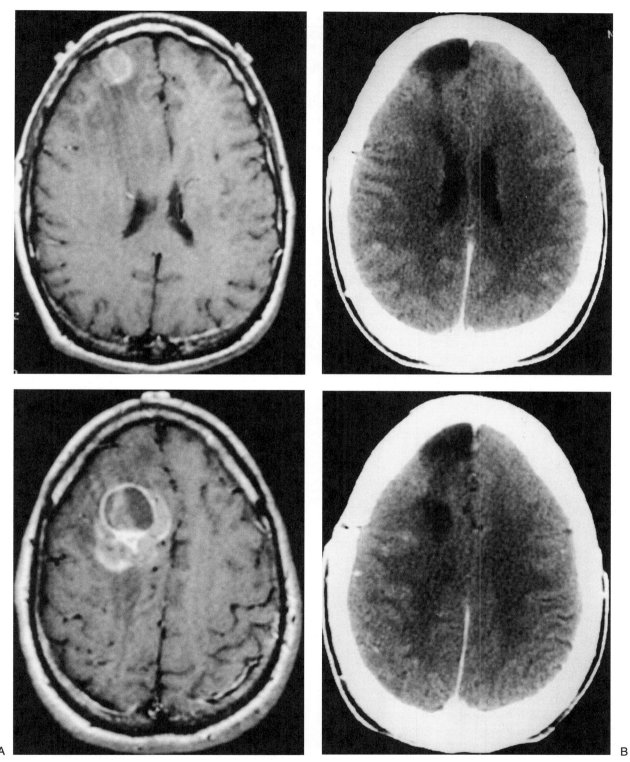

FIG. 4. A 57-year-old man with multiple right frontal metastases evident on magnetic resonance imaging with a short TR and contrast **(A)**. He underwent resection of all lesions through a single approach with gross total resection, as evident on a contrasted CT scan performed 3 weeks after surgery **(B)**.

TABLE 8. *Morbidity and mortality associated with resection of intracranial metastases*

Author	Years[a]	No. patients	% morbidity	% mortality[b]
Bindel et al. (32)	1984–1992	56	8%	2%
Wronski et al. (59)	1976–1991	231	17%	1.3%
Vecht et al. (22)	1985–1991	66	Surgery[c] 28% Radiation[d] 29%	9%
Patchell et al. (21)	1985–1988	48	Surgery 8% Radiation 17%	4%
Kelly et al. (13)	1980–1987	45	9%	0%
DeAngelis et al. (61)	1978–1985	98		6.6%
Badalament et al. (65)	1976–1986	22		9%
Sundaresan and Galicich (57)	1978–1983	50	12%	2%
Patchell et al. (23)	1978–1982	86	20%	2%
Mandell et al. (53)	1978–1980	104	31%	2%

[a]Years during which resections were performed.
[b]Mortality within 30 days of operation.
[c]Morbidity and mortality associated with surgical resection with postoperative radiation.
[d]Thirty-day morbidity and mortality in patients who did not undergo surgical resection.

mately become the treatment of choice even for solitary, easily accessible lesions in appropriately selected patients. On the other hand, for situations in which histologic diagnosis of a superficial lesion is needed or in which the patient is rapidly deteriorating neurologically because of local mass effect, open surgical resection remains a cost-effective and therapeutically appropriate alternative to radiosurgery.

Brachytherapy

Stereotactic placement of high-activity iodine-125 implants into a metastasis can deliver a high dose of radiation to the tumor while minimizing the exposure of surrounding brain (69,70). Typical radiation doses within the tumor range from 3500 to 13,000 cGy delivered over a 5-day period. After 5 days, the implants are removed under local anesthesia. Median survival for patients undergoing brachytherapy for CNS metastases ranges from 8 to 18.5 months (68,69). This technique is typically used in patients with recurrent metastases who cannot tolerate additional whole-brain radiation (68).

CONCLUSION

Many surgeons regard open surgical resection of solitary metastases as the treatment of choice in patients with stable extracranial disease. In addition, tumors that are imminently life threatening or causing significant neurologic dysfunction from edema and mass effect despite corticosteroid therapy should be resected if the patient has a reasonable life expectancy. Postoperative radiation is beneficial in patients with stable extracranial disease. Radiosurgery is likely superior to open resection in patients with deep, multiple, or recurrent metastases. Radiation therapy alone is indicated in patients with highly radiosensitive metastases and those

that are not amenable to either surgical or radiosurgical intervention.

REFERENCES

1. Parker SL, Tong T, Bolden S, Wingo PA. Cancer statistics, 1996. *CA Cancer J Clin* 1996;65:5–27.
2. Aronson SM, Garcia JH, Aronson BE. Metastatic neoplasms of the brain:their frequency in relation to age. *Cancer* 1964;17:558–563.
3. Pickren JW, Lopez G, Tsukada Y, Lans WW. Brain metastases: an autopsy study. *Cancer Treat Symp* 1983;2:295–313.
4. Posner JB, Chernik NL. Intracranial metastases from systemic cancer. *Advances in Neurology* 1978;19:579–592.
5. Takakura K, Sano K, Hojo S, Hirano A. *Metastatic tumors of the central nervous system.* Tokyo: Igaku-Shoin; 1982:5–12.
6. Cairncross JG, Posner JB. The management of brain metastases. In: Walker MD, ed. *Oncology of the nervous system.* Boston: Martinus Nijhoff; 1983:341–377.
7. Walker AE, Robins M, Weinfeld FD. Epidemiology of brain tumors: the national survey of intracranial neoplasms. *Neurology* 1985;35:219–226.
8. Kofman S, Garvin JS, Nagamani D, Taylor SG. Treatment of cerebral metastases from breast carcinoma with prednisolone. *JAMA* 1957;163:1473–1476.
9. Horton J, Baxter DH, Olson KB. The management of metastases to the brain by irradiation and corticosteroids. *AJR Am J Roentgenol* 1971;111:334–336.
10. Ruderman NB, Hall TC. Use of glucocorticoids in the palliative treatment of metastatic brain tumors. *Cancer* 1965;18:298–306.
11. Deutsch M, Parsons JA, Mercado R. Radiotherapy for intracranial metastases. *Cancer* 1974;34:1607–1611.
12. Black P. Brain metastasis: current status and recommended guidelines for management. *Neurosurgery* 1979;5:617–631.
13. Kelly PJ, Kall BA, Goerss SJ. Results of computed tomography-based computer-assisted stereotactic resection of metastatic intracranial tumors. *Neurosurgery* 1988;22:7–17.
14. Alexander E, Moriarty TM, Davis RB, et al. Stereotactic radiosurgery for the definitive, noninvasive treatment of brain metastases. *J Natl Cancer Inst* 1995;87:34–40.
15. Kihlstrom L, Karlsson B, Lindquist C. Gamma knife surgery for cerebral metastases: implications for survival based on 16 years experience. *Stereotact Funct Neurosurg* 1993;61(Suppl 1):45–50.
16. Kelly PJ. *Tumor stereotaxis.* Philadelphia: WB Saunders; 1991:358–369.
17. Wright DC. Surgical treatment of brain metastases. In: *Surgical treatment of metastatic cancer.* Philadelphia: JB Lippincott; 1987:165–222.
18. Routh A, Khansur T, Hickman BT, Bass D. Management of brain metastases: past, present, and future. *South Med J* 1994;87:1218–1226.
19. Zimm S, Wampler GL, Stablein D, Hazra T, Young HF. Intracerebral metastases in solid-tumor patients: natural history and results of treatment. *Cancer* 1981;48:384–394.

20. Noordijk EM, Vecht CJ, Haaxma-Reiche H, et al. The choice of treatment of single brain metastasis should be based on extracranial tumor activity and age. *Int J Radiat Oncol Biol Phys* 1994;29:711–717.

21. Patchell RA, Tibbs PA, Walsh JW, et al. A randomized trial of surgery in the treatment of single metastases to the brain. *N Engl J Med* 1990; 322:494–500.

22. Vecht CJ, Haaxma-Reiche H, Noordijk EM, et al. Treatment of single brain metastasis: radiotherapy alone or combined with neurosurgery? *Ann Neurol* 1993;33:583–590.

23. Patchell RA, Cirrincione C, Thaler HT, Galicich JH, Kim JH, Posner JB. Single brain metastases: surgery plus radiation or radiation alone. *Neurology* 1986;36:447–453.

24. O'Neill BP, Buckner JC, Coffey RJ, Dinapoli RP, Shaw EG. Brain metastatic lesions. *Mayo Clin Proc* 1994;69:1062–1068.

25. Galicich JH, Sundaresan N, Arbit E, Passe S. Surgical treatment of single brain metastasis: factors associated with survival. *Cancer* 1980;45: 381–386.

26. Yardeni D, Reichenthal E, Zucker G, et al. Neurosurgical management of dingle brain metastasis. *Surg Neurol* 1984;21:377–384.

27. Sundaresan N, Galicich JH. Surgical treatment of brain metastases: clinical and computerized tomography evaluation of the results of treatment. *Cancer* 1985;55:1382–1388.

28. Black PM. Solitary brain metastases: radiation, resection, or radiosurgery? *Chest* 1993;103:367S–369S.

29. Coia LR, Aaronson N, Linggood R, Loeffler J, Priestman T. A report of the consensus workshop panel on the treatment of brain metastases. *Int J Radiat Oncol Biol Phys* 1992;23:223–227.

30. Galicich JH, Arbit E, Wronski M. Metastatic brain tumors. In: Wilkins RH, Rengachary SS, eds. *Neurosurgery*. New York: McGraw-Hill; 1996:807–821.

31. Ransohoff J. Surgical therapy of brain metastases. In: Weiss L, Gilbert HA, Posner JB, eds. *Brain metastases*. Boston: GK Hall; 1978:380–389.

32. Bindal RK, Sawaya R, Leavens ME, Lee JJ. Surgical treatment of multiple brain metastases. *J Neurosurg* 1993;79:210–216.

33. Hazuka MB, Burleson WD, Stroud DN, Leonard CE, Lillehei KO, Kinzie JJ. Multiple brain metastases are associated with poor survival in patients treated with surgery and radiotherapy. *J Clin Oncol* 1993;11: 369–373.

34. Somaza S, Kondziolka D, Lunsford LD, Kirkwood JM, Flinkinger JC. Stereotactic radiosurgery for cerebral metastatic melanoma. *J Neurosurg* 1993;79:661–666.

35. DeAngelis LM. Management of brain metastases. *Cancer Invest* 1994; 12:156–165.

36. Fernandez E, Maira G, Puca A, Vignati A. Multiple intracranial metastases of malignant melanoma with long-term survival. *J Neurosurg* 1984;60:621–624.

37. Posner JB. Management of brain metastases. *Rev Neurol (Paris)* 1992; 148:477–487.

38. Bindal RK, Sawaya R, Leavens ME, Hess KR, Taylor SH. Reoperation for recurrent metastatic brain tumors. *J Neurosurg* 1995;83:600–604.

39. Sundaresan N, Sachdev VP, DiGiacinto GV, Hughes JEO. Reoperation for brain metastases. *J Clin Oncol* 1988;6:1625–1629.

40. Little JR, Dale AJD, Okazaki H. Meningeal carcinomatosis. *Arch Neurol* 1974;30:138–143.

41. Olson ME, Chernik NL, Posner JB. Infiltration of the leptomeninges by systemic cancer. *Arch Neurol* 1974;30:122–137.

42. Wasserstrom WR, Glass JP, Posner JB. Diagnosis and treatment of leptomeningeal metastases from solid tumors: experience with 90 patients. *Cancer* 1982;49:759–772.

43. Little JR, Frankel A. Meningeal carcinomatosis. In: Wilkins RH, Rengachary SS, eds. *Neurosurgery*. New York: McGraw-Hill; 1996:829–832.

44. Akeson P, Larsson EM, Kristoffersen DT, Jonsson E, Holtas S. Brain metastases: comparison of gadodiamide injection-enhanced MR imaging at standard and high dose, contrast-enhanced CT and non-contrast-enhanced MR imaging. *Acta Radiol* 1995;36:300–305.

45. Yuh WTC, Fisher DJ, Runge VM, et al. Phase III multicenter trial of high-dose gadoteridol in MR evaluation of brain metastases. *AJNR Am J Neuroradiol* 1994;15:1037–1051.

46. Yuh WTC, Tali ET, Nguyen HD, Simonson TM, Mayr NA, Fisher DJ. The effect of contrast dose, imaging time, and lesion size in the MR detection of intracerebral metastasis. *AJNR Am J Neuroradiol* 1995;16:373–380.

47. Young B, Patchell RA. Surgery for a single brain metastasis. In: Wilkins RH, Rengachary SS, eds. *Neurosurgery*. New York: McGraw-Hill; 1996:823–828.

48. Cohen N, Strauss G, Lew R, Silver D, Recht L. Should prophylactic anticonvulsants be administered to patients with newly-diagnosed cerebral metastases? A retrospective analysis. *J Clin Oncol* 1988;6:1621–1624.

49. Kondziolka D, Lunsford LD. Brain metastases. In: Apuzzo MLJ, ed. *Brain surgery: complication avoidance and management*. New York: Churchill Livingstone; 1993:615–641.

50. Salcman M. Intracranial hemorrhage caused by brain tumor. In: Kaufman HH, ed. *Intracerebral hematomas*. New York: Raven Press; 1992: 95–107.

51. Graus F, Rogers LR, Posner JB. Cerebrovascular complications in patients with cancer. *Medicine* 1985;64:16–35.

52. Young B, Patchell RA. Metastatic tumors. In: Rengachary SS, Wilkins RH, eds. *Principles of neurosurgery*. London: Wolfe; 1994:27.1–27.6.

53. Mandell L, Hilaris B, Sullivan M, et al. The treatment of single brain metastasis from non-oat cell lung carcinoma: surgery and radiation versus radiation therapy alone. *Cancer* 1986;58:641–649.

54. Stevens G, Firth I, Coates A. Cerebral metastases from malignant melanoma. *Radiother Oncol* 1992;23:185–191.

55. Rosenstein M, Wallner K, Scher H, Sternberg CN. Treatment of brain metastases from bladder cancer. *J Urol* 1993;149:480–483.

56. DiStefano A, Yap HY, Hortobagyi GN, Blumenschein GR. The natural history of breast cancer patients with brain metastases. *Cancer* 1979; 44:1913–1918.

57. Sundaresan N, Galicich JH. Surgical treatment of single brain metastases from non-small-cell lung cancer. *Cancer Invest* 1985;3:107–113.

58. White KT, Fleming TR, Laws ER. Single metastasis to the brain: surgical treatment in 122 consecutive patients. *Mayo Clin Proc* 1981;56: 424–428.

59. Wronski M, Arbit E, Burt M, Galicich JH. Survival after surgical treatment of brain metastases from lung cancer: a follow-up study of 231 patients treated between 1976 and 1991. *J Neurosurg* 1995;83: 605–616.

60. Hagen NA, Cirrincione C, Thaler HT, DeAngelis LM. The role of radiation therapy following resection of single brain metastasis from melanoma. *Neurology* 1990;40:158–160.

61. DeAngelis LM, Mandell LR, Thaler HT, et al. The role of postoperative radiotherapy after resection of single brain metastases. *Neurosurgery* 1989;24:798–805.

62. Smalley SR, Laws ER, O'Fallon JR, Shaw EG, Schray MF. Resection for solitary brain metastasis: role of adjuvant radiation and prognostic variables in 229 patients. *J Neurosurg* 1992;77:531–540.

63. Smalley SR, Schray MF, Laws ER, O'Fallon JR. Adjuvant radiation therapy after surgical resection of solitary brain metastasis: association with pattern of failure and survival. *Int J Radiat Oncol Biol Phys* 1987; 13:1611–1616.

64. Armstrong JG, Wronski M, Galicich J, Leibel SA, Burt M. Postoperative radiation for lung cancer metastatic to the brain. *J Clin Oncol* 1994; 12:2340–2344.

65. Badalament RA, Gluck RW, Wong GY, et al. Surgical treatment of brain metastases from renal cell carcinoma. *Urology* 1990;36:112–117.

66. Gutin PH, Wilson CB. Radiosurgery for malignant brain tumors. *J Clin Oncol* 1990;8:571–573.

67. Loeffler JS, Kooy HM, Wen PY, et al. The treatment of recurrent brain metastases with stereotactic radiosurgery. *J Clin Oncol* 1990;8:576–582.

68. Rutigliano MJ, Lunsford LD, Kondziolka D, Strauss MJ, Khanna V, Green M. The cost effectiveness of stereotactic radiosurgery versus surgical resection in the treatment of solitary metastatic brain tumors. *Neurosurgery* 1995;37:445–455.

69. Bernstein M, Cabantog A, Laperriere N, Leung P, Thomason C. Brachytherapy for recurrent single brain metastasis. *Can J Neurol Sci* 1995;22:13–16.

70. Prados M, Leibel S, Barnett CM, Gutin P. Interstitial brachytherapy for metastatic brain tumors. *Cancer* 1989;63:657–660.

CHAPTER 14

Radiosurgery of Brain Metastases

John C. Flickinger, Douglas Kondziolka, and L. Dade Lunsford

> The tool used by the surgeon must be adapted to the task, and where the human brain is concerned the tool cannot be too refined.
>
> —*Lars Leksell*

BACKGROUND

For several reasons, the brain is one region of the body where tumor metastasis heralds a poor outcome. First, metastatic disease to the brain can be quite disabling, with symptoms that impinge on quality of life and basic function. These symptoms include (depending on size and location) decreased mental status, hemiparesis, aphasia, ataxia/imbalance, seizure, severe headache, and nausea. Second, brain metastases usually cannot be treated effectively with conventional systemic chemotherapy or immunotherapy, despite their relative efficacy elsewhere in the body. Most chemotherapy agents cannot penetrate the blood–brain barrier in sufficient concentrations to be effective. Brain metastases pose even a greater problem with immunotherapy because the danger of increasing peritumoral edema makes IL-2–based therapy contraindicated in this setting. The management of brain metastases is, therefore, restricted to regional therapies (surgery and radiation). Lastly, median survival is limited to months before diagnosis. At least 100,000 cancer patients develop brain metastases each year in the United States alone (1,2).

The frequency and distribution of brain metastases is well described in the series of Pickren and associates (3). They reported on the autopsy results of 10,916 cancer patients. This population represented 95% of the in-hospital deaths at Roswell Park Memorial Institute from 1959 to 1979. The overall incidence of brain metastases in this autopsy series was 8.7% (67% had systemic metastases with no brain metastases and 24% had no metastatic disease). This study found considerable variation in the incidence of brain metastases with primary site. The rate of brain disease was considerably higher than average for the following primary sites: skin (28%), lung (23%), and unknown primary sites (21%). Figure 1 shows the distribution of the number of brain metastases identified. Most patients had only a limited number of brain metastases even at the end of their lives. When tumors were present in the brain, solitary metastases were present in 39% of patients, two or fewer in 54%, and four or fewer in 74%.

Unfortunately, only 3.4% of patients with metastases to the brain had this as the only metastatic site identified at autopsy. It is in this small group of patients that aggressive regional therapy to the brain may have the greatest impact on survival. In the remaining 97% of patients, regional

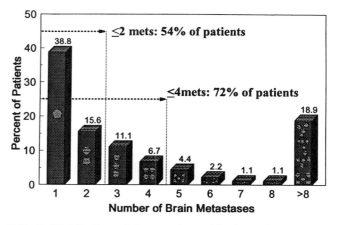

FIG. 1. Distribution of the number of brain metastases at autopsy in 954 brain metastases patients studied by Pickren and associates (3).

J. C. Flickinger and D. Kondziolka: Departments of Neurological Surgery and Radiation Oncology, University of Pittsburgh Medical Center, Pittsburgh, Pennsylvania 15213.

L. D. Lunsford: Department of Neurosurgery, Presbyterian University Hospital, Pittsburgh, Pennsylvania 15213-2582.

therapy can still improve survival and quality of life, because the local impact of a metastasis can lead to symptoms and earlier death. Unfortunately, in many patients the optimal therapy of brain metastases does not significantly extend survival due to progression of extracranial disease.

ALTERNATIVE APPROACHES

Conservative Medical Management

The average survival for patients with brain metastases who are not treated is about 1 month after diagnosis in historical series (4,5). Medical management consists chiefly of corticosteroids and anticonvulsant therapy when appropriate. Corticosteroids alone (with no surgery or radiation) can at best prolong survival another month on the average. Corticosteroids are indicated in patients with brain metastases that are symptomatic from local mass effect (headache, nausea, or any persistent neurologic deficit).

The practice of prescribing corticosteroids to all patients with brain metastases should be discouraged. Patients with asymptomatic brain metastases and those who present with limited seizures that are subsequently controlled with anticonvulsants do not need corticosteroids unless symptoms due to a local mass effect develop. Although some physicians are concerned that radiation therapy will lead to increased edema that will cause symptoms in previously asymptomatic patients, it is debatable whether this ever occurs from standard fractionated radiotherapy doses. The development of cushingoid features in most patients on long-term, high-dose corticosteroids (steroid myopathy, leg edema, sleep disturbances, personality changes including occasional steroid psychosis, gas, occasional cases of intractable hiccups, gastric/duodenal irritation, ulceration, or hemorrhage) are all good reasons to avoid corticosteroid therapy whenever possible and to look for therapies that will allow symptomatic patients to be tapered from corticosteroids.

Although some (6) have recommended withholding anticonvulsants until seizures are documented, we and most physicians prescribe anticonvulsant therapy for any patient at significant risk for seizure. This includes patients with subcortical supratentorial metastases and any patient with a transient neurologic symptom that could be suspected as a seizure, regardless of tumor location. Patients with cerebellar, brain stem, or diencephalic metastases are considered at low risk for seizures. Anticonvulsant blood levels must be checked in all patients to ensure drug doses are proper (6).

Radiation Therapy Alone

Fractionated whole-brain radiotherapy has been considered the standard treatment for brain metastases for at least the last 40 years. The average survival in large series of unselected patients is about 4 to 6 months (7,8). The side effects of conventional whole-brain radiotherapy are relatively minor. Skin redness and dryness is usually mild and normally occurs at the end of treatment. More pronounced skin redness that occurs during the first week of radiotherapy is usually an early sign of a phenytoin allergy in patients taking this medication. Hair loss usually begins at the end of treatment and becomes fairly complete, with significant hair regrowth occurring about 3 months after radiotherapy. This regrowth is usually complete, although some patients have permanent baldness or thinning of the hair in the midline after radiotherapy that gives the appearance of male-pattern baldness. This is from the tangential effect of the radiation beams at midline, where the thinner thickness of tissue to attenuate the radiation leads to higher doses at the scalp. For good prognosis patients, it is usually worthwhile to prevent permanent hair loss by using a scalp block (Fig. 2).

Historically, the rationale for irradiating the whole brain to treat a solitary intracerebral metastasis has been unassailable. Before the development of computed tomographic (CT) scanning and more recently magnetic resonance imaging (MRI), identification of the extent and location of metastatic disease was difficult. Because standard doses of whole-brain irradiation (eg, 30 Gy in 10 fractions) were thought to have little or no effect on subsequent cognitive function (which is now known to be untrue) (9–11), not only was there no interest in limiting radiation fields for established metastases, but prophylactic whole-brain irradiation was indiscriminately used in small cell lung cancer and was proposed for use in nonsmall cell cancer. Another reason for giving radiation to the whole brain when only one metastasis was present was the fear that other metastases could appear at the

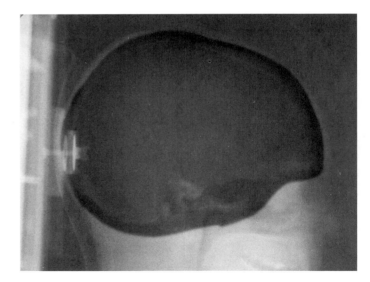

FIG. 2. High-energy (6 MV) x-ray, double-exposure, portal film of a patient receiving whole-brain radiotherapy for brain metastasis using a scalp protection block to prevent permanent midline hair loss.

edge of the radiation treatment field and that overlap with a new external beam field would lead to radiation injury. This is less of a contraindication to localized irradiation now, because current radiosurgery fields present fewer overlap problems. There is recent information that the brain can repair more radiation injury over time than was previously appreciated (12). The possibility that whole-brain irradiation might prevent the subsequent development of new brain metastases (from the irradiation of subclinical microscopic disease) is the chief reason whole-brain radiation is still standard therapy for solitary tumors.

The Radiation Therapy Oncology Group investigated different radiation fractionation schedules of whole-brain irradiation for brain metastases in 1,830 patients (9,13). No differences in median survival were detected among the five different treatment schedules that were evaluated: 20 Gy in five fractions, 30 Gy in 10 or 15 fractions, and 40 Gy in 15 or 20 fractions. Because of a concern that the larger dose-fractions with 20 Gy in five fractions could lead to delayed neurologic deterioration, most radiotherapists in the United States have settled on 30 Gy in 10 fractions as the standard dose for whole-brain radiotherapy. Ambulatory patients with no systemic metastases had the greatest median survival (28 weeks) compared to other patients (11 weeks).

The extent to which solitary brain metastases eventually regrow after conventional radiotherapy has not always been appreciated, as many patients succumb to progression of extracranial metastases. Patchell and colleagues demonstrated actuarial recurrence rates exceeding 80% after whole-brain radiotherapy using 30 Gy in 10 fractions for patients with solitary brain metastasis (14). For this reason, conventional fractionated whole-brain radiotherapy alone is inadequate treatment in patients with limited or slowly progressive extracranial metastasis.

Surgical Resection of Brain Metastases

Surgery for brain metastases is discussed in detail in Chapter 13. Because of the poor long-term control rates of brain metastases with conventional radiotherapy, resection of solitary brain metastases has been advocated in good prognosis patients (8,14,15). Patients with good functional status and no other systemic metastases benefit most (15). Randomized trials by Patchell and more recently by Noordijk and coworkers (16) have shown not only superior tumor control but also superior survival in patients undergoing surgical resection plus radiotherapy compared to radiotherapy alone. Although these studies established the inferiority of conventional radiotherapy alone compared to surgical resection followed by whole-brain irradiation, surgical resection is not generally considered feasible for patients with deeply located tumors or those with extensive comorbidity. The use of surgical

resection in the management of multiple brain metastases was recently evaluated by Sawaya and associates (17). Although resection of multiple brain metastases is possible in some patients, most neurosurgeons feel that the morbidity is not justified in these patients because of their poor prognosis.

RADIOSURGERY

Background

Radiosurgery is a term coined by the brilliant and innovative Swedish neurosurgeon Lars Leksell, who originally defined it in 1951 as the single-session, closed-skull destruction of a stereotactically defined intracranial target with high-dose ionizing external beam irradiation with relative sparing of surrounding normal tissue (18). Leksell used "-surgery" as part of the term because he intended it to be a substitute for open surgical resection. This early vision of superseding open surgical resection with a closed-skull, noninvasive, high-tech procedure was revisited in the movie *Star Trek IV*, in which the concept of craniotomy was considered barbaric. Although most of the initial uses of radiosurgery were for benign targets (eg, arteriovenous malformations, benign neoplasms, and normal brain or cranial nerves for functional radiosurgery), it was soon realized that these techniques could be substituted for the resection of brain metastases, particularly solitary tumors.

Detailed Methodology

Modern radiosurgery began with the development of the gamma knife by Leksell and his colleagues at the Karolinska Institute. After initially working with orthovoltage radiation and then proton beam irradiation, they designed a machine with a hemispherical array of highly collimated small cobalt-60 beams they called the gamma knife (a name chosen to present this as a new or more evolved type of surgical procedure). The gamma knife models currently in use have 201 cobalt-60 beams capable of accurately producing spherical radiation dose distributions with 4-, 8-, 14-, or 18-mm collimators (Figs. 3 and 4). Nonspherical radiation distributions are produced by computer-planned combinations of treatments to different numbers of isocenters. The dramatic success of gamma knife radiosurgery in treating arteriovenous malformations and acoustic neuromas stimulated the development of methods to imitate these radiation distributions with modified linear accelerators (linac radiosurgery) by using a single radiation source with multiple arcs (19,20). Advantages of the gamma knife include greater efficiency and reliability, which facilitate the use of multiple isocenters to shape the radiation treatment volume optimally to

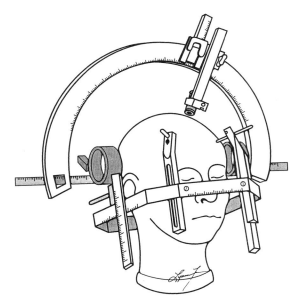

FIG. 3. Stereotactic frame (Leksell G) with coronal arc attachments for stereotactic needle biopsy.

Technique

A radiosurgical procedure (whether gamma knife or linac) begins with application of a stereotactic frame. The stereotactic frame is a rectangular or circular frame usually made of precisely machined, nonferromagnetic, imaging-compatible metal. It is usually secured to the skull by a series of screws (usually four) that puncture the skin (see Fig. 3). A coordinate system can be read on the subsequent radiologic images. Any target in the brain can be identified by its coordinates. Using local anesthesia, pain medication, and sedation, patients can tolerate the frame with minimal discomfort. After radiologic imaging is complete (usually CT, MRI, or both), computerized treatment planning is used to match a radiosurgery treatment volume exactly to the targeted brain metastasis. At our institution, therapy is coordinated by a radiosurgery team, which includes a neurosurgeon, radiotherapist, and radiation physicist. After treatment (see Fig. 4), the stereotactic frame is removed, and the patient can usually go home after several hours of observation. The only acute side effects anticipated are mild headache from the frame, a small chance of nausea, and slightly greater chance of seizure in patients with subcortically located tumors. Hair loss occurs only when larger tumors that are close to the surface of the brain are treated (and the hair loss is then limited to a small overlying area). Delayed effects include permanent brain injury or reversible edema, developing 3 to 24 months after radiosurgery in a few patients. This is sometimes difficult to distinguish from tumor regrowth on CT or MRI.

the target volume. Radiosurgery optimization assumes greater importance in treating irregular or nonspherical targets. The chief advantage of linac radiosurgery over gamma knife radiosurgery is that the equipment (the linear accelerator) is already in use at most hospitals, decreasing its up-front cost.

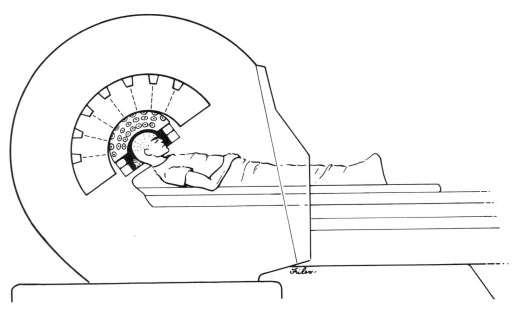

FIG. 4. Drawing of a patient in the gamma knife. The coronal arc from Fig. 3 is replaced by the collimator helmet and cobalt-60 sources. The stereotactic frame, although present, was not drawn in this figure.

TABLE 1. *Results of radiosurgery for brain metastases*

Institution	No. mets	Min. dose (median)	Median survival	% Local control	% Necrosis
Harvard JCRT2 (2)	421	15.0 Gy	9 mo	65*	7*
Karolinska (21)	235	30.0 Gy	NS	94	NS
Heidelberg (22)	124	17.0 Gy	6 or 12 mo†	94	3
Gamma Knife Users (23)	112	16.0 Gy	11 mo	67*	4
Stanford (24)	52	25.0 Gy	NS	94	4
U. Wisconsin (25)	47	18.0 Gy	8.5 mo	73	0

NS: Not stated
*Actuarial
†6 months disseminated disease, 12 months no extracerebral disease

Clinical Results

In general, the results of radiosurgery equal or exceed those reported for surgical resection followed by whole-brain irradiation. Table 1 lists several large representative series of patients treated by radiosurgery for brain metastases (2,21–25). A representative response to radiosurgery is shown in Figure 5.

The Gamma Knife Users' Group series was made up entirely of patients treated for solitary brain metastases (23). Radiosurgery was part of initial treatment in 71 patients, and an additional 45 patients were treated for recurrent tumors after prior whole-brain radiotherapy. Minimum radiosurgery tumor doses varied from 8 to 30 Gy (mean 17.5 Gy), with 51 patients receiving radiosurgery alone (usually for recurrent disease) and 65 as combined treatment with whole-brain radiotherapy (mean dose 34 Gy). As shown in Table 1, the actuarial median survival without radiosurgery was 11 months and 20 months after diagnosis. Patients with recurrent tumors survived 43 months from diagnosis, as compared to 14 months for patients treated with radiosurgery at initial presentation. Multivariate analysis of post-radiosurgery survival identified histology as the only significant vari-

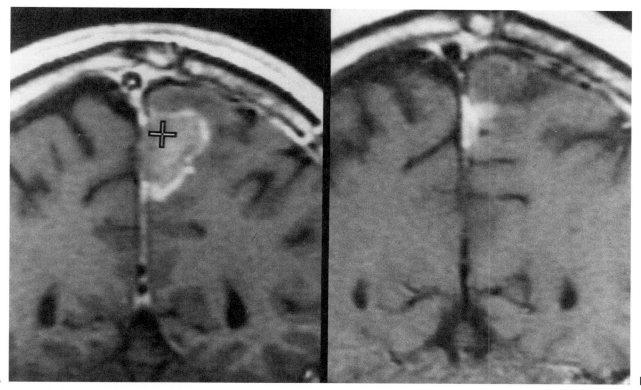

FIG. 5. Coronal MRI scan **(A)** before and **(B)** 6 weeks after radiosurgery. This patient had whole-brain radiotherapy and craniotomy 9 months before in this same location. Radiosurgery was used to treat the local recurrence.

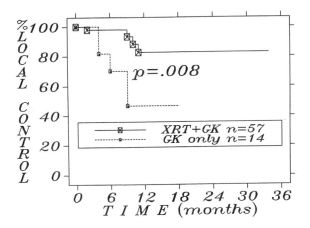

FIG. 6. Comparison of actuarial local tumor control between the subsets of solitary brain metastasis patients in the Gamma Knife Users' Group studies receiving initial treatment with radiosurgery alone (median minimum tumor dose 17 Gy) versus whole-brain radiotherapy (median dose 30 Gy/12 fractions) combined with radiosurgery (median minimum tumor dose 16 Gy) (23).

able (p=0.041), with better survival for breast cancer and worse for melanoma and renal cell cancer. The excellent tumor control with radiosurgery for "radioresistant" tumors such as malignant melanoma in this study (and also in the report by Somaza and associates) is impressive compared to fractionated radiotherapy results (26,27). The overall actuarial tumor control rate was 85% at 2 years. Univariate and multivariate analysis identified significantly improved tumor control in patients who received combined radiosurgery and whole-brain radiotherapy compared to radiosurgery alone ($p \leq 0.011$) as shown in Fig. 6 and for patients with melanoma or renal cell carcinoma ($p \leq 0.0006$). Two-year actuarial rates for developing radiation necrosis requiring surgical resection and symptomatic edema were 4% and 11% respectively. Radiosurgery could not entirely prevent the development of tumor hemorrhage, which occurs naturally, particularly with malignant melanoma and renal cell carcinoma metastases.

The 2-year actuarial rate of tumor hemorrhage after radiosurgery was 8%. This may be explained by the fact that vascular obliteration after radiosurgery appears to be a slow process that takes 6 months to 3 years with arteriovenous malformations.

In the Harvard Joint Center series of over 250 patients treated with linac radiosurgery for brain metastases, multivariate analysis revealed that survival was significantly associated with the lack of any active systemic disease and age <60 (2). They reported actuarial tumor control rates that were similar to those in the Gamma Knife Users' Group study (85% at 1 year, 65% at 2 years). Multivariate analysis of local failure identified it to be significantly associated with recurrent tumors and infratentorial location, but not histology. The greater local failure rate with infratentorial tumors may be from inadequate imaging of the posterior fossa, where CT scans may show bone artifacts, leading to inadequate targeting of the radiation. Complications were limited to mass effect requiring surgery in 7% of patients and cranial neuropathies developing in 1% of patients.

CHOICE OF THERAPY

Table 2 lists standard treatment strategies for dealing with brain metastases and optimal patient groups for different approaches. Patients with small solitary brain metastases could be treated with radiosurgery alone if they have a good prognosis (no systemic disease), particularly if they have a tumor such as melanoma that is relatively resistant to conventional doses of whole-brain irradiation. In these patients, whole-brain irradiation, with its resultant hair loss and possible late effects on cognitive function, could be withheld until other brain metastases develop, at which time radiosurgery could also be considered. We offer patients with solitary brain metastases participation in our randomized trial of radiosurgery alone (minimum tumor dose 20 Gy) versus radiosurgery to 16 Gy plus 30 Gy whole-brain irradiation. The higher radiosurgery dose in the group to receive radiosurgery alone should overcome the lower tumor control rates reported in the Gamma Knife Users' Group study for radiosurgery alone (where the median dose was only 17 Gy compared to 16 Gy for radiosurgery) when given with 30 Gy irradiation. The use of initial radiosurgery in patients with multiple metastases is also controversial. We have undertaken a prospective trial that randomizes patients with two to four metastases to whole-brain irradiation to 30 Gy with either

TABLE 2. *Treatment strategies for brain metastases*

Initial therapy	Treatment for recurrence	Patient characteristics
Radiosurgery alone	Radiosurgery or surgery and/or whole-brain XRT	Solitary metastasis <3 cm; no active systemic disease
Radiosurgery and whole-brain XRT	Radiosurgery or surgery	Solitary metastasis <3 cm; no active systemic disease
Surgical resection and whole-brain XRT	Radiosurgery	Resectable solitary brain metastasis with mass effect >3 cm; no active systemic disease
Whole-brain XRT	Radiosurgery, repeat XRT, or supportive care	Active systemic disease and/or multiple brain metastases

immediate radiosurgery to follow or radiosurgery as a salvage treatment if tumor progression develops. The latter option is the only one offered to patients who do not want to participate.

Patients with significant mass effect from solitary metastasis >3 cm in diameter are better managed with surgical resection and postoperative radiotherapy than radiosurgery. This is because tumor shrinkage may take several months to occur after radiosurgery, and the risks of radiation injury are greater in patients with tumors >3 cm in diameter.

Despite achieving controlled or eradicated brain disease, the average survival for patients with brain metastases is about 10 to 12 months. Progression of systemic disease is the most common reason for death. As improvements in systemic care match improvements in regional brain treatment, we can anticipate further significant improvements in survival.

REFERENCES

1. Wingo P, Tong T, Bolden S. Cancer statistics, 1995 [published erratum appears in *CA Cancer J Clin* 1995;45(2):127–128]. *CA Cancer J Clin* 1995;45(1):8–30.
2. Loeffler JS, Shrieve DC. What is appropriate therapy for a patient with a single brain metastasis? *Int J Radiat Oncol Biol Phys* 1994;29(4):915–917.
3. Pickren JW, Lopez G, Tzukada Y, Lane WW. Brain metastases. An autopsy study. *Cancer Treat Symp* 1983;2:295–313.
4. DiStefano A, Yap HY, Hortobagi GN, Blumenschein GR. The natural history of breast cancer patients with brain metastases. *Cancer* 1979;44:1913–1918.
5. Lang EF, Slater J. Metastatic brain tumor: results of surgical and nonsurgical treatment. *Surg Clin North Am* 1964;44:865.
6. Cohen N, Strauss G, Lew R, Silver D, Recht L. Should prophylactic anticonvulsants be administered to patients with newly-diagnosed cerebral metastases? A retrospective analysis. *J Clin Oncol* 1988;6(10):1621–1624.
7. Egawa S, Tukiyama I, Akine Y, et al. Radiotherapy of brain metastases. *Int J Radiat Oncol Biol Phys* 1986;12:1621–1625.
8. Mandell L, Hilaris B, Sullivan M, et al. The treatment of single brain metastasis from non–oat cell lung carcinoma; surgery and radiation vs. radiation alone. *Cancer* 1986;58:641–649.
9. Borgelt B, Gelber R, Kramer S, et al. The palliation of brain metastases: the final results of the first two studies by the radiation therapy oncology group. *Int J Radiat Oncol Biol Phys* 1980;6:1–9.
10. Fleck JF, Einhorn LH, Lauer RC, Schultz SM, Miller ME. Is prophylactic cranial irradiation indicated in small-cell lung cancer? *J Clin Oncol* 1990;8:209–214.
11. Lishner M, Feld R, Payne DG, et al. Late neurological complications after prophylactic cranial irradiation in patients with small-cell lung cancer: the Toronto experience. *J Clin Oncol* 1990;8:215–221.
12. Flickinger JC, Deutsch M, Lunsford LD. Repeat megavoltage irradiation of pituitary and suprasellar tumors. *Int J Radiat Oncol Biol Phys* 1989;17:171–175.
13. Gelber R, Larson M, Borget BB, Kramer S. Equivalence of radiation schedules for the palliative treatment of brain metastases in patients with favorable prognosis. *Cancer* 1981;48:1749–1753.
14. Patchell RA, Tibbs PA, Walsh JW, et al. A randomized trial of surgery in the treatment of single metastases to the brain. *N Engl J Med* 1990;322:494.
15. Smalley SR, Laws ER, O'Fallon JR, Shaw EG, Schray MF. Resection for solitary brain metastasis: role of adjuvant radiation and prognostic variables in 229 patients. *J Neurosurg* 1992;77:531–540.
16. Noordijk EM, Vecht CJ, Haaxma-Reiche H, et al. The choice of treatment of single brain metastasis should be based on extracranial tumor activity and age. *Int J Radiat Oncol Biol Phys* 1994;29:711–717.
17. Bindal RK, Sawaya R, Leavens ME, et al. Surgical treatment of multiple brain metastases. *J Neurosurg* 1993;79:210–216.
18. Leksell L. The stereotaxic method and radiosurgery of the brain. *Acta Chir Scand* 1951;102:316–319.
19. Steiner L. Treatment of arteriovenous malformations by radiosurgery. In: Wilson CB, Stein BM, eds. *Intracranial arteriovenous malformations*. Baltimore: Williams & Wilkins, 1984:295–313.
20. Lutz W, Winston KR, Maleki PV. A system for stereotactic radiosurgery with a linear accelerator. *Int J Radiat Oncol Biol Phys* 1988;14:373–381.
21. Kihlstrom L, Karlsson B, Lindquist C. Gamma knife surgery for cerebral metastasis: implications for survival based on 16 years experience. *Stereotactic and Functional Neurosurgery* 1993;61(suppl. 1)1:45–50.
22. Engenhart R, Kimmig BN, Hover KH, et al. Long-term follow-up for brain metastases treated by percutaneous stereotactic single high-dose irradiation. *Cancer* 1993;71(4):1353–1361.
23. Flickinger JC, Kondziolka D, Lunsford LD, et al. A multi-institutional experience with stereotactic radiosurgery for solitary brain metastasis. *Int J Radiat Oncol Biol Phys* 1994;28(4):797–802.
24. Fuller BG, Kaplan ID, Adler J, et al. Stereotaxic radiosurgery for brain metastases: the importance of adjuvant whole brain irradiation. *Int J Radiat Oncol Biol Phys* 1992;23:413–418.
25. Mehta MP, Rozental JM, Levin AB, et al. Defining the role of radiosurgery in the management of brain metastases. *Int J Radiat Oncol Biol Phys* 1992;24(4):619–625.
26. Somaza S, Kondziolka D, Lunsford LD, Kirkwood J, Flickinger J. Stereotactic radiosurgery for cerebral metastatic melanoma. *J Neurosurg* 1993;79:661–666.
27. Vlock DR, Kirkwood JM, Leutzinger C, Kapp DS, Fischer JJ. High-dose fraction radiation therapy for intracranial metastases of malignant melanoma. *Cancer* 1982;49:2289–2294.

CHAPTER 15

Perfusional Therapy of Brain Metastases

William C. Welch and Paul L. Kornblith

Brain metastases can be a devastating complication of systemic cancer. They usually occur in patients with disseminated systemic disease and are often felt by the patient and physician alike to be the final step in the uncontrolled progression of the patient's malignancy.

—*DeAngelis (1)*

BACKGROUND

Brain metastases occur in 25% to 40% of patients with systemic cancer (2). Their intracranial distribution is proportional to the relative regional cerebral blood flow (3). These lesions are most commonly found in the cerebral hemispheres (85%) followed by the cerebellum (10%–15%) and lastly in the brain stem (1%–2%) (Table 1) (4–6). The most common metastatic tumors found in the brain are of lung, breast, gastrointestinal, and genitourinary origin (5–7). The incidence is greatest in patients who are 50 to 70 years old. The overall frequency of metastatic brain tumors appears to be increasing (8).

Metastatic tumor cells that successfully implant in the cerebral hemispheres have spread via hematogenous dissemination after separating from the primary site (1). The cells travel through the systemic bloodstream and enter the intracranial circulation. The cells invade cerebral blood vessels and normal brain tissue through the production of proteases (9). Alternatively, venous plexuses may provide a path for metastatic spread (10).

Successful metastatic tumor cell implants must actively recruit and develop an adequate blood supply to maintain cellular growth (11). The tumors produce a series of peptide growth factors (12) and vascular permeability factors

W. C. Welch: Department of Neurological Surgery, Orthopedic Surgery, University of Pittsburgh School of Medicine, Presbyterian University Hospital, Pittsburgh, Pennsylvania 15213.

P. L. Kornblith: Institute for Transfusion Medicine, Pittsburgh, Pennsylvania 15213.

that stimulate tumor angiogenesis and promote increased capillary permeability (2). The increased capillary permeability causes a breakdown of the blood–brain barrier (BBB), identified on contrast-enhanced computed tomographic (CT) and magnetic resonance imaging (MRI) scans as areas of peritumoral edema and increased contrast uptake (13,14).

Small metastatic deposits can be readily identified by technologically advanced imaging methods such as CT and MRI scanning (15,16). These studies are usually performed with iodinated contrast agents for CT and paramagnetic agents such as gadolinium diethyemetriamine pentaacetic acid (GdDPTA) for MRI. These contrast agents identify both pathologic and normal (physiologic) areas of breakdown in the BBB and increase the sensitivity of tumor detection.

The metastatic spread of tumor cells to the leptomeninges with associated neurologic findings is defined as meningeal carcinomatous or carcinomatous meningitis. This occurs in about 15% of patients with metastatic disease (17) and may represent the initial presentation of patients with cancer (18). Leptomeningeal spread may occur as a result of metastatic cells depositing on the leptomeninges through hematogenous routes or spread from the choroid plexus, subependyma, or adjacent bony struc-

TABLE 1. *Approximate distribution of intracranial metastases (8,25,26)*

Location	Approximate distribution (%)
Supratentorial	
Frontal	20
Parietal	45
Temporal	10
Occipital	10
Total	85
Infratentorial	
Cerebellum, brain stem, spinal cord	15

tures (19,20). Numerous samplings of cerebrospinal fluid (CSF) may be required to establish the diagnosis (21). Adenocarcinoma is the most common type of secondary tumor with leptomeningeal spread. Other common primary sources include lung, breast, and gastrointestinal cancer, as well as lymphoma and leukemia (15). Because most systemically administered chemotherapeutic agents achieve low CSF concentrations (22), intrathecal delivery of chemotherapy is frequently used (23,24).

Systemic chemotherapy has not proven to be effective therapy for metastatic brain tumors (1,3,25–28). Factors that govern the distribution and uptake of chemotherapeutic agents into metastatic brain tumors underlie this lack of efficacy. Delivery variables include the amount and type of drug administered, the rate and method of drug injection, and host metabolic factors. Other factors include the rate of blood-to-brain exchange (extraction fraction), the rate of tissue perfusion, and the ability of the tumor and brain tissue to take up the drug (partition coefficient) (29). Blood flow through the tumor-feeding vessels also influences drug delivery (30). Greater extraction fractions, tissue perfusion, and tumor uptake result in more effective drug delivery to tumor.

Drug-specific variables include molecular size and charge, pH, lipid solubility (28,31), availability of specific transport mechanisms (32), drug half-life, and binding to proteins and other intravascular components (27). Smaller molecular sizes, high lipid solubility, low molecular ionization at physiologic pH, minimal protein binding, and availability of transport mechanisms all increase the ability of an agent to enter the CSF, brain, and brain tumors. Extended drug half-life will improve tumoricidal/tumoristatic effects.

An important tissue-specific factor is the BBB. The BBB is maintained by tight cellular junctions of the brain's vascular endothelial cells and astrocytic foot processes (31,33). This unique anatomy also partially isolates the CNS from systemic immune surveillance (34). Exceptions include the pituitary gland, the subfornical and commissural organs, the pineal body, the tuber cinereum, the wall of the optic recess, the area postrema, and the choroid plexus (35,36).

Pathophysiologic conditions that disrupt the BBB include infections (meningitis, abscess), tumor, trauma, vasculitis, and radiation. Corticosteroids help preserve the BBB by stabilizing cellular membranes (37). The BBB can be disrupted with the intra-arterial injection of hyperosmolar agents such as iodinated contrast agents (38), mannitol (39), and others.

Other tissue-specific factors include the blood–tumor barrier (40), tumor vascularity, luminal surface of the capillaries (41), intrinsic tumor heterogeneity and increased hydrostatic pressure of the tumor matrices (42,43), chemosensitivity of the tumor, and the time course of drug metabolism. Tumor vascularity and the potential difficulty for agents crossing tumor capillaries and entering the

tumor cells make up the blood–tumor barrier. Poorly maintained endothelial cell junctions may permit an increased uptake of chemotherapeutic or other agents. Intrinsic tumor heterogeneity and increased hydrostatic pressure in the tumor matrices may prevent chemotherapeutic agents from achieving an effective concentration and uniform distribution within the tumor.

The interplay of these variables determines the uptake and efficacy of the chemotherapeutic agent selected (22,30). Although some of the variables, such as tissue vascularity, tumor heterogeneity, and vascularity, are fixed and not easily altered by the clinician, other variables can be modified. Examples include transient opening of the BBB through the intra-arterial injection of hyperosmolar agents and modifying drug delivery techniques so as to increase the partition coefficient.

PATIENT SELECTION

The mainstay of treatment for patients with metastatic CNS neoplasms includes corticosteroid therapy followed by radiation therapy, usually whole-brain irradiation. Patients with isolated or several metastases may undergo surgical resection if the lesions are approachable. Alternatively, focused radiotherapy may be considered (44). The use of regional perfusional therapy is most clearly defined for patients with meningeal carcinomatous. These patients are frequently afforded symptomatic relief with intraventricular chemotherapy, and this type of therapy can be considered a standard of care. Intra-arterial perfusion techniques, extracorporeal hemoperfusion, intratumoral injections, and the use of monoclonal antibodies (MABs) and BBB disruption are investigational treatment options. Ongoing clinical trials will help determine both the effectiveness of these techniques and appropriate selection criteria for patients with metastatic intracranial neoplasms.

METHODS

Intra-arterial Perfusion

The development of advanced intravascular catheters that can be guided has enabled clinicians to deliver therapeutic agents to the brain with extreme selectivity. The complications of intra-arterial chemotherapy include those associated with catheter insertion (described below), ipsilateral blindness, transient visual disturbances, transient and permanent neurologic deficits, nausea and vomiting, myelosuppression (45,46), leukoencephalopathy (47,48), and others (49). Intra-arterial chemotherapy can be used in both the carotid and vertebral arteries (50). Most studies have used intracarotid placement only, and we will limit our discussion to this.

The process of intra-arterial injection incorporates the Seldinger technique of catheter placement in the femoral artery. Fluoroscopic guidance enables the clinician to guide the flexible catheter into the carotid or vertebral arteries. Nonionic contrast is injected at intervals throughout catheter placement to identify relevant anatomy and potential complicating factors such as carotid artery stenosis or plaques. The tip of the catheter is routinely placed above the ophthalmic artery to avoid the well-described complications associated with the flow of chemotherapeutic agents into this vessel (46,47,51). Superselective arterial catheter placement can also be considered (52). The major morbidity rate of catheter placement is about 1% (53). Complications include vessel lacerations, intimal tears, groin hematoma, fixed neurologic deficits, and others (54).

Once the catheter tip is successfully placed, the intra-arterial chemotherapeutic agent is injected as a bolus or with continuous infusion. Diastole-phased pulsatile administration has been suggested to reduce intravascular streaming of chemotherapy and, potentially, to reduce the complications associated with intra-arterial delivery (55). As noted by Eckman (56) and Fenstermacher (29) and their coworkers, the advantage of intra-arterial perfusion usually exists only during the infusion and first passage of the drug.

Chemotherapeutic agents that have been infused intra-arterially for the treatment of cerebral malignancy (30, 57,58) include methotrexate, vincristine, vinblastine, mechlorethamine, melphalan, carmustine (BCNU) (30, 50,57), numustine (ACNU) (30), PCNU (45), HECNU (46), etoposide (VP-16) (59), teniposide (VM-26) and cisplatin (50), carboplatin (60), bleomycin (61), and AZQ (62). Most of these studies did not examine patients with metastatic disease exclusively, but also included patients who had malignant, primary glial neoplasms.

An interesting and novel approach to reduce systemic toxicity has been the use of extracorporeal removal of arterially infused chemotherapy (63). More specifically, the hemoperfusion of jugular drainage after the intra-arterial administration of the chemotherapeutic agent BCNU (64) has been performed in patients with malignant glial neoplasms. Doppman and colleagues also described a similar technique for use with cisplatinum (cisplatin) therapy (65).

These techniques involved the placement of an intracarotid artery catheter via a femoral artery puncture. The arterial catheter was preferentially positioned above the ophthalmic artery on the side of the brain to be infused. An angiogram was performed to outline the cerebral circulation and cerebral venous drainage. A venous catheter was then inserted into the femoral vein and guided to the jugular venous bulb on the selected side, usually the side to be perfused. Indocyanine green dye was injected into the arterial catheter as the jugular catheter was aspirated. This allowed the researchers to confirm that efficient blood recovery was obtained and that little arterially injected drug escaped into the systemic circulation. The patients were anticoagulated and the chemotherapeutic agent was infused. Extracorporeal perfusion through hemoperfusion cartridges or dialysis units removed the chemotherapeutic agents (Fig. 1). This technique was experimentally applied to monkeys before human use and was remarkably effective at removing intra-arterially infused carmustine (BCNU) from the systemic circulation.

The combination of BBB disruption and intra-arterial selective injection has been shown to augment the effects of regional perfusion by directing higher doses of agent to the specific tumor site (31,39,57).

MABs have been examined as a technique to localize drug delivery on tumor cells while potentially reducing associated toxicities. The antibodies are raised against tumor-associated antigens and can be used as carriers for chemotherapeutic agents (66). MABs conjugated with immunotoxins or radionuclides may be useful clinically (Table 2) (67,68). The antibodies can also be bispecific in design so as to bind to both tumor antibodies and immune cells (69). These techniques are still in the early stages of development and could potentially be combined with other techniques such as BBB disruption to provide increased MAB concentrations. Major drawbacks to this design are the lack of specific tumor antigens for MAB binding, the relatively low binding activity of the antibody, and nonspecific binding of the MAB.

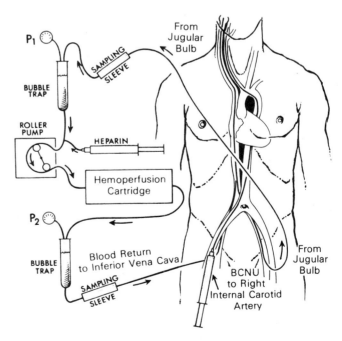

FIG. 1. Diagram of intra-arterial perfusion technique using extracorporeal hemoperfusion. (Doppman JL, Dedrick RL, Shook DR, et al. Glioblastoma: catheter techniques for isolated chemotherapy perfusion. *Radiology* 1986;159:477, with permission).

TABLE 2. *Clinical studies using monoclonal antibodies (MABs) directed against CNS tumors*

Author	Number of patients	MAB directed against	MAB conjugated to	Location of MAB injection	Outcome
Epenetos (77)	1	oncofetal neuroblast antigen	radiolabel	CSF	marked clinical improvement
Coakham (76)	1	epidermal growth factor receptor	radiolabel	intracarotid	tumor decreased in size
Kemshead (78)	2	neuroectoderm	radiolabel	CSF	1 patient improved; 1 patient continued to decline
Behnke (68)	1	melanoma antigen MCI-14	radiolabel	CSF	clinical improvement
Moseley (74)	7	human milk fat globule (HMFG1)	radiolabel	CSF	4 patients, no response; 2 patients, partial response; 1 patient died
Nitta (69)	10	bispecific glioma (NE150) and immune cell (CD3)	-	tumor resection bed	8 patients free from tumor recurrence at 10–18 months; 2 patients died from pneumonia
Lashford (105)	5	tumor type	radiolabel	CSF	4 patients improved; 1 patient deteriorated

Intrathecal Delivery

The intrathecal injection of chemotherapeutic agents has a limited cytotoxic effect on metastatic lesions within the brain parenchyma. Leptomeningeal deposits are spread within the CSF, however, and are often amenable to intraventricular drug infusion. Leptomeningeal spread of tumor can frequently be identified with radiographic imaging (Fig. 2). Lumbar puncture and cytologic evaluation of any cells present is used to confirm CSF spread when the diagnosis is in doubt (21).

Access to the subarachnoid space is obtained via lumbar puncture or through the insertion of a permanent catheter into the lumbar subarachnoid space or ventricular cavity. The Ommaya reservoir (Baxter Heyer Schulte, Baxter Healthcare Corporation, Deerfield, IL), a standard apparatus used for repeated ventricular access, consists of a mushroom-shaped reservoir that is secured to the periosteum immediately beneath the scalp. The reservoir is connected to intraventricular tubing that traverses the brain parenchyma and resides in the ventricular system (Fig. 3). The tip of the tubing has perforations that allow instilled chemotherapeutic agents to enter the CSF circulation. The reservoir can be inserted using local anesthesia. Occasionally, stereotactic guidance is required to place the catheter in a patient with small lateral ventricles. CSF flow is often assessed with a ventriculogram before reservoir use because of the potential for CSF flow abnormalities and unequal distribution of injected agent (70).

Several chemotherapeutic agents have been instilled into the subarachnoid spaces as treatment for leptomeningeal carcinomatosis. Agents with limited ability to enter the brain and spinal cord parenchyma are more appropriate for use in this space than lipid-soluble agents. Specifically, chemotherapeutic agents with good brain parenchymal uptake may be absorbed to the point that CNS toxicity occurs. Also, absorbed agents do not remain in contact with the meningeal deposits as long as nonab-

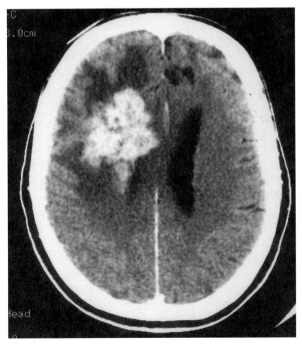

FIG. 2. Contrast-enhanced CT scan demonstrating a malignant primary tumor extending into the ventricular system.

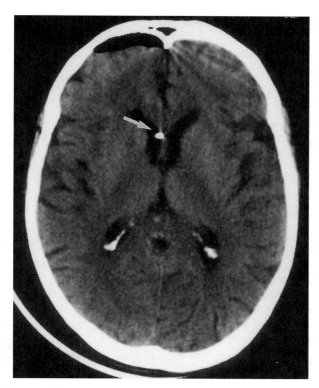

FIG. 3. Midventricular CT scan image of a ventricular catheter placed for the intraventricular administration of chemotherapy.

sorbable agents. Methotrexate is, therefore, a commonly used agent. Other chemotherapy agents undergoing clinical trials or currently in use include ACNU (71), melphalan (72), and thiotepa (73).

Both immunotoxins and radionuclides linked to MABs directed against tumor antigens have also been used for intrathecal injection; see Table 2 (74–78). The MAB studies have shown limited but promising results and are undergoing clinical trials.

Intratumoral and Local Delivery of Therapeutic Agents

The intratumoral delivery of chemotherapeutic, viral, and immunologic agents is intriguing and is undergoing clinical trials. Methods to achieve intratumoral delivery include the intratumoral placement of drug-impregnated biodegradable polymers (79,80), the use of intratumoral catheters for the instillation of cytokines and cells (81), and microinfusion pumps (82,83) for the continuous infusion of chemotherapeutic agents.

Successful, slow release and delivery of chemotherapeutic agents into a tumor bed might increase the effective kill of tumor cells while reducing systemic toxicity. Technical difficulties with regard to both drug and polymer development have limited the practical application of this type of intratumoral drug-impregnated polymer place-

ment. Initial polymers developed for sustained release of agents were not biodegradable and might require removal (84). Biodegradable polyanhydride polymers have been developed and used in a phase 1–2 clinical trial in patients with malignant primary glial tumors (79). The polymer was dissolved with BCNU, spray-dried into microspheres, and pressed into wafers. The wafers were placed in the tumor bed after resection and were shown to release the BCNU safely (79). No systemic toxicity was noted. A phase 3 trial is currently underway. Alternatively, microspheres may be used to release agents such as cytokines (85). These microspheres can be stereotactically placed into the region of interest, thereby potentially avoiding a craniotomy (80).

Intratumoral injection of antineoplastic agents has been performed with chemotherapeutic agents and lymphokine-activated killer (LAK) cells. The chemotherapeutic agents that have been injected directly into tumors include methotrexate, BCNU, and fluorouracil (57). These agents have been used in the treatment of malignant primary glial neoplasms, but their use may be limited due to tissue distribution (82,83).

The treatment of patients with primary malignant glial neoplasms using LAK cells has been evaluated (81, 86–88). This treatment involves removing peripheral blood lymphocytes and culturing them with interleukin-2 (IL-2). These activated cells are then infused into the tumor cavity through direct injection or via an Ommaya reservoir or indwelling catheter after tumor resection. IL-2 itself can also be injected into the tumor bed to activate in situ lymphocytes. Side effects include brain swelling, fever, confusion, and others, especially when high doses of IL-2 are used (81). This mode of therapy has not been extensively tested in metastatic tumors and is still being developed. The major limiting factor has been achieving satisfactory delivery of the LAK cells to the tumor.

Recently, intratumoral gene therapy has been examined for potential efficacy against primary malignant glial tumors (89). One experimental study used the direct tumor inoculation of thymidine kinase-negative attenuated herpes simplex virus-1 to cause tumor regression (90). Other studies have used adenovirus to transduce glioma cells and render them sensitive to antiviral agents (91). Ram and colleagues have also explored the possibility of increasing cytokine production in tumors as a means of immune enhancement (92). Human studies are being performed to assess the role of genetic therapy in glial tumors (93).

CLINICAL RESULTS

Intra-arterial Perfusion

The intra-arterial administration of chemotherapeutic agents for patients with metastatic disease has not been fully explored, and the data supporting this type of admin-

TABLE 3. *Clinical studies using intra-arterial agents for metastatic brain tumors*

Author	No. of patients with brain metastasis	Agent	Outcome
Iwadate (41)	64	ACNU, CCDP±mannitol	Patients who received mannitol had longer median survival times (MST); average MST for both groups, 40 wk
Feun (61)	5	CCDP+bleomycin	4 patients stable or improved
Stewart (96)	13	Mitomycin-C	6 patients responded
Stewart (60)	4	Carboplatin	3 patients stable or responded
Feun (95)	23	CDDP±BCNU or bleomycin	7 patients improved; 3 stabilized; 13 progressed
Feun (59)	12	VP-16	4 patients, no change; 8 patients, no response

ACNU, numustine; BCNU, carmustine; CDDP, cisplatin

istration and the use of these agents are limited (94). A few studies have shown promising results (Table 3). Feun and colleagues demonstrated a 30% objective radiologic improvement, 13% stabilization, and a 57% failure rate in patients with metastatic melanoma treated with intra-arterial cisplatin (95). Iwadate and coworkers randomized 64 patients with brain metastases to receive cisplatin and ACNU after brain radiotherapy (41). Both groups received common carotid injections of the chemotherapy agents. Group A patients also received 50 mL of 20% mannitol injected into the common carotid artery at a rate of 50 mL/min before the chemotherapy. The patients who received the intra-arterial mannitol had greater response rates and longer median times to tumor progression. Group A patients also survived longer and had fewer deaths due to neurologic causes. Stewart and associates treated 13 patients with brain metastases using intra-arterial mitomycin-C (96) and noted a 46% response rate. Feun (61) and Stewart (60) and their colleagues used platinum-based therapies to treat patients with metastatic disease with good results. VP-16 has also been used, with 4 of 12 patients demonstrating no change and the remaining 8 patients demonstrating no response (59).

Intrathecal Delivery

Methotrexate is the most commonly used chemotherapeutic drug, and it is frequently used in conjunction with cytosine arabinoside. The reported methotrexate dosage is 7 mg/m², and the frequency of treatment depends on clinical response (Table 4) (97).

Wasserstrom and colleagues examined 90 patients with carcinomatous meningitis treated with radiation therapy and methotrexate, with or without cytosine arabinoside (98). Median survival time for patients was 5.8 months after diagnosis and 8 months in patients with disease limited to the nervous system. Grossman and colleagues evaluated over 50 patients with carcinomatous meningitis (73). The patients were treated with either methotrexate or thiotepa. Neither therapy resulted in significant patient improvement, although 12 patients remained stable. ACNU has been shown to have a therapeutic effect in over 50% of patients with disseminated primary CNS tumors (71). Methotrexate is used with good success in the treatment of children with acute leukemia (99,100) and has provided symptomatic improvement in patients with carcinomatous meningitis when used alone or with cytosine arabinoside (101).

Numerous complications have been reported following the administration of intrathecal chemotherapy agents. Ascending myelitis and encephalopathy has occurred after methotrexate and cytosine injections (102). Other complications include demyelination of spinal roots and leptomeningeal fibrosis after methotrexate prophylaxis against non-Hodgkin's lymphoma (103), as well as myelopathy following intrathecal injection (104,105).

TABLE 4. *Clinical studies using intrathecal agents for carcinomatous meningitis*

Author	No. patients	Agent	Results
Wasserstrom (98)	90	MTX±Ara-C	Median survival 5.8 mo after diagnosis and 8 mo in patients with disease limited to the CNS
Nakagawa (101)	29	MTX+Ara-C	3 patients died early in treatment; 21 showed improvement, survival 11–485 d
Kochi (71)	11	ACNU	6 patients had a therapeutic response
Grossman (73)	59	MTX or thiotepa	52 patients assessable: 0 improved, 12 remained stable, 39 progressed

MTX, methotrexate; Ara-C, cytosine arabinoside

Intratumoral and Local Delivery of Therapeutic Agents

Little information is available on the results of treatment of metastatic spine lesions using this type of therapy.

PATIENT ASSESSMENT AND CARE CONSIDERATIONS

The assessment and care of patients with CNS metastases can be difficult because of their often-tenuous medical condition due to the underlying malignant processes. The initial assessment includes the establishment of an accurate diagnosis. This is performed through a detailed general and neurologic history, followed by appropriate imaging studies as outlined above. Patients are frequently placed on dexamethasone to reduce the cerebral edema associated with mass lesions of the brain, and anticonvulsants are often instituted. One must evaluate both treatment options and the timing of intervention in light of the patient's medical course to date, the expected outcome based on knowledge of the natural history of the disease, the availability of effective treatments, psychosocial constructs, and family support.

Patients require adequate pain management throughout their treatment course. Care from multiple subspecialists should be closely coordinated with a central physician. Close observations must be maintained for the development of neurologic and systemic complications such as the progression of disease due to treatment failure, development of CNS infection, hydrocephalus, leptomeningeal or spinal metastatic involvement, intracranial hematoma due to bone marrow suppression, seizures, pneumonia, deep venous thrombosis, and others. Early detection of these events and appropriate treatment can improve the patient's quality of life and survival. Ultimately, quality-of-life issues must be considered, as do the patient's desires with regard to continued treatment.

PATIENT INFORMATION

Your physician has selected a localized type of treatment to help kill the cancer cells that have spread to your brain. This treatment may effectively kill the cancer cells or slow their growth while avoiding the side effects associated with more generalized treatments (such as chemotherapy by vein). You should discuss the exact type of treatment, risks, benefits, and surgery required with your physician. The following outline may help give you a broader idea of the different types of treatment.

Intra-arterial Chemotherapy

Chemotherapy involves the administration of drugs that kill or injure cancer cells or make the cells sensitive to other treatments such as radiation therapy. Chemotherapy is usually given by vein. When given this way, it spreads throughout the body and may injure normal cells. This can cause diarrhea, hair loss, and other side effects. Also, the chemotherapy may not be adequately absorbed by the brain cancer cells.

Intra-arterial chemotherapy means that the chemotherapy is given into an artery. This artery is usually the carotid artery, which supplies the brain with blood. By giving the chemotherapy through this artery, more chemotherapy is delivered to the brain and brain tumor, where it is needed most. The risks of this include pain, disturbances in vision, numbness, weakness, and others.

You will be taken to the x-ray department and the radiologists will numb your groin. They will insert a catheter into your femoral artery and position the artery at the base of your brain using x-ray. The chemotherapy will be given through the catheter and the catheter will be removed. You will be observed and should report any pain, numbness, weakness, or visual difficulties to your physician or the nurse. This procedure may need to be repeated in the future to control tumor growth.

Intraventricular Chemotherapy

Your physicians have determined that the most effective way to treat tumor cells that have spread to the center of your brain is to put the chemotherapy into your cerebrospinal fluid (CSF). CSF is the fluid that is in and around your brain. Your physician may have surgeons insert a permanent catheter into the fluid-filled spaces of your brain and connect this to a plastic reservoir under your scalp. Alternatively, your physician may perform lumbar punctures ("spinal taps") when the chemotherapy is to be given. The risks of this type of chemotherapy include headache, numbness, weakness, infection (meningitis), visual disturbances, and others. After the instillation of the chemotherapy, your physician will ask you to stay in a certain position for a time to best direct the drug. Should you have pain, weakness, numbness, fevers, sweats, or chills, experience a seizure, or have other problems, please contact the nurse or your physician.

Intratumoral Delivery

Your physicians have determined that the most effective treatment for your brain tumor is to put chemotherapy or other agents directly into the tumor or onto the tumor bed after the brain tumor is removed. If your physicians have determined that direct injection of chemotherapy or other agents into the tumor will provide you with the greatest chance of tumor control, you will have a frame placed around your head. This frame will be solidly attached to the outer part of your skull using four screws. One or several small holes will be drilled into your skull and catheters will be placed into the tumor using CT guidance. The appropriate agents will be injected into the tumor while you remain awake. Your physicians may choose to leave a catheter in your tumor and connect it to a permanent plastic reservoir that will remain under your scalp.

If your physicians have determined that placing chemotherapeutic or other agents onto the area of brain adjacent to the tumor is most appropriate, you will undergo surgery (craniotomy) and most of the visible tumor will be removed. The chemotherapy or other agents will be placed on the area of brain that was adjacent to the tumor. The bone will be replaced and the skin closed. This operation will be performed with you asleep (general anesthesia).

These treatments are investigational and have specific risks associated with them. These risks include seizures, strokes, blood clot formation, infection, and others. You should discuss the exact type of treatment you are to receive and alternative treatments with your physician.

REFERENCES

1. DeAngelis LM. Management of brain metastases. *Cancer Invest* 1994;12:156.
2. Strugar J, Rothbart D, Harrington W, Criscuolo GR. Vascular permeability factor in brain metastases: correlation with vasogenic brain edema and tumor angiogenesis. *J Neurosurg* 1994;81:560.
3. Tikhtman AJ, Patchell RA. Brain metastases. In: Morantz RA, Walsh JW, eds. *Brain tumors: a comprehensive text*. New York: Marcel Dekker, 1994:553.
4. Delattre JY, Krol G, Thaler HT, Posner JB. Distribution of brain metastases. *Arch Neurol* 1988;45:741.
5. Merchut MP. Brain metastases from undiagnosed systemic neoplasms. *Arch Intern Med* 1989;149:1076.
6. Zimm S, Wampler GL, Stablein D, Hazra T, Young HF. Intracerebral metastases in solid-tumor patients: natural history and results of treatment. *Cancer* 1981;48:384.
7. Walker AE, Robins M, Weinfeld FD. Epidemiology of brain tumors: the national survey of intracranial neoplasms. *Neurology* 1985;35:219.
8. Radhakrishnan K, Bohnen NI, Kurland LT. Epidemiology of brain tumors. In: Morantz RA, Walsh JW, eds. *Brain tumors: a comprehensive text*. New York: Marcel Dekker, 1994:1.
9. Gottesman M. The role of proteases in cancer. *Semin Cancer Biol* 1990;1:97.
10. Batson OV. The function of the vertebral veins and their role in the spread of metastases. *Ann Surg* 1940;112:138.
11. Jahroudi N, Greenberger J. The role of endothelial cells in tumor invasion and metastasis. *J Neurooncol* 1995;23:99.
12. Folkman J. Tumor angiogenesis: a possible control point in tumor growth. *Ann Intern Med* 1975;82:96.
13. Osborn AG. *Introduction to cerebral angiography*. Philadelphia: Harper & Row, 1980:276.
14. Batnitzky S, Eckard DA. The radiology of brain tumors: general considerations and neoplasms of the posterior fossa. In: Morantz RA, Walsh JW, eds. *Brain tumors: a comprehensive text*. New York: Marcel Dekker, 1994:213.
15. Batnitzky S, Eckard DA. The radiology of brain tumors: supratentorial neoplasms. In: Morantz RA, Walsh JW, eds. *Brain tumors: a comprehensive text*. New York: Marcel Dekker, 1994:273.
16. Yuh WTC, Engelken JD, Muhonen MG, Mayr NA, Fisher DJ, Erhardt JC: Experience with high-dose gadolinium MR imaging in the evaluation of brain metastases. *AJNR* 1992;13:335.
17. Azar Kia B. Intracranial neoplasms. In: Sarwar M, Azar Kia B, Batnitzky S, eds. *Basic neuroradiology*. St. Louis: Warren H. Green, 1983: 535.
18. Lilienfeld F, Benda C. Fall von merastischer Karcinose der Neiven und Hirnhaute. *Berl Klin Wochenschr* 1901;38:729.
19. Russell DS, Rubinstein LJ. Secondary tumours of the nervous system. In: *Pathology of tumours of the nervous system*. Baltimore: Williams & Wilkins, 1989:838.
20. Little JR, Hanson MR. Meningeal carcinomatous. In: Wilkins RH, Rengachary SS, eds. *Neurosurgery*. New York: McGraw-Hill, 1985:610.
21. Olson ME, Chernik NL, Posner JB. Infiltration of the leptomeninges by systemic cancer: a clinical and pathologic study. *Arch Neurol* 1974; 30:122.
22. Donelli MG, Zucchetti M, D'Incalci M. Do anticancer agents reach the tumor target in the human brain? *Cancer Chemother Pharmacol* 1992;30:251.
23. Dyck P. Lumbar reservoir for intrathecal chemotherapy. *Cancer* 1985; 55:2771.
24. Sundaresan N, Suite NDA. Optimal use of the Ommaya reservoir in clinical oncology. *Oncology* 1989;3:15.
25. Cairncross JG, Posner JB. The management of brain metastases. In: Walker MD, ed. *Oncology of the nervous system*. Boston: Martinus Nijhoff, 1983:341.
26. Greig NH. Chemotherapy of brain metastases: current status. *Cancer Treat Rev* 1984;11:157.
27. Greig NH, Soncrant TT, Shetty HU, Momma S, Smith QR, Rapoport SI. Brain uptake and anticancer activities of vincristine and vinblastine are restricted by their low cerebrovascular permeability and binding to plasma constituents in rat. *Cancer Chemother Pharmacol* 1990; 26:263.
28. Siegers HP. Chemotherapy for brain metastases: recent developments and clinical considerations. *Cancer Treat Rev* 1990;17:63.
29. Fenstermacher JD, Cowles AL. Theoretic limitations of intracarotid infusions in brain tumor chemotherapy. *Cancer Treat Rep* 1977;61:519.
30. Loew F, Papavero L. The intraarterial route of drug delivery in the chemotherapy of malignant brain tumors. *Adv Tech Stand Neurosurg* 1988;16:51.
31. Scheld WM. Drug delivery to the central nervous system: general principles and relevance to therapy for infections of the central nervous system. *Rev Infect Dis* 1989;11:S1669.
32. Friden PM. Receptor-mediated transport of therapeutics across the blood-brain barrier. *Neurosurgery* 1994;35:294.
33. Salcman M, Broadwell RD. The blood-brain barrier. In: Salcman M, ed. *Neurobiology of brain tumors*. Baltimore: Williams & Wilkins, 1991, Chapter 13.
34. Young HF, Merchant RE, Apuzzo MLJ. Immunocompetence of patients with malignant glioma. In: Salcman M, ed. *Neurobiology of brain tumors*. Baltimore: Williams & Wilkins, 1991, Chapter 12.
35. Brightman MW, Reese TS. Junctions between intimately apposed cell membranes in the vertebrate brain. *J Cell Biol* 1969;40:648.
36. Sage MR. Blood-brain barrier: phenomenon of increasing importance to the imaging clinician. *AJR* 1982;138:887.
37. Marshall LF. Treatment of brain swelling and brain edema in man. *Adv Neurol* 1980;28:459.
38. Broman T, Olsson O. Experimental study of contrast media for cerebral angiography with reference to possible injurious effects of the cerebral blood vessels. *Acta Radiol* 1949;31:321.
39. Neuwelt EA, Dahlborg SA. Chemotherapy administered in conjunction with osmotic blood-brain barrier modification in patients with brain metastases. *J Neurooncol* 1987;4:195.
40. Blasberg RG, Groothuis DR. Chemotherapy of brain tumors: physiological and pharmacokinetic considerations. *Semin Oncol* 1986;13(1): 70.
41. Iwadate Y, Namba H, Saegusa T, Sueyoshi K. Intra-arterial mannitol infusion in the chemotherapy for malignant brain tumors. *J Neurooncol* 1993;15:185.
42. Jain RK. Barriers to drug delivery in solid tumors. *Sci Am* 1994;271: 58.
43. Steen RG, Kromhout-Schiro S, Graham MM. Relationship of perfusion to edema in the 9L gliosarcoma. *J Neurooncol* 1993;16:81.
44. Welch WC, Oestreich HM, del Rowe J, Hirshfeld A, Kao MS,

Michelsen WJ. Radiosurgery: a non-invasive method to treat lesions within the brain. *Einstein Quart J Biol Med* 1993;11:2.

45. Stewart DJ, Grahovac Z, Russell NA, et al. Phase I study of intra-arotid PCNU. *J Neurooncol* 1987;5:245.

46. Poisson M, Chiras J, Fauchon F, Debussche C, Delattre JY. Treatment of malignant recurrent glioma by intra-arterial, infra-ophthalmic infusion of HECNU 1-(2-chloroethyl)-1-nitroso-3-(2-hydroxyethyl) urea-a phase II study. *J Neurooncol* 1990;8:255.

47. Johnson DW, Parkinson D, Wolpert SM, et al. Intra-carotid chemotherapy with 1,3-bis(2-chloroethyl)-1-nitrosourea (BCNU) in 5% dextrose in water in the treatment of malignant glioma. *Neurosurgery* 1987;20:577.

48. Kleinschmidt-DeMasters BK, Geier JM. Pathology of high-dose intraarterial BCNU. *Surg Neurol* 1989;31:435.

49. Kapp JP, Vance RB. Supraophthalmic carotid infusion for recurrent glioma: rationale, technique, and preliminary results for cisplatin and BCNU. *J Neurooncol* 1985;3:5.

50. Stewart DJ, Grahovac Z, Hugenholtz H, Russell N, Richard M, Benoit B. Combined intra-arterial and systemic chemotherapy for intracerebral tumors. *Neurosurgery* 1987;21:207.

51. Mahaley MS Jr, Whaley RA, Blue M, Bertsch L. Central neurotoxicity following intracarotid BCNU chemotherapy for malignant gliomas. *J Neurooncol* 1986;3(4):297.

52. Stewart DJ. Novel modes of chemotherapy administration. *Prog Exp Tumor Res* 1984;28:32.

53. Mani RL, Eisenberg RL, McDonald EJ, et al. Complications of catheter cerebral angiography: analysis of 5000 procedures. I. Criteria and incidence. *AJR* 1978;131:861.

54. Osborn AG. *Introduction to cerebral angiography.* Philadelphia: Harper & Row, 1980:1.

55. Saris SC, Blasberg RG, Carson RE, et al. Intravascular streaming during carotid artery infusions. *J Neurosurg* 1991;74:763.

56. Eckman WW, Patlak CS, Fenstermacher JD. A critical evaluation of the principles governing the advantage of intra-arterial infusions. *J Pharmacokinet Biopharm* 1974;2:257.

57. Gumerlock MK, Neuwelt EA. Chemotherapy of brain tumors: innovative approaches. In: Morantz RA, Walsh JW, eds. *Brain tumors: a comprehensive text.* New York: Marcel Dekker, 1994:763.

58. Welch WC, Kornblith PL. Chemotherapy of brain tumors: fundamental principles. In: Morantz RA, Walsh JW, eds. *Brain tumors: a comprehensive text.* New York: Marcel Dekker, 1994:717.

59. Feun LG, Lee YY, Yung WK, Savaraj N, Wallace S. Intra-carotid VP-16 in malignant brain tumors. *J Neurooncol* 1987;4:397.

60. Stewart DJ, Belanger JMEG, Grahovac Z, et al. Phase I study of intracarotid administration of carboplatin. *Neurosurgery* 1992;30:512.

61. Feun LG, Savaraj N, Lee YY, et al. A pilot clinical and pharmacokinetic study of intracarotid cisplatin and bleomycin. *Sel Cancer Ther* 1991;7:29.

62. Greenberg HS, Ensminger W, Layton P, et al. A phase I-II evaluation of intra-arterial diaziquone (AZQ) for malignant tumors of the central nervous system [abstract]. *Proc Annu Meet Am Soc Clin Oncol* 1984;3:256.

63. Dedrick RL, Oldfield EH, Collins JM. Arterial drug infusion with extracorporeal removal. I. Theoretic basis with particular reference to the brain. *Cancer Treat Rep* 1984;68:373.

64. Oldfield EH, Dedrick RL, Chatterji DC, et al. Reduced systemic drug exposure by combining intracarotid chemotherapy with hemoperfusion of jugular drainage. *Surg Forum* 1983;34:535.

65. Doppman JL, Dedrick RL, Shook DR, et al. Glioblastoma: catheter techniques for isolated chemotherapy perfusion. *Radiology* 1986;159:477.

66. Uadia P, Blair AH, Ghose T, Ferrone S. Uptake of methotrexate linked to polyclonal and monoclonal anti-melanoma antibodies by a human melanoma cell line. *J Natl Cancer Inst* 1985;74:29.

67. Gilliland DG, Steplewski Z, Collier RJ, Mitchell KF, Chang TH, Koprowski H. Antibody-directed cytotoxic agents: use of monoclonal antibody to direct the action of toxin A chains to colorectal carcinoma cells. *Proc Natl Acad Sci USA* 1980;77:4539.

68. Behnke J, Coakham HB, Mach JP, Carrel S, de Tribolet N. Monoclonal antibodies in the diagnosis and therapy of brain tumors. In: Kornblith PL, Walker MD, eds. *Advances in neuro-oncology.* Mt. Kisco, NY: Futura Publishing Co, 1988:255.

69. Nitta T, Sato K, Yagita H, Okumura K, Ishii S. Preliminary trial of specific targeting therapy against malignant glioma. *Lancet* 1990;335:368.

70. Grossman SA, Trump DL, Chen DCP, Thompson G, Camargo EE. Cerebrospinal fluid flow abnormalities in patients with neoplastic meningitis: an evaluation using Indium-DTPA ventriculography. *Am J Med* 1982;73:641.

71. Kochi M, Kuratsu J, Mihara Y, et al. Ventriculolumbar perfusion of 3-[(4-amino-2-methyl-5-pyrimidinyl)methyl]-1-(2-chloroethyl)-1-nitrosourea hydrochloride. *Neurosurgery* 1993;33:817.

72. Friedman HS, Archer G, Bigner DD. Re: Toxicity of intrathecal melphalan [letter; comment]. *J Natl Cancer Inst* 1994;86(11):870.

73. Grossman SA, Finkelstein DM, Ruckdeschel JC, Trump DL, Moynihan T, Ettinger DS. Randomized prospective comparison of intraventricular methotrexate and thiotepa in patients with previously untreated neoplastic meningitis. Eastern Cooperative Oncology Group. *J Clin Oncol* 1993;11:561.

74. Moseley RP, Benjamin JC, Ashpole RD. Carcinomatous meningitis: antibody-guided therapy with I-131 HMFG1. *J Neurol Neurosurg Psychiatry* 1991;54:260.

75. Holladay FP, Griffitt WE, Wood GW. Immunology and immunotherapy of brain tumors. In: Morantz RA, Walsh JW, eds. *Brain tumors: a comprehensive text.* New York: Marcel Dekker, 1994:779.

76. Coakham HB, Richardson RB, Bourne S, Davies AG, Kemshead JT. Antibody-guided radiolocalisation and therapy of neoplastic meningitis. *Br J Cancer* 1985;52:655.

77. Epenetos AA, Courtenay-Luck N, Pickering D, Hooker G, et al. Antibody-guided irradiation of brain glioma by arterial infusion of radioactive monoclonal antibody against epidermal growth factor receptor and blood group A antigen. *Br Med J (Clin Res Ed)* 1985;290 (6480):1463.

78. Kemshead JT, Jones DH, Lashford L, et al. [131]I coupled to monoclonal antibodies as therapeutic agents for neuroectodermally derived tumors. Fact or fiction. *Cancer Drug Deliv* 1986;3(1):25.

79. Brem H, Mahaley MS Jr, Vick NA, et al. Interstitial chemotherapy with drug polymer implants for treatment of recurrent gliomas. *J Neurosurg* 1991;74:441.

80. Menei P, Benoit JP, Boisdron-Celle M, Fournier D, Mercier P, Guy G. Drug targeting into the central nervous system by stereotactic implantation of biodegradable microspheres. *Neurosurgery* 1994;34:1058.

81. Blancher A, Roubinet F, Grancher AS, et al. Local immunotherapy of recurrent glioblastoma multiforme by intracerebral perfusion of interleukin-2 and LAK cells. *Eur Cytokine Netw* 1993;4:331.

82. Kroin JS, Penn RD. Intracerebral chemotherapy: chronic microinfusion of cisplatin. *Neurosurgery* 1982;10:349.

83. Penn RD, Kroin JS, Harris JE, Chiu KM, Braun DP. Chronic intratumoral chemotherapy of a rat tumor with cisplatin and fluorouracil. *Appl Neurophysiol* 1983;46:240.

84. Langer R, Folkman J. Polymers for sustained release of proteins and other macromolecules. *Nature* 1976;263:797.

85. Yamasaki T, Kikuchi H, Moritake K, et al. A morphological and ultrastructural investigation of normal mouse brain tissue after intra-cerebral injection of tumor necrosis factor. *J Neurosurg* 1992;65:659.

86. Jacobs SK, Wilson DJ, Kornblith PL, Grimm EA. Interleukin-2 or autologous lymphokine-activated killer cell treatment of malignant glioma: Phase I trial. *Cancer Res* 1986;46:2101.

87. Jacobs SK, Wilson DJ, Melin G, et al. Interleukin-2 and lymphokine activated killer (LAK) cells in the treatment of malignant glioma: clinical and experimental studies. *Neurol Res* 1986;8:81.

88. Merchant RE, Merchant LH, Cook SHS, McVicar DW, Young HF. Intralesional infusion of lymphokine-activated killer (LAK) cells and recombinant interleukin-2 (rIL-2) for the treatment of patients with malignant brain tumor. *Neurosurgery* 1988;23:725.

89. Kornblith PL, Welch WC, Bradley MK. The future of therapy for glioblastoma. *Surg Neurol* 1993;39:538.

90. Martuza RL, Malik A, Markert JM, Ruffner KL, Coen DM. Experimental therapy of human glioma by means of a genetically engineered virus mutant. *Science* 1991;252:854.

91. Chen SH, Shine HD, Goodman JC, Grossman RG, Woo SLC. Gene therapy for brain tumors: regression of experimental gliomas by adenovirus-mediated gene transfer in vivo. *Proc Natl Acad Sci USA* 1994;91:3054.

92. Ram Z, Walbridge S, Heiss JD, Culver KW, Blaese RM, Oldfield EH. In vivo transfer of the human interleukin-2 gene: negative tumoricidal results in experimental brain tumors. *J Neurosurg* 1994;80:535.

93. Oldfield EH, Culver KW, Ram Z, Blaese RM. A clinical protocol: gene therapy for the treatment of brain tumors using intratumoral

transduction with the thymidine kinase gene and intravenous ganciclovir. *Hum Gene Ther* 1993;4:39.

94. Stewart DJ. Pros and cons of intra-arterial chemotherapy. *Oncology* 1989;3:20.

95. Feun LG, Lee YY, Plager C, et al. Intracarotid cisplatin-based chemotherapy in patients with malignant melanoma and central nervous system (CNS) metastases. *Am J Clin Oncol* 1990;13:448.

96. Stewart DJ, Grahovac Z, Hugenholtz H, et al. Intra-arterial mitomycin-C for recurrent brain metastases. *Am J Clin Oncol* 1987;10(5):432.

97. Cairncross JG. Carcinomatous meningitis. In: Wittes RE, ed. Part V. Regional therapy for metastatic disease. *Manual of oncologic therapeutics.* Philadelphia: JB Lippincott, 1989:419.

98. Wasserstrom WR, Glass JP, Posner JB. Diagnosis and treatment of leptomeningeal metastases from solid tumors. *Cancer* 1982;49:759.

99. Tubergen DG, Gilchrist GS, O'Brien RT, et al. Improved outcome with delayed intensification for children with acute lymphoblastic leukemia and intermediate presenting features: a Children's Cancer Group phase III trial. *J Clin Oncol* 1993;11:527.

100. Choudhry VP, Krishnamurthy L, Rath GK, Arya LS, Pati H, Saraya AK. Efficacy of intrathecal methotrexate with and without cranial radiotherapy in preventing central nervous system relapses in acute lymphocytic leukemia. *Indian Pediatr* 1992;29:843.

101. Nakagawa H, Murasawa A, Kubo S, et al. Diagnosis and treatment of patients with meningeal carcinomatosis. *J Neurooncol* 1992;13:81.

102. Ozon A, Topaloglu H, Cila A, Gunay M, Cetin M. Acute ascending myelitis and encephalopathy after intrathecal cytosine arabinoside and methotrexate in an adolescent boy with acute lymphoblastic leukemia. *Brain Dev* 1994;16:246.

103. Nowacki P, Dolinska D, Honczarenko K, Potemkowski A. Impairment of vertebral canal nervous structures after intrathecal prophylaxis in non-Hodgkin's lymphomas. *Neuropatol Pol* 1992;30:325.

104. McLean DR, Clink HM, Ernst P, et al. Myelopathy after intrathecal chemotherapy. A case report with unique magnetic resonance imaging changes. *Cancer* 1994;73:3037.

105. Lashford LS, Davies AG, Richardson RB, et al. A pilot study of ^{131}I monoclonal antibodies in the therapy of leptomeningeal tumors. *Cancer* 1988;61:857.

CHAPTER 16

Abdominopelvic Imaging in Cancer Patients

Michael P. Federle

Such as for their bellies' sake
Creep and intrude, and climb into the fold.

—*John Milton,* Lycidas, 1637

BACKGROUND

As a result of the rapid advances in radiologic techniques over the past two decades, imaging studies play an increasingly important role in the evaluation of cancer patients. Accurate assessment of the local and distant extension of cancer is crucial if the innovative medical and surgical techniques discussed in this book are to have optimal efficacy. The radiologist can play an important role in the staging and classification of tumors to aid the clinicians in planning therapy, to assist in the evaluation of the results of therapy, to give an indication of prognosis, and to facilitate the exchange of information among treatment centers (1).

The most widely used system for staging of cancer is the TNM classification coordinated by the International Union Against Cancer (UICC). The most recently published revision (1987) of the TNM classification incorporates important changes based on imaging methods that were unavailable when prior editions were formulated (2). The 1987 revision also eliminated differences between the UICC version and that of the American Joint Committee on Cancer. One important revision is the application of endosonography for staging of esophageal, gastric, and rectal carcinomas. Advances in computed tomography (CT) and magnetic resonance imaging (MRI) have not been formally incorporated into all staging systems in recognition of the lack of universal availability and in an attempt to establish a common ground for comparisons among treatment centers internationally. Nevertheless, where available, CT and MRI can provide valuable assistance in the clinical staging of cancer.

The relative accuracy of various imaging techniques in cancer staging is surprisingly difficult to assess. Prospective, controlled trials with an adequate gold standard of proof and sufficient numbers of cases to achieve significant results have been reported rarely. The National Institutes of Health has addressed this deficiency by sponsoring multi-institutional trials targeted at individual cancer types, called the Radiological Diagnostic Oncology Group (RDOG) trials. The results of the RDOG trials are now being published in various scientific journals, but even these have not met with universal acclaim or acceptance.

Studies that compare imaging modalities are also difficult to interpret due to the rapid evolution of imaging technology. Frequently, specific CT and MRI techniques have been rendered obsolete by the time an investigation has been completed and reported. Recent advances in MRI imaging that may have profound effects on diagnosis have been realized as a result of improved magnets, computer software, imaging sequences, and the availability of intravascular and oral contrast media. Important recent innovations in CT scanning include the routine use of rapid intravascular administration of contrast material by a mechanical injector during scanning, which has been shown to provide more accurate results than the widely practiced drip infusion technique (2–4). Helical (spiral) CT scanners permit large anatomic areas such as the chest or abdomen to be scanned during the optimal phase of vascular and parenchymal contrast enhancement.

Despite the ongoing evolution in imaging technology, consensus regarding the general principles of good CT and MRI imaging of the abdomen and pelvis has been reached. These include:

Imaging sequences or the use of oral and vascular contrast media to distinguish bowel and blood vessels, respectively, from pathologic processes.

M. P. Federle: Department of Radiology, University of Pittsburgh Medical Center, Pittsburgh, Pennsylvania 15213-2582.

Techniques to minimize or eliminate artifacts from physiologic motion or other sources.

Use of rapid intravascular infusion of contrast media during dynamic CT or MRI scanning to optimize tumor detection and differentiation, particularly for hepatic neoplasms.

IMAGING MODALITIES

Radiography

The role of plain radiographs in cancer evaluation is limited mainly to the chest and skeleton, where the inherently high contrast between lung or cortical bone and malignant processes may render them apparent. Barium studies of the gastrointestinal (GI) tract retain an important role even in the age of endoscopy, especially in portions of the gut that may be inaccessible due to physiologic or pathologic factors (eg, redundancy, stenosis). Excretory or retrograde pyelography maintains similar advantages in evaluating the urinary system and uroepithelial neoplasms, although parenchymal tumors are much better demonstrated by cross-sectional imaging.

Ultrasonography

Ultrasonography is versatile and plays an important screening and ancillary role for a variety of abdominal malignancies and may have a primary role in the evaluation of pelvic tumors, as discussed below. Endoscopic ultrasound combines endoscopy for visual inspection and sonography for evaluating lesions arising in or near the GI tract. It accurately stages esophageal and rectal tumors, demonstrating the depth of wall invasion, and has excellent spatial resolution in defining masses such as pancreatic tumors that lie close to the ultrasound transducer placed into the stomach or duodenum.

Radionuclide Scintigraphy

Radionuclide scintigraphy has a well-established but evolving role in oncologic imaging. Radionuclide imaging is limited by relatively poor spatial resolution but provides physiologic and functional information that can be valuable in specific settings. Bone scintigraphy and gallium scanning are in common use, and radiolabeled octreotide scanning is emerging as an important adjunct. Specific applications, such as monoclonal antibody imaging and positron emission tomography (PET), are discussed below.

The use of bone scintigraphy in the evaluation of patients with suspected osseous metastatic disease dates back to the 1960s. The current radiopharmaceuticals, Tc-99m diphosphonates, localize in bone in proportion to the amount of blood flow and osteoblastic activity. The most common oncologic use of bone scintigraphy is evaluation of patients with carcinomas of the breast or prostate, although it is useful in selective evaluation of other tumors that metastasize to bone, including lung cancer and non-Hodgkin's lymphoma. Even in the evaluation of patients with breast or prostate cancer, bone scanning should be used selectively. Patients with prostate carcinoma, for instance, who have clinical evidence of limited disease, no skeletal symptoms, and a serum prostate-specific antigen (PSA) level of <10 μg/L rarely have bone metastases and probably do not require radionuclide evaluation. Breast cancer patients with clinical stage III or IV disease warrant bone scintigraphy, especially those who are symptomatic but whose plain radiographs are normal or equivocal. The routine use of bone scintigraphy in following patients with malignancies is no longer advisable and should be limited primarily to patients who are symptomatic or have rising tumor markers (eg, PSA), and in whom therapy might be altered by the results of the test.

Gallium-67 citrate was discovered to localize in soft-tissue tumors in the 1960s. It is excreted by the urinary and GI tracts, interfering somewhat with the ability to distinguish tumors from normal abdominal contents within the first 24 hours after injection. Bowel cleansing regimens and repeated imaging can aid in tumor detection. Gallium can also have altered biodistribution in oncologic patients. Examples include increased salivary gland activity following radiation or chemotherapy, persistent renal activity in patients with compromised renal or hepatic function, and increased lung activity in patients with pneumonitis due to radiation, chemotherapy, or infections.

The major oncologic uses of gallium scanning are in evaluating patients with lymphoma or melanoma. The primary modality in staging lymphoma is usually CT; gallium scanning is valuable in detecting recurrent or residual disease. The accuracy of CT staging of lymphoma generally exceeds that of gallium scanning, although scintigraphy has been found to have variable results relating to tumor subtypes, anatomic sites, and tumor size. The sensitivity for detection and accurate staging of Hodgkin's disease (80%–90%) exceeds that for non-Hodgkin's lymphoma (60%–80%) (5). The use of single photon emission computed tomography (SPECT) can improve accuracy as well as anatomic localization when compared with planar imaging (6). Gallium scanning is especially valuable in evaluating patients with CT evidence of residual masses following treatment, with persistently increased gallium activity having a high predictive value for viable tumor (7–9).

Gallium-67 citrate scanning may also be useful in evaluating patients with malignant melanoma. Sensitivity averages about 75% (range 50%–80%) and specificity is very high (about 90%–95%) (10). CT and MRI have assumed the primary role of the staging and evaluation of therapeutic results, as discussed on the next page.

An analog of somatostatin, indium-111 labeled octreotide, has been approved recently for clinical use in the evaluation of patients with various neuroendocrine tumors. A recent study reported excellent results of more than 1,000 patients with various hormonally active tumors, including pituitary, islet cell, carcinoid, pheochromocytoma, and small cell lung cancer (11). The sensitivity of tumor detection for these tumor types varied from 70% to 100%. Octreotide scanning may also have a role in the evaluation of other tumors, including lymphoma and meningioma, but this has not yet been established.

Computed Tomography

For the comprehensive evaluation of multiple organ systems in the cancer patient, CT remains the pre-eminent imaging test. Modern scanners with powerful computer platforms can image the thorax, abdomen, and pelvis within 10 minutes, and rapid scan times essentially eliminate artifacts due to respiratory or other physiologic motion. These are practical but important considerations in cancer patients, who are often relatively debilitated and in pain. The single set of axial sections can be manipulated later to demonstrate optimally bone, soft tissue, or lung detail (Fig. 1) and can be reconstructed by computer programs into sagittal, coronal, or even three-dimensional images (indirect or simulated multiplanar imaging). None of these manipulations requires extra scanning time or radiation exposure for the patient. Proper use of oral and intravenous contrast material obviates most problems in distinguishing bowel or blood vessels from masses.

Helical (spiral) CT is a recent modification of the scanner hardware, allowing uninterrupted acquisition of scan data by continuously rotating the x-ray table and detectors as the table carrying the patient is moved through the CT gantry. The entire thorax or liver can now be scanned in a single or several breath-holds, eliminating misregistration errors from breathing and allowing optimal timing in the delivery of vascular contrast media. There are no

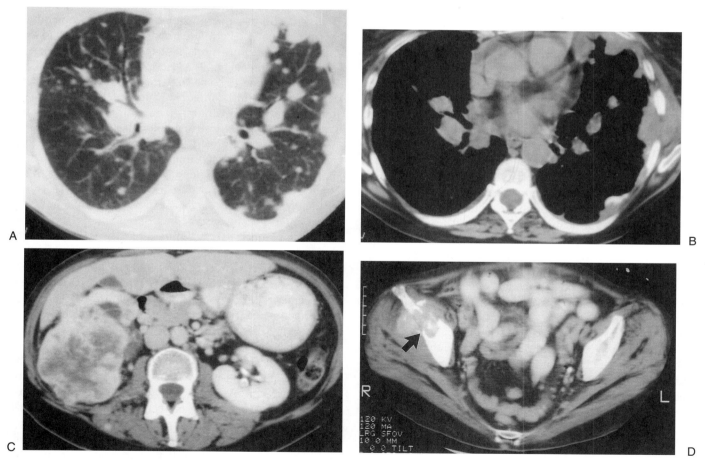

FIG. 1. Renal cell carcinoma with widespread metastases. CT can demonstrate the full extent of metastases on a series of axial sections through the chest, abdomen, and pelvis. **(A)** Chest section photographed at "lung windows" shows multiple pulmonary lesions. **(B)** The same section photographed on "soft-tissue windows" demonstrates nodal, pleural, and chest wall metastases. **(C)** An abdominal section shows the primary tumor and regional lymphadenopathy. **(D)** A pelvic section shows a lytic lesion in the right iliac wing (*arrow*).

significant drawbacks to the technique, and most U.S. hospitals will have upgraded to this equipment within a few years.

Magnetic Resonance Imaging

MRI is a powerful and rapidly evolving imaging tool. MRI has advantages over CT in tissue-contrast resolution, direct high-resolution multiplanar imaging, and lack of ionizing radiation. The excellent tissue-contrast resolution makes MRI the primary modality for imaging the brain, spine, and musculoskeletal system and makes it competitive with CT in evaluation of the liver (2,3, 12–16). Its multiplanar capability and contrast resolution also make MRI valuable in evaluating primary pelvic masses. Problems with MRI include its considerable cost and lack of general availability. MRI is less useful than CT in evaluating thoracic lymphadenopathy and pulmonary parenchymal metastases due to inferior spatial resolution and the inherently low MRI signal intensity of lung parenchyma. MRI imaging times are decreasing in general, but a comprehensive examination of the abdomen and pelvis is still beyond practical consideration. Even focused examinations of the liver or pelvis often require sedation of very young or elderly patients, and some patients are intolerant of the claustrophobic sensation of confinement within the magnet bore. The lack of an acceptable contrast agent for marking bowel has proved to be a persistent limitation in MRI evaluation of the abdomen and pelvis. In studies from multiple institutions, CT consistently has been found superior to MRI in recognition and characterization of extrahepatic abdominal, thoracic, and pelvic disease in the comprehensive evaluation of cancer patients (2,16).

The excellent tissue-contrast resolution of MRI makes it very sensitive in distinguishing normal from diseased tissue. Unfortunately, both tumors and inflammatory processes generally cause an increase in tissue water, appearing as dark signal in T1-weighted MRI images and bright signal on T2-predominant sequences. Most organs and muscle have low signal intensity, and invasion by tumor is usually apparent. MRI is inherently well suited for evaluating pelvic masses, where tumors are well delineated from low-signal pelvic organs and high-signal surrounding fat (16). Distinguishing recurrent or residual tumor from fibrosis or granulation tissue in the MRI evaluation of posttherapy patients has proved difficult.

IMAGING OF SPECIFIC ORGAN SYSTEMS

Gastrointestinal

For colorectal cancer, the TNM classification has never been as widely used as various modifications of the Dukes system, although criteria such as depth of invasion and local and distant extension still are applied. CT has relatively low sensitivity for nodal metastases (22%–73%) and local tumor invasion (50%–75%) (17–21), although staging accuracy increases with more advanced tumor stages. MRI shares many of the same shortcomings, although multiplanar imaging and the availability of endorectal MRI coils have shown promise of substantial improvements over prior staging, with a reported accuracy of about 75% (22–24). MRI with endorectal coils has achieved detection of perirectal spread of tumor with sensitivities of 67% to 96% and regional lymphadenopathy of 50% to 57%. The ability to show advanced disease, particularly by coronal MRI depiction of involvement of the levator ani muscles, may have an important impact on sphincter preservation surgery or full-dose preoperative radiation therapy.

Endoscopic ultrasonography has had a significant impact on the clinical staging of cancer of the luminal GI tract. Earlier staging schemes emphasized factors well defined by barium studies, such as tumor size, circumferential involvement, and presence of obstruction. More recently, however, depth of tumor infiltration has been found to be a more pertinent criterion. Endoscopic ultrasonography has been found to be very accurate in assessing the "T" stage of tumors of the esophagus, stomach, and colorectum (Fig. 2) (17,25,26). Problems may be encountered due to prior surgery, biopsy, radiation therapy, or ongoing inflammation. Failure of the endoscope to traverse a stenosing tumor is a limitation, but this may be overcome by newer instruments with smaller diameters, sometimes requiring sacrifice of the optical portion of the endoscope. Obstructing impassable tumors are usually deeply invasive, and CT and MRI have been found to be valuable in staging such tumors. Although CT has relatively poor sensitivity for local extension or nodal involvement in most esophageal and intestinal tumors, it remains useful in preoperative recognition of liver metastases and large nonresectable nodal masses (17,26–28). It also provides an objective record of the tumor before systemic therapy, if indicated. Finally, it is often necessary for the percutaneous biopsy of masses to establish a diagnosis.

Detection of recurrent colorectal cancer remains a controversial issue. Both CT and MRI can detect recurrent disease in asymptomatic patients while tumor markers such as CEA are still normal. This is especially valuable in patients who have had abdominoperineal resection with colostomy, in whom endoscopic evaluation is limited. Nevertheless, recurrent tumor is very difficult to distinguish from granulation tissue, hemorrhage, or fibrosis by CT or MRI. Serial CT studies following a baseline study 2 to 4 months after surgery have been found useful in detecting recurrent disease, and resection of limited recurrences can prolong survival in selected cases (18).

The current inability of morphologic imaging studies such as CT or MRI to distinguish recurrent rectal tumor

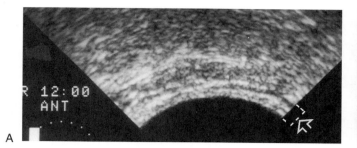

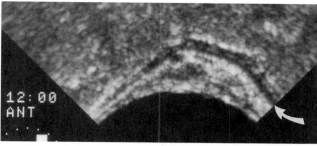

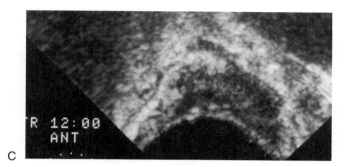

FIG. 2. Rectal carcinoma. Endoscopic ultrasonography. **(A)** With the transducer applied to the right anterolateral wall, the normal five-layered structure of the rectal wall is evident as alternating bright and dark lines (*arrows+brackets*). These represent mucosa, muscularis mucosa, submucosa, muscularis propria, and serosa. **(B)** A mass along the left anterior rectal wall displaces the dark line representing the muscularis propria (*arrow*). **(C)** Closer to the anus, the mass invades through the muscularis propria into the perirectal fat, making this a T4 lesion.

from various benign inflammatory conditions has been addressed in several ways. We use CT-guided biopsies of persistent or recurrent perirectal masses. Imaging with radiolabeled monoclonal antibodies (MoAbs) may provide tissue-specific information. MoAbs can be developed to bind selectively to oncofetal proteins and tumor-associated antigens (eg, CEA) and theoretically should function like Erlich's "magic bullets" to detect primary and metastatic colorectal cancer (29–31). Practical problems have delayed widespread application of this technique, however, such as the formation of antibodies against the mouse-derived MoAbs, which results in decreased availability of target MoAbs to image and an increased risk of allergic reactions. SPECT enhances the detection of tumor uptake. The inability to recognize anatomic landmarks on SPECT MoAb studies has been approached in an innovative fashion by "fusing" (matching and aligning data from various modalities) the functional information provided by SPECT MoAb with the anatomic detail provided by CT or MRI (Fig. 3) (31). Radiolabeled MoAbs have also been used as part of "radioimmunoguided surgery," in which a hand-held gamma detecting probe is used. This may prove useful in identifying hepatic and nonregional lymph node metastases that may escape routine preoperative diagnosis and would not have been excised as part of the usual surgical resection.

PET also offers physiologic or functional analysis that may prove useful in distinguishing recurrent rectal carcinoma from inflammation or fibrosis. PET radiopharmaceuticals allow accurate localization and measurement of regional glucose and oxygen uptake as indicators of viable tumor metabolism (Fig. 4). Fusion of MRI, CT, and PET information has been described for planning

narrow-beam radiation therapy in primary brain tumors (32). The superimposition of metabolic and anatomic measurements afforded by the various modalities has defined better the viable tumor target.

If standard intravenous contrast-enhanced CT demonstrates potentially resectable hepatic metastases from colorectal carcinoma, further evaluation is necessary before surgery. The most sensitive imaging test available is CT arterial portography, in which rapid CT sections of the liver are performed during the injection of contrast material through a catheter placed into the superior mesenteric or splenic artery (33–35). CT portography detects about 90% of all colorectal hepatic metastases, generally missing only lesions less than a few millimeters in diameter. Only intraoperative ultrasonography has comparable accuracy. Although it is very sensitive, CT portography is technically challenging to perform and interpret, and various flow artifacts and benign lesions may simulate metastases.

Much effort is currently directed toward the development of liver-specific MRI contrast agents. Agents have been designed to target hepatocytes or Kupffer cells with paramagnetic agents that cause normal liver to either enhance or become very dark, while nonhepatic tissues (eg, metastases) become more conspicuous (36–38). These selectively enhanced MRI scans will probably replace invasive studies such as CT portography for the preoperative evaluation of potentially resectable liver tumors.

Pancreas

Evaluation of patients with suspected pancreatic carcinoma has been greatly simplified by CT scanning. Fewer than 15% of patients are found to have resectable tumors at the time of initial presentation, and even patients whose

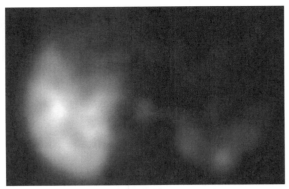

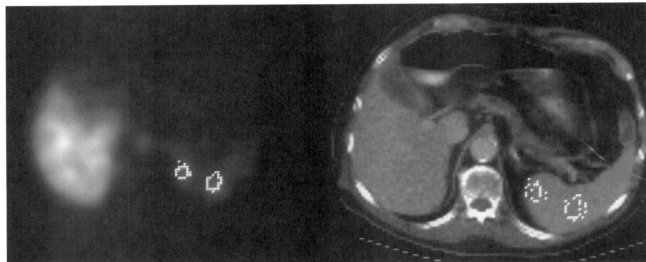

FIG. 3. Colorectal carcinoma, "fusion" image. This 57-year-old man had a known metastatic lesion in the spleen from colon carcinoma. Radioimmunodetection was performed to evaluate suspected progression while on therapy. **(A)** Seventy-two hours after the intravenous administration of 5 mCi of indium-111 labeled IVPZCE025, a CEA-directed murine monoclonal antibody (Hybritech, Inc., San Diego, CA), single photon emission computed tomography (SPECT) of the upper abdomen was obtained. This shows two foci of uptake in the spleen. **(B)** Image fusion of the SPECT and CT was performed using *qsh* software on a SUN computer work station (SUN Microsystems, Sunnyvale, CA). Regions of interest were generated on the SPECT abnormalities and then warped onto the corresponding CT slice. The more medial focus of uptake on the SPECT corresponds to the known lesion on CT, but the more lateral focus of uptake on SPECT corresponds to a site of tumor in the spleen that was not previously identified on CT. (Courtesy of Elissa Lipcon Kramer, M.D., and Marilyn Noz, M.D., New York University Medical Center)

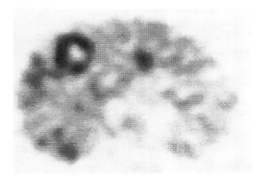

FIG. 4. Colorectal carcinoma metastatic to liver. Positron emission tomography (PET scan) demonstrates multiple foci of increased uptake of labeled fluorodeoxyglucose (FDG) representing increased glucose metabolism in the malignant lesions. The largest lesion has a target appearance due to central necrosis.

tumors are "resectable for cure" survive surgery by an average of only 10 to 20 months (39,40). In over 90% of cases, a well-performed CT scan demonstrates the pancreatic tumor itself, along with ancillary signs such as dilated pancreatic and bile ducts (Fig. 5). Thin (3–7 mm) CT sections improve recognition of small morphologic features, including blood vessels and the pancreatic duct. Automated bolus delivery of 100 to 150 mL of intravenous contrast medium at 2 to 3 mL/sec produces a high concentration of iodine in the circulating blood as well as the hepatic and pancreatic parenchyma and improves recognition of the typically hypovascular primary and secondary tumor.

CT is highly accurate for determining resectability. In one large series, 92% of patients were judged unre-

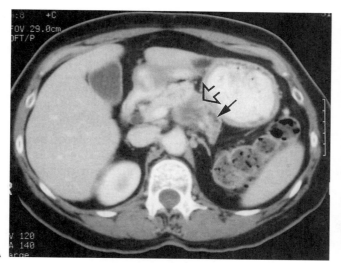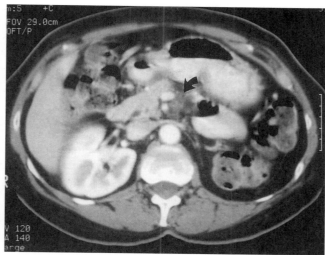

FIG. 5. Pancreatic carcinoma. **(A)** CT demonstrates a hypodense mass in the body of the pancreas (*open arrow*), causing a dilated pancreatic duct (*arrow*). **(B)** Section at the level of the pancreatic head demonstrates infiltration of fat planes around the superior mesenteric vessels (*arrow*), establishing non-resectability. Splenic vein occlusion was also evident on other sections.

sectable by CT criteria (eg, liver metastases, vascular invasion, adjacent organ invasion) (41). No patients were denied potentially curative surgery due to false-positive CT findings, and many patients were spared the additional morbidity and expense of futile surgery.

In current practice, endoscopic retrograde cholangiopancreatography (ERCP) usually plays a supplementary role in evaluating patients suspected of having pancreatic carcinoma. ERCP may help differentiate duodenal or ampullary tumors from cancer of the pancreatic head. Carcinoma of the pancreatic head classically results in a "double duct" sign, demonstrated on ERCP by abrupt obstruction of adjacent portions of the pancreatic and

common bile ducts. Endoscopy is also used to place endoprostheses to relieve biliary obstruction.

The role of angiography in the diagnosis and evaluation of pancreatic carcinoma has diminished markedly. Good-quality CT reveals vascular involvement with an accuracy equal to or greater than that of angiography in 95% of cases (41).

Although the vast majority of pancreatic neoplasms prove to be adenocarcinoma of duct cell origin, other epithelial and nonepithelial tumors of the pancreas occur. In most cases the imaging features, together with relevant clinical information, indicate that the lesion is probably something other than ductal carcinoma. Occasionally,

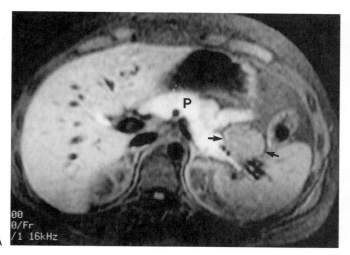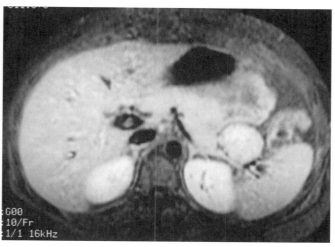

FIG. 6. Insulinoma. This 25-year-old woman had episodic dizziness, confusion, and seizures related to hypoglycemia. **(A)** Fat-suppressed T1-weighted spin echo MR image of pancreas (*P*). A low-intensity mass (*arrows*) is identified in the tail of the pancreas. **(B)** After intravenous infusion of Gd-DTPA, the mass enhances dramatically, reflecting its hypervascular nature.

however, some of these less common neoplasms, such as primary pancreatic lymphoma or nonfunctioning islet cell tumor, may be indistinguishable from ductal adenocarcinoma.

Functioning islet cell tumors are often clinically evident while still very small due to endocrinopathy. Both CT and MRI have proved useful in diagnosis, particularly when dynamic bolus-enhanced studies are performed to take advantage of the typically hypervascular nature of these neoplasms (Fig. 6). Endoscopic or even intraoperative sonography may be necessary to detect small, multiple islet cell tumors.

Several rare types of pancreatic neoplasms may be manifested as cystic masses. These may be difficult to distinguish from pancreatic pseudocysts by imaging criteria alone, and the absence of a prior history of trauma or other insult to the pancreas is often key. Serous (microcystic) adenoma is a benign tumor that may be confidently diagnosed when the typical features of central septa with calcification and numerous small cystic spaces (<2 cm) are identified. Mucinous (macrocystic) neoplasms are regarded as malignant or premalignant. The cysts in these tumors are typically larger (>2 cm) and fewer, and the cyst contents are higher than water density and intensity on CT and MRI, respectively.

Percutaneous thin-needle image-guided (CT or ultrasound) biopsy of pancreatic masses is an important adjunct to diagnosis. Pancreatic ductal adenocarcinoma is typically found to be unresectable at the time of diagnosis, and percutaneous biopsy is an effective means of confirming the diagnosis without exploratory laparotomy. Biopsy techniques vary depending on personal preferences and available cytopathologic services. Thin needles with cutting tips make it possible to obtain tissue cores suitable for histologic and cytologic diagnosis. Experienced cytopathologists can often make an immediate microscopic confirmation, enabling the radiologist to limit the number of needle passes. Needle biopsy can help distinguish ductal carcinoma from other rare types of pancreatic neoplasms or focal pancreatitis.

The safety and efficacy of pancreatic biopsy are well established. Rare cases of seeding of tumor cells along the needle path have been reported (42), leading some authorities to recommend that the procedure be performed only in patients who are not considered to have potentially resectable tumors. Rare cases of postbiopsy pancreatitis have also been reported, although no fatal cases of pancreatitis have been encountered in patients who eventually proved to have pancreatic cancer (43).

Genitourinary

For renal tumors, CT is the primary imaging modality for diagnosis and staging (44–46). Masses may be detected by excretory urography or ultrasonography, but additional information is usually necessary to characterize the lesions. CT can occasionally render a specific diagnosis, for instance by detecting small amounts of fat that characterize the benign tumor angiomyolipoma. Most solid renal masses are renal cell carcinomas, and in almost all patients CT provides the necessary preoperative information, including the size of the tumor, involvement of adjacent organs, lymphadenopathy, and bone involvement (see Fig. 1). Scans performed with an adequate bolus of intravenous contrast material (2–5 mL/sec) accurately detect extension into the renal vein or inferior vena cava, obviating the need for angiography and venography (Fig. 7). CT can distinguish stage I/II renal carcinoma from stage III or IV with an accuracy of 96% (45).

MRI is unreliable for detecting small renal carcinomas, as the signal intensity of tumors is variable and often similar to normal parenchyma on standard imaging sequences (41–47). However, if intravenous iodinated contrast material cannot be given for proper CT evaluation, MRI becomes a valuable alternative. Gadolinium-based MRI contrast agents are handled physiologically like iodinated compounds but appear to be safe in patients with allergies to iodine-based agents or renal insufficiency. MRI scans obtained before and after contrast enhancement are very accurate for the detection and characterization of renal tumors (46–48).

We rarely perform percutaneous biopsies of solid renal masses thought to represent primary renal carcinoma, as the diagnosis is rarely in doubt, there is a real danger of seeding the needle track with tumor, and surgical excision is the standard therapy even in advanced cases. An exception to this policy is the very useful role of biopsy in patients with renal masses who have a separate primary malignancy or who are at high risk of lymphoma (eg, AIDS patients, recipients of solid organ transplantation). Although surgery is used as primary therapy for almost all renal carcinomas, different surgical approaches may be used for early (stages I/II) and advanced (III/IV) tumors. The accurate staging provided by CT also has an important influence on prognosis. The two lower stages combined have a markedly higher 5-year survival rate (71%) than do the two higher stages combined (12%) (49). In some patients, the CT demonstration of extensive lymph node or liver metastases may preclude radical surgery, and image-guided biopsy of the primary or metastatic focus may be indicated and adequate to initiate systemic therapy.

The adrenal glands are relatively common sites of metastatic tumor, particularly from melanoma and lung and renal cell carcinoma. The presence of an adrenal mass in a patient with a known cancer cannot be presumed to represent metastases, however, because benign adrenal adenomas are common neoplasms. In autopsy series and large series of patients undergoing CT with no known malignancy or adrenal disease, adrenal adenomas 0.5 to 1 cm in size are found in 1% to 3% (50). These "incidentalomas" usually represent nonhyperfunctioning adenomas.

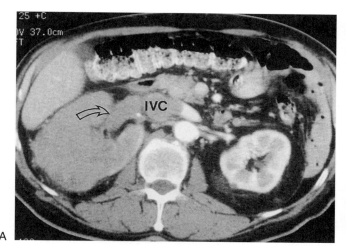

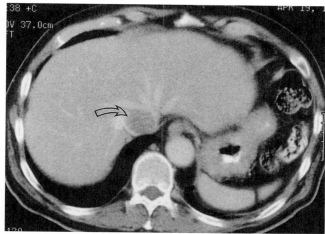

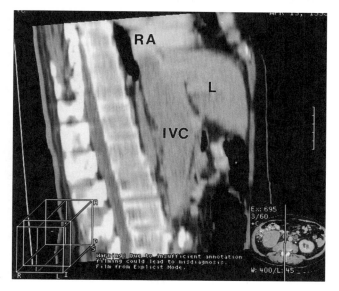

FIG. 7. Renal cell carcinoma with vena cava invasion. **(A)** A large tumor replaces most of the right kidney and invades the renal vein (*curved arrow*), inferior vena cava (*IVC*), and distal left renal vein. **(B)** The tumor thrombus (*arrow*) extends upward through the intrahepatic portion of the IVC. Note the enhancing hepatic veins. **(C)** A sagittal re-formation of the axial CT sections shows the extension of the tumor throughout the suprarenal vena cava (*IVC*). The thrombus extends to, but not into, the right atrium (*RA*). *L*, liver.

When an adrenal mass is the only finding suspicious of metastatic disease in an oncologic patient, confirmation of its nature may be crucial in determining whether curative therapy is warranted. Even in patients with lung cancer, an adrenal mass is more likely to be an adenoma than a metastasis.

Typical CT features of adenoma are small size, homogeneous low density (less than water density on unenhanced images), and lack of significant enhancement with intravenous contrast media. Metastases tend to appear larger and more heterogeneous, with areas of irregular enhancement. In an individual case, however, CT findings are usually not definitive. Percutaneous CT-guided biopsy is effective in distinguishing metastasis from adenoma, but it is invasive and technically difficult due to the anatomic position of the adrenals.

There has been extensive investigation of the use of MRI in differentiating among adrenal masses. Initial studies suggested that adrenal adenomas had a lower sig-

nal intensity on T2-weighted images than did metastatic lesions. Subsequent studies showed the separation between the two groups was not complete, with an overlap of 20% to 30% (51,52). More recent studies have focused on MRI enhancement patterns and "chemical shift imaging." After intravenous bolus administration of Gd-DTPA, adenomas show only mild enhancement and quick washout; malignant lesions typically show strong enhancement and slower washout (52). Because adrenal adenomas, unlike metastases, almost always contain small amounts of lipid, MRI sequences, such as lipid-sensitive chemical shift, can help in the evaluation of adrenal masses (Fig. 8). Mitchell and colleagues reported that 26 of 27 benign adrenal adenomas displayed a visible loss of signal on at least one chemical shift image; all 12 metastases did not (53). If these results can be confirmed by other investigators, biopsy and aggressive follow-up of some adrenal masses might be obviated.

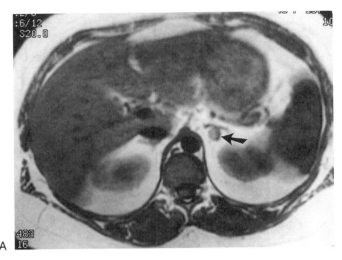

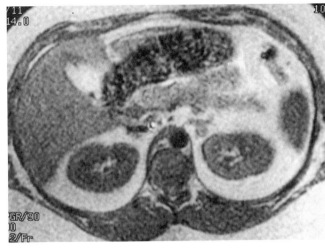

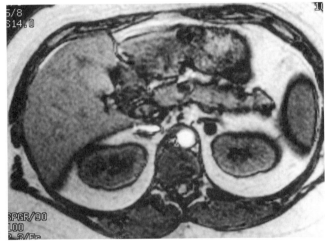

FIG. 8. Adrenal adenoma. **(A)** Standard T1-weighted spin echo MR image demonstrates a 1-cm nodular mass (*arrow*) in the left adrenal gland. **(B)** The adrenal mass remains of relatively bright intensity on "in phase" gradient echo imaging. **(C)** On "out of phase" imaging, which suppresses the signal from tissues that contain both lipid and water, the adrenal mass is markedly diminished in intensity compared with other soft tissues. This confirms that it is a benign adenoma rather than a metastasis.

Gynecologic Neoplasms

The evaluation of primary pelvic masses in women remains a somewhat complex and controversial issue. Ultrasound is the primary modality, and the refinements of transvaginal probes and color Doppler allow superb spatial resolution and characterization of vascularity and morphology. Cystic masses with complex morphologic features (eg, mural nodularity) or evidence of a low-resistance vascular supply (low resistive index and low pulsatility index) are considered suspicious for malignancy (54). Most obstetric and benign gynecologic conditions are accurately evaluated by ultrasound alone, with the added benefits of low cost and lack of ionizing radiation. The role of CT scanning is mainly for ovarian carcinoma; MRI will probably supplant CT and ultrasound for endometrial, cervical, and vaginal carcinomas.

Neither CT nor other imaging tests have a major role in the initial staging of patients with ovarian carcinoma (55,56). Standard therapy calls for surgical removal of all macroscopic disease, followed by intravenous chemotherapy and perhaps intraperitoneal chemotherapy. CT has been found valuable in detecting residual or recurrent macroscopic disease and can obviate repeat surgery, especially when residual tumor is confirmed by percutaneous needle biopsy of suspicious masses or loculated fluid collections (Fig. 9) (56–58). Excellent CT technique is mandatory, including dynamic bolus scanning of the liver and upper abdomen, bowel opacification, and thin sections. The intraperitoneal instillation of contrast material ("CT peritoneography") has been found to increase substantially the detection rate of ovarian metastases (59). Although no imaging test is likely to detect the tiny peritoneal and omental deposits so frequent in ovarian cancer (thus limiting their role in primary staging), gross peritoneal tumor is usually evident by nodular, reticular, or solid omental lesions or loculated ascites (57). The presence of an omental "cake" is virtually specific for malignancy (Fig. 10).

MRI offers several compelling advantages in the evaluation of pelvic masses (60). It is noninvasive and nonionizing and demonstrates blood vessels (as distinct from lymph nodes) without the use of intravenous contrast medium. Direct imaging in sagittal and coronal planes

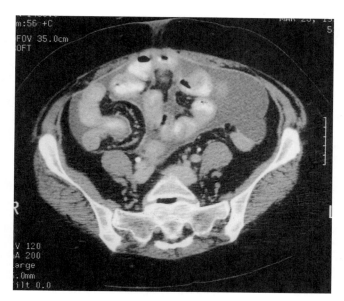

FIG. 9. Recurrent ovarian carcinoma. CT 7 years after hysterectomy and chemotherapy demonstrates loculated ascites and peritoneal thickening. Paracentesis confirmed carcinomatosis.

and unsurpassed contrast resolution are provided, along with a larger field of view than ultrasound.

The prognosis and treatment of cervical and endometrial carcinomas are highly dependent on accurate staging. Precise knowledge of tumor size and location affects the therapeutic decision between surgery and radiation therapy. The International Federation of Gynecology and Obstetrics (FIGO) has limited the clinical staging of cervical and endometrial cancer to findings from physical examination, colposcopy, cystoscopy, sigmoidoscopy, excretory urography (IVP), and barium enema. These studies, however, are often inaccurate and sometimes redundant or obsolete. In a 1980 report on cases of cervical carcinoma staged surgically, errors in the FIGO clinical staging were found in 23% of stage IIB tumors and 64.4% of Stage IIIB (61).

The criteria advocated for MRI staging of cervical/ endometrial carcinoma parallel those recommended by FIGO. The size of the tumor and its relation to the vagina, bladder, pelvic side walls, and so forth are all clearly displayed. Endometrial carcinoma demonstrates a higher signal intensity than myometrium, cervix, and vagina on T2-predominant images, allowing accurate assessment of tumor volume, depth of myometrial invasion, and tumor extension into or beyond the corpus. T1-predominant images are useful in assessing invasion of pelvic fat (Fig. 11) (62).

MRI is not needed in every patient with cervical or endometrial carcinoma. It is not indicated in early-stage small lesions in which tumor volume is not a factor in treatment planning. The value of MRI rises in proportion to the volume and stage of the disease and the presence of concomitant lesions (63). Lingering problems include the impracticality of MRI screening of the upper abdomen and thorax along with the pelvis, and the inability of MRI to depict the ureters. All these factors suggest a role for CT, although further advances and experience with MRI may supplant the use of CT (56).

Prostate

The diagnosis and therapy of prostate cancer have become matters of intense debate in the medical and lay

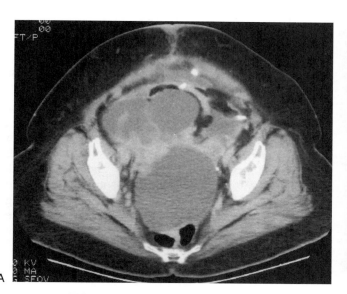

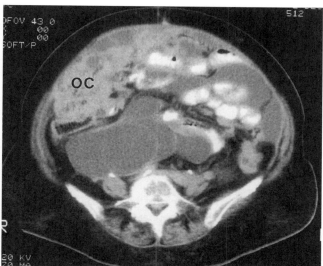

FIG. 10. Recurrent ovarian carcinoma. **(A)** A complex cystic and solid mass is found in the pelvis. **(B)** Along with loculated ascites, an omental "cake" (*OC*) is found, representing a solid mass of tissue lying between the abdominal wall and bowel loops.

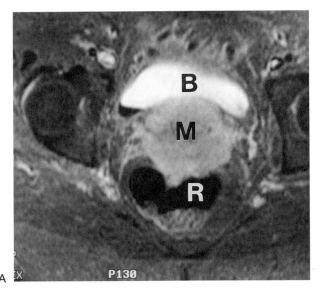

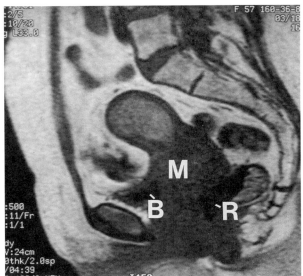

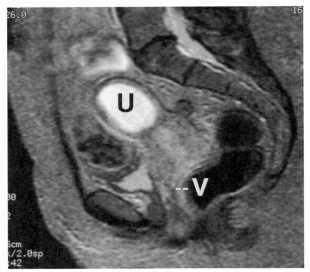

FIG. 11. Invasive cervical carcinoma. **(A)** Axial image after intravenous gadolinium shows a large enhancing cervical mass (*M*) that invades the rectum (*R*) and displaces the bladder (*B*). **(B)** T1-weighted sagittal image demonstrates best the full extent of the cervical mass (*M*), which appears low intensity before contrast administration. **(C)** T2-weighted sagittal image shows loss of the fat plane between the mass and the posterior bladder wall. The obstructed cervical os is reflected by the fluid-distended uterine cavity (*U*). The tumor extends well into the vagina (*V*) and appears relatively high in intensity due to increased water content relative to normal viscera or muscle.

press. Treatment options vary depending on the extent of disease and various patient comorbid factors. Radical surgery is often recommended for tumor confined to the prostate; palliative therapy is usually offered for more advanced disease. Serum tumor markers such as PSA and radionuclide bone scanning play important roles in staging (64,65). In a review of more than 2,000 patients with newly diagnosed, untreated prostate cancer, no patient who had a PSA value of 8 μg/L or less had an abnormal bone scan, and the positive bone scan rate with a PSA value of 10 μg/L or less was only 0.5% (66). Thus, a staging radionuclide bone scan appears to be unnecessary for newly diagnosed prostate tumors when the serum PSA is 10 μg/L or less and no skeletal symptoms are present.

Both clinical staging (67) and CT (68) are inaccurate, with only about 50% sensitivity in detecting spread beyond the prostatic capsule. We generally reserve CT for two situations: simulation for radiation therapy programs,

and evaluating patients suspected to have advanced disease who are poor operative risks. In the latter group, CT-guided lymph node (or other metastatic focus) biopsy has been advocated (69).

There has been a great deal of interest in transrectal ultrasound and MRI as aids in staging prostate cancer. In a 1990 report of a multi-institutional study, the overall staging accuracy of transrectal ultrasound was 58% and that of MRI was 69% (70). Both ultrasound and MRI had significant error rates in overstaging and understaging disease. The performance of MRI can be improved by the use of intrarectal MRI coils, but staging accuracy has not been established in large prospective trials.

Lyphoreticular

Because the lymphatics and lymph nodes are among the most common avenues of malignant spread, detection of these remains a critical test of any imaging modality. To date, all imaging tests have shown disappointing limitations in this task. Spread of tumor outside the capsule of an organ may be demonstrated by streaky densities or subtle infiltration of the surrounding fat on CT or MRI, but these findings are neither sensitive nor specific. Microscopic or macroscopic involvement of lymph nodes by tumor is undetectable as an alteration of CT or MRI appearance; we are limited to using size criteria and establishing threshold values for various nodal groups, while acknowledging a substantial overlap between benign and malignant nodal sizes. Human trials are underway of an intravenously administered MRI contrast agent that would selectively enhance thoracic and abdominal lymph nodes (71,72).

In a consecutive series of 160 patients with abdominal lymphadenopathy, 45% of cases were attributable to lymphoma, 49% to metastatic carcinomas, and 6% to various benign conditions such as tuberculosis, Crohn's disease, and mastocytosis (73). Ancillary imaging findings are often useful and essentially diagnostic in the proper clinical setting, such as the presence of localized bowel wall and mesenteric abnormalities in patients with Crohn's disease. Other criteria, including size, location, confluence, density, contour, and presence of mass effect, are not of value in distinguishing benign from malignant lymph nodes. Biopsy is often needed for definitive diagnosis, although short-term follow-up may be adequate. For example, CT is a standard tool in evaluating patients with testicular neoplasms and accurately reflects the status of abdominal and mediastinal lymph nodes, along with pulmonary and visceral metastases (74). CT evaluation of abdominal lymphadenopathy has even been found to be valuable in evaluating patients with small cell carcinoma of the lung (75). Initial staging by CT has demonstrated abdominal metastases (visceral or nodal) in over half of patients with extensive thoracic tumor, and these patients had a poorer prognosis than those without abdominal involvement.

In the past, lymphangiography (LAG) was widely used for evaluating lymphomas and pelvic tumors. This is a technically demanding procedure, requiring a surgical incision and cannulation of lymphatics on the dorsum of the feet. Radiopaque oil (Ethiodol) is slowly injected over minutes to hours, and abdominal and pelvic radiographs are obtained. Interpretation of the radiographs is also challenging, with the goal of distinguishing among normal, tumor-bearing, and inflamed nodes. In experienced hands, LAG has been reported to have >90% accuracy in staging lymphomas (76). However, beyond the technical failures, LAG frequently fails to opacify medial pelvic, upper abdominal, and mesenteric lymph nodes. Even in the best hands, LAG misses abdominal involvement in over 30% of patients with Hodgkin's disease and underestimates the extent of nodal involvement in non-Hodgkin's lymphoma (77,78). LAG offers some theoretical advantages, including detecting tumor in normal-size nodes and distinguishing a cluster of normal nodes from enlarged nodes. Nodes may remain opacified for many months, allowing simple follow-up by plain radiography and percutaneous biopsy of nodes under fluoroscopic control.

There are variable reports on the relative accuracy and advantages of CT and LAG. Investigators from the Roswell Park Cancer Institute studied almost 100 patients with thoracic Hodgkin's disease and concluded that neither LAG nor radionuclide gallium scanning offered substantial improvement over CT alone in detecting abdominal involvement (79). From a practical standpoint, LAG seems to be dying out, as fewer radiologists are trained to perform and interpret the study. Improvements in CT and MRI and the availability of various serum tumor markers seem to have supplanted LAG in most centers (80). In addition, the histology of testicular tumors and non-Hodgkin's lymphoma appears to have a greater influence on prognosis and initial treatment than traditional staging schemes (81). Bone marrow biopsy frequently demonstrates a more advanced pathologic stage of disease in lymphoma patients than that suggested by clinical staging or imaging. The major role for CT (or LAG) in patients with non-Hodgkin's lymphoma is the detection of otherwise unsuspected disease, especially in patients with limited clinical signs of disease and "negative" bone marrow biopsy results (81).

Melanoma

Malignant melanoma is an increasingly common and very aggressive malignancy for which imaging plays an important role. The depth of skin invasion (the Clark stage) correlates well with the incidence of metastases, ranging from 46% for relatively superficial lesions to 84% for deep lesions (82). Overall, metastases are discovered in about 60% of patients, with an even higher incidence when the primary melanoma is in the orbit or other head or neck sites. Metastases can affect virtually any part of the body and may occur up to 15 to 20 years after initial discovery and treatment. As previously noted, the role of gallium scanning in the evaluation of patients with melanoma is controversial. In a study of 222 patients with melanoma, gallium scanning had a sensitivity of 74% and a specificity of 94% (10). Nevertheless, these investigators concluded that gallium imaging provided little information that affected either staging or management. They recommended that it be used only in conjunction with CT evaluation of the chest and abdomen. The ease of screening multiple organ systems as well as the various fat planes makes CT the current imaging modality of choice in melanoma. No imaging study may be needed in cases of very superficial melanoma lesions with normal liver function tests. Nodes that are enlarged by CT criteria (>1.5 cm) in melanoma patients are almost always involved with tumor, and CT demonstrates multiorgan sites of involvement in almost 50% of patients (83).

ACKNOWLEDGMENT

The author thanks Manny Brown, M.D., for his input regarding radionuclide imaging.

REFERENCES

1. Sobin LH, Ros PR. Radiology and the new TNM classification of tumors: the future. *Radiology* 1990;176:1–4.
2. Chezmar JL, Rumancik WM, Megibow AJ, et al. Liver and abdominal screening in patients with cancer: CT versus MRI imaging. *Radiology* 1988;168:43–47.
3. Glazer GM, Aisen AM, Francis IR, et al. Evaluation of focal hepatic masses: a comparative study of MRII and CT. *Gastrointest Radiol* 1986;11:263–268.
4. Burgener FA, Hamlin DJ. Contrast enhancement of hepatic tumors in CT: comparison between bolus and infusion techniques. *AJR* 1983;140:291–295.
5. Tumeh SS, Rosenthal DS, Kaplan WD, English RJ, Holman BL. Lymphoma: evaluation with Ga-67 SPECT. *Radiology* 1987;164:111–114.
6. Front D, Israel O, Epelbaum R, et al. Ga-67 SPECT before and after treatment of lymphoma. *Radiology* 1990;175:515–519.
7. Front D, Ben-Hairn S, Israel O, et al. Lymphoma: predictive value of Ga-67 scintigraphy after treatment. *Radiology* 1992;182:359–363.
8. Hagemeister FB, Fesus SM, Lamki LM, Heyuie TP. Role of the gallium scan in Hodgkin's disease. *Cancer* 1990;65:1090–1096.
9. Kaplan WD. Editorial: Residual mass and negative gallium scintigraphy in treated lymphoma: when is the gallium scan really negative? *J Nucl Med* 1990;31:369–371.
10. Kagen R, Well T, Bines S, Mesleh G, Ecinomoa S. Gallium scanning for malignant melanoma. *Cancer* 1989;61:272–274.
11. Krenning EP, Kwekkeboom DJ, Baker WH, et al. Somatostatin receptor scintigraphy with [^{111}In–DTPA–D–Phe^1] and [^{123}I–Tyr^3] octeotide: the Rotterdam experience with more than 1000 patients. *Eur J Nucl Med* 1993;20:716–731.
12. Boechat MI, Kangarloo H. MRI imaging of the abdomen in children. *AJR* 1989;152:1245–1250.
13. Brant-Zawadzki M. MRI imaging of the brain. *Radiology* 1988;166:1–10.
14. Ehman RL, Berquist TH, McLeod RA. MRI imaging of the musculoskeletal system: A 5-year appraisal. *Radiology* 1988;166:313–320.
15. Kangarloo H, Dietrich RB, Taira RT, et al. MRI imaging of the bone marrow in children. *J Comput Assist Tomogr* 1986;10:205–209.
16. Aisen AM. Body MRI imaging and the local staging of neoplasms. *Radiology* 1990;176:617–619.
17. Rifkin MD, Erlich SM, Marks G. Staging of rectal carcinoma: Prospective comparison of endorectal US and CT. *Radiology* 1989;170:319–322.
18. Thoeni RF. Colorectal cancer: cross-sectional imaging for staging of primary tumor and detection of local recurrence. *AJR* 1991;156:909–915.
19. Thompson WM, Halvorsen RA, Foster WL, et al. Preoperative and postoperative CT staging of rectosigmoid carcinoma. *AJR* 1986;146:703–710.
20. Freeny PC, Marks WM, Ryan JA, et al. Colorectal carcinoma evaluation with CT: preoperative staging and detection of postoperative recurrence. *Radiology* 1986;158:347–353.
21. Balthazar EJ, Megibow AJ, Hulnick D, et al. Carcinoma of the colon: detection and preoperative staging by CT. *AJR* 1988;150:301–306.
22. deLange EE, Fechner RE, Edge SB, Spaulding CA. Preoperative staging of rectal carcinoma with MRI imaging: surgical and histopathologic correlation. *Radiology* 1990;176:623–628.
23. Butch RJ, Stark DD, Wittenberg J. Staging rectal cancer by MRI and CT. *AJR* 1986;146:1155–1160.
24. Guinet C, Buy JN, Ghossain MA, et al. Comparison of magnetic resonance imaging and computed tomography in the preoperative staging of rectal cancer. *Arch Surg* 1990;125:385–388.
25. Tio TL, Coene PPLO, Schouwink MH, Tytgat GNJ. Esophagogastric carcinoma: preoperative TNM classification with endosonography. *Radiology* 1989;173:411–417.
26. Vilgrain V, Mompoint D, Palazzo L, et al. Staging of esophageal carcinoma: comparison of results with endoscopic sonography and CT. *AJR* 1990;155:277–281.
27. van Overhagen H, Lameris JS, Berger MY, et al. CT assessment of resectability prior to transhiatal esophagectomy for esophageal/gastroesophageal junction carcinoma. *J Comput Assist Tomogr* 1993;17:367–373.
28. Sussman SK, Halvorsen RA Jr, Illescas FF, et al. Gastric adenocarcinoma: CT versus surgical staging. *Radiology* 1988;167:335–340.
29. Babaian RJ, Sayer J, Podoloff DA, et al. Radioimmunoscintigraphy of pelvic lymph nodes with ^{111}Indium-labeled monoclonal antibody CYT-356. *J Urol* 1994;152:1952–1955.
30. Goldenberg DM, DeLand F, Kirn E, et al. Use of radiolabeled antibodies to carcinoembryonic antigen for the detection and localization of diverse cancers by external photoscanning. *N Engl J Med* 1978;298:1384–1387.
31. Scott AM, Macapinlac HA, Divgi CD, et al. Clinical validation of SPECT and CT/MRII image registration in radiolabeled monoclonal antibody studies of colorectal carcinoma. *J Nucl Med* 1994;35:1976–1984.
32. Schad LR, Boesecke R, Schlegel W, et al. Three-dimensional image correlation of CT, MRI, and PET studies in radiotherapy treatment planning of brain tumors. *J Comput Assist Tomogr* 1987;11:948–954.
33. Baron RL. Understanding and optimizing use of contrast material for CT of the liver. *AJR* 1994;163:323–331.
34. Nelson RP, Chezmar JL, Sugarbaker PH, Bernardino ME. Hepatic tumors: comparison of CT during arterial portography, delayed CT and MRI imaging for preoperative evaluation. *Radiology* 1989;172:27–34.
35. Matsui O, Takashima T, Kadoya M, et al. Liver metastases from colorectal cancers: detection with CT during arterial portography. *Radiology* 1987;165:65–69.
36. Fretz C, Stark DD, Metz CE, et al. Detection of hepatic metastases: comparison of contrast-enhanced CT, unenhanced MRI imaging, and iron oxide–enhanced MRI imaging. *AJR* 1990;155:763–770.
37. Hamm B, Vogl TJ, Branding JG, et al. Focal liver lesions: MRI imaging with Mn-DPDP: initial clinical results in 40 patients. *Radiology* 1992;182:167–174.
38. Rofsky NM, Weinreb JC, Bernardino ME, et al. Hepatocellular tumors: characterization with Mn-DPDP-enhanced MRI imaging. *Radiology* 1993;188:53–59.
39. Edis AJ, Kiernan PD, Taylor WF. Attempted curative resection of ductal carcinoma of the pancreas: review of Mayo Clinic experience, 1951–1975. *Mayo Clinic Proc* 1981;55:531–536.
40. Mannell A, van Heerden JA, Weiland LH, Ilstrup DM. Factors influencing survival after resection for ductal adenocarcinoma of the pancreas. *Ann Surg* 1986;203:403–407.
41. Freeny PC, Marks WM, Ryan JA, Traverso LW. Pancreatic ductal adenocarcinoma: diagnosis and staging with dynamic CT. *Radiology* 1988;166:125–133.
42. Rasleigh-Belcher HJC, Russell RCG, Lees WR. Cutaneous seeding of pancreatic carcinoma by fine needle aspiration biopsy. *Br J Radiol* 1986;59:59–60.
43. Smith E. Complications of percutaneous fine-needle biopsy. *Radiology* 1991;128:253–256.
44. Benson MA, Haaga JR, Resnick MI. Staging renal carcinoma: what is sufficient? *Ann Surg* 1989;123:71–73.
45. Johnson CD, Dunnick NR, Cohan RH, Illescas FF. Renal adenocarcinoma: CT staging of 100 tumors. *AJR* 1987;148:59–63.
46. Fein AB, Lee JKT, Balfe DM, et al. Diagnosis and staging of renal cell carcinoma: a comparison of MRI imaging and CT. *AJR* 1987;148:749–753.
47. Hricak H, Thoeni RJ, Canoll PR, et al. Detection and staging of renal neoplasms: a reassessment of MRI imaging. *Radiology* 1988;166:643–649.
48. Rofsky NM, Weinreb JC, Bosniak MA, et al. Renal lesion characterization with gadolinium-enhanced MRI imaging: efficacy and safety in patients with renal insufficiency. *Radiology* 1991;180:85–89.
49. Bottiger LE. Prognosis in renal carcinoma. *Cancer* 1970;20:780–787.
50. Copeland PM. The incidentally discovered adrenal mass. *Ann Intern Med* 1983;98:940–945.
51. Baker ME, Blinder R, Spritzer C, et al. MRI evaluation of adrenal masses at 1.5 T. *AJR* 1989;153:307–312.
52. Krestin GP, Steinbrick W, Friedmann G. Adrenal masses: evaluation

with fast gradient-echo MRI imaging and GdDTPA-enhanced dynamic studies. *Radiology* 1989;171:675–680.

53. Mitchell GD, Crovello M, Matteucci RD, et al. Benign adrenocortical masses: diagnosis with chemical shift MRI imaging. *Radiology* 1992; 185:345–351.

54. Brown DL, Frates MC, Laing FC, et al. Ovarian masses: can benign and malignant lesions be differentiated with color and pulsed Doppler US? *Radiology* 1994;190:333–336.

55. Chang YCF, Hricak H. Gynecologic tumor imaging. *Semin Ultrasound CT MRI* 1989;10:29–42.

56. Walsh JW. Computed tomography of gynecologic neoplasms. *Radiol Clin North Am* 1992;30:817–830.

57. Megibow AJ, Bosniak MA, Ho AG, et al. Accuracy of CT in detection of persistent or recurrent ovarian carcinoma: correlation with second-look laparotomy. *Radiology* 1988;166:341–345.

58. Silverman PM, Osborne M, Dunnick NR, Bandy LC. CT prior to second-look operation in ovarian cancer. *AJR* 1988;150:829–832.

59. Halvorsen RA Jr, Panushka C, Oakley GJ, et al. Intraperitoneal contrast material improves the CT detection of peritoneal metastases. *AJR* 1991; 157:37–40.

60. Heiken JP, Lee JKT. MRI imaging of the pelvis. *Radiology* 1988;166: 11–16.

61. Lagasse LD, Creasman WT, Shingleton HM, et al. Results and complications of operative staging in cervical cancer: experience of the Gynecologic Oncology Group. *Gynecol Oncol* 1980;9:90–98.

62. Hricak H, Lacey CG, Sandless LG, et al. Invasive cervical carcinoma: comparison of MRI imaging and surgical findings. *Radiology* 1988; 166:623–631.

63. Hricak H, Stern JL, Fisher MRI, et al. Endometrial carcinoma staging by MRI imaging. *Radiology* 1987;162:297–305.

64. Partin AW, Yoo J, Carter HB, et al. The use of prostate specific antigen, clinical stage and Gleason score to predict pathological stage in men with localized prostate cancer. *J Urol* 1993;150:110–114.

65. Bluestein DL, Bostwick DG, Bergstralk EJ, Oesterling JE. Eliminating the need for bilateral pelvic lymphadenectomy in select patients with prostate cancer. *J Urol* 1994;151:1315–1320.

66. Oesterling JE, Martin SK, Bergstralk EJ, Lowe FC. The use of prostate-specific antigen in staging patients with newly diagnosed prostate cancer. *JAMA* 1993;269:57–60.

67. Lange PH, Narayan P. Understaging and undergrading of prostate cancer. *Urology* 1983;21:113–118.

68. Platt JF, Bree RL, Schwab RE. The accuracy of CT in the staging of carcinoma of the prostate. *AJR* 1987;149:315–318.

69. van Poppel H, Ameye F, Oyen R, et al. Accuracy of combined computerized tomography and fine needle aspiration cytology in lymph node staging of localized prostatic carcinoma. *J Urol* 1994;151: 1310–1314.

70. Rifkin MD, Zerhouni EA, Gatsonis CA, et al. Comparison of magnetic resonance imaging and ultrasonography in staging early prostate cancer: results of a multi-institutional cooperative trial. *N Engl J Med* 1990;323:621–626.

71. Guimaraes R, Clemet O, Bittoun J, Carnot F, Friga G. MRI lymphography with superparamagnetic iron nanoparticles in rats: pathologic basis for contrast enhancement. *AJR* 1994;162:201–207.

72. Vassallo P, Matei C, Heston WDW, et al. AMI-227-enhanced MRI lymphography: usefulness for differentiating reactive from tumor-bearing lymph nodes. *Radiology* 1994;193:501–506.

73. Deutch SJ, Sandler MA, Alpern MB. Abdominal lymphadenopathy in benign diseases: CT detection. *Radiology* 1987;163:335–338.

74. Williams MP, Naik G, Heron CW, Husband JE. Computed tomography of the abdomen in advanced seminoma: response to treatment. *Clin Radiol* 1987;38:629–633.

75. Mirvis SE, Whitley NO, Aisner J, et al. Abdominal CT in the staging of small-cell carcinoma of the lung. *AJR* 1987;148:845–847.

76. Castellino RA, Billingham M, Dorfman RF. Lymphographic accuracy in Hodgkin's disease and malignant lymphoma with a note on the "reactive" lymph node as a cause of most false-positive lymphograms. *Invest Radiol* 1990;25:412–422.

77. Gamble JF, Fuller LM, Martin RG, et al. Influence of staging celiotomy in localized presentations of Hodgkin's disease. *Cancer* 1975;35: 817–825.

78. Heifetz LJ, Fuller LM, Rogers RW, et al. Laparotomy findings in lymphangiogram-staged I and II non-Hodgkin's lymphomas. *Cancer* 1980; 45:2778–2786.

79. Stomper PC, Cholewinski SP, Park J, Bakshi SP, Barcos MP. Abdominal staging of thoracic Hodgkin disease: CT-lymphangiography-Ga 67 scanning correlation. *Radiology* 1993;187:381–386.

80. North LB, Lindell MM, Jing BS, Wallace S. Current use of lymphography for staging lymphomas and genital tumors. *AJR* 1992;158:725–728.

81. Pond GD, Castellino RA, Horning S, Hoppe RT. Non-Hodgkin lymphoma: influence of lymphography, CT, and bone marrow biopsy on staging and management. *Radiology* 1989;170:159–164.

82. Patel JK, Didolkar MS, Pickren JW, et al. Metastatic pattern of malignant melanoma. *Am J Surg* 1978;135:807–810.

83. Shirkhoda A, Albin J. Malignant melanoma: correlating abdominal and pelvic CT with clinical staging. *Radiology* 1987;165:75–78.

CHAPTER 17

Abdominal and Pelvic Procedures

Laparoscopic Resection

José M. Dominguez and Heidi Nelson

The scientist in searching for the truth must ever be guided by the cold logic of facts, and be animated by scientific imagination.
—*William J. Mayo, M.D.*

BACKGROUND

Since its introduction in 1988, laparoscopic cholecystectomy has rapidly gained favor with patients, surgeons, and healthcare providers and has become the preferred manner of cholecystectomy (1). By reducing subjective and objective measures of pain (2) and reducing length of postoperative ileus by 21 hours (2), hospital stay by 2 to 4 days (2–6), recovery and time to work by 31 to 35 days (3,5,6), laparoscopic cholecystectomy has met with widespread patient satisfaction (7). For patients and surgeons alike, it is appealing to believe that we may lessen the stress, trauma, and pain associated with oncologic surgery by expanding the indications for laparoscopic surgery to include malignancy.

At this time, the overall role of laparoscopic surgery in malignancy has not yet been determined. It has not been established whether laparoscopic surgery offers special advantages or unique risks to the cancer patient. Because different tumor types and tumor sites manifest distinct biologic behavior and provide unique opportunities and challenges, it may be impossible to draw universal conclusions regarding the role of laparoscopic surgery in cancer. We, therefore, have chosen to examine the merits

and risks of each tumor site independently. This chapter reviews the results to date on the intra-abdominal tumor sites and types that are under investigation, including cancers of the colon, rectum, pancreas, and adrenal as well as lymphomas.

COLON TUMORS

Background

The widespread acceptance of laparoscopic cholecystectomy, together with rapid advancements in laparoscopic equipment, techniques, and experience, has led to the application of laparoscopy for increasingly complex bowel resections (8–24). Laparoscopic colon resection offers several unique technical challenges, including the necessity of viewing and working in multiple operative fields, the requirement for using a two-handed technique, and the need to ligate a large vascular pedicle, perform resection and anastomosis, and deliver a large specimen. Although numerous technical descriptions for laparoscopic colon resection have been published, there are only two fundamental approaches, the complete or intracorporeal laparoscopic colectomy (13) and the laparoscopic-assisted colectomy (24).

The complete laparoscopic colectomy is performed using exclusively intracorporeal techniques, including intracorporeal mobilization, vascular ligation, resection, and anastomosis. Specimens are retrieved through large cannulae or per anus. This approach is technically more advanced, requiring extensive laparoscopic suturing experience, provides challenges of specimen removal, and is associated with higher complication rates. Phillips and colleagues reported an 18% anastomotic leak rate for

J. M. Dominguez and H. Nelson: Division of Colon and Rectal Surgery, Mayo Clinic and Foundation, Rochester, Minnesota 55905

intracorporeal laparoscopic colectomy versus 8% using open colectomy (13). In contrast, laparoscopic-assisted colectomy uses the same laparoscopic techniques of mobilization and vascular ligation, but the resection and anastomosis are completed and the specimen, therefore, is delivered through a small abdominal incision, rendering it less difficult and less risky. By using the assisted technique, the anastomosis can be performed in the same fashion as for open colectomy. Because the laparoscopic-assisted approach is simpler and safer, is more commonly performed, and is associated with patient-related benefits, this chapter will focus principally on laparoscopic-assisted colectomy.

Selection of Patients

No rigid criteria have been described for the selection of patients and diseases best suited for laparoscopic-assisted colectomy. However, overall patient suitability should include an assessment of whether the patient can fully understand that this is a relatively new application of laparoscopy and that long-term results are not available. Full disclosure regarding the potential benefits and risks, including the risk of conversion to an open procedure, is essential.

Indications

Indications for laparoscopic colon resection include colon cancer (8–14,16,23), rectal cancer (9,10,12,13,17, 18), colonic polyps (8,10–13,16,18,19), diverticular disease (8,9,13,16,18), volvulus (10,13,18), the need for fecal diversion (9), rectal prolapse (10,11,16), endometriosis (10,13,18), lipomas (12,20), and inflammatory bowel disease (9–12), as well as pathology requiring total abdominal colectomy (9–12,21,22) such as ulcerative colitis, familial adenomatous polyposis, and colonic inertia. Because the only prospective investigation reported for laparoscopic total abdominal colectomy demonstrated no patient-related advantage for the laparoscopic compared to the open procedure, laparoscopic total abdominal colectomy is not currently recommended (21). Technical advancements may encourage surgeons to reevaluate this procedure in the future.

Contraindications

Although no absolute contraindications have been identified, the presence of advanced organ diseases, such as liver failure with coagulopathy and cardiac failure, with no margin for hemodynamic fluctuations, should dissuade most surgeons from performing laparoscopic colectomy. Common sense should be applied to any clinical condition where surgical risk may be increased or potential benefits decreased. As an example, cases requiring extraction of a large tumor or inflammatory phlegmon, and therefore an exaggerated incision, will probably not provide much advantage for the patient. The presence of obstruction with dilated loops of proximal bowel makes abdominal entry risky and also compromises intra-abdominal visualization. Further, such bowel may be difficult to handle, with risk of fecal contamination.

The only preoperative factor that has been reliably associated with a significantly greater conversion rate is obesity. In the Mayo Clinic series of 122 patients, those weighing over 90 kg had a conversion rate of 75% (23). It would similarly be anticipated that procedures performed in patients who have undergone previous abdominal surgery would be technically more challenging and more likely to require conversion. Although the first statement may be true, the second statement has not been confirmed. At least two studies have shown that a history of previous abdominal surgery does not increase the rate of conversion to open colectomy (9,23). Obese patients or patients with known abdominal adhesions from multiple prior surgeries can be considered as candidates but should be counseled on the high risk of conversion.

Finally, whether the laparoscopic resection of curable colon cancer is contraindicated is hotly debated (discussed below).

Pretreatment Evaluation

Although the preoperative evaluation for laparoscopic resection is generally identical to that performed for an open procedure, a few differences deserve special consideration. Because it is impossible to perform manual palpation of the intra-abdominal contents, the operating surgeon must be confident of the exact location of the colonic pathology. If the diagnosis is established using endoscopic techniques, the degree of confidence is based on whether the lesion is in close proximity to anatomic landmarks such as the ileocecal valve or the junction of the rectum and sigmoid, as even the best endoscopist can misjudge scope position. For any uncertainty, either a barium contrast study can be obtained or India ink can be locally injected into the lesion endoscopically. Rigid proctoscopy is a simple and inexpensive method of ensuring that the pathology is colonic rather than rectal. If a colonic malignancy is being considered for laparoscopic resection, it is reasonable to obtain a preoperative abdominal computed tomography (CT) scan for staging purposes. The CT scan will reveal whether the primary tumor is locally advanced or adherent to adjacent structures and will supplement the intraoperative visual assessment of the liver for metastases, as discussed below.

Detailed Methodology

Laparoscopic-assisted right (Figs. 1–4) and sigmoid (Figs. 5–7) colectomies are performed as illustrated (24). Preoperative preparation is essentially identical to that for open colectomy, including the mechanical and antibiotic

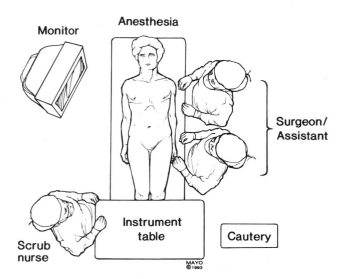

FIG. 1. Right hemicolectomy. With the patient supine, the monitor is positioned on the same side of the pathology and the surgeon/assistant on the opposite side of the pathology. Pneumoperitoneum is established and four cannulae (10- to 12-mm) are placed (periumbilical, left upper and lower paramedian, and right mid-paramedian). Cannula placement should be adjusted for each patient to maximize the ability to reach multiple fields and minimize cross-field interference.

bowel preparation. To minimize the risk of injury and improve intra-abdominal visualization, the stomach and bladder should be decompressed with a nasogastric tube and Foley catheter, respectively. Patients should be well secured to the table to prevent unwanted shifting during

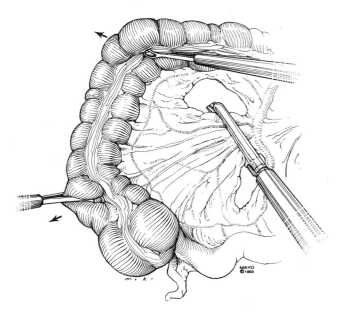

FIG. 3. Intracorporeal vascular ligation can be accomplished with the use of a linear vascular stapler, clips, or endoloops. Full cecal and hepatic flexure mobilization, followed by intracorporeal vascular pedicle ligation, facilitates the extracorporeal delivery of the right colon.

intraoperative table manipulations. Pneumoperitoneum can be accomplished using the Veress needle or Hasson technique (25), depending on the risk of adherent bowel or other complicating factors. It is simplest to use 10- to 12-mm cannulae with stability threads for all port positions:

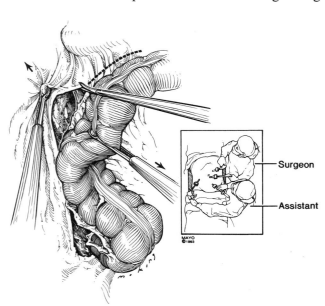

FIG. 2. After thorough abdominopelvic exploration, the cecum and ascending colon are mobilized using colon traction, peritoneal countertraction, and scissor dissection. Trendelenburg and left-side-down table manipulations position the small bowel out of the operative field, thereby providing optimal cecal exposure. The hepatic flexure is approached by reversing the Trendelenburg as well as the surgeon, assistant, and camera positions.

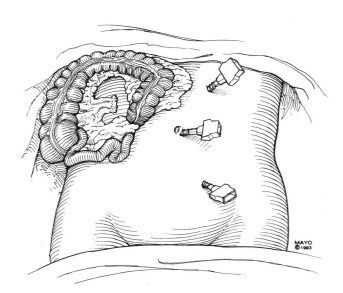

FIG. 4. The bowel is delivered through a 4- to 6-cm incision, and a standard resection and anastomosis are performed. For malignant disease, specimen isolation, wound protection, or both is advised.

this ensures that the camera, Babcocks, stapling devices, and clip applicators can readily be inserted at any site. Inexpensive adaptors can be used to introduce smaller instruments. Although port placements are typically positioned as illustrated in Figs. 2 and 5 for right and sigmoid colon resections, these may be individualized according to the patient's body habitus. In a patient with a long torso, the ports may need to be brought closer together so that the instruments will readily reach all operative fields. In a patient with a short torso, the ports may be adjusted outward so as to avoid cross-field interference.

Once the abdominal cavity is entered, a thorough laparoscopic exploration should be carried out, including an inspection of the peritoneal surfaces, liver, and ovaries and uterus in female patients. In the future, laparoscopic ultrasound probes may facilitate a parenchymal examination of the liver to complement the visual inspection, as discussed below. For malignant disease, the tumor should not be directly handled. If direct extension to an adjacent organ is detected during laparoscopy, the case should be converted to ensure that a complete, en bloc resection is performed.

The equipment list for laparoscopic-assisted colectomy includes many of the same basic tools used in other

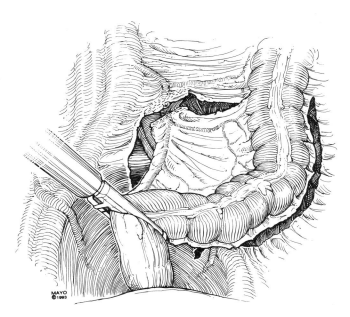

FIG. 6. A combination of Trendelenburg and two-point traction on the sigmoid, with lateral countertraction on the peritoneum, allows sigmoid dissection and ureteral identification. Mesenteric windows are developed, the vascular pedicle is divided, and the distal bowel is prepared for linear stapler division. The splenic flexure is mobilized if required.

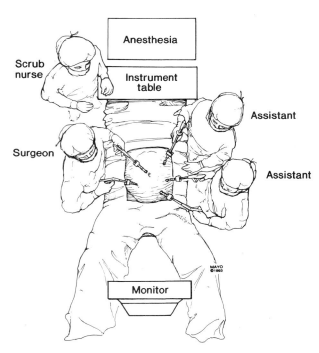

FIG. 5. Sigmoid colectomy. With the patient in legs-up position, a monitor is placed between the legs. Two assistants stand on the patient's left side and the surgeon and nurse stand on the patient's right side. Five cannulae (10- to 12-mm) positions include the camera in the left upper quadrant, grasping instruments in the left middle, left lower, and periumbilical, and the scissor/dissector in the right lower quadrant.

laparoscopic abdominal procedures, such as a 30° laparoscope, grasping instruments, and clip appliers. Exclusive use of 10- to 12-mm cannulae with 5-mm adaptors is recommended, as this simplifies the repositioning of instruments, many of which are 10 to 12 mm in size. Stability threads for the cannulae add little additional cost but greatly facilitate two-handed laparoscopic surgery and minimize pneumoperitoneal leakage. For tissue handling, reusable Babcocks, with functional ends comparable to those used in open surgery, are available. Babcocks should be at least 36 to 38 cm long. Although cauterizing scissors are illustrated here, any dissecting tool can be used, based on the surgeon's experience and familiarity. Linear staplers should be available for vascular pedicle ligation (30-mm vascular stapler) and for bowel transection.

The left colon is removed using the same techniques as for the right colon, only using opposite positions and approaches. Due to the technical challenges associated with having to mobilize the omentum and the hepatic and splenic flexure, transverse colon tumors are not considered suitable for laparoscopic resection.

Morbidity/Mortality

As with any new and particularly complex procedure, safety and feasibility must be top concerns. To date, mor-

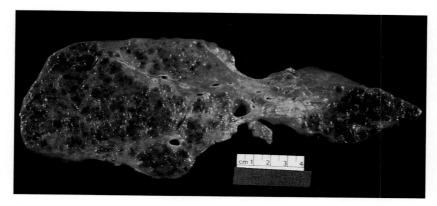

COLOR PLATE 1. Pathologic specimen after liver transplantation shows the capsular retraction with underlying replacement of liver parenchyma by homogenous yellow fibrous tissue, corresponding to the CT scan shown in Fig. 13A, page 84. (See also Fig. 13B, page 84.)

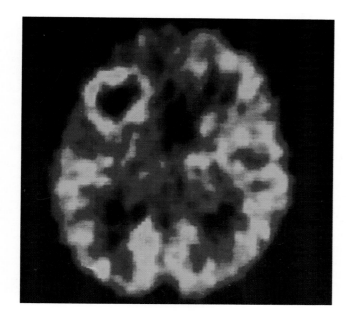

COLOR PLATE 2. Metastatic brain tumor studied with positron emission tomography with fluorodexoxyglucose (PET-FDG). PET-FDG study shows increased glucose comsumption in the periphery of the lesion, representing viable tumor. There is no activity in the necrotic center. (Courtesy of Dr. Ramesh Raman.) (See also Fig. 9B, page 161.)

COLOR PLATE 3. Functional magnetic resonance imaging using the blood oxygen level-dependent technique. Parasagittal image of the left cerebral hemisphere obtained during repetitive movements of the right hand. The activated motor cortex demonstrates increased signal. (Courtesy of Dr. Lucie Pannier.) (See also Fig. 10, page 162.)

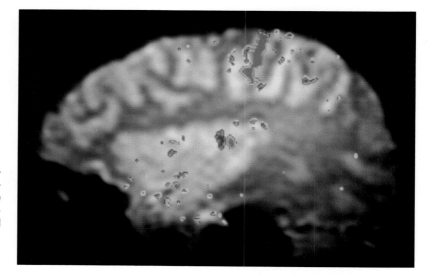

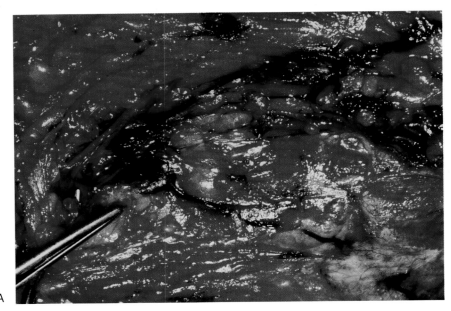

A

B

COLOR PLATE 4. A: Blue dye highlights the path of lymphatics in the inguinal basin draining a primary cutaneous melanoma on the lower back. Forceps point to the blue-staining sentinel node. (Reprinted with permission from Morton DL, Wen D-R, Wong JH, et al. Technical details of intraoperative lymphatic mapping for early stage melanoma. *Arch Surg* 1992;127:392) B: Blue dye stains skin around a primary melanoma on the cheek (*top left*) incision over the cervical basin reveals blue-staining sentinel node (*bottom right*) adjacent to the superficial lobe of the parotid gland. (Reprinted with permission from Morton DL, Wen D-R, Foshag LJ, Essner R, Cochran A. Intraoperative lymphatic mapping and selective cervical lymphadenectomy for early-stage melanomas of the head and neck. *J Clin Oncol* 1993; 11:1751.) (See also Figs. 2A,B, page 295.)

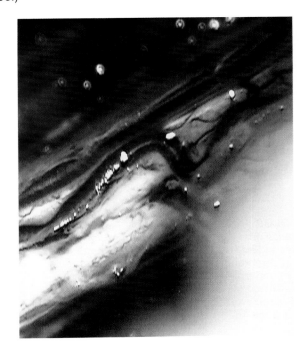

COLOR PLATE 5. Commissural myelotomy. Intraoperative photograph obtained through the operating microscope demonstrating longitudinal medial splitting of three segments of the thoracolumbar spinal cord. (See also Fig. 10, page 410.)

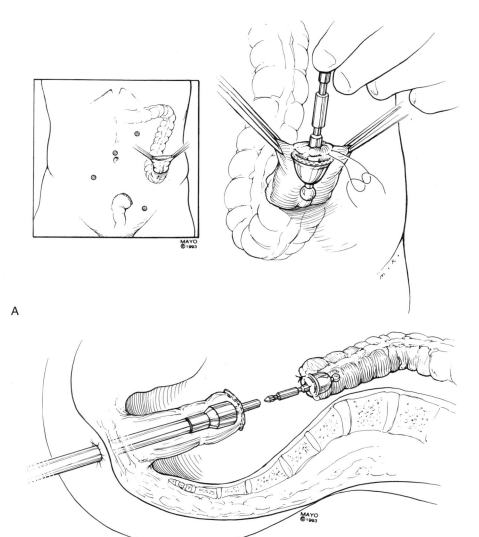

A

B

FIG. 7. The left midabdominal cannula site is extended into a 4- to 6-cm incision, and the proximal bowel is readily exteriorized and resected. The anvil of a circular stapler is secured within the bowel with a purse-string and the bowel is returned to the abdominal cavity. With the wound closed, pneumoperitoneum is reestablished and the shaft of the stapler in the rectum is connected with the proximal anvil. After the stapler is fired, the donuts are inspected for defects.

tality and complication rates for laparoscopic-assisted colectomy have been comparable to those for standard open colectomy. Mortality rates vary from 0% to 3.6%, morbidity rates from 0% to 30% (Table 1) (9,10,12,13,16, 18,23,26). The overall mortality, 0.6%, in this group of

TABLE 1. *Laparoscopic colectomy: mortality and morbidity rates*

Author, year	No. patients	Morbidity (%)	Mortality (%)
Jacobs, 1991 (18)	20	30	—
Phillips, 1992 (13)	51	8	2
Falk, 1993 (9)	66	24	0
Peters, 1993 (12)	28	13	3.6
Senagore, 1993 (16)	38	15	—
Dean, 1994 (23)	122	11	0
Hoffman, 1994 (10)	80	23	0
Lacy, 1995 (26)	21	9.5	—

347 patients in which mortality is specifically reported is very similar to that reported for open colectomy. The Mayo Clinic series of 122 patients showed no mortality and an 11% major morbidity rate (23). In this same report, seven intraoperative complications (atrial fibrillation, ureteral injury, bowel rotation, enterotomy [3], and hemorrhage) and six postoperative complications (prolonged ileus [3], small bowel obstruction, urinary retention, and recurrent prolapse) were reported. Neither the rate nor the severity of complications appears unique to laparoscopic-assisted colectomy.

Clinical Results

The feasibility of laparoscopic-assisted colectomy has been evaluated in terms of operative time and rate of conversion to open surgery. In early reports, operative times for both completed and converted laparoscopic-assisted

TABLE 2. *Laparoscopic colectomy: operative times and conversion rates*

Author, year	No. patients	Operative times (min)			Conversion rates (%)
		Laparoscopic	Converted	Open	
Senagore, 1993 (16)	38	174	204	126	32
Peters, 1993 (12)	28	136	—	77*	14
Dean, 1994 (23)	122	143	114	—	48
Hoffman, 1994 (10)	80	221	244	183	23
Lacy, 1995 (26)	21	153	—	117	—

*Data for right colectomy. For sigmoid resection, operative times were reported as 193 min for laparoscopic resection and 94 min for open.

colectomy tended to be longer than for standard open surgery (Table 2) (9,10,12,13,16,18,23,26). Although most authors report that converted cases take longer to perform than completed cases, the Mayo Clinic series reported that converted cases were quicker, reflecting an initial policy of rapid assessment and rapid conversion when indicated (23). As is often true for new surgical procedures, laparoscopic colectomy is associated with a significant learning curve. That operative time decreases significantly with increasing experience has been repeatedly described. The plateau effect most often occurs somewhere between 10 and 20 cases (9,12).

Like operative times, conversion rates, which vary from 14% to 48%, are also inversely related to experience (see Table 2) (10,13,16,23,26). Hoffman and colleagues reported a decrease in the conversion rate to open colectomy from 22.5% to 15% when comparing the first and second half of his series of 80 patients (10). In an attempt to examine preoperative selection factors, the early Mayo experience included a diverse population of patients and diseases. In this series of 122 patients, obesity (specifically, weight exceeding 90 kg) was the only factor that reliably predicted conversion (75%) (23). Although adhesions are a common indication for conversion, and conversion rates are generally lower when patients with previous surgery are excluded, surprisingly, a history of previous abdominal surgery is not predictive for conversion.

Conversion to an open colectomy may be necessary for any number of reasons. Technical reasons may include prohibitive adhesions, inability to localize primary tumor, instrumentation difficulties, prolonged surgical times, or variation in anatomy. Primary tumor factors such as the presence of a large bulky tumor or

adherence to adjacent structures or intraoperative complications such as bleeding, bowel injury, or surgical misadventure may also lead to conversion. Conversion to an open colectomy should be regarded as the application of sound surgical judgment rather than as a complication or failure. Increased experience, improved techniques, and refined instrumentation are likely to affect safety, operative times, and conversion rates.

Many of the same patient-related advantages described for laparoscopic cholecystectomy may be realized with laparoscopic colectomy. Patients undergoing laparoscopic colectomy experience reductions in the length of ileus, with more rapid return of flatus, bowel movement, and tolerance of oral intake (Table 3) (10,12,14,16,23, 26). The reasons for shortened postoperative ileus are not yet clear, but possible explanations include associated reductions in postoperative pain, narcotic requirements, and operative bowel manipulations. Reductions in the length of hospital stay compared to open colectomy have been reported (Table 4) (9,10,12,16,23). In some cases, a cosmetic advantage may be accomplished, due to the limited size or strategic location of the scar.

The reduction in the duration of postoperative ileus and the length of hospital stay has led to the evaluation of costs with laparoscopic-assisted colectomy. Costs have been analyzed in three reports totaling 135 laparoscopic colectomy patients (9,14,16). When total hospital costs for all laparoscopic colectomies, completed plus converted ($27,387), are compared to the costs for open colectomies ($24,219), the laparoscopic procedures appear more expensive (14). However, when completed and converted procedures are independently examined, completed laparoscopic colectomies ($12,131±612)

TABLE 3. *Laparoscopic colectomy: return of bowel function (days)*

Author, year	No. patients	Laparoscopic	Converted	Open	Parameter
Senagore, 1993 (16)	38	3	4.3	4.9	oral intake
Vayer, 1993 (14)	38	3.2	—	5.5	flatus
Peters, 1993 (12)	28	2.3	—	4.6	flatus
		2.3	—	3.7	oral intake
Dean, 1994 (23)	122	2.3	4.8	—	oral intake
Hoffman, 1994 (10)	80	2	3	4	flatus
		3	5	5	regular diet

TABLE 4. *Laparoscopic colectomy: length of hospital stay (days)*

Author, year	No. patients	Laparoscopic	Converted	Open
Falk, 1993 (9)*	66	5	8	8
Senagore, 1993 (16)	38	6	9.3	9.9
Peters, 1993 (12)	28	4.8	—	8.2
Dean, 1994 (23)	122	5.7	8.4	—
Hoffman, 1994 (10)	80	5.2	6.5	7.8
Lacy, 1995 (26)	21	6.0	—	8.4

*Length of stay estimated from Fig. 3, right and sigmoid colectomy combined.

appear to be less costly than converted laparoscopic colectomies ($17,583±173) and are cost-competitive with open colectomies ($14,449±696) (9,16). Hoffman and colleagues, who reported that laparoscopic completed and converted procedures were slightly more expensive than open colectomy ($12,464, $13,956, and $10,213, respectively), examined the components of cost and noted that the cost savings from reduced length of stay were offset by increased operating room expenses—operating room charges were $7,351, $7,148, and $3,990 for laparoscopic completed, converted, and open procedures, respectively (10). In the future, improvements in patient selection, surgical experience, operative times, and conversion rates, and the availability of better reusable instruments are likely to decrease the costs associated with laparoscopic colectomy.

Another potential advantage of laparoscopic-assisted colectomy is that it may decrease operative stress. Animal data demonstrate that with laparoscopy, the immunosuppressive effects of surgery are less dramatic. Evidence that surgical stress is lessened after laparoscopic colectomy comes from studies of serum cortisol and interleukin 6 (IL-6), both of which normally rise in proportion to the degree of surgical trauma. When preoperative and postoperative serum cortisol and IL-6 levels were compared between laparoscopic and open colectomy patients, cortisol levels were similar but IL-6 levels were significantly decreased in the laparoscopic colectomy group (27). It is premature to judge the clinical relevance of these immunologic data as well as other favorable physiologic indicators, but these findings represent at least theoretical advantages for laparoscopy. Further support for these theoretical advantages comes from animal models where laparotomy compared to pneumoperitoneum is associated with more of a systemic tumor-permissive effect (28). Additional studies are indicated to examine local and systemic factors and to expand the model to include a laparoscopic-assisted resective procedure. Taken together, it is possible that patients undergoing laparoscopy may benefit from a faster recovery and earlier administration of adjuvant therapy or from immunologic advantages. The latter requires further investigation, however.

Finally, laparoscopic colectomy may reduce the number of postoperative adhesions, as demonstrated for laparoscopic appendectomy. In a prospective randomized trial, the occurrence of late adhesion formation was significantly lower in patients who underwent laparoscopic appendectomy (10%) compared to those who underwent open appendectomy (80%) (15). This reduction in adhesions may also be relevant for patients undergoing laparoscopic-assisted colectomy. Because late postoperative bowel obstruction affects 5% to 15% of patients, reducing adhesions may have a significant impact on late surgical complications and overall patient satisfaction.

Although most would agree that palliative laparoscopic procedures are reasonable in patients with stage IV colorectal cancer, the appropriateness of laparoscopic resection for surgically curable colon cancer remains controversial. Ultimately, the appropriateness of laparoscopic colectomy for colon cancer will be measured by its impact on recurrence and survival rates. Prospective randomized trials are underway to provide such important data, but in the meantime several essential issues demand thoughtful consideration:

Can a comparable exploration be performed laparoscopically, with or without additional imaging modalities, such as CT or hepatic ultrasound, external or intraoperative?

Are laparoscopic cancer resections comparable to open resections?

Is staging with laparoscopy comparable to staging with open surgery?

Are patterns of recurrence altered with the laparoscopic technique?

Concern regarding the adequacy of laparoscopic exploration comes from the fact that laparoscopic hepatic evaluation is limited to visual inspection. Supplementing the laparoscopic examination with a preoperative abdominal CT scan, with a negative predictive value of 90% (29) and sensitivity of 100% compared to surgery (30), may resolve this limitation. Combining preoperative abdominal CT with laparoscopic exploration is likely to detect most, if not all, synchronous hepatic metastases. A CT scan also may visualize the primary tumor and detect adjacent structure invasion, which would mandate laparotomy. Other findings, such as the presence of duplicate ureters, would be helpful when mobilization is undertaken.

With the intent of improving or assisting laparoscopic exploration, laparoscopic ultrasound probes have been developed. No data are available with respect to the potential improvement of liver evaluation in the setting of colon carcinoma. John and colleagues reported a series of 50 patients, 43 of whom underwent laparoscopy and laparoscopic ultrasound to evaluate the liver before hepatic resection (31). Laparoscopic ultrasound identified tumors not visualized by laparoscopy in 14 patients (33%) and provided additional information not derived from laparoscopy alone in 18 patients (42%). With the use of laparoscopy and laparoscopic ultrasound, resectability rates were increased to 93%, compared to 58%. These data demonstrate great promise for the use of laparoscopic hepatic ultrasound.

As to the adequacy of resection and nodal staging, reports to date suggest that both margins of resection and mesenteric resections are comparable for laparoscopic and open colectomy. In a series of 80 patients undergoing laparoscopic colectomy, with 38 performed for cancer, Hoffman and colleagues reported that the closest margins for open colectomy (6.7 cm) were comparable to those for laparoscopic colectomy (5.8 cm) (10). Similarly, with few exceptions, the number of nodes resected with open colectomy is not significantly different from the number resected with laparoscopic colectomy (Table 5) (9,10,12, 26,32). With adequate experience, a comparable resection can be carried out laparoscopically. Proponents of laparoscopic colectomy advocate that a standard resection with proximal mesenteric resection and at least 5- to 10-cm margins should be performed for cancer cases. Laparoscopic resections should be *identical* to corresponding open procedures.

Even if laparoscopic colon resections are identical to open colectomy, the issue of whether laparoscopic techniques alter patterns of recurrence must be addressed. Wound and trocar site recurrences after laparoscopic colectomy—13 cases to date—raise concern that tumor cell dissemination may be enhanced by the seepage of pneumoperitoneal gases through operative cannulae or by the passage of large tumors through small surgical wounds. Although data from controlled trials are not yet available, the best estimate of wound recurrence after laparoscopic colectomy, from a registry reported by

Ramos and colleagues, is 1.4% (33). This figure reasonably matches the incidence of such wound recurrences after open colectomy—0.8% (34) to 2.5% (35). A direct prospective comparison is essential to address this concern objectively, and at least one phase 3 trial is in progress. A consortium of surgeons with laparoscopic colectomy experience has been established and, using an intergroup mechanism (including CALGB, ECOG, NCCTG, RTOG, and SWOG), is performing a prospective randomized trial to compare laparoscopic and open colectomy. A patient accrual of 1,200 will be required to test the primary hypothesis, that disease-free and overall survival rates are equivalent, whether patients receive laparoscopic or open colectomy.

In summary, laparoscopic colectomy is an important new technique that can be performed with acceptable morbidity and mortality. Advantages such as decreases in postoperative ileus, pain, and hospital stay are reported but must be documented in controlled trials. Although there are theoretical advantages to applying laparoscopic techniques to colon tumors, the lack of long-term recurrence and survival data precludes the wide application of these procedures at this time for curable colon tumors.

Patient Care Considerations

After laparoscopic colon surgery, patient recovery is managed in a manner similar to open colectomy, only generally at a faster pace. The nasogastric tube is removed in the recovery room or the next morning. For abdominal colectomies, the urinary catheter can be removed as soon as the patient can use a urinal or restroom. For pelvic procedures, return of bladder function is often delayed, and urinary catheter drainage is useful until there is evidence of the return of bowel function, usually at 4 to 6 days. Same-day or next-day ambulation can be accomplished in most patients. Pain is managed initially with intravenous patient-controlled analgesia and subsequently with oral analgesics. Dietary intake is regulated using the same principles as patient-controlled analgesia. Patients are offered a liquid diet the morning after surgery and allowed to advance as tolerated.

Hospital discharge can be considered when the patient can maintain hydration and nutritional support through oral intake. Although some objective evidence of colonic function, such as passage of flatus, is generally present by the time the patient is enterally self-sufficient, it is unnecessary to delay dismissal for complete function (ie, passage of stool). The patient may be discharged before the passage of a bowel movement, provided close contact is maintained and hospital services for potential complications are readily available. Outpatient follow-up and initiation of adjuvant therapies are performed as customary for open colectomy. Although patients are often strong enough to return to unrestricted activities within a few weeks of laparo-

TABLE 5. *Mesenteric lymph node harvest for laparoscopic versus open colectomy*

Author, year	No. lymph nodes	
	Laparoscopic	Open
Peters, 1993 (12)	9.0*	8.5*
	7.3†	4.7†
Falk, 1993 (9)	14*	9*
	9†	5†
Ota, 1994 (32)	8.8*	18.8*
Hoffman, 1994 (10)	8.0	6.1
Lacy, 1995 (26)	12.7	12.8

*Right hemicolectomy; †sigmoid colectomy

scopic surgery, they should be encouraged to avoid strenuous lifting, as incisional hernias may develop.

RECTAL TUMORS

Detailed Methodology

Most of the conclusions reached for colon tumors probably apply as well to rectal tumors. Indeed, many of the clinical reports include "colorectal" procedures. The techniques for performing laparoscopic abdominoperineal resection have many similarities to laparoscopic colectomy, particularly for the abdominal phase of the operation. The left colon is mobilized and the vascular pedicle ligated using the techniques previously described (24). The rectum is then mobilized, the proximal bowel divided, and a colonic stoma created. The perineal phase of the operation is performed as for a standard abdominoperineal resection. In experimental models, laparoscopic abdominoperineal resection provides a resection equivalent to open abdominoperineal resection (36).

Clinical Results

Decanini and colleagues examined the thoroughness of laparoscopic abdominoperineal resection in a series of 11 abdominoperineal resections performed on fresh cadavers (36). After the laparoscopic procedure, laparotomy was performed to examine the completeness of the procedure. Based on this series, they concluded that laparoscopic abdominoperineal resection could be performed according to standard oncologic principles, including proximal vascular ligation, wide clearance of the pelvic side wall, and complete mesorectal excision.

The technical similarities between laparoscopic colectomy and laparoscopic abdominoperineal resection will probably translate into similar outcomes and benefits. Unfortunately, separate analyses for laparoscopic abdominoperineal resection are rare, with only a few reports published to date. Dodson and colleagues reported three laparoscopic abdominoperineal resections (17). In this small series, there was one mortality; the other 2 patients experienced shorter hospital stays than historical controls. Kumar and colleagues reported and compared five laparoscopic abdominoperineal resections to 18 conventional abdominoperineal resections (37). No differences in operative times, blood loss, extent of tumor resection, or lymph node dissection were identified. Larger experiences and more controlled evaluations will be required before definitive conclusions can be drawn.

Despite numerous similarities between laparoscopic rectal resections and laparoscopic colon resections, several distinctions deserve attention. The first is the risk of wound or trocar recurrences. It has been suggested that due to the extraperitoneal position of rectal tumors, there is no risk of intraperitoneal tumor contamination and, therefore, no risk of altering patterns of recurrence with laparoscopic abdominoperineal resection. Theoretically, viable tumor cells should not be present in the abdominal cavity with rectal malignancies, below the peritoneal reflection. Whether dissection of the rectum at or below the level of the tumor introduces viable tumor cells into the peritoneal cavity has not been determined. Therefore, laparoscopic abdominoperineal resection may or may not have the same theoretical risks as laparoscopic colectomy. Further studies are essential. Perhaps equally important is the question of whether maximal efforts at sphincter preservation can be achieved using the laparoscopic approach.

Recent emphasis has focused on sphincter-preserving procedures, including the coloanal anastomosis and the application of neoadjuvant therapy for the purposes of reducing tumor size and maximizing the length of tumor-free margins. In most cases of low-lying rectal tumors (within 5 cm of the dentate line), the determination as to whether the sphincter can be preserved or must be sacrificed is made intraoperatively. It is not yet known whether the same intraoperative assessment can be accomplished with laparoscopy. For lesions that directly involve the sphincters, where the abdominal dissection does not violate the site of the tumor, laparoscopic abdominoperineal resection probably offers advantages without significant risks.

Patient Care Considerations

Patient management after laparoscopic rectal procedures differs only minimally from that described for laparoscopic-assisted colectomy. As described above, urinary catheter drainage should be maintained for 4 to 6 days. For abdominal perineal resections, perineal drains are maintained on suction until the output has diminished, usually to <30 cc/day. If the patient is otherwise ready for dismissal but high drain output persists, then the perineal drains can be managed on bulb suction as an outpatient. Adaptation to a new stoma may present the greatest impediment to early hospital discharge. The time required for proper adjustment must be acknowledged by healthcare providers. If outpatient enterostomal support services are readily accessible on a frequent basis, it may be physically and psychologically possible for the patient to manage and accept the stoma despite an early dismissal.

PANCREATIC TUMORS

Background

Pancreatic cancer, the fifth leading cause of cancer deaths in the United States, is curative in at most 10% to 15% of patients. Although laparoscopic resective procedures such as distal pancreatectomy and Whipple have been described (38,39), probably the more important question is whether laparoscopic staging or palliative techniques can improve the quality of life for these patients with limited life expectancy. For example, if accurate laparoscopic staging can preclude the need for full laparotomy in patients with technically unresectable pancreatic cancer, this may minimize morbidity and convalescence in patients who have few months to live.

Laparoscopic staging includes visual inspection of the parietal peritoneal surfaces, visceral peritoneum, and liver. Small tumor implants, not identified using conventional imaging techniques, can frequently be detected and biopsied with laparoscopy. The pancreas can be visualized using the supragastric approach, through an opening in the gastrocolic omentum, or the infracolic approach, through an opening in the transverse mesocolon. Laparoscopic ultrasound probes may further enhance pancreatic visualization, establishing the location of a tumor or vascular structure (40,41).

Laparoscopic staging has been advocated as a prelude for more radical resective procedures (42–45). Cuschieri reported a series of 73 patients undergoing laparoscopy for pancreatic cancer (42). Fifty-one patients had laparoscopy immediately before laparotomy. Forty-two of the 51 were correctly judged to be inoperable. Four of the 9 patients judged to be resectable by laparoscopy were in fact resectable. Warshaw and colleagues studied the accuracy of preoperative staging of pancreatic cancer in 88 patients using CT scan, magnetic resonance imaging, angiography, and laparoscopy (45). Laparoscopy detected liver and peritoneal metastases in 22 of 23 cases, with an overall accuracy of 98%. Seventy-eight percent of pancreatic head carcinomas were resectable if CT, angiogram, and laparoscopy were negative. If any single test was positive, only 5% were resectable. Based on these early reports, laparoscopy is likely to play an important role in the staging of pancreatic cancer.

Detailed Methodology

Laparoscopic interventions may similarly be useful in the palliation of unresectable pancreatic carcinomas. Both biliary-enteric (46–49) and gastroenteric (49–51) bypass procedures have been described for biliary and duodenal obstruction, respectively. Although endoscopically and percutaneously placed biliary stents have been shown to have lower complication rates than open surgical decompression (52,53), such stents are associated with significant problems, such as stent occlusion, recurrent jaundice, and cholangitis. By using laparoscopic techniques, the complication rates from surgery may be reduced and the success of long-term palliation improved.

Biliary decompression using a laparoscopic cholecystojejunostomy technique has been described using both stapled and sutured anastomoses (46–49). A disease-free gallbladder is required to perform the anastomosis, and evidence of chronic cholelithiasis makes this technique undesirable. A loop of jejunum is identified near the ligament of Treitz and anastomosed to the gallbladder. Before anastomosis, a cholangiogram is required to document that tumor does not encroach on the cystic/common bile duct junction. With a needle inserted into the fundus of the gallbladder, contrast is injected and fluoroscopy performed.

Clinical Results

Although no large series are available to evaluate results from biliary decompression using laparoscopic cholecystojejunostomy conclusively, Shimi and colleagues have reported five cases of laparoscopic cholecystojejunostomy (46). Four of the patients had rapid relief of their jaundice; the fifth patient required a laparoscopic reevaluation with eventual successful biliary decompression. Potential benefits of laparoscopic cholecystojejunostomy, including reduced ileus, pain, and hospital stay, can probably be realized. Hawasli (47) and Fletcher and Jones (48) have reported cases of laparoscopic cholecystojejunostomies with early oral intake and early discharge. Whether or not this laparoscopic application is better than endoscopic stenting or open bypass remains to be proven.

Laparoscopic decompression of duodenal obstruction has also been described (49–51). The technique is similar to laparoscopic cholecystojejunostomy. A loop of jejunum near the ligament of Treitz is anastomosed to the anterior surface of the stomach. Combining endoscopic stenting and laparoscopic gastrojejunostomy has been advocated by Mouiel and colleagues (50). Such an approach would obviate the need for laparotomy, but the success and therefore the role of this form of bypass remain to be defined.

In summary, the role of laparoscopy in the management of pancreatic cancer requires further experience and evaluation. Evidence suggests that preoperative staging can be improved with laparoscopy, thereby sparing patients the need for a laparotomy. Laparoscopic palliative procedures, if proven to be effective, have great potential for improving quality of life in patients with a limited life expectancy. Finally, laparoscopic resection techniques may become more feasible with future refinements.

ADRENAL TUMORS

Background

Although laparoscopic resection for malignant adrenal tumors is frequently impossible or inappropriate due to the size of these tumors at presentation, unilateral and bilateral laparoscopic adrenalectomies for benign hormone-producing tumors are increasingly being attempted. Due to the retroperitoneal location and close proximity to major vascular structures, laparoscopic adrenalectomy is difficult, particularly on the right. Direct comparisons between laparoscopic and open adrenalectomy are not simple due to the many and varied technical approaches.

Detailed Methodology

Traditional open surgical approaches to adrenalectomies include transabdominal, thoracoabdominal, flank, and posterior incisions. The transabdominal approach allows complete abdominal exploration and generous exposure for vascular control. The thoracoabdominal approach has the same benefits as the transabdominal approach, with the addition of better thoracic exposure, which is ideal for large tumors and if a portion of diaphragm must be resected. Morbidities associated with the laparotomy and thoracotomy can be avoided by using the flank or posterior approach. The flank incision, a retroperitoneal approach, decreases the amount of bowel manipulation and potentially decreases the postoperative ileus; however, complete abdominal exploration is impossible, and rib resection may be required. The posterior approach requires a rib resection and does not permit abdominal exploration. Recovery time is quickest using the posterior approach.

The best technique for laparoscopic adrenalectomy has not been determined (39,54–57). Factors making laparoscopic adrenalectomy challenging include the gland's retroperitoneal location and abundant surrounding adipose tissue. It is a fragile gland, is difficult to grasp, and resides in close proximity to other organs and vascular structures. Most laparoscopic adrenalectomies reported use a transabdominal approach with the patient in the lateral position. Four trocars are placed along the flank, allowing exposure to the retroperitoneal adrenal gland. Mobilization and vascular ligation are then accomplished, allowing resection.

Clinical Results

A series of 21 laparoscopic adrenalectomies was reported by Gagner and colleagues with a mean operative time of 2.3 hours (39). Left laparoscopic adrenalectomies averaged 1.8 hours, right adrenalectomies 2.7 hours. A single patient was converted to an open procedure. The median hospital stay was 4 days. Suzuki and colleagues reported a series of 12 laparoscopic adrenalectomies and compared them to 11 open procedures (55). Laparoscopic adrenalectomy was associated with significantly prolonged operative times, but reduced times to first oral intake, ambulation, and return to preoperative activities.

Three laparoscopic cases in one report were complicated by "massive" bleeding intraoperatively.

The use of laparoscopic techniques in adrenal surgery is technically possible, but the potential use in malignant tumors is unknown. Many malignant adrenocortical carcinomas are very large at presentation, making laparoscopic removal unsafe using current techniques. Laparoscopic adrenalectomy will probably find a role in the resection of benign, relatively small tumors.

LYMPHOMA

Background

Casirola and colleagues advocated the use of laparoscopic evaluation of the liver in Hodgkin's lymphoma as early as 1973, but this option has only recently been seriously reconsidered (58). The staging laparotomy, consisting of an abdominal exploration, liver biopsy, lymph node sampling, splenectomy, and in some cases oophoropexy, has been the tradition in staging for select cases of Hodgkin's lymphoma (59–61). If laparoscopic staging is to replace staging laparotomy, results of each must be compared.

The classic staging laparotomy is associated with a low rate of morbidity and mortality. Taylor and colleagues, in a series of 825 staging laparotomies performed at Stanford University Hospital, reported only one mortality (60). A 9.6% major complication rate was reported; most of the complications were related to the wound or respiratory tract. The clinical stage was altered as a result of the laparotomy in 43.2% of cases. The average postoperative hospital stay was 6.5 days.

Detailed Methodology

Due to refinements in laparoscopic technology, most if not all components of the staging laparotomy for Hodgkin's lymphoma can now be performed laparoscopically. There are reported cases of complete staging laparoscopy, including splenectomy, using both laparoscopic and laparoscopic-assisted techniques (62–64). Laparoscopic evaluations of the liver are well described and not technically demanding. Part of the hepatic surface can be inspected laparoscopically, and percutaneous core needle biopsies may be obtained with hemostasis achieved with electrocautery under direct vision. Lefor and Flowers have described a technique of laparoscopic hepatic wedge biopsy using an endoscopic stapling device (65).

The need to perform splenectomy as part of a staging laparotomy is controversial. The technique of laparoscopic splenectomy is evolving, and techniques are described for both complete laparoscopic and laparoscopic-assisted procedures (66–70). In cases of Hodgkin's lymphoma where splenectomy is desirable, pathologists prefer to receive an intact spleen, where the structural anatomy has been preserved and the histologic architecture can be assessed. This precludes the use of endoscopic morcellating devices and mandates the use of a minilaparotomy for specimen extraction.

Clinical Results

Preoperative splenic artery embolization has been described as a technique to minimize blood loss (67,68). Early results with laparoscopic splenectomy are limited. Poulin and colleagues, in a series of 22 laparoscopic splenectomies, reported a conversion rate of 9%, a mean operative time of 3 hours and 35 minutes, and a mean postoperative stay of 3.9 days (68). All patients but 2 were back to normal activities within 2 weeks of surgery. Data such as these show the feasibility and potential advantages of laparoscopic splenectomy.

The laparoscopic sampling of lymph nodes has been described for staging purposes in genitourinary and gynecologic malignancies (71,72). Para-aortic lymphadenectomy, which is technically most challenging, has also been described (73,74). This experience is being incorporated into the laparoscopic staging of lymphomas (62). The role of laparoscopic staging of lymphoma is yet to be defined. Although the individual components of a classical staging laparotomy can be performed using laparoscopic techniques, a formal comparison or critical appraisal has not been reported. Further innovations, such as more practical and efficient laparoscopic ultrasound probes, may improve the diagnostic yield of laparoscopic staging of lymphoma.

REFERENCES

1. NIH Consensus Conference. Gallstones and laparoscopic cholecystectomy. *JAMA* 1993;269:1018.
2. Attwood SEA, Hill ADK, Mealy K, Stephens RB. A prospective comparison of laparoscopic versus open cholecystectomy. *Ann R Coll Surg Engl* 1992;74:397.
3. Stoker ME, Vose J, O'Mara P, Maini BS. Laparoscopic cholecystectomy: a clinical and financial analysis of 280 operations. *Arch Surg* 1992;127:589.
4. Grace PA, Quereshi A, Coleman J, et al. Reduced postoperative hospitalization after laparoscopic cholecystectomy. *Br J Surg* 1991;78:160.
5. Kelley JE, Burrus RG, Burns RP, Graham LD, Chandler KE. Safety, efficacy, cost, and morbidity of laparoscopic versus open cholecystectomy: a prospective analysis of 228 consecutive patients. *Am Surg* 1993;59:23.
6. Sanabria JR, Clavien PA, Cywes R, Strasberg SM. Laparoscopic versus open cholecystectomy: a matched study. *CJS* 1993;36:330.
7. Donohue JH, Farnell MB, Grant CS, et al. Laparoscopic cholecystectomy: early Mayo Clinic experience. *Mayo Clin Proc* 1992;67:449.
8. Corbitt JD Jr. Preliminary experience with laparoscopic-guided colectomy. *Surg Laparoscopy Endosc* 1992;2:79.
9. Falk PM, Beart RW Jr, Wexner SD, et al. Laparoscopic colectomy: a critical appraisal. *Dis Colon Rectum* 1993;36:28.
10. Hoffman GC, Baker JW, Fitchett CW, Vansant JH. Laparoscopic-assisted colectomy: initial experience. *Ann Surg* 1994;219:732.
11. Milsom JW, Lavery IC, Church JM, Stolfi VM, Fazio VW. Use of laparoscopic techniques in colorectal surgery: preliminary study. *Dis Colon Rectum* 1994;37:215.
12. Peters WR, Bartels TL. Minimally invasive colectomy: are the potential benefits realized? *Dis Colon Rectum* 1993;36:751.
13. Phillips EH, Franklin M, Carroll BJ, Fallas MJ, Ramos R, Rosenthal D. Laparoscopic colectomy. *Ann Surg* 1992;216:703.
14. Vayer AJ Jr, Larach SW, Williamson PR, Ferrara A, Salomon M. Cost effectiveness of laparoscopic assisted colectomy. *Dis Colon Rectum* 1993;36:34A.
15. DeWilde RL. Goodbye to late bowel obstruction after appendectomy. *Lancet* 1991;338:1012.
16. Senagore AJ, Luchtefeld MA, MacKeigan JM, Mazier WP. Open colectomy versus laparoscopic colectomy: are there differences? *Am Surg* 1993;59:549.
17. Dodson RW, Cullado MJ, Tangen LE, Bonello JC. Laparoscopic-assisted abdominoperineal resection. *Contemp Surg* 1993;42:42.
18. Jacobs M, Verdeja JC, Goldstein HS. Minimally invasive colon resection (laparoscopic colectomy). *Surg Laparoscopy Endosc* 1991;1:144.
19. Scoggin SD, Frazee RC, Snyder SK, et al. Laparoscopic-assisted bowel surgery. *Dis Colon Rectum* 1993;36:747.
20. Saclarides TJ, Ko ST, Airan M, Dillon C, Franklin J. Laparoscopic removal of a large colonic lipoma: report of a case. *Dis Colon Rectum* 1991;34:1027.
21. Wexner SD, Johansen OB, Nogueras JJ, Jagelman DG. Laparoscopic total abdominal colectomy: a prospective trial. *Dis Colon Rectum* 1992;35:651.
22. Peters WR. Laparoscopic total proctocolectomy with creation of ileostomy for ulcerative colitis: report of two cases. *J Laparoendosc Surg* 1992;2:175.
23. Dean PA, Beart RW Jr, Nelson H, Elftmann TD, Schlinkert RT. Laparoscopic-assisted segmental colectomy: early Mayo Clinic experience. *Mayo Clin Proc* 1994;69:834–840.
24. Elftmann TD, Nelson H, Ota DM, Pemberton JH, Beart RW Jr. Laparoscopic-assisted segmental colectomy: surgical techniques. *Mayo Clin Proc* 1994;69:825.
25. Hasson HM. Open laparoscopy vs. closed laparoscopy: a comparison of complication rates. *Adv Planned Parenthood* 1978;13:41.
26. Lacy AM, Garciá-Valdecasas JC, Delgado S, et al. Laparoscopic versus conventional surgery in colon cancer: preliminary results of a prospective randomized trial. *Surg Endosc* 1995;9:216.
27. Harmon G, Senagore AJ, Kilbride M, Luchtefeld M, MacKeigan J, Warzynski M. Cortisol and IL-6 response attenuated following laparoscopic colectomy. *Surg Endoscopy* 1993;7:121A.
28. Allendorf JD, Kayton M, Libutti S, Whelan R, Bessler M. The effect of laparotomy vs. insufflation on tumor establishment and growth. *Dis Colon Rectum* 1994;37:11.
29. Cance WG, Cohen AM, Enker WE, Sigurdson ER. Predictive value of a negative computed tomographic scan in 100 patients with rectal carcinoma. *Dis Colon Rectum* 1991;34:748.
30. Fisher KS, Zamboni WA, Ross DS. The efficacy of preoperative computed tomography in patients with colorectal carcinoma. *Am Surg* 1990;56:339.
31. John TG, Greig D, Crosbie JL, Miles WFA, Garden OJ. Superior staging of liver tumors with laparoscopy and laparoscopic ultrasound. *Ann Surg* 1994;220:711.
32. Ota DM, Nelson H, Weeks JC. Controversies regarding laparoscopic colectomy for malignant diseases. *Curr Op Gen Surg* 1994:208.
33. Ramos JM, Gupta S, Anthone GJ, Ortega AE, Simons AJ, Beart RW Jr. Laparoscopy and colon cancer: is the port site at risk? A preliminary report. *Arch Surg* 1994;129:897.
34. Hughes ESR, McDermott FT, Polglase AL, Johnson WR. Tumor recurrence in the abdominal wall scar tissue after large-bowel cancer surgery. *Dis Colon Rectum* 1983;26:571.
35. Cass AW, Million RR, Pfaff WW. Patterns of recurrence following surgery alone for adenocarcinoma of the colon and rectum. *Cancer* 1976;37:2861.
36. Decanini C, Milsom JW, Böhm B, Fazio VW. Laparoscopic oncologic abdominoperineal resection. *Dis Colon Rectum* 1994;37:552.
37. Kumar RR, Ballantyne GH, Thornton S, McMillen MA. Laparoscopic abdominoperineal resection. *Surg Endosc* 1995;9:216.
38. Gagner M, Pomp A. Laparoscopic pylorus-preserving pancreatoduodenectomy. *Surg Endosc* 1994;8:408.
39. Gagner M, Lacroix A, Bolté E, Pomp A. Laparoscopic adrenalectomy: the importance of a frank approach in the lateral decubitus position. *Surg Endosc* 1994;8:135.
40. Murugiah M, Paterson-Brown S, Windsor JA, Miles WFA, Garden OJ.

Early experience of laparoscopic ultrasonography in the management of pancreatic carcinoma. *Surg Endosc* 1993;7:177.

41. Pietrabissa A, Shimi SM, Vander Velpen G, Cuschieri A. Localization of insulinoma by laparoscopic infragastric inspection of the pancreas and contact ultrasonography. *Surg Oncol* 1993;2:83.
42 Cuschieri A. Laparoscopy for pancreatic cancer: does it benefit the patient? *Eur J Surg Oncol* 1988;14:41.
43. del Castillo CF, Warshaw AL. Laparoscopy for staging in pancreatic carcinoma. *Surg Oncol* 1993;2:25.
44. del Castillo CF, Warshaw L. Peritoneal metastases in pancreatic carcinoma. *Hepato-Gastroenterology* 1993;40:430.
45. Warshaw AL, Gu Z, Wittenberg J, Waltman AC. Preoperative staging and assessment of resectability of pancreatic cancer. *Arch Surg* 1990;125:230.
46. Shimi S, Banting S, Cuschieri A. Laparoscopy in the management of pancreatic cancer: endoscopic cholecystojejunostomy for advanced disease. *Br J Surg* 1992;79:317.
47. Hawasli A. Laparoscopic cholecysto-jejunostomy for obstructing pancreatic cancer: technique and report of two cases. *J Laparoendo Surg* 1992;2:351.
48. Fletcher DR, Jones RM. Laparoscopic cholecystojejunostomy as palliation for obstructive jaundice in inoperable carcinoma of pancreas. *Surg Endosc* 1992;6:147.
49. Nathanson LK. Laparoscopic cholecysto-jejunostomy and gastroenterostomy for malignant disease. *Surg Oncol* 1993;2:19.
50. Mouiel J, Katkhouda N, White S, Dumas R. Endolaparoscopic palliation of pancreatic cancer. *Surg Laparosc Endosc* 1992;2:241.
51. Rangraj MS, Mehta M, Zale G, Maffucci L, Herz B. Laparoscopic gastrojejunostomy: a case presentation. *J Laparoendosc Surg* 1994;4:81.
52. Smith AC, Dowsett JF, Hatfield ARW, et al. Prospective randomised trial of bypass surgery vs endoscopic stenting in patients with malignant obstructive jaundice. *Gut* 1989;30:A1513.
53. Bornman PC, Harries-Jones EP, Tobias R, Van Stiegmann G, Terblanche J. Prospective controlled trial of transhepatic biliary endoprosthesis versus bypass surgery for incurable carcinoma of head of pancreas. *Lancet* 1986;1:69.
54. Rassweiler JJ, Henkel TO, Potempa DM, Coptcoat M, Alken P. The technique of transperitoneal laparoscopic nephrectomy, adrenalectomy, and nephroureterectomy. *Eur Urol* 1993;23:425.
55. Suzuki K, Kageyama S, Veda D, et al. Laparoscopic adrenalectomy: clinical experience with 12 cases. *J Urol* 1993;150:1099.
56. Fernández-Cruz L, Benarroch G, Torres E, Astudillo E, Saenz A, Taura P. Laparoscopic approach to the adrenal tumors. *J Laparoendosc Surg* 1993;3:541.
57. Gagner M, Lacroix A, Bolté E. Laparoscopic adrenalectomy in Cushing's syndrome and pheochromocytoma. *N Engl J Med* 1992;327:1003.
58. Casirola G, Ippoliti G, Marini G. Laparoscopy in Hodgkin's disease. *Acta Haemat* 1973;49:1.
59. Martin JK Jr, Clark SC, Beart RW Jr, et al. Staging laparotomy in Hodgkin's disease. Mayo Clinic experience. *Arch Surg* 1982;117:586.
60. Taylor MA, Kaplan HS, Nelsen TS. Staging laparotomy with splenectomy for Hodgkin's disease: the Stanford experience. *World J Surg* 1985;9:449.
61. Glatstein E, Guernsey JM, Rosenberg SA, Kaplan HS. The value of laparotomy and splenectomy in the staging of Hodgkin's disease. *Cancer* 1969;24:709.
62. Lefor AT, Flowers JL, Heyman MR. Laparoscopic staging of Hodgkin's disease. *Surg Oncol* 1993;2:217.
63. Kusminsky RE, Tiley EH, Lucente FC, Boland JP. Laparoscopic staging laparotomy with intra-abdominal manipulation. *Surg Laparosc Endosc* 1994;4:103.
64. Childers JM, Balserak JC, Kent T, Surwit EA. Laparoscopic staging of Hodgkin's lymphoma. *J Laparoendosc Surg* 1993;3:495.
65. Lefor AT, Flowers JL. Laparoscopic wedge biopsy of the liver. *J Am Coll Surg* 1994;178:307.
66. Thibault C, Mamazza J, Létourneau R, Poulin E. Laparoscopic splenectomy: operative technique and preliminary report. *Surg Laparosc Endosc* 1992;2:248.
67. Poulin E, Thibault C, Mamazza J, Girotti M, Côté G, Renaud A. Laparoscopic splenectomy: clinical experience and the role of preoperative splenic artery embolization. *Surg Laparosc Endosc* 1993;3:445.
68. Poulin EC, Thibault C, Mamazza J. Laparoscopic splenectomy. *Surg Endosc* 1995;9:172.
69. Lobe TE, Presbury GJ, Smith BM, Wilimas JA, Wang WC. Laparoscopic splenectomy. *Ped Ann* 1993;22:671.
70. Carroll BJ, Phillips EH, Semel CJ, Fallas M, Morgenstern L. Laparoscopic splenectomy. *Surg Endosc* 1992;6:183.
71. Burney TL, Campbell EC Jr, Naslund MJ, Jacobs SC. Complications of staging laparoscopic pelvic lymphadenectomy. *Surg Laparosc Endosc* 1993;3:184.
72. Flowers JL, Feldman J, Jacobs SC. Laparoscopic pelvic lymphadenectomy. *Surg Laparosc Endosc* 1991;1:62.
73. Childers JM, Surwit EA. Laparoscopic para-aortic lymph node biopsy for diagnosis of a non-Hodgkin's lymphoma. *Surg Laparosc Endosc* 1992;2:139.
74. Childers JM, Hatch KD, Tran A, Surwit EA. Laparoscopic para-aortic lymphadenectomy in gynecologic malignancies. *Obstet Gynecol* 1993;82:741.

CHAPTER 18

Surgical Treatment of Pelvic Recurrence

Michael P. Vezeridis and Harold J. Wanebo

There must be a final limit to the development of manipulative surgery; the knife cannot always have fresh fields for conquest, and although methods of practice may be modified and varied and even improved to some extent, it must be within a certain limit. That this limit has nearly, if not quite, been reached will appear evident if we reflect on the great achievements of modern operative surgery. Very little remains for the boldest to devise or the most dexterous to perform.

—*Sir John Erichsen, The Lancet, 1873*

BACKGROUND

Recurrence rates after curative resection of colorectal carcinoma range from 5% to 70%, depending on the site and stage of the primary tumor. In a review of 350 patients with colorectal cancer, the sites of first recurrence were liver in 33%, lung in 22%, intra-abdominal in 18%, and retroperitoneal in 10% (1). Carcinomas of the colon were associated with a significantly higher incidence of retroperitoneal recurrences; carcinomas of the rectum had a significantly higher incidence of local, regional, and pulmonary recurrences (Fig. 1).

Local or regional tumor recurrence is defined as recurrence in the previous operative field after a presumed curative resection. The extent of local recurrences can range from small isolated failures in the anastomosis to diffuse involvement of the peritoneal cavity, pelvis, or perineum. About 10% to 20% of all recurrences after colectomy or low anterior resection are small isolated failures in the anastomosis (2–4). An anastomotic recurrence on the luminal aspect of the anastomosis may escape detection until it becomes large enough to present with associated extramural disease. Conversely, an anastomotic recurrence may have originated outside the intestinal wall with tumor seedings and spread inward to

reach the mucosal surface. Extramural regional recurrence is more common and consists of involvement of perirectal fat, regional mesentery, adjacent pelvic structures, or perineum as a result of an inadequate initial operation or microinvasion at the time of resection. Local-regional recurrence is the most common pattern of recurrence from rectal cancer. The incidence of isolated local recurrence after curative resection of rectal carci-

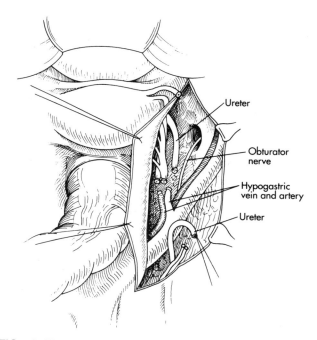

FIG. 1. The hypogastric artery and vein are clamped, divided, and ligated distal to the bifurcation of the common iliac vessels. The ureter is cut in the pelvis, the distal end is tied, and the proximal end is tagged with a suture for later identification and use. (Koness RJ, Wanebo HJ. Pelvic exenteration for advanced rectal cancer. In Bauer JJ, ed. *Colorectal surgery illustrated.* St. Louis: Mosby-Yearbook, 1993:233, with permission)

M. P. Vezeridis and H. J. Wanebo: Department of Surgery, Brown University School of Medicine, Roger Williams Medical Center, Providence, Rhode Island 02908.

235

noma in the literature ranges from 7% to 33%; the incidence of combined local and systemic recurrence ranges from 7% to 30% (Table 1) (5–10). The high incidence of local recurrence may be attributed to the inability to achieve adequate margins of resection in the pelvis and also to the diffuse rich lymphatic channels in the mesorectum. The site of the recurrence from a rectal cancer depends on the location of the primary lesion, with local recurrence predominating in low and mid-rectal lesions and systemic recurrence being more prevalent in upper rectal cancers (8). The incidence of local recurrence ranges from 12% to 32% after abdominosacral resection and from 14% to 43% after low anterior resection (11). The pattern of recurrence is also related to the initial operation. After abdominoperineal resection, only 10% of patients with a local recurrence have no evidence of pelvic side wall or combined side wall with anterior-posterior involvement; after low anterior resection, recurrences are more frequently nonfixed and therefore have greater potential for surgical resection (8).

Without surgery, the 5-year survival rate for patients with locoregional recurrence is <4%, with most patients dying with isolated disease. In one series, recurrence of pelvic disease or initial inoperability resulted in a median life expectancy of 7 months, with 50% of patients dying from disease confined to the pelvis (6). In a review of 105 patients with pelvic recurrence of rectal cancer, at the close of the study 89% were dead of their disease, 7% were alive with disease, and only 3.8% were clinically free of disease. Of all patients without pelvic recurrence, 22% were dead of disease, 22% were dead of other causes, and 56% were alive without evidence of recurrence (8). These reports underscore the dire prognosis associated with unresected locally recurrent disease, even in otherwise healthy patients.

METHODOLOGY

Preoperative Evaluation

Determination of resectability, exclusion of metastatic disease, and assessment of the patient's general medical status are the main objectives of the preoperative evaluation. A complete clinical examination should include a detailed assessment of the neuromuscular function of the lower extremities, with documentation of any existing deficits. Rectal and vaginal examinations are helpful in assessing the extent of the tumor, its fixation to the lateral pelvic wall, and possible involvement of pelvic viscera.

Essential imaging studies include computed tomography (CT) scanning of the abdomen and pelvis, x-ray studies of the chest and lumbosacral bones, bone scanning, and in selected cases magnetic resonance imaging (MRI). The CT scan defines the local extent of the tumor, and it may reveal enlarged periaortic nodes and liver metastases (12,13). If the physician observes suspicious findings, laparoscopy can provide direct visualization and access for biopsy. On CT scan it may be difficult to differentiate a recurrence from postoperative changes, particularly if only one scan is taken (14,15). A series of pelvic CT scans is more helpful because masses due to postoperative fibrosis will not change or may actually decrease in size, but recurrent tumors will enlarge or become less defined (15). A baseline postoperative CT 6 to 8 weeks after the initial operation, followed by repeat scans at regular intervals, may increase the detection of pelvic recurrences. CT-guided fine-needle aspiration cytology usually confirms the diagnosis of pelvic recurrence.

MRI has been found to be very useful in the diagnosis of pelvic side wall recurrences and metastatic lymphadenopathy, although its sensitivity is decreased in irradi-

TABLE 1. *Mortality, morbidity, and survival after pelvic exenteration for recurrent cancer*

Series	Year	No. patients	Operative morbidity (%)	Operative mortality (%)	5-year survival (%)
*Ketcham (39)	1970	94	—	22	28
*Galante & Hill (40)	1971	41	41.5	2.4	34
*Symmonds (41)	1975	161	—	8	32
†Jakowatz (26)	1985	104	77	8.7	27
†Lindsey (42)	1985	68	—	4.4	33§
*Stanhope & Symmonds (43)	1985	44‡	—	6.8	17
*Morley (44)	1989	100	49	2	61
*Soper (45)	1989	57	46	7.2	48
*Hatch (46)	1990	31	32	0	38
*Stanhope (47)	1990	72	39	4.2	52
†Hafner (48)	1992	21	50	4.2	20
*Matthews (49)	1992	63	38	11	46
†Zincke (50)	1992	30	53	3	—

*Gynecologic cancers
†Colorectal and other cancers
‡Palliative pelvic exenteration
§Survival of patients who had curative pelvic exenteration

ated patients (16). MRI is also helpful in identifying tumor extension into the bladder and rectum, even when endoscopic findings are negative (16). Arteriography is performed only in patients with extensive tumors. A plain chest radiograph is usually sufficient to exclude pulmonary metastases, although a chest CT scan may be useful in the presence of suspicious or equivocal findings. In patients with recurrent rectal cancer, evaluation of the colon with colonoscopy or barium enema is important because of the possibility of metachronous lesions.

Preoperative cystoscopy is useful in evaluating the presence and extent of involvement of the urinary bladder. Limited involvement of the dome of the bladder may allow the performance of a partial cystectomy only with preservation of bladder function. We place ureteral catheters immediately before the operation.

Assessment of the patient's medical status is of vital importance, because operations of this magnitude impose a heavy burden on the reserves of the various organ systems and may cause significant disturbance to the patient's homeostasis. All major organ systems are carefully assessed. Respiratory, cardiac, and renal functions are evaluated and optimized. Chronic metabolic disorders, if present, are studied and controlled. Hematologic parameters should be studied and optimized. The patient's coagulation status is evaluated, and any abnormalities found should be investigated and corrected. Assessment of the patient's nutritional status is of great importance because existing nutritional deficits may impede healing and predispose to infectious complications. Such deficiencies, if present, are corrected preoperatively with enteral or parenteral alimentation.

Assessment of the patient's mental and psychological status is also of critical importance. The major functional alterations resulting from radical operations for pelvic recurrence, such as pelvic exenteration or abdominosacral resection, may have profound psychological effects on the patient. Coping with both the physiologic and psychological effects of these radical operations requires capability of adjustment, motivation for self-care, and potential for rehabilitation. Severe mental or psychological impairment may be a contraindication to such operations. Preoperative teaching and psychosocial preparation are of great importance. The surgical team must establish very satisfactory lines of communication with the patient and family. The participation of the patient's family in discussions regarding the operation and other related issues is very important. All the major elements of the procedure, including risks, complications, and functional sequelae, should be discussed in detail with the patient. The patient is seen by an enterostomal therapist who will mark the appropriate site(s) for the stoma(s) and will start teaching about stoma care.

Patients who did not have an abdominoperineal resection at the time of initial cancer surgery are started on a clear liquid diet 48 hours before the operation. The day

before, they receive a bowel preparation consisting of an 8-oz glass of polyethylene glycol taken orally every 10 to 15 minutes until the rectal effluent becomes clear. In addition to this mechanical lavage, oral neomycin and erythromycin base are given. Intravenous hydration and electrolyte replacement are important. A broad-spectrum antibiotic covering gram-negative and anaerobic bacteria is given intravenously 30 minutes before the operation.

Pelvic Exenteration

The patient is placed in the lithotomy position using padded Allen stirrups. Pneumatic sequential compression stockings are placed on the legs for deep venous thrombosis prophylaxis. A folded blanket is placed under the buttocks to elevate the pelvis and to protect the sciatic nerve. The entire abdomen, perineum, and genitalia are prepped. Ureteral catheters are placed cytoscopically just before the operation.

The abdomen is entered through a lower midline incision extending from the pubic symphysis to 10 cm above the umbilicus. A thorough abdominal exploration should establish the absence of metastasis to the liver, peritoneum, omentum, and mesenteric, portal, and periaortic nodes. Proper exposure of the lower abdomen and pelvis is obtained by placing the patient in the Trendelenburg position, packing the small intestine in the upper abdomen, and using a self-retaining retractor. The posterior peritoneum is incised below the terminal ileum and cecum to expose the common iliac vessels bilaterally. In women, the round ligaments are divided at the pelvic wall and ligated. The ureters are identified and teased away, safely avoiding injury to them. Pelvic node dissection begins at the level of the aortic bifurcation and continuous downward along the iliac arteries and veins. The adipose tissue overlying these vessels is dissected sharply and reflected medially, and the external and internal iliac vessels are skeletonized bilaterally. After identification of the obturator nerve bilaterally, dissection is carried along the nerve into the obturator space. The obturator vessels are divided and ligated, but the nerve is protected. Adipose tissue and nodes are swept away from the nerve medially. The hypogastric artery and vein are clamped, divided, and ligated distal to the bifurcation of the common iliac vessels. The ureters are divided in the pelvis, their distal ends are tied, and the proximal ends are tagged with sutures for later identification (see Fig. 1).

If the rectum is still in place, the sigmoid colon is mobilized by incising the lateral parietal peritoneum along the white line of Toldt and separating the ureter from the mesocolon. The incision in the lateral parietal peritoneum is extended down into the pelvis. The site of transection of the sigmoid colon is selected and the peritoneum of the medial aspect of the mesosigmoid is incised, from the chosen point of transection to the root of the mesocolon to meet the previously performed peritoneal incision, below the terminal ileum and cecum. The mesosigmoid is serially stamped, divided, and ligated down to the level of the sacral promontory. The sigmoid is transected using the linear gastrointestinal stapler. The retrorectal space is entered and sharp dissection is carried down to the tip of the coccyx. The lateral stalks of the rectum are divided with the electrocautery and visualized vessels are clamped and ligated (Fig. 2).

The bladder is separated from the pubic symphysis and the pubic rami. The space of Retzius is entered and the bladder is freed by sharply dividing the anterior and lateral peritoneal attachments (Fig. 3). Attention to hemostasis is essential, as this is a very vascular area. The dissection is markedly facilitated by laying a hand flat on the bladder and using the fingers to pull upward and backward, continually readjusting as the dissection continues down to the urethra. In men, the dorsal vessels of the penis must be suture-ligated carefully. The endopelvic fascia is divided bilaterally by clamping and tying on the pelvic side wall. The lateral attachments of the bladder to the pelvic wall contain a plexus of hypogastric vessels and lymph node-bearing tissue, which is included in the specimen. The anterior dissection finishes at the levator ani muscles.

At this point, with the specimen fully mobilized anteriorly, laterally, and posteriorly, the only remaining attachments are the urethra, the vagina, and the rectum, and the perineal part of the procedure begins. An elliptical incision is made from the tip of the coccyx to a point anterior to the urethral orifice in women and to the bulb of the penis in men. The distance of the skin incision lateral to the anal margin is determined by the proximity of the tumor to the anal canal. For very low-lying lesions, a

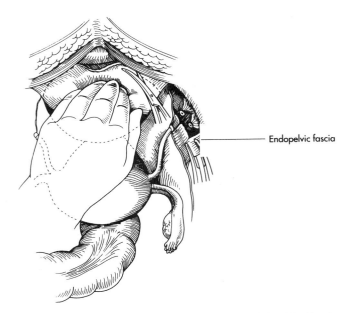

Endopelvic fascia

FIG. 3. The space of Retzius is entered and the bladder is freed by dividing the lateral peritoneal attachments bilaterally. (Koness RJ, Wanebo HJ. Pelvic exenteration for advanced rectal cancer. In Bauer JJ, ed. *Colorectal surgery illustrated.* St. Louis: Mosby-Yearbook, 1993:236, with permission)

wide excision of perianal skin is needed, removing ischiorectal fat and transecting the levator ani muscles at the pelvic wall. The subcutaneous tissue is divided with electrocoagulation, the tip of the coccyx is identified by palpation, the anococcygeal raphe is divided, and the presacral space is entered. The levator ani muscles are divided to the ischial tuberosity using the electrocautery (Fig. 4). A few absorbable ties or suture-ligatures are required to control inferior hemorrhoidal and internal pudendal vessels. The dissection is completed anteriorly at the pubic symphysis and the specimen is removed en bloc through the abdominal incision. After satisfactory hemostasis is ascertained, closed-suction drains are placed in the pelvis and brought out through stab wound incisions in the perineal skin. The perineal incision is closed using interrupted 3-0 absorbable sutures for the subcutaneous tissue and staples for the skin.

At this point, attention is focused on the formation of an ileal conduit for urinary diversion. A stay suture is placed on the terminal ileum about 10 cm from the ileocecal valve, proximal to the ileocecal vascular arcade. A segment of terminal ileum including one or two clear-cut vascular arcades is chosen for the formation of the ileal conduit. The mesentery is divided enough to allow the distal end to reach through the abdominal wall. The site of the proximal bowel division is selected by measuring the distance from the sacral promontory to the skin of the abdominal wall, and the mesentery is divided for a short distance at this point. Before dividing the bowel, the selected arcade is reexamined to ensure adequate vascu-

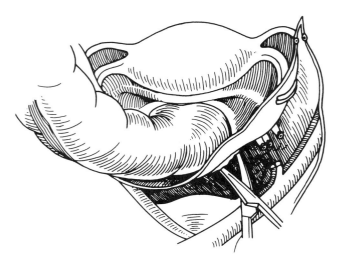

FIG. 2. The rectal stalks are divided and the visualized vessels are clamped and ligated. (Koness RJ, Wanebo HJ. Pelvic exenteration for advanced rectal cancer. In Bauer JJ, ed. *Colorectal surgery illustrated.* St. Louis: Mosby-Yearbook, 1993:235, with permission)

The proximal end of the ileal sites for the ureteral anastomosis are selected to allow anastomosis without tension. The anastomosis may be performed over the ureteral catheters, already in place, or a No. 8 pediatric feeding tube may be inserted into the ileal segment (outside in), brought out through two small stab wounds, and passed retrograde up the ureters to the kidney. Mucosal to mucosal sutures are placed with 5-0 polyglycolic monofilament thread (usually six sutures are needed) (see Fig. 5). A second row of 5-0 serosal silk sutures is placed to bolster the anastomosis. The ureteral catheters are brought out through the stoma and sutured to the skin so as to permit the stoma appliance to be placed. The closed end of the ileal loop is sutured to the periosteum of the sacral promontory to prevent twisting of the mesentery. The distal end of the ileal loop and the divided end of the sigmoid, if an end colostomy is not already present, are exteriorized through openings at preselected areas of the abdominal wall. The abdominal incision is closed in layers. Before this closure, an omental J-flap can often be moved down into the pelvis and sutured to the pelvic side walls to help keep the small bowel out of the true pelvis and to provide additional blood supply to previously irradiated pelvic tissue. After the closure of the abdominal incision, the stomas are matured with 4-0 Vicryl sutures. The ureteral stents are transfixed to the skin surrounding the stoma of the ileal loop, are left in place for 5 to 7 days, and are removed only after anastomotic integrity is confirmed by a retrograde contrast study.

For the abdominal part of the abdominosacral resection procedure, the patient is placed in the supine position, after placement of ureteral catheters, and the abdomen is prepped and draped. The abdomen is entered through a midline incision as described for the previous procedure and a complete abdominal exploration is performed. After extrapelvic disease is excluded, exposure of the pelvis is obtained by placing the patient in the Trendelenburg position, using a self-retaining retractor, and packing the small bowel in the upper abdomen.

If the rectum is still in place and must be resected, the site of transection of the sigmoid colon is selected by tak-

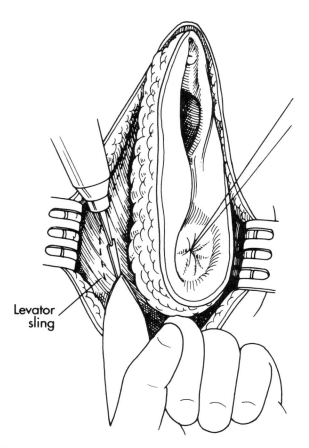

FIG. 4. The surgeon's index finger is inserted above the levator sling and the muscle is divided into the ischial tuberosity on both sides. (Koness RJ, Wanebo HJ. Pelvic exenteration for advanced rectal cancer. In Bauer JJ, ed. *Colorectal surgery illustrated.* St. Louis: Mosby-Yearbook, 1993:237, with permission)

lar supply. The bowel is then divided at the selected points of transection, and continuity of the small bowel is reestablished by an end-to-end anastomosis (Fig. 5). Irradiated ileum must be avoided. If the terminal ileum is irradiated, a more proximal segment of ileum or transverse colon should be used.

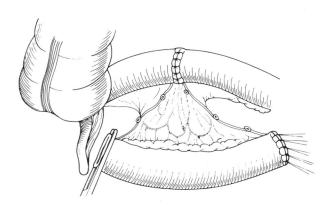

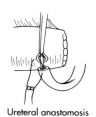

Ureteral anastomosis

FIG. 5. The small bowel is divided at the selected points of transection and continuity is reestablished by an end-to-end anastomosis. Ureteral anastomoses are performed over ureteral catheters or No. 8 pediatric feeding tubes. The closed end of the ileal loop is sutured to the periosteum of the sacral promontory; the distal end is exteriorized through the abdominal wall to create the stoma. (Koness RJ, Wanebo HJ. Pelvic exenteration for advanced rectal cancer. In Bauer JJ, ed. *Colorectal surgery illustrated.* St. Louis: Mosby-Yearbook, 1993 239, with permission)

ing into consideration the adequacy of the length and blood supply of the remaining left colon for forming a permanent colostomy without tension or ischemia. The mesocolon is serially clamped, divided, and ligated from the selected transection site to the level of the sacral promontory, and the sigmoid is transected with a linear gastrointestinal stapler. The upper rectum is mobilized with sharp dissection. To avoid jeopardizing a curative resection, dissection must be avoided in the area where the tumor appears to invade the sacrum.

Aortoiliac node dissection is started at the level of the aortic bifurcation and continues along the common and external iliac arteries; it includes the internal iliac, the obturator, and the hypogastric nodes. The lymph nodes are submitted for histopathologic study separately from the main specimen. Extensive nodal involvement in the lower pelvis generally precludes continuing the resection, but the presence of enlarged but easily resectable obturator nodes does not. If the ureters are free of tumor, they are dissected and fixed anteriorly to the lateral pelvic wall just below the external iliac artery and vein to prevent injury during the posterior dissection. If the bladder and pelvic ureters are involved but considered resectable, the ureters are divided, the bladder is dissected from the pelvic wall, and an ileal conduit is constructed using the same technique described above.

Pelvic devascularization is accomplished by transecting and ligating with sutures the internal iliac arteries and veins (Fig. 6). An effort should be made to ligate the internal iliac artery beyond its first branch to provide better vascularization of the skin and muscle flaps to be used for closure of the posterior wound. The middle sacral artery and vein and individual branches are divided if found in the plane of dissection. The peritoneal floor is restored with Vicryl mesh, an omental pedicle, or a local peritoneal flap. The closed end of the ileal loop is sutured to paravertebral tissues proximal to the periosteum of the sacral promontory to prevent twisting of the mesentery. Before closure of the abdominal incision, the distal end of the ileal loop and the divided end of the sigmoid colon are exteriorized through openings at the preselected areas of the abdominal wall. The ureteral catheters are also brought out.

After satisfactory hemostasis has been achieved, the abdominal incision is closed. If oozing persists despite meticulous hemostasis, the pelvis is packed with laparotomy sponges, which are removed during the sacral part of the procedure. After closure of the abdominal incision, the stomas are matured with interrupted 4-0 Vicryl sutures. The ureteral stents are transfixed to the skin surrounding the stoma of the ileal loop and left in place for 5 to 7 days; they are removed only after anastomotic integrity has been documented by means of retrograde contrast study.

The sacral stage of the procedure is usually done about 48 hours after the abdominal operation. The patient is

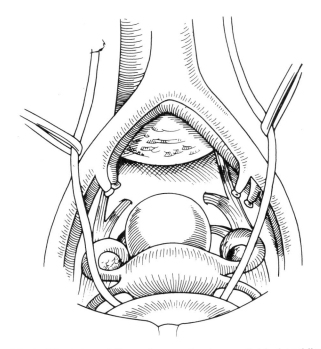

FIG. 6. The internal iliac artery and vein are divided and ligated with sutures bilaterally to accomplish devascularization of the pelvis. (Wanebo HJ, Turk PS. Abdominosacral resection for recurrent cancer of the rectum. In Bauer JJ, ed. *Colorectal surgery illustrated.* St. Louis: Mosby-Yearbook, 1993: 243, with permission)

placed in the prone position. A posterior sacral incision is made from the spinous process of L5 to the perineum. The lower part of the incision has an elliptical course so that it can include the anus and urethra, depending on which pelvic organs are to be removed (Fig. 7). Full-thickness flaps are raised at the level of the sacral periosteum to the lateral extent of the sacrum. The gluteus maximus and medius muscles are dissected from their sacral origins, with maintenance of a fascial cuff on the muscles for the subsequent midline wound closure (Fig. 8).

The sciatic nerve is located by retracting the gluteus maximus and underlying piriformis muscles superiorly and at the lateral aspect of the middle portion of the sacrum. The nerve lies superficial to the obturator internus and gemelli muscles as it courses inferolaterally midway between the ischial tuberosity and the greater trochanter. During the dissection, it is encircled with a vessel loop for ease of identification (see Fig. 8). The sacrotuberous and sacrospinous ligaments are incised at the level of their attachments to the ischial tuberosity and ischial spine. A finger is then inserted medially to the sciatic nerve and advanced deeply, beneath the piriformis muscles and through the underlying endopelvic fascia (Fig. 9). With this maneuver, the surgeon breaks through the endopelvic fascia to reach the anterior surface of the sacrum in the area of the pelvic dissection performed during the abdominal procedure. This approach directs the subsequent sacral osteotomy and

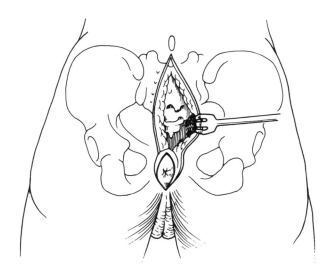

FIG. 7. A posterior sacral incision is made from the spinous process of L5 to the perineum and the flaps are raised to the level of the sacral periosteum. (Wanebo HJ, Turk PS. Abdominosacral resection for recurrent cancer of the rectum. In Bauer JJ, ed. *Colorectal surgery illustrated*. St. Louis: Mosby-Yearbook, 1993:244, with permission)

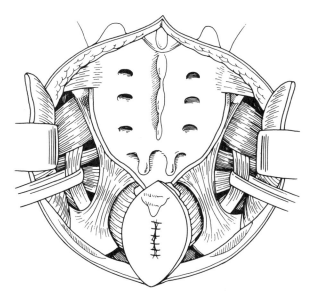

FIG. 8. After dissection of the gluteus maximus and medius muscles from their sacral origins, the sciatic nerve is identified bilaterally and encircled with a vessel loop. (Wanebo HJ, Turk PS. Abdominosacral resection for recurrent cancer of the rectum. In Bauer JJ, ed. *Colorectal surgery illustrated*. St. Louis: Mosby-Yearbook, 1993:245, with permission)

ensures an adequate margin proximal to the tumor. Further dissection is carried out around the sacrum by incising the piriformis muscles and the soft tissues surrounding the sciatic nerve.

A laminectomy is performed to the planned level of sacral transection, usually between L5 and S1, to ligate the terminal end of the dural sac (Fig. 10). The proximal sacral roots are identified and an effort is made to preserve them by dissecting them free of the portion of the sacrum to be resected. After the resection line on both

sides of the sacrum is determined, an osteotome or oscillating saw is used to transect the bone while the surgeon's finger is positioned anteriorly to protect the intra-abdominal contents (Fig. 11). For resections above the level of S3, the line of resection is continued through the sacroiliac joints laterally. Care is taken not to injure the lumbar component of the sciatic nerve. The sacral components of the nerve are dissected if necessary. The sacrum, pelvic

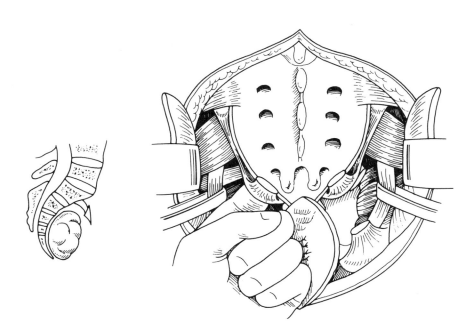

FIG. 9. The surgeon's finger is inserted anteriorly from the medial aspect of the sciatic nerve and advanced deeply beneath the piriformis muscle through the underlying endopelvic fascia to reach the anterior surface of the rectum. (Wanebo HJ, Turk PS. Abdominosacral resection for recurrent cancer of the rectum. In Bauer JJ, ed. *Colorectal surgery illustrated*. St. Louis: Mosby-Yearbook, 1993: 245, with permission)

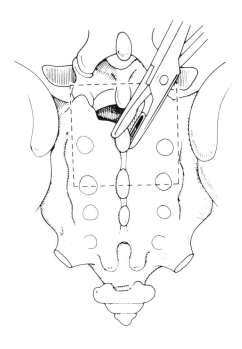

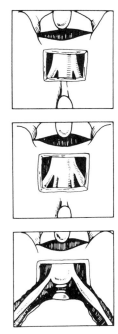

FIG. 10. A laminectomy is performed to the planned level of sacral transection to ligate the terminal end of the dural sac. If possible, the proximal sacral roots are identified and an effort is made to preserve them by dissecting them free from the portion of the sacrum to be resected. (Wanebo HJ, Turk PS. Abdominosacral resection for recurrent cancer of the rectum. In Bauer JJ, ed. *Colorectal surgery illustrated*. St. Louis: Mosby-Yearbook, 1993:246, with permission)

side wall, and tumor-bearing structures are removed en bloc (Fig. 12).

Hemostasis is obtained after initial packing of the wound to gain temporary control of bleeding. The region is examined carefully and any residual tumor or devital-ized tissue removed. If the presence of residual tumor at the resection margins is suspected, the margins are examined histologically by frozen-section study. If tumor is found, additional margins are obtained. Confirming that margins are free of tumor depends on repeated frozen-

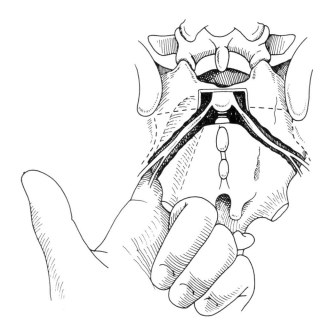

FIG. 11. The sacrum is divided with an osteotome or an oscillating saw; the surgeon's finger is positioned anteriorly to protect the underlying intra-abdominal contents. (Wanebo HJ, Turk PS. Abdominosacral resection for recurrent cancer of the rectum. In Bauer JJ, ed. *Colorectal surgery illustrated*. St. Louis: Mosby-Yearbook, 1993:247, with permission)

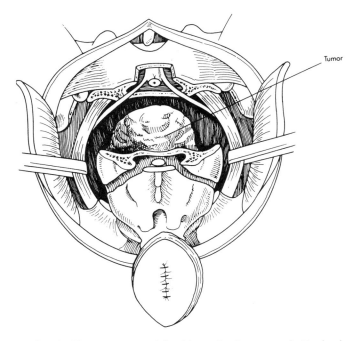

FIG. 12. The sacrum, pelvic side walls, tumor, and attached pelvic structures are removed en bloc. (Wanebo HJ, Turk PS. Abdominosacral resection for recurrent cancer of the rectum. In Bauer JJ, ed. *Colorectal surgery illustrated*. St. Louis: Mosby-Yearbook, 1993:248, with permission)

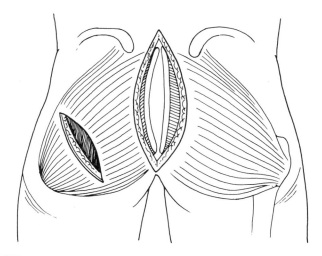

FIG. 13. The muscles are approximated in the midline. The lateral insertion of the gluteus maximus may have to be incised to allow medial advancement of the muscle. (Wanebo HJ, Turk PS. Abdominosacral resection for recurrent cancer of the rectum. In Bauer JJ, ed. *Colorectal surgery illustrated*. St. Louis: Mosby-Yearbook, 1993:249, with per-

section evaluations. It is important to examine the specimen carefully with the pathologist and do frozen-section assessments on close margins. It is also helpful to perform biopsies at the periphery of the resection sites that correspond to the higher-risk areas observed on examination of the specimen.

Closed-suction drains are placed bilaterally and the sacral wound is closed. If the fascial origin of the gluteus maximus has been preserved, the muscles are approximated in the midline with a heavy, nonabsorbable monofilament suture, thereby forming a new pelvic floor. A relaxing incision at the level of the lateral insertion of the gluteus maximus on the greater trochanter may be necessary to allow additional medial advancement of the muscle (Fig. 13). The subcutaneous tissue is approximated with interrupted absorbable sutures and the skin with staples.

Mortality and Morbidity

The potential complications of radical surgery for pelvic recurrence cover the entire spectrum of morbidity related to major abdominal surgery. In addition, complications unique to the urinary diversion, the stomas, and the sacral resection occur. The prolonged anesthesia and operative time and the associated major blood loss, requiring massive replacement with crystalloids and blood products, may present an overwhelming challenge to the patient. Therefore, close intra- and postoperative hemodynamic monitoring are of paramount importance. We routinely use autotransfusion for major pelvic resections where the potential for major and rapid blood loss is

great. Severe postoperative hemorrhage leading to death has been reported (17–20). Mortality from uncontrolled bleeding should be preventable in most cases by proper handling of the pelvic vasculature during the operation and achievement of satisfactory hemostasis before the end of the procedure. When satisfactory hemostasis cannot be accomplished, as in the case of dilutional coagulopathy, a safe and effective approach is packing the pelvis and returning the patient to the operating room for removal of the pack 48 hours later, after coagulation has been normalized.

Cardiopulmonary complications are likely to occur after procedures of this magnitude and have been reported (18–22). Massive fluid shifts, rapid administration of large volumes of crystalloids intraoperatively, and significant continuing losses in the immediate postoperative period make these patients particularly prone to cardiac complications. Essential to the prevention of such complications is close hemodynamic monitoring, with proper replacement of fluids and correction of electrolyte imbalances. Adequate urine output is a good index of adequate hydration and renal function, as well as evidence of the integrity and patency of the ureteral anastomoses.

Wound infections have been reported (20–23) and were a significant cause of morbidity in earlier series (19). In abdominosacral resections, wound infection and flap separation are markedly more common after resections for recurrent disease, occurring exclusively in patients who had been heavily irradiated (23).

Intestinal obstruction, a rather common early postoperative complication (19–23), may lead to significant morbidity if not diagnosed on a timely basis and treated properly (17.) The main factors predisposing to this serious complication are the empty deperitonealized pelvis and the presence and position of the urinary diversion conduit (19,24–26). The former factor also predisposes to the formation of enteroperineal fistula (26–29). Delaying the surgical management of early postoperative intestinal obstruction entails the risk of entering the pelvis after the formation of adhesions, substantially increasing the surgical morbidity and mortality (17). Sound clinical judgment dictates that if the bowel cannot be safely dissected free from the pelvis, the obstruction should be relieved by an intestinal bypass procedure (19,27,29,30). The incidence of this complication is significantly higher in patients who had preoperative radiation treatment, particularly those who did not undergo pelvic reconstruction with omental or myocutaneous flaps or colonic advancement (24,26). It is, therefore, advisable to perform a pelvic reconstruction using these techniques in patients who have been irradiated before surgery. Obliteration of the pelvic defect with omentum or muscles should also be considered in patients who did not have preoperative radiation but are likely candidates for postoperative radiation. Such obliteration prevents the small intestine from descending into the lower part of the pelvis, which results in exposure to radiation and its associated complications (31). Gracilis, rectus abdominis, tensor fascia lata, and inferior gluteal flaps have been used successfully for filling pelvic defects (32–34).

Dehiscence of intestinal and ureteral anastomoses has been reported (19,21,22) and appears to be more common after preoperative radiation. It can be minimized by using nonirradiated ileum or, if necessary, colon for the formation of the ileal conduit (19). Other reported complications include fecal and urinary fistulae, urinary tract infections, hydronephrosis, retraction or separation of the stomas, thrombophlebitis, pulmonary embolism, evisceration, psychosis, cerebrovascular accident, prolonged ileus, atelectasis, and pneumonia (19–24,26,35).

Late complications occur quite often, making evident the importance of continued surgical follow-up of these patients. Late intestinal obstruction and enteroperineal fistula formation have been reported, and their surgical management entails a significant surgical risk (19). The surgical management is the same as that described for the early postoperative complications. Again, if the risk associated with dissection of the small intestine from the pelvis is high, an intestinal bypass procedure should be performed. Although it is very unlikely that an enteroperineal fistula will close after a bypass procedure, leaving a draining fistula in the perineum may be the proper choice if the risk of dissecting the small intestine from the pelvis is prohibitive (19). Extensive resections of the small bowel should be avoided, as they may lead to short bowel syndrome, which will compromise the patient's quality of life.

Pyelonephritis occurs as a late complication and is usually easily controlled with proper antibiotics if there is no mechanical obstruction at the ureteral anastomosis causing stasis. However, if obstruction is present, it should be corrected surgically. Extensive dissection of the ureters in the irradiated patient incurs the risk of ischemic damage to the ureter, with the hazard of ureteral fibrosis, fistula, or both. An acute episode of ureteral obstruction in such a patient may be managed by percutaneous nephrostomies to permit controlled urinary decompression. This will allow time to assess the problem and plan reconstruction at an elective future date. Other late complications include perineal, paracolostomy, and incisional hernia (19,20); these are usually amenable to surgical repair with conventional techniques, the use of synthetic mesh, or the use of myocutaneous flaps (19,36–38).

The morbidity rates after pelvic exenteration for recurrent pelvic cancer range from 32% to 77%. Operative mortality rates range from 0% to 22% (see Table 1) (26,39–50). The mortality rates in the series reported after 1970 (26,40–50) ranged from 0% to 11%, a significant decline from the mortality rates of 22% to 33% reported in earlier series (39,51,52). This decline in operative mortality can be attributed to improved patient selection, refinement of surgical techniques, and advancements in perioperative patient care (18,24,41,53–55).

Abdominosacral resection is a procedure associated with considerable morbidity. In our most recent series of abdominosacral resection in patients with recurrent rectal cancer, the mean operative blood loss was 11,700 ml for the second half of this patient population, and the mean operative time was 20 hours for this group (56). Perioperative mortality was 8.5%. Complications were common and included cardiopulmonary, sepsis, fistula, deep vein thrombosis, arterial ischemia, peroneal nerve palsy, wound infections, and flap separations (Table 2). Sepsis, wound infection, and flap separation were the most frequent complications. Peroneal nerve palsy occurred in 6 patients and resolved in all cases. Although 5 patients had documented deep venous thrombosis, no recognized episodes of pulmonary embolism occurred.

CLINICAL RESULTS

Five-year survival rates after pelvic exenteration for recurrent cancer are summarized in Table 1 and range from 20% to 61% when the procedure is performed with curative intent. The results of abdominosacral resection performed for cure of recurrent rectal cancer are shown

TABLE 2. *Pelvic resection—morbidity and mortality in 47 patients*

Perioperative mortality	4 (8.5%)
Complications	
Cardiovascular	
Myocardial ischemia arrhythmia	2
Pneumonia	2
Pulmonary insufficiency (prolonged intubation/ARDS)	9
Intraoperative coagulopathy	1
Postoperative hemorrhage	6
Fistula	
Small bowel/large bowel	6
Bladder/ureteral	3
Infection	
Sepsis	16
Urinary tract	6
Wound complications	
Wound infection	9
Posterior wound infection/flap separation	18
Bowel/urinary dehiscence	
Small bowel obstruction	4
Renal failure	7
Hydronephrosis, ureteral stricture	2
Bowel/urinary dehiscence	
Urinary incontinence	4
Vascular/nerve	
Ileal conduit leak	1
Perineal nerve palsy	6
Deep venous thrombosis	5
Arterial transection/ischemia	2
Myonecrosis	1
Hepatic failure	1

TABLE 3. *Recurrent rectal carcinoma: abdominal sacral resections for cure*

Series	Year	No. patients	Results
Takagi (58)	1986	7	4 patients NED; one LWD at 32 mo
Schiessel (57)	1986	9	3-y survival, approx 30%
Pearlman (62)	1987	8	3 patients NED; 1 patient dead of other causes at 46 mo
Touran (60)	1990	12	12-mo survival, 62%; 24-mo survival, 14%
Temple & Ketcham (59)	1992	9	Local control, 45%; 5-y disease-free survival, 18%
Maetani (61)	1992	23	5-y survival, 23%
Wanebo (56)	1994	47	Medial overall survival, 39 mo (43 operative survivors); 5-y estimated survival, 33%

NED, no evidence of disease; LWD, living with disease.

in Table 3. The estimated 5-year survival in our most recent series was 33%, and our results are similar to those reported by others (56–62). Takagi and colleagues (58) reported on abdominosacral resections in 7 patients with localized recurrence of rectal cancer. Three of the patients died of recurrent disease, 2 were alive with recurrent disease in the lungs and pelvic wall, and 2 were alive without evidence of recurrence. Schiessel and associates (57) reported a 3-year survival of about 30%. Pearlman and colleagues (62) performed sacropelvic resections for cure in 8 patients. Four of them subsequently had no evidence of cancer: 3 were alive and 1 had died from other causes at 46 months. Temple and Ketcham (59) performed single-stage abdominosacral resections in 12 patients (9 of whom had rectal cancer) and reported a median disease-free survival time of 24 months and a 5-year disease-free survival rate of 18%. Maetani and colleagues (61) reported a 5-year survival of 23% in 23 patients who underwent aggressive en bloc resection of regionally recurrent carcinoma of the rectum.

An important objective of resection of recurrent pelvic tumors is relief from the unrelenting symptoms they cause. The results achieved with respect to this goal have been very satisfactory. In a series reported by Wanebo and coworkers (23), 97% of the patients with long-term follow-up (>6 months) experienced relief of pain originating from the mass, fistulae, perineum, or lower back. Takagi and colleagues (58) reported pain relief in all 7 patients they treated with abdominosacral resection for localized recurrence of rectal cancer. Appreciable pain relief was reported by Pearlman and colleagues in 7 of 12 patients after sacropelvic resection.(62). Touran and asso-

ciates (60) reported good palliation in all 12 patients who had abdominosacral resection. Temple and Ketcham (59) also observed excellent palliation of pelvic pain in all 9 of their patients who underwent curative resection for local recurrence.

The patient's functional capacity after resection depends on the extent and level of the sacral resection. We found that those who had sacral resections at or distal to the level of S3 retained normal anorectal function. Bilateral resections above the S3 level compromised both anorectal and urogenital function. In general, for anatomic reasons, female patients were less likely to have urinary retention. Patients with resection at the S1/S2 level could manage urologic function by practicing the Credé method at defined times. Male patients with high sacral resections (through the S1 level) also required periodic catheterization. In some patients, treatment with ephedrine lessened incontinence. Placement of a periurethral device for control of persistent incontinence was necessary in 1 patient after resection of a sacral chondrosarcoma. A penile implant can be placed in men with impotence.

Twelve of 34 patients (35%) had persistent postoperative pain, typically new phantomlike pain or causalgia, and local symptoms related to delayed wound healing. In 7 of the 12 patients, the symptoms improved during ensuing months, often with administration of amitriptyline or carbamazepine. Although long-term neurologic sequelae were unusual, many patients did have short-term lower extremity symptoms, including unsteadiness, diminished lower leg strength, and sensory deficits in the foot. Serious locomotive dysfunction was evident only in those who had resections involving the S1 and S2 roots bilaterally. Overall, 66% of the patients returned to their previous lifestyle, and 43% returned to work. In general, function was impaired for only about 3 months. All patients were referred for rehabilitation and usually required aggressive outpatient therapy.

Although radical resections for recurrent pelvic cancer are associated with substantial morbidity, in properly selected patients, treated in centers where the necessary expertise is available, the perioperative mortality should not exceed 10% and the anticipated 5-year survival should be 20% or higher. These radical resections, as a general rule, should be undertaken with curative intent. However, their use for palliation on specific occasions may significantly improve the patient's quality of life by providing relief from the unrelenting symptomatology of advanced pelvic tumors (63). Sound clinical judgment should be exercised in the selection of patients for palliative radical pelvic resections, because the probability of disastrous consequences is significant if the selection is not proper. Incomplete resection or transection through tumor invariably leads to rapid recurrence, resulting in severe compromise of the quality of life because of refractory and unbearable symptomatology.

PATIENT CARE CONSIDERATIONS

The importance of careful follow-up of patients after radical surgery for recurrent pelvic cancers cannot be overemphasized. A significant percentage of these patients will develop another pelvic recurrence or distant metastases. In addition, late complications related to the operation may occur, and psychological or marital problems may arise. The surgeon should have a major role in the coordination of the follow-up and the management of the patient's problems. Despite the profound anatomic, physiologic, and functional changes caused by radical pelvic surgery, with the proper support and rehabilitation the patient can adjust and live a meaningful, productive life.

REFERENCES

1. Galandiuk S, Wieand HS, Moertel CG, et al. Patterns of recurrence after curative resection of carcinoma of the colon and rectum. *Surg Gynecol Obstet* 1992;174:27–32.
2. Vassilopoulos PP, Yoon JM, Ledesma EJ, Mittelman A. Treatment of recurrence of adenocarcinoma of the colon and rectum at the anastomotic site. *Surg Gynecol Obstet* 1981;152:777–780.
3. Pihl E, Hughes ES, McDermott FT, Price AB. Recurrence of carcinoma of the colon and rectum at the anastomotic suture line. *Surg Gynecol Obstet* 1981;153:495–496.
4. Welch JP, Donaldson GA. Detection and treatment of recurrent cancer of the colon and rectum. *Am J Surg* 1978;135:505–511.
5. Berge T, Ekelund G, Mellner C, Pihl B, Wenckert A. Carcinoma of the colon and rectum in a defined population. *Acta Chir Scand* 1973;438 (Suppl):1–84.
6. Gunderson LL, Sosin H. Areas of failure found at reoperation following curative surgery for adenocarcinoma of the rectum. *Cancer* 1974;34:1278–1292.
7. Rao AR, Kagan AR, Chan PM, Gilbert HA, Nussbaum H, Hintz BL. Patterns of recurrence following curative resection alone for adenocarcinoma of the rectum and sigmoid colon. *Cancer* 1981;48:1354–1362.
8. Pilipshen SJ, Heilweil M, Quan SH, Sternberg SS, Enker WE. Patterns of pelvic recurrence following definitive resections of rectal cancer. *Cancer* 1984;53:1354–1362.
9. McDermott FT, Hughes ESR, Pihl E, Johnson WR, Price AB. Local recurrence after potentially curative resection for rectal cancer in a series of 1,008 patients. *Br J Surg* 1985;72:34–37.
10. Carlsson U, Lasson A, Ekelund G. Recurrence rates after curative surgery for rectal carcinoma with special reference to their accuracy. *Dis Colon Rectum* 1987;30:431–434.
11. Pilipshen S. Cancer of the rectum: local recurrence. In: Fazio VW, ed. *Current therapy in colon and rectal surgery*. Toronto: Brian C. Decker, 1990:137–149.
12. Feigen M, Crocker EF, Read J, et al. The value of lymphoscintigraphy, lymphangiography and computed tomography scanning in the preoperative assessment of lymph nodes involved by pelvic malignant conditions. *Surg Gynecol Obstet* 1987;165:107–112.
13. Nicholls RJ, Mason AY, Morson BC, et al. The clinical staging of rectal cancer. *Br J Surg* 1982;69:404–406.
14. Butch RJ, Wittenberg J, Mueller PR, et al. Presacral masses after abdominoperineal resection for colorectal carcinoma: the need for needle biopsy. *Am J Roentgenol* 1985;144:309–312.
15. Kelvin FM, Korobkin M, Heaston DK, et al. The pelvis after surgery for rectal carcinoma: serial CT observations with emphasis on nonneoplastic features. *Am J Roentgenol* 1983;141:959–962.
16. Popovich MJ, Hricak H, Sugimura K, et al. The role of MR imaging in determining surgical eligibility for pelvic exenteration. *Am J Roentgenol* 1993;160:525–528.
17. Kiselow M, Butcher HR, Bricker EM. Results of the radical surgical treatment of advanced pelvic cancer: A fifteen-year study. *Am Surg* 1967;166:428–432.
18. Boey J, Wong J, Ong GB. Pelvic exenteration for locally advanced colorectal carcinoma. *Ann Surg* 1982;195:513–518.
19. Bricker EM, Kraybill WG, Lopez MJ, et al. The current role of ultra-radical surgery in the treatment of pelvic cancer. *Curr Probl Surg* 1986;23:871–927.
20. Kraybill WG, Lopez MJ, Bricker EM. Total pelvic exenteration as a therapeutic option in advanced malignant disease of the pelvis. *Surg Gynecol Obstet* 1988;166:259–264.
21. Eldar S, Kemeny MM, Terz JJ. Extended resections for carcinoma of the colon and rectum. *Surg Gynecol Obstet* 1985;161:319–322.
22. Eisenberg SB, Kraybill WB, Lopez MJ. Long-term results of surgical resection of locally advanced colorectal carcinoma. *Surgery* 1990;108:779–786.
23. Wanebo HJ, Koness RJ, Turk PS, Cohen SI. Composite resection of posterior pelvic malignancy. *Ann Surg* 1992;215:685–695.
24. Lopez MJ, Kraybill WG, Downey RS, et al. Exenterative surgery for locally advanced rectosigmoid cancers: is it worthwhile? *Surgery* 1987;102:644–671.
25. Jaffe BM, Bricker EM, Butcher HR Jr. Surgical complications of ileal segment urinary diversion. *Ann Surg* 1968;167:367–376.
26. Jakowatz JG, Porudominsky D, Riihimaki DU, et al. Complication of pelvic exenteration. *Arch Surg* 1985;120:1261–1265.
27. Lifshitz S, Johnson R, Roberts JA, et al. Intestinal fistula and obstruction following pelvic exenteration. *Am J Obstet Gynecol* 1983;145:325–332.
28. Devereaux DF, Sears HF, Ketcham AS. Intestinal fistula following pelvic exenteration surgery: predisposing causes and treatment. *J Surg Oncol* 1980;14:227–232.
29. Polk HC, Butcher HR Jr, Bricker EM. Perineal fecal fistula following pelvic exenteration. *Surg Gynecol Obstet* 1966;123:308–312.
30. Wheeless CR Jr. Small bowel bypass for complications related to pelvic malignancy. *Obstet Gynecol* 1973;42:661–666.
31. Devine RM, Dozois RR. Surgical management of locally advanced adenocarcinoma of the rectum. *World J Surg* 1992;16:486–489.
32. Palmer JA, Vernon CP, Cummings BJ, et al. Gracilis myocutaneous flap for reconstructing perineal defects resulting from radiation and radical surgery. *Can J Surg* 1983;26:510–512.
33. Temple WJ, Ketcham AS. The closure of large pelvic defects by extended compound tensor fascia lata and inferior gluteal myocutaneous flaps. *Am J Clin Oncol* 1982;5:573–577.
34. Miller LB, Steele G, Cady B, et al. Resection of tumors in irradiated fields with subsequent immediate reconstruction. *Arch Surg* 1987;122:461–466.
35. Ledesma EJ, Bruno S, Mittelman A. Total pelvic exenteration in colorectal disease. *Ann Surg* 1981;194:701–703.
36. Ego-Aguirre E, Spratt JS Jr, Butcher HR Jr, et al. Repair of perineal hernias developed subsequent to pelvic exenteration. *Ann Surg* 1964;159:66–71.
37. Leuchter RS, Lagasse LD, Hacker NF, et al. Management of postexenteration perineal hernias by myocutaneous axial flaps. *Gynecol Oncol* 1982;14:15–22.
38. Powell WJ, Parsons L. Perineal hernia repair with nylon mesh. *Surgery* 1958;43:447–451.
39. Ketcham AS, Deckers PJ, Sugarbaker EV, et al. Pelvic exenteration for carcinoma of the uterine cervix: a 15-year experience. *Cancer* 1970;26:513–521.
40. Galante M, Hill EC. Pelvic exenteration: a critical analysis of a ten-year experience with the use of the team approach. *Am J Obstet Gynecol* 1971;110:180–189.
41. Symmonds RE, Pratt JH, Webb MJ. Exenterative operations: experience with 198 patients. *Am J Obstet Gynecol* 1975;121:907–918.
42. Lindsey WF, Wood DK, Briele HA, et al. Pelvic exenteration. *J Surg Oncol* 1985;30:231–234.
43. Stanhope CR, Symmonds RE. Palliative exenteration—what, when and why? *Am J Obstet Gynecol* 1985;152:12–16.
44. Morley GW, Hopkins MP, Lindenauer SM, et al. Pelvic exenteration: University of Michigan: 100 patients at 5 years. *Surg Obstet Gynecol* 1989;74:934–942.
45. Soper JT, Berchuck A, Creasman WT, et al. Pelvic exenteration: factors associated with major surgical morbidity. *Gynecol Oncol* 1989;35:93–98.
46. Hatch KD, Gelder MS, Soong S-J, et al. Pelvic exenteration with low rectal anastomosis: survival, complications and prognostic factors. *Gynecol Oncol* 1990;38:462.
47. Stanhope CR, Webb MJ, Padrantz KC. Pelvic exenteration for recurrent cervical cancer. *Clin Obstet Gynecol* 1990;33:897.
48. Hafner GH, Herrera L, Petrelli NJ. Morbidity and mortality after pelvic exenteration for colorectal adenocarcinoma. *Ann Surg* 1992;215:63–67.

49. Matthews CM, Morris M, Burke TW, et al. Pelvic exenteration in the elderly patient. *Obstet Gynecol* 1992;79:773–777.
50. Zincke H. Radical prostatectomy and exenterative procedures for local failure after radiotherapy with curative intent: comparison of outcomes. *J Urol* 1992;147:894-899.
51. Appleby LH. Proctocystectomy. The management of colostomy with ureteral transplants. *Am J Surg* 1950;79:57–60.
52. Brintnall ES, Flocks RH. En masse pelvic viscerectomy with ureterointestinal anastomosis. *Arch Surg* 1950;61:851–864.
53. Rutledge FN, Smith JP, Wharton JT, et al. Pelvic exenteration: analysis of 296 patients. *Am J Obstet Gynecol* 1977;129:881–887.
54. Eckhauser FE, Lindenauer SM, Morley GW. Pelvic exenteration for advanced rectal carcinoma. *Am J Surg* 1979;138:411–414.
55. Takagi H, Morimoto T, Yasue M, et al. Total pelvic exenteration for advanced carcinoma of the lower colon. *J Surg Oncol* 1985;28:59–62.
56. Wanebo HJ, Koness RJ, Vezeridis MP, et al. Pelvic resection of recurrent rectal cancer. *Ann Surg* 1994;220:586–597.
57. Schiessel R, Wunderlick M, Herbst F. Local recurrence of colorectal cancer: effect of early detection and aggressive surgery. *Br J Surg* 1986;72:342–344.
58. Takagi H, Morimoto T, Hara S, et al. Seven cases of pelvic exenteration combined with sacral resection for locally recurrent rectal cancer. *J Surg Oncol* 1986;32:184–188.
59. Temple WJ, Ketcham AS. Sacral resection for control of pelvic tumors. *Am J Surg* 1992;163:370–374.
60. Touran T, Frost DB, O Connell TX. Sacral resection: operative technique and outcome. *Arch Surg* 1990;125:911–913.
61. Maetani S, Nishikawa T, Yasnynki I, et al. Extensive en bloc resection of regionally recurrent carcinoma of the rectum. *Cancer* 1992;69:2876–2883.
62. Pearlman NW, Donohue RE, Steigman GV, et al. Pelvic and sacropelvic exenteration for locally advanced or recurrent anorectal cancer. *Arch Surg* 1987;122:537–541.
63. Deckers PJ, Olssom C, Williams LA, et al. Pelvic exenteration as palliation of malignant disease. *Am J Surg* 1976;131:509–515.

CHAPTER 19

Visceral and Parietal Peritonectomy Procedures

Paul H. Sugarbaker

Patience and persistence are the supreme surgical virtues.

BACKGROUND

Peritoneal carcinomatosis from gastrointestinal malignancy has always been regarded as a lethal clinical condition. Recently, a new strategy for treatment of established tumor implants within the abdominal cavity has been reported. A rationale for these treatments, based on the stepwise progression of gastrointestinal cancer, has been presented (1–12). An interpretation of the tumor biology that regulates the distribution of cancer deposits within the abdominal cavity has been proposed (13). A pharmacologic basis for intraperitoneal chemotherapy infusion as adjuvant therapy in the early postoperative period has been established (14–16). The prognostic features that would allow better patient selection have been recorded (17). These studies show clearly that the lesser the extent of peritoneal carcinomatosis and the lower its invasive capability, the better the results of treatment. The cytoreductive approach combining surgery and intraperitoneal chemotherapy as integrated strategy has been described (7,16–18). To optimize these treatments, one attempts to achieve maximal cytoreductive effects of surgery and combine these with the maximal cytoreductive effects of intraperitoneal chemotherapy used intraoperatively and in the early postoperative period. The morbidity (37%) and mortality (2%) has been described and the problems encountered with fistula formation have been analyzed (19–21). A new approach using induction intraperitoneal chemotherapy has been presented (22).

P. H. Sugarbaker: Department of Surgical Oncology, The Washington Cancer Institute, Washington Hospital Center, Washington, DC 20010.

This chapter presents the techniques required to complete six different peritonectomy procedures that are used to resect cancer from visceral intra-abdominal surfaces or to strip implants from parietal peritoneal surfaces. One or all six of these procedures may be required, depending on the distribution and volume of peritoneal carcinomatosis. This approach has been used in colorectal, appendiceal, gastric, pancreatic, ovarian, and small bowel adenocarcinoma. These procedures may also be of benefit to patients with mesothelioma and peritoneal sarcomatosis (23,24).

PRETREATMENT EVALUATION

An important concept in the modern treatment of malignancy is dose intensity (25,26). In the cytoreductive approach presented here, the maximal effects of surgery are combined with the maximal effects of chemotherapy at the same time and at the same anatomic location. This results in maximal dose intensity and treatment success in selected patients with peritoneal carcinomatosis. Surgical attempts to cure peritoneal carcinomatosis have never been successful in the past. Palliative attempts to remove even limited quantities of peritoneal carcinomatosis have always resulted in rapid recurrence of tumor within the abdominal cavity. Also, intraperitoneal chemotherapy alone has been singularly unsuccessful in treating large volumes of intra-abdominal cancer. Only when the combined treatments are used have treatment successes been reported.

Six different peritonectomy procedures are reported that may be required for maximal surgical cytoreduction. It is unusual for all six of these procedures to be needed in a single patient if low-volume disease is being treated. When all six procedures are used, patients usually have grade I cystadenocarcinoma of appendiceal origin. Also, mesothelioma patients may require all the peritonectomy procedures.

The pelvic peritonectomy may be the most frequently performed procedure. It may be used in the treatment of primary ovarian malignancy with peritoneal spread. Also, advanced rectal and rectosigmoid colon cancers with full-thickness penetration of the bowel wall and peritoneal seeding in the pelvis should have a pelvic peritonectomy. If a large volume of grade I cancer is present within the abdomen, the pelvis often has the largest volume of disease.

The right and left upper quadrant peritonectomy also is frequently required in appendiceal, colon, and ovarian cancer patients. Lymphatic lacuna (large peritoneal pores) exist on the undersurface of the diaphragm. These open lymphatic channels accept tumor cells into the superficial layer of the diaphragm's undersurface (27,28). These tumor cells then grow as a sheet of cancer adherent to the undersurface of the hemidiaphragm. As tumor beneath the diaphragm progresses, this malignancy may involve the dome of the right or left lobes of the liver. Complete removal of this tumor requires stripping of the undersurface of the diaphragm and an electrosurgical dissection of Glisson's capsule away from liver parenchyma.

Greater omentectomy usually is combined with splenectomy to achieve a complete cytoreduction. Of course, if the spleen is free of tumor, it is left in situ. The same is true when performing a lesser omentectomy. If the gallbladder is not involved by tumor, it can be preserved.

Perhaps the most difficult peritonectomy is the lesser omentectomy with stripping of the omental bursa. Vital structures here are of great density, and mistakes in dissection can lead to life-endangering hemorrhage or severe loss of function. The left gastric artery is the most commonly traumatized vessel. Its loss may result in the need for total gastrectomy. Ligation of the coronary vein may cause gastric portal hypertension. The left hepatic vein or left inferior subphrenic vein are thin-walled and may be damaged inadvertently by sudden and unpredictable diaphragmatic contractions stimulated by electrosurgical dissection. The left gastric artery, if arising from the left hepatic artery, will be encased by tumor and tends to obscure visualization of the vena cava, the crus of the right hemidiaphragm, and the origin of the left gastric artery.

METHODOLOGY

Position and Incision (Fig. 1)

The patient is in a supine position with the gluteal folds advanced to the break in the operating table to allow full access to the perineum during the surgical procedure. This modified lithotomy position is achieved with the legs extended in St. Mark's leg holders (AMSCO, Erie, PA). Proper positioning is essential to avoid intraoperative myonecrosis. The weight of the legs must be directed to the bottom of the feet by positioning the footrests so

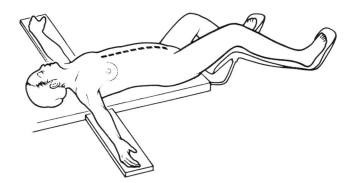

FIG. 1. Position and incision. (Sugarbaker PH. *Ann Surg* 1995;221:29–42)

that minimal weight is borne by the calf muscle. Myonecrosis within the posterior compartment of the leg may occur unless the legs are protected properly. All surfaces of the St. Mark's stirrups are protected by egg-crate foam padding. The thigh and legs are surrounded by alternating-pressure boots (SCB Compression Boots, Kendall Co., Boston, MA). These should be operative before the start of anesthesia for maximal protection against venothrombosis. A heating/cooling blanket is placed over the chest and arms of the patient (Bair Hugger Upper Body Cover, Augustine Medical, Eden Prairie, MN 55344) and also beneath the torso (Cincinnati Sub-Zero, Cincinnati, OH).

Abdominal skin preparation is from mid-chest to mid-thigh. The external genitalia are prepared in the male and a vaginal preparation used in females. The Foley catheter is placed in position after the surgical preparation. An 18-gauge nasogastric tube is placed within the stomach (Argyle Salem Sump Tube, Sherwood Medical, St. Louis, MO).

Abdominal Exposure, Greater Omentectomy, and Splenectomy (Fig. 2)

The abdomen is opened from xiphoid to pubis, and the xiphoid is excised using a rongeur. Generous abdominal exposure is achieved through the use of a Thompson Self-Retaining Retractor (Thompson Surgical Instruments, Inc., Traverse City, MI). The standard tool used to dissect tumor on peritoneal surfaces from the normal tissues is a ball-tipped electrosurgical handpiece (Valleylab, Boulder, CO). The ball-tipped instrument is placed at the interface of tumor and normal tissues. The focal point for further dissection is placed on strong traction. The electrosurgical generator is used on pure cut at high voltage. The 2-mm ball-tipped electrode is cautiously used for dissecting on visceral surfaces, including the stomach, small bowel, and colon. Dissection on parietal peritoneal surfaces presents less risk for heat necrosis.

Using ball-tipped electrosurgery on pure cut creates a large volume of plume because of the electroevaporation

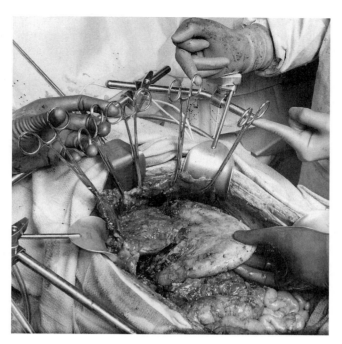

FIG. 2. Abdominal exposure, greater omentectomy and splenectomy.

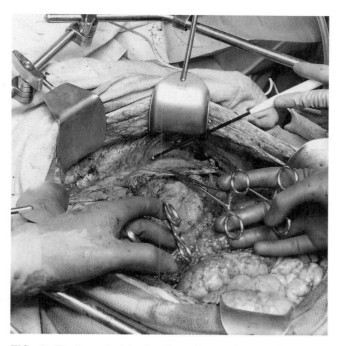

FIG. 3. Peritoneal stripping from beneath the left hemidiaphragm.

of tissue. To maintain visualization of the operative field and to preserve a smoke-free atmosphere, a smoke filtration unit is used (Stackhouse Inc., El Segunda, CA). The vacuum tip is maintained 2" to 3" from the field of dissection whenever electrosurgery is in use.

To free to mid-abdomen a large volume of tumor, a complete greater omentectomy is performed. The greater omentum is elevated and then separated from the transverse colon using electrosurgery. This dissection continues beneath the peritoneum that covers the transverse mesocolon so as to expose the pancreas. The gastroepiploic vessels on the greater curvature of the stomach are clamped, ligated, and divided. Also, the short gastric vessels are transected. The mound of tumor that covers the spleen is identified. With traction on the spleen, the peritoneum anterior to the pancreas is elevated from the gland using ball-tipped electrosurgery. This freely exposes the splenic artery and vein at the tail of the pancreas. These vessels are ligated in continuity and proximally suture-ligated. This allows the greater curvature of the stomach to be reflected anteriorly from the pylorus to the gastroesophageal junction.

Peritoneal Stripping from Beneath the Left Hemidiaphragm (Fig. 3)

To begin exposure of the left upper quadrant, the peritoneum that constitutes the edge of the abdominal incision is stripped off the posterior rectus sheath. To secure this peritoneal layer, large clamps are positioned about every 10 cm. This allows strong traction to be exerted on the tumor specimen throughout the left upper quadrant.

The left upper quadrant peritonectomy involves a stripping of all tissue from beneath the left hemidiaphragm to expose the diaphragmatic muscle, the left adrenal gland, the superior aspect of the pancreas, and the superior half of Gerota's fascia. To achieve exposure in the left upper quadrant, the splenic flexure is severed from the left abdominal gutter and moved medially by dividing the peritoneum along Toldt's line. The dissection beneath the hemidiaphragm must be performed with ball-tipped electrosurgery, not by blunt dissection. Numerous blood vessels between the diaphragm muscle and its peritoneal surface must be electrocoagulated before their transection or unnecessary bleeding will occur. Generally, tissues are transected using the ball-tipped electrosurgery on pure cut, but all blood vessels are electrocoagulated before their division.

Left Upper Quadrant Peritonectomy Completed (Fig. 4)

When the left upper quadrant peritonectomy is completed, the stomach may be reflected medially. Numerous ligated branches of the gastroepiploic arteries are evident. The left adrenal gland, pancreas, and left Gerota's fascia are visualized completely, as is the anterior peritoneal surface of the transverse mesocolon. Occasionally, tumor in and along the cephalad border of the pancreas requires small branches of the left gastric artery to be ligated and divided. However, with all the peritonectomy procedures, the surgeon must avoid the left gastric artery and coronary vein to preserve the sole remaining vascular supply to the stomach.

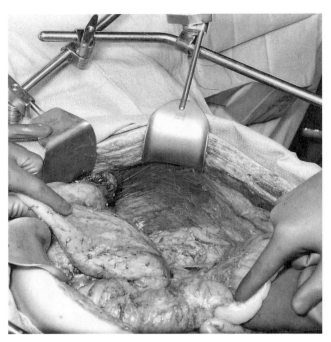

FIG. 4. Left upper quadrant peritonectomy, completed dissection.

Peritoneal Stripping From Beneath the Right Hemidiaphragm (Fig. 5)

Peritoneum is stripped from the right posterior rectus sheath to begin the peritonectomy in the right upper quadrant of the abdomen. Large clamps are placed on the

tumor and strong traction is used to elevate the hemidiaphragm into the operative field. Again, ball-tipped electrosurgery on pure cut is used to dissect at the interface of tumor and normal tissue. Coagulation current is used to divide the blood vessels as they are encountered to minimize problems with postoperative hemorrhage.

The stripping of tumor from the undersurface of the diaphragm continues until the bare area of the liver is encountered. At that point, tumor on the anterior surface of the liver is electroevaporated until the liver surface is encountered. With both blunt and ball-tipped electrosurgical dissection, the tumor is lifted off the dome of the liver by moving through or beneath Glisson's capsule. Hemostasis is achieved as the dissection proceeds, using coagulation electrosurgery on the liver surface. Isolated patches of tumor on the liver surface are electroevaporated with the distal 2 cm of the ball tip bent and stripped of insulation ("hockey-stick" configuration). Ball-tipped electrosurgery is also used to extirpate tumor from in and around the falciform ligament, round ligament, and umbilical fissure of the liver.

Removal of Tumor From Beneath the Right Hemidiaphragm, From Right Subhepatic Space, and From the Surface of the Liver (Fig. 6)

Tumor from beneath the right hemidiaphragm, from the right subhepatic space, and from the surface of the liver forms an envelope as it is removed en bloc. The dissection is greatly facilitated if the tumor specimen can be

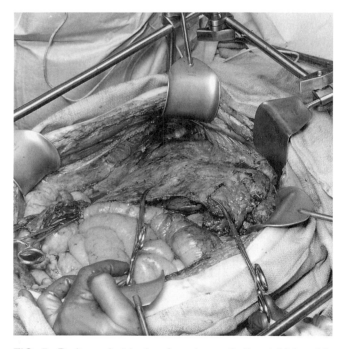

FIG. 5. Peritoneal stripping from beneath the right hemidiaphragm.

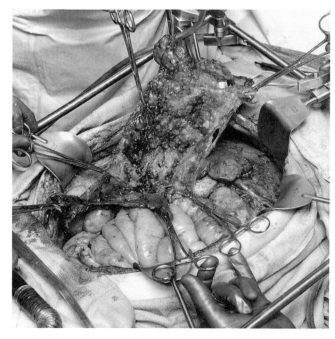

FIG. 6. Removal of tumor from beneath the right hemidiaphragm, from the right subhepatic space, and from the surface of the liver.

maintained intact. The dissection continues laterally on the right to encounter Gerota's fascia covering the right kidney. Also, the right adrenal gland is visualized as tumor is stripped from Morrison's pouch (right subhepatic space). Care is taken not to traumatize the vena cava or to disrupt the caudate lobe veins that pass between the vena cava and segment 1 of the liver.

Completed Right Upper Quadrant Peritonectomy Including Stripping of the Right Subhepatic Space (Fig. 7)

With strong traction on the right costal margin and medial displacement of the right liver, one can visualize the completed right upper quadrant peritonectomy. The anterior branches of the phrenic artery and vein are seen and have been preserved. The right hepatic vein and the vena cava below have been exposed. The right adrenal gland and Gerota's fascia covering the right kidney constitute the base of the dissection.

Frequently, tumor is densely adherent to the tendinous central portion of the left or right hemidiaphragm. If this occurs, the tissue infiltrated by tumor must be resected. This usually requires an elliptical excision of a portion of the hemidiaphragm on either the right or the left. The defect in the diaphragm is closed with interrupted sutures.

Lesser Omentectomy and Cholecystectomy (Fig. 8)

The gallbladder is removed in a routine fashion from its fundus toward the cystic artery and cystic duct. These

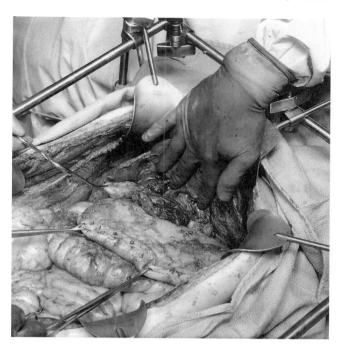

FIG. 8. Lesser omentectomy and cholecystectomy. Cholecystectomy completed.

structures are ligated and divided. The hepatoduodenal ligament that covers the porta hepatis is usually heavily layered with tumor. Using strong traction, the cancerous tissue that coats the structure is stripped from the base of the gallbladder bed toward the duodenum. In this dissection, the ball-tipped electrosurgery may be excessively traumatic. The delicate structures of the porta hepatis, especially the left hepatic artery, are dissected free of tumor by the spreading action of a clamp. Blade electrosurgery on coagulation current is used to divide tissues above the clamp. To continue resection of the lesser omentum, one proceeds along the gastrohepatic fissure that divides liver segments 2, 3, and 4 from segment 1. One goes back to ball-tipped electrosurgery for this maneuver and for electroevaporation of tumor from the anterior surface of the left caudate process. Great care is taken not to traumatize the caudate process, for this can result in excessive and needless blood loss. The segmental blood supply to the caudate lobe is located on the anterior surface of this segment of the liver, and hemorrhage may occur with only superficial trauma. Also, a replaced left hepatic artery may arise from the left gastric artery and cross through the hepatogastric fissure. If this occurs, one dissects with a spreading clamp along this vessel to isolate it from the surrounding tumor and localize the left gastric artery.

Stripping of the Omental Bursa (Fig. 9)

As one clears the left part of the caudate liver segment of tumor, the vena cava is visualized directly beneath. To

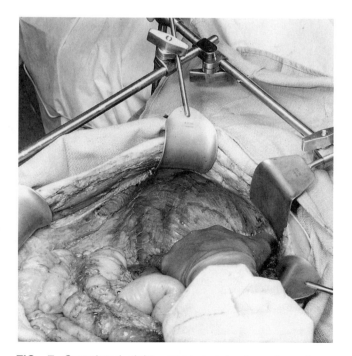

FIG. 7. Completed right upper quadrant peritonectomy, including stripping of the right subhepatic space.

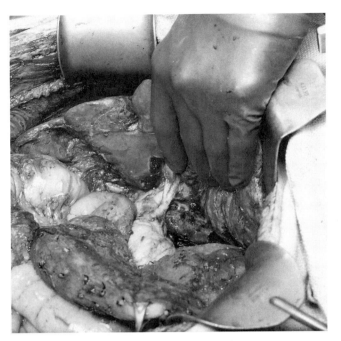

FIG. 9. Stripping of the omental bursa completed.

begin to strip the omental bursa, strong traction is maintained on the tumor and ball-tipped electrosurgery is used to divide the loose fibrous tissue above the vena cava. The crus of the right hemidiaphragm is skeletonized. The common hepatic artery and the left gastric artery are skeletonized and avoided. A spreading clamp with blade electrosurgery is used to identify the cephalad and cau-

dad branching of the left gastric artery and the coronary vein. Dissection of lesser omental fat by compressing tissue between the thumb and index finger helps identify the major branches of the left gastric artery. They are preserved to ensure adequate blood supply to the stomach. At least two major branches of the left gastric artery are required to provide blood supply to the stomach.

The surgeon dissects in a clockwise direction along the lesser curvature of the stomach. Care is taken to preserve as much omental fat as possible; only tumor tissue is removed. The multiple branches of the vagus nerve to the antrum of the stomach are divided. Finally, dissection through the celiac lymph nodes allows the specimen to be released.

A pyloroplasty or gastrojejunostomy must be performed to allow the stomach to empty. In the absence of a gastric drainage procedure, gastric stasis will occur because of the vagotomy.

Pelvic Peritonectomy (Fig. 10)

To begin the pelvic peritonectomy, the tumor-bearing peritoneum is stripped from the posterior surface of the lower abdominal incision, exposing the rectus muscle. The muscular surface of the bladder is seen, as ball-tipped electrosurgery strips peritoneum and preperitoneal fat from this structure. The urachus must be divided and then elevated as the leading point for this dissection. The round ligaments are divided as they enter the internal inguinal ring on both the right and left in the female.

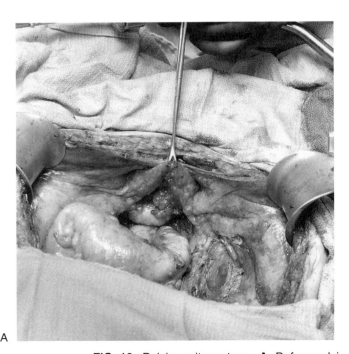

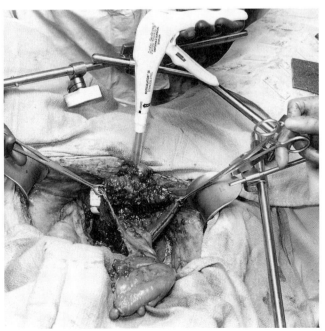

A   B

FIG. 10. Pelvic peritonectomy. **A:** Before pelvic stripping. **B:** Centripetal dissection completed.

The peritoneal incision around the pelvis is completed by dividing the peritoneum along the pelvic brim. The right and left ureters are identified and preserved. In women, the right and left ovarian veins are ligated and divided. A linear stapler is used to divide the sigmoid colon in its midportion. The vascular supply of the distal portion of bowel is traced back to its origin on the aorta. The inferior mesenteric artery is ligated and divided. This allows one to pack all the viscera, including the proximal sigmoid colon, in the upper abdomen.

Resection of Rectosigmoid Colon Beneath Peritoneal Reflection (Fig. 11)

Ball-tipped electrosurgery is used to dissect beneath the mesorectum. The surgeon works in a centripetal fashion to free the entire pelvis. Extraperitoneal ligation of the uterine arteries is performed just above the ureter and close to the base of the bladder. In women, the bladder is moved gently off the cervix and the vagina is entered. The vaginal cuff anterior and posterior to the cervix is transected using ball-tipped electrosurgery, and the perirectal fat inferior to the posterior vaginal wall is encountered. Ball-tipped electrosurgery is used to divide the perirectal fat beneath the peritoneal reflection. This ensures that all tumor that occupies the cul de sac is removed intact with the specimen. The midportion of the rectal musculature is skeletonized using ball-tipped electrosurgery. A roticulator stapler (Autosuture, Norwalk, CT) is used to staple the rectal stump closed.

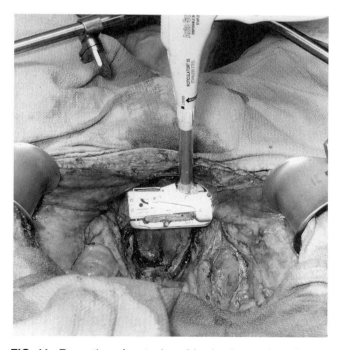

FIG. 11. Resection of rectosigmoid colon beneath peritoneal reflection.

Vaginal Closure and Colorectal Anastomosis

Interrupted sutures are used to close the vaginal cuff. A circular stapling device is passed into the rectum, and the trochar penetrates the staple line. A monofilament suture placed in a purse-string fashion is used to secure the staple anvil in the proximal sigmoid colon. The body of the circular stapler and anvil are mated and the stapler is activated to complete the low colorectal anastomosis (Intraluminal Stapler 33, Ethicon, Sommerville, NJ).

A requirement for a complication-free low colorectal anastomosis is absence of tension on the suture line. Adequate mobilization of the entire left colon is needed, and several steps may be required to accomplish this. The inferior mesenteric artery is ligated on the aorta, and then its individual branches are ligated as they arise from this vascular trunk. This allows for great stretching of the left colic mesentery. The inferior mesenteric vein is divided as it courses around behind the duodenum. The mesentery of the transverse colon and splenic flexure are completely elevated from Gerota's fascia. Taking care to avoid the left ureter, the surgeon divides the left colon mesentery from all its attachments. These maneuvers allow the junction of the sigmoid and descending colon to reach to the low rectum or anus for a tension-free anastomosis.

To ensure a safe colorectal anastomosis, the proximal and distal tissue rings are examined for completeness. Air is insufflated into the rectum with a water-filled pelvis to check for an airtight anastomosis. A hand is passed beneath the sigmoid colon to ensure there is no tension on the stapled anastomosis. A rectal examination is done to check for staple-line bleeding at the anastomosis.

Antrectomy (Fig. 12)

The gastric antrum, along with other intra-abdominal structures that have restricted peristalsis, may be surrounded so densely by tumor that resection rather than peritoneal stripping is required for complete tumor removal (13). The right gastric artery is divided and the first portion of the duodenum is separated from the pancreas. A stapler (Ethicon PLC 75, Cincinnati, OH) is used to close off and transect the duodenum just below the last visible evidence of tumor. Similarly, a stapler (Ethicon TA 90, Cincinnati, OH) divides the stomach proximally above the tumor.

Gastric Reconstruction

The duodenal and gastric staple lines are inverted with interrupted sutures. A side-to-side gastrojejunostomy is performed. A large-bore Malincott tube is secured through the side of the duodenum with purse-string

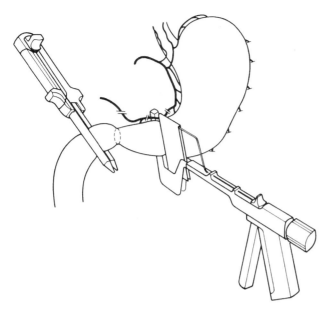

FIG. 12. Antrectomy.

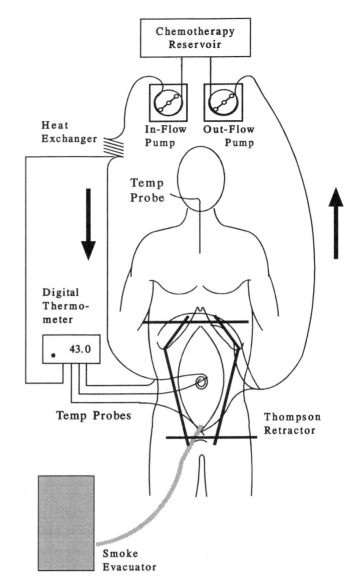

FIG. 13. Tubes and drains required for intraoperative and early postoperative intraperitoneal chemotherapy.

sutures. Plication of the Malincott tube within the wall of the duodenum prevents leakage around the tube.

Tubes and Drains Required for Intraoperative and Early Postoperative Intraperitoneal Chemotherapy (Fig. 13)

Closed-suction drains are placed in the dependent portions of the abdomen. This includes the right subhepatic space, the left subdiaphragmatic space, and the pelvis. A Tenckhoff catheter (Quinton spiral peritoneal catheter, Quinton, Inc., Seattle, WA) is placed through the abdominal wall and positioned beneath the loops of small bowel. All transabdominal drains and tubes are secured in a watertight fashion with a purse-string suture at the peritoneal level. Temperature probes are placed at the inflow (Tenckhoff catheter) and at a remote site. They are removed after the intraoperative chemotherapy is completed. Right-angle thoracostomy tubes (Deknatel, Floral Park, NY) are inserted on both the right and left to prevent fluid accumulation in the chest as a result of intraperitoneal chemotherapy.

As soon as the abdomen is closed, irrigation of the abdomen with 1.5% dextrose dialysis solution (Dianeal, Abbott Laboratories, Chicago, IL) is begun. Standardized orders for early postoperative intraperitoneal lavage and for early postoperative intraperitoneal chemotherapy administration are instituted (16).

Specimens

Figure 14A shows the specimen recovered from the greater omentectomy/splenectomy/stripping of the left

hemidiaphragm. In this patient, a potential resection of the greater omentum had occurred at a prior operation. The greater omentum was resected from the left lateral aspect of the greater curvature of the stomach; this tissue (along with the spleen, peritoneum from the undersurface of the left hemidiaphragm, and tumor), which fixed three structures together, was submitted to the pathologist as an intact specimen.

Figure 14B shows the specimen recovered from stripping the right hemidiaphragm. The mucinous tumor is resected from the undersurface of the diaphragm, from the right subhepatic space, and from all surfaces of the liver. The result is an envelope of tumor tissue that is submitted to the pathologist.

Figure 14C shows the specimen recovered from the lesser omentectomy/cholecystectomy. All tumor from

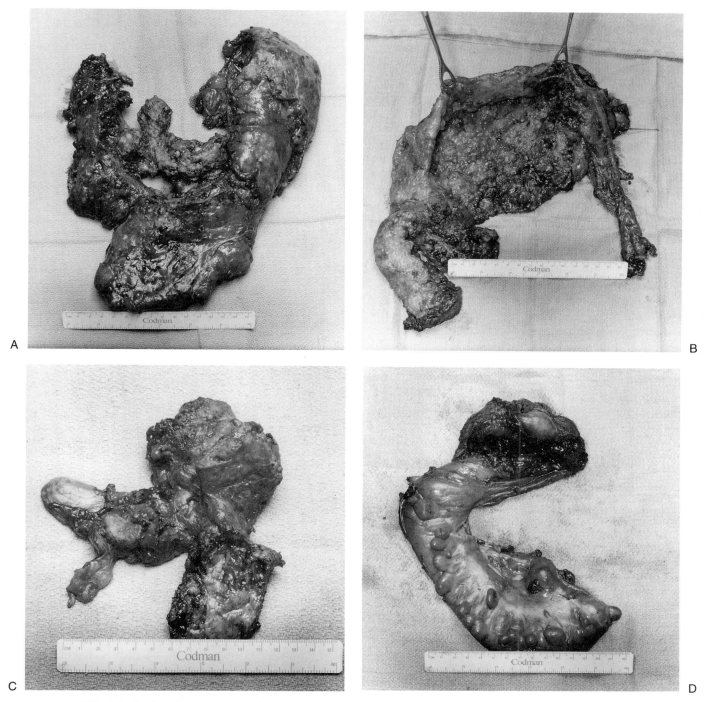

FIG. 14. A: Specimen recovered from greater omentectomy/splenectomy/stripping of the left hemidiaphragm. **B:** Specimen recovered from stripping the right hemidiaphragm. **C:** Specimen recovered from lesser omentectomy/cholecystectomy. **D:** Specimen recovered from pelvic peritonectomy/rectosigmoid resection.

the visceral surface of the liver, omental bursa, hepatogastric ligament, and hepatoduodenal ligament is included. Usually the gallbladder is included. In advanced disease, the antrum of the stomach is part of this specimen.

Figure 14D shows the specimen recovered from the pelvic peritonectomy/rectosigmoid resection. This tissue includes a complete removal of the cul de sac of Douglas. Occasionally, the complete stripping of tumor from the pelvis can occur without removal of the rectosigmoid colon, uterus, ovaries, and fallopian tubes.

SUMMARY

Decisions regarding the treatment of cancer depend on the anatomic location of the malignancy and the biologic aggressiveness of the disease. Some patients may have isolated intra-abdominal seeding of malignancy of limited extent or of low biologic grade. In the past, these clinical situations have been regarded as lethal. The cytoreductive approach may require six peritonectomy procedures to resect or strip cancer from all intra-abdominal surfaces: greater omentectomy/splenectomy, left upper quadrant peritonectomy, right upper quadrant peritonectomy, lesser omentectomy/cholecystectomy with stripping of the omental bursa, pelvic peritonectomy with sleeve resection of the sigmoid colon, and antrectomy.

Peritonectomy procedures and preparation of the abdomen for intraoperative and early postoperative intraperitoneal chemotherapy were described. We have used the cytoreductive approach to achieve long-term disease-free survival in selected patients with peritoneal carcinomatosis, peritoneal sarcomatosis, or mesothelioma.

REFERENCES

1. Sugarbaker PH. Cancer of the appendix and pseudomyxoma peritonei. In Fazio VW, ed. *Current therapy in colon and rectal surgery.* Philadelphia: BC Decker, 1989.
2. Sugarbaker PH, Cunliffe W, Belliveau JF, et al. Rationale for perioperative intraperitoneal chemotherapy as a surgical adjuvant for gastrointestinal malignancy. *Regional Cancer Treat* 1988;1:66–79.
3. Sugarbaker PH. Surgical treatment of peritoneal carcinomatosis. *Can J Surg* 1989;32:164–170.
4. Sugarbaker PH. Management of peritoneal carcinomatosis. *Progress in Regional Cancer Therapy, Acta Medica Austriaca* 1989;3/4:57–60.
5. Sugarbaker PH, Cunliffe WJ, Belliveau JF, et al. Rationale for integrating early postoperative intraperitoneal chemotherapy (EPIC) into the surgical treatment of gastrointestinal cancer. *Sem Oncol* 1989;16:83–97.
6. Sugarbaker PH, Landy D, Pascal R. Intraperitoneal chemotherapy for peritoneal carcinomatosis from colonic or appendiceal cystadenocarcinoma. Rationale and results of treatment. In Ragaz J, ed. *Effects of therapy on biology and kinetics of surviving tumor.* New York: Liss, 1991.
7. Sugarbaker PH. Cytoreductive surgery and intraperitoneal chemotherapy with peritoneal spread of cystadenocarcinoma. *Eur J Surg* 1991 (suppl);561:75–82.
8. Sugarbaker PH. The natural history of large bowel cancer, surgical implications. *J Exp Clin Cancer Res* 1989;8:41–43.
9. Vidal-Jove J, Sugarbaker PH. Curative approach to abdominal mesothelioma. Case report and review of the literature. *Reg Cancer Treat* 1991; 3:269–274.
10. Sugarbaker PH. Rule of least margins. Rationale for surgical treatment planning in gastrointestinal cancer. *Reg Cancer Treat* 1991;4:116–120.
11. Sugarbaker PH. Mechanisms of release for colorectal cancer. Implications for intraperitoneal chemotherapy. *J Surg Oncol* 1991;2:36–41.
12. Jacquet P, Vidal-Jove J, Zhu B, Sugarbaker PH. Peritoneal carcinomatosis from gastrointestinal malignancy. Natural history and new prospects for management. *Acta Belgica Chirurgica* 1994;94:191–197.
13. Sugarbaker PH. Observations concerning cancer spread within the peritoneal cavity and concepts supporting an ordered pathophysiology. In Sugarbaker PH, ed. *Peritoneal carcinomatosis, diagnosis and treatment.* Boston: Kluwer, 1995.
14. Speyer JL, Sugarbaker PH, Collins JM, Dedrick RL, Klecker RW Jr, Meyers CE. Portal levels and hepatic clearance of 5-fluorouracil after intraperitoneal administration in humans. *Cancer Res* 1981;41: 1916–1922.
15. Sugarbaker PH, Landy D, Pascal R, Jaffe G. Histologic changes induced by intraperitoneal chemotherapy in patients with peritoneal carcinomatosis from cystadenocarcinoma of the large bowel. *Cancer* 1990;65:1495–1501.
16. Sugarbaker PH. *Intraperitoneal chemotherapy and cytoreductive surgery, a manual for physicians and nurses.* Grand Rapids: Ludann, 1993.
17. Sugarbaker PH, Jablonski KA. Prognostic features of 51 colorectal and 130 appendiceal cancer patients with peritoneal carcinomatosis treated by cytoreductive surgery and intraperitoneal chemotherapy. *Ann Surg* 1995;221:124–132.
18. Sugarbaker PH, Kern K, Lack E. Malignant pseudomyxoma of colonic origin. Natural history and presentation of a curative approach to treatment. *Dis Colon Rectum* 1987;30:772–779.
19. Fernandez-Trigo V, Sugarbaker PH. Diagnosis and management of postoperative gastrointestinal fistula. A kinetic analysis. *J Exp Clin Cancer Res* 1994;13:233–241.
20. Esquivel J, Vidal-Jove J, Steves MA, Sugarbaker PH. Morbidity and mortality of cytoreductive surgery and intraperitoneal chemotherapy. *Surgery* 1993;113:631–636.
21. Morena E, Sugarbaker PH. Gastrointestinal fistula following cytoreductive procedures for peritoneal carcinomatosis. Incidence and outcome. *J Exp Clin Cancer Res* 1993;12:153–158.
22. Sugarbaker PH, Steves MA, Hafner GH. Treatment of peritoneal carcinomatosis from colon or appendiceal cancer with induction intraperitoneal chemotherapy. *Reg Cancer Treat* 1993;4:183–187.
23. Auerbach AM, Sugarbaker PH. Peritoneal mesothelioma: treatment approach based on natural history. In: Sugarbaker PH (ed). *Peritoneal carcinoma: drugs and diseases.* Boston: Kluwer, 1996.
24. Sugarbaker PH, Schillinx MET, Chang D, Koslowe P, Meyenfeldt MV von. Peritoneal carcinomatosis from adenocarcinoma of the colon. *World J Surg* 1996;20:585–592.
25. Hryniuk WM. Average relative dose intensity and the impact on design of clinical trials. *Semin Oncol* 1987;14:65–74.
26. DeVita VT, Hubbard SM, Longo DL. The chemotherapy of lymphomas: looking back, moving forward. *Cancer Res* 1987;47:5810–5824.
27. Torres IG, Litterest CL, Guarino AM. Transport of model compounds across the peritoneal membrane in the rat. *Pharmacology* 1987;17: 330–340.
28. Feldman GB, Knapp RI. Lymphatic drainage of the peritoneal cavity and its significance in ovarian cancer. *Am J Obstet Gynecol* 1974;119: 991–994.

CHAPTER 20

Intraperitoneal Chemotherapy

Paul H. Sugarbaker

Diseases desperate grow by desperate appliance are relieved, or not at all.
    —*Shakespeare, Hamlet, IV, iii, 9.*

BACKGROUND

Most cancers that occur within the abdomen or pelvis will disseminate by three different routes: hematogenous metastases, lymphatic metastases, and implants of peritoneal surfaces. In many patients, surgical treatment failure that is isolated to the resection site or to peritoneal surfaces may occur. This leads us to postulate that the elimination of peritoneal surface spread may affect the survival of these cancer patients and that a prominent cause of death in patients with intra-abdominal malignancy is peritoneal carcinomatosis or sarcomatosis. Before the use of intraperitoneal chemotherapy, these conditions were uniformly fatal, eventually resulting in intestinal obstruction over the course of months or years. Occasionally, patients with low-grade malignancies survived long term, but all end result reportings show a fatal outcome with spread of intra-abdominal cancer.

The devised techniques allow for the administration of intraperitoneal chemotherapy as an integrated part of a surgical procedure for cancer. This approach involves two conceptual changes in chemotherapy administration. The intraperitoneal route ensures uniform distribution of a high concentration of anticancer therapy at the peritoneal surfaces. This can be achieved because the surgeon intraoperatively manually manipulates the intestines to distribute the chemotherapy uniformly. Secondly, the timing for the chemotherapy administration is such that all the malignancy, except microscopic residual disease, will have been removed before the chemotherapy treatments.

P. H. Sugarbaker: Department of Surgical Oncology, The Washington Cancer Institute, Washington Hospital Center, Washington, DC 20010.

This means that the limited penetration of chemotherapy (about 1 mm into tissues) will be adequate to eradicate all tumor cells. Also, the chemotherapy is used before the construction of any anastomoses. This means that suture line recurrences should also be eliminated.

This chapter discusses the methods for treatment and prevention developed for peritoneal carcinomatosis and sarcomatosis over the last 12 years.

Peritoneal–Plasma Barrier

Intraperitoneal chemotherapy gives high response rates within the abdomen because the peritoneal–plasma barrier provides dose-intensive therapy (1). Figure 1 shows that large-molecular-weight substances, such as mitomycin, are confined to the abdominal cavity for long periods (2). This means that the exposure of peritoneal surfaces to pharmacologically active molecules can be increased considerably by giving the drugs via the intraperitoneal (IP) route as opposed to the intravenous (IV) one.

For the chemotherapy agents used to treat peritoneal carcinomatosis or peritoneal sarcomatosis, the area under the curve (AUC) ratios of IP to IV exposure are favorable. Table 1 presents the AUC IP/IV for the drugs in routine clinical use in patients with peritoneal seeding (2,3). In our studies, these include 5-fluorouracil, mitomycin, doxorubicin (Adriamycin), and cisplatin.

Tumor Cell Entrapment

My colleagues and I have advanced the "tumor cell entrapment" hypothesis to explain the high incidence of peritoneal seeding in patients who undergo the surgical treatment of intra-abdominal adenocarcinoma or sarcoma. This theory relates the high incidence of tumor implantation to:

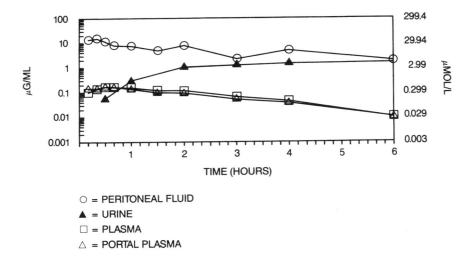

FIG. 1. Early postoperative administration of intraperitoneal mitomycin. Large-molecular-weight compounds, when instilled into the peritoneal cavity, are sequestered at that site for long periods. The physiologic barrier to the release of intraperitoneal drugs is called the peritoneal–plasma barrier. In this experiment, 15 mg of mitomycin was infused into the cavity as rapidly as possible. Intraperitoneal, intravenous, portal venous, and urine mitomycin concentrations were determined by HPLC assay. (Sugarbaker PH, Graves T, DeBruijn EA, et al. Rationale for early postoperative intraperitoneal chemotherapy [EPIC] in patients with advanced gastrointestinal cancer. *Cancer Res* 1990;50:5790–5794, with permission)

Free intraperitoneal tumor emboli as a result of serosal penetration by cancer

Leakage of malignant cells from lymphatics

Dissemination of malignant cells from trauma as a result of surgical dissection

Fibrin entrapment of intra-abdominal tumor emboli on traumatized peritoneal surfaces

Tumor promotion of these entrapped cells through growth factors involved in the wound healing process.

Change in the Route and Timing of Chemotherapy Administration

To interrupt this widespread implantation of tumor cells on intra-abdominal and pelvic surfaces, the abdominal cavity is flooded with chemotherapy by a large volume of fluid before surgery (induction chemotherapy), during surgery (heated intraoperative intraperitoneal chemotherapy) and in the postoperative period (early postoperative intraperitoneal chemotherapy). Some patients with a poor

TABLE 1. *Area under the curve ratios of peritoneal surface exposure for drugs used to treat intra-abdominal cancer*

Drug	Molecular weight	Area under the curve ratio
5-fluorouracil	130	250
Mitomycin	334	75
Adriamycin	544	500
Cisplatin	300	20

prognosis may be recommended for adjuvant intraperitoneal and systemic chemotherapy (4–7).

Therefore, the strategy for treatment and prevention of peritoneal carcinomatosis and sarcomatosis involves not only a change in the route, but also a change in the timing of chemotherapy administration. This new approach to the surgical treatment of intra-abdominal malignancy begins in the operating room after a complete resection of a primary cancer or after the complete cytoreduction of peritoneal carcinomatosis or peritoneal sarcomatosis. Proper placement of tubes and drains and temperature probes is needed before initiating intraperitoneal chemotherapy. (Before abdominal closure, the temperature probes are removed, but the tubes and drains are left in place for early postoperative intraperitoneal lavage and chemotherapy.)

Heated Intraoperative Intraperitoneal Chemotherapy Administration

In the operating room, heated intraperitoneal chemotherapy is used. Heat is part of the optimizing process and is used to bring as much dose intensity to the abdominal and pelvic surfaces as possible. Hyperthermia with intraperitoneal chemotherapy has several advantages. First, heat by itself has more toxicity for cancerous tissue than for normal tissue. This predominant effect on cancer increases as the vascularity of the malignancy decreases. Second, hyperthermia increases the penetration of chemotherapy into tissues. As tissues soften in response to heat, the elevated interstitial pres-

TABLE 2. *Benefits of using heated intraoperative intraperitoneal chemotherapy*

Heat increases drug penetration into tissue.
Heat increases the cytotoxicity of selected chemotherapy agents.
Heat has antitumor effect by itself.
Intraoperative chemotherapy allows manual distribution of drug and heat uniformly to all surfaces of the abdomen and pelvis.
Renal toxicities of chemotherapy given in the operation room can be avoided by careful monitoring of urine output during chemotherapy perfusion.
The time that elapses during the heated perfusion allows a normalization of many functional parameters (e.g., temperature, blood clotting, hemodynamics).

sure of a tumor mass may decrease, allowing improved drug penetration. Third, and probably most important, heat increases the cytotoxicity of selected chemotherapy agents. This synergism occurs only at the interface of heat and body tissue, at the peritoneal surface. The reasons for using heated chemotherapy as a surgically directed modality in the operating room are listed in Table 2.

In the immediate postoperative period, an abdominal lavage removes tissue debris and blood products from the abdominal cavity so there is little or no fibrin accumulation. Tumor cells that remain in the abdominal cavity can be destroyed by the pharmacologic concentrations of intraperitoneal chemotherapy instilled on postoperative days 1 through 5. The timely use of intraperitoneal chemotherapy in the early postoperative period eliminates tumor cells from the abdomen before they are fixed within the scar tissue that results from wound healing.

The chemotherapy not only directly destroys tumor cells, but it also eliminates viable platelets, white blood cells, and monocytes from the peritoneal cavity. This diminishes the promotion of tumor growth associated with the wound healing process. Consequently, the results from use of intraperitoneal chemotherapy show a reduction in local recurrence and peritoneal surface recurrence in patients with intra-abdominal cancer. Removal of the leukocytes and monocytes also decreases the ability of the abdomen to resist an infectious process. For this reason, strict aseptic technique is imperative when administering the chemotherapy or handling abdominal tubes and drains.

SELECTION OF PATIENTS BY PROGNOSTIC GROUPS

The prognostic features that control the results of treatment in patients with peritoneal carcinomatosis have been determined. Prognostic indicators include the grade of the malignant tumor, the presence or absence of lymphatic or hematogenous metastases, and the completeness of the surgical removal of cancer from the abdomen and pelvis. Table 3 presents the prognostic groups for peritoneal carcinomatosis from colon cancer, rectal cancer, and appendiceal cancer now being used clinically to predict outcome. Unfortunately, the grade of these tumors is not easily determined, and much confusion exists among pathologists. A complete cytoreduction indicates that no nodules of cancer >2.5 mm in diameter remain after surgery.

Large-Volume, Low-Grade Adenocarcinoma and Sarcoma

Table 4 presents the current indications for the use of intraperitoneal chemotherapy. Adenocarcinoma or sarcoma of low malignant potential may arise from many different intra-abdominal sites and seed the abdominal or pelvic cavity extensively. Most of these noninvasive malignancies can be eradicated from the abdomen. Cytoreductive surgery followed by intraperitoneal chemotherapy should be considered the standard therapy for patients with malignant pseudomyxoma peritonei of colonic, appendiceal, or ovarian origin. Also, these treatments have demonstrated benefits for patients with peritoneal surface disease from grade I sarcoma and mesothelioma.

Moderate- to High-Grade Adenocarcinoma

Higher-grade adenocarcinomas of colonic or appendiceal origin are selectively treated with induction intraperitoneal chemotherapy followed by cytoreductive surgery (7). In patients with large-volume, high-grade cancer, only palliative treatments for peritoneal carcinomatosis should be considered. In patients with low-volume, high-grade peritoneal seeding, three cycles of intraperitoneal chemotherapy are routinely used before definitive cytoreductive surgery. About 10% of patients with colon and rectal cancer have peritoneal seeding documented at the time of resection of the primary cancer. This merits induction intraperitoneal chemotherapy

TABLE 3. *Prognostic groups of peritoneal carcinomatosis patients*

Group	Histology	Metastases	Cytoreduction	N	3-year survival (%)
I	Grade 1	None	Complete	76	99
II	Grades 2–3	None	Complete	23	65
III	Any	Present	Complete	24	66
IV	Any	Any	Incomplete	58	20

TABLE 4. *Indications for intraperitoneal chemotherapy*

Large-volume, low-grade peritoneal carcinomatosis or
  sarcomatosis after definitive cytoreductive surgery
Low-volume peritoneal seeding of moderate- or high-grade
  cancer
Perforated gastrointestinal cancers
Cancers adherent to adjacent organs or structures
Tumor spill intraoperatively
Stage IIb or greater primary ovarian cancer after definitive
  cytoreductive surgery
Chemotherapy-resistant, recurrent ovarian cancer after
  definitive cytoreductive surgery
Gastrointestinal or ovarian cancer with positive
  intraperitoneal cytology
Abdominal mesothelioma after definitive cytoreductive
  surgery

and cytoreductive surgery. Figure 2 presents current treatment options for peritoneal carcinomatosis from gastrointestinal cancer.

Importance of Tumor Volume and Distribution in Patient Selection

Tumor volume and tumor distribution are the fundamental criteria for the selection of patients for treatment with intraperitoneal chemotherapy. The treatment of bulk disease from moderate to high grade or cancer in the abdominal cavity by intraperitoneal chemotherapy must be avoided: only patients with low-volume, high-grade peritoneal surface cancer should be treated with intraperitoneal chemotherapy. Small-lesion peritoneal seeding with limited distribution on peritoneal surfaces should be expected to respond and is an indication for induction chemotherapy. If large-volume, low-grade disease is present, a complete surgical cytoreduction must precede intraperitoneal chemotherapy (7). Figure 3 shows the effect of lesion size of peritoneal nodules on the long-term survival of patients with peritoneal carcinomatosis from colon cancer (8).

Prevention of Peritoneal Carcinomatosis

A major role for intraperitoneal chemotherapy is the prevention of subsequent peritoneal carcinomatosis or sarcomatosis. Virtually every patient who has a free intra-abdominal perforation of gastrointestinal cancer through the malignancy itself develops peritoneal carcinomatosis. We recommend intraoperative and early postoperative intraperitoneal chemotherapy for all patients with perforated gastrointestinal cancers.

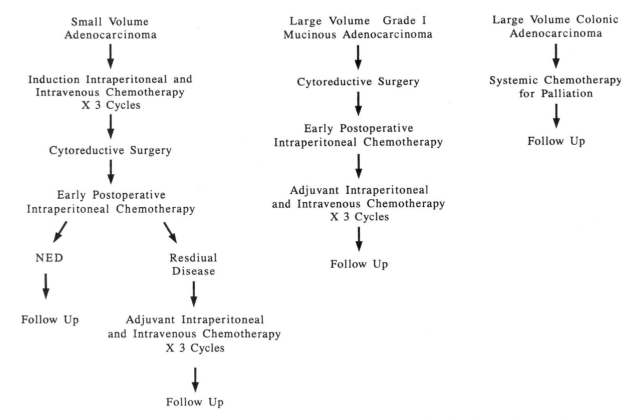

FIG. 2. Treatment options for patients with peritoneal carcinomatosis. Small-volume adenocarcinoma is defined as implants <5 cm in diameter with no confluence of disease at any anatomic site. A matting together of organs by cancer is scored as large-volume disease and will not profit from induction chemotherapy. (Esquivel J, Vidal-Jove J, Steves MA, Sugarbaker PH. Morbidity and mortality of cytoreductive surgery and intraperitoneal chemotherapy. *Surgery* 1993;631–636).

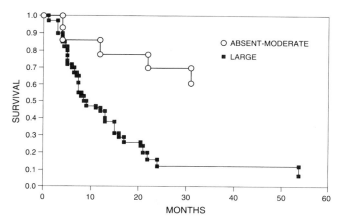

FIG. 3. Lesion size was assessed in patients with peritoneal carcinomatosis from colon cancer who were treated by cytoreductive surgery and intraperitoneal chemotherapy. Survival was plotted by the Kaplan-Meier method and statistically analyzed by the log-rank test. The size of the peritoneal implants before cytoreduction was estimated as follows: absent (complete response to induction chemotherapy), minimal (nodules <0.5 cm in greatest dimension), moderate (nodules 0.5–5.0 cm), and large (nodules >5.0 cm). The differences in survival are significant (*p*<0.0001). (Sugarbaker PH, Schellinx MET, Chang D, Koslow P, Meyenfeldt M von. Peritoneal carcinomatosis from adenocarcinoma of the colon [*World J Surg* 1996;20:585–592]).

Not infrequently, patients who are undergoing the resection of a large intra-abdominal tumor have a tumor spill. This is extremely common with advanced primary or recurrent rectal malignancy and recurrent colonic cancer. It occurs almost routinely in resection of advanced gastric cancer. If there is a tumor spill, we recommend the use of intraperitoneal chemotherapy to prevent subsequent development of peritoneal carcinomatosis or sarcomatosis. Limited peritoneal seeding, perforation, and tumor spill are considered absolute indications for the use of intraperitoneal chemotherapy.

Treatment Options for Ovarian Cancer

Intraperitoneal chemotherapy is an important treatment option for ovarian malignancy. An essential feature of this approach is the use of the early postoperative period for chemotherapy. If peritoneal or pelvic seeding is documented with a primary ovarian cancer, then intraperitoneal chemotherapy with Adriamycin and cisplatin is recommended. In patients with recurrent ovarian cancer who have systemic cisplatin chemotherapy, cytoreduction is followed by intraperitoneal chemotherapy with mitomycin and 5-fluorouracil.

PRETREATMENT EVALUATION

Computed tomography (CT) scanning has been regarded as an inaccurate way to quantitate peritoneal carcinomatosis from adenocarcinoma. The malignant tissue progresses on the peritoneal surfaces and its shape conforms to the normal contours of the abdominopelvic structures. This is quite different from the metastatic process in the liver or lung, which progresses as three-dimensional tumor nodules.

CT has been of greater help in locating and quantitating mucinous adenocarcinoma within the peritoneal cavity (9). These tumors produce a copious colloid material that is readily distinguished by shape and density from normal structures. Using two new and distinctive radiologic criteria, patients with resectable mucinous peritoneal carcinomatosis can be selected from those with nonresectable malignancy. This keeps patients who are unlikely to benefit from reoperative surgery away from cytoreductive surgical procedures.

The two radiologic criteria found to be most useful are segmental obstruction of bowel and the presence of tumor >5 cm in greatest dimension on small bowel or directly adjacent to small bowel mesentery. These criteria reflect radiologically the biology of the mucinous adenocarcinoma. The obstructed segments of bowel signal an invasive character of malignancy that would be unlikely to be completely cytoreduced. The mucinous cancer on small bowel and small bowel mesentery indicates that the mucinous cancer is no longer redistributed. This means that small bowel surfaces or small bowel mesentery will have residual disease after cytoreduction, for these surfaces are impossible to peritonectomize (Figs. 4 and 5).

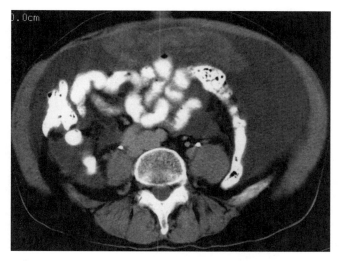

FIG. 4. Patient with grade 1 mucinous adenocarcinoma of appendiceal origin (pseudomyxoma peritonei) who had a complete cytoreduction and remains disease-free 2 years postoperatively. The mucinous tumor is very extensive, but the small bowel loops are of normal caliber and are not distended by air. Also, the small bowel has become compartmentalized by the mucinous tumor. The small bowel surfaces and small bowel mesentery remain tumor-free.

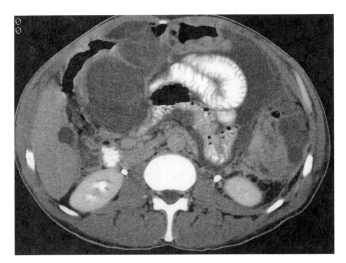

FIG. 5. Patient with grade 2 mucinous adenocarcinoma that has recurred after extensive prior cytoreductive surgery. Small bowel loops are slightly distended and contain small volumes of air, and the mesenteric surface is coated by mucinous tumor nodules. This patient has a less than 5% likelihood of a complete cytoreduction.

METHODS

Immediate Postoperative Abdominal Lavage

To keep the catheters for drug instillation and abdominal drainage clear of blood clots and tissue debris, an abdominal lavage is begun in the operating room. This requires tubes and drains to be positioned before closure of the abdomen. We have used large volumes of fluid rapidly infused and then drained from the abdomen after a short dwell time. The standard orders for immediate postoperative lavage are given in Table 5. All intra-abdominal catheters are withdrawn before the patient is discharged from the hospital.

TABLE 5. *Immediate postoperative abdominal lavage*

Day of Operation
1. Run in 1000 mL 1.5% dextrose peritoneal dialysis solution as rapidly as possible. Warm to body temperature before instillation. Clamp all abdominal drains during infusion.
2. No dwell time.
3. Drain as rapidly as possible through Tenckhoff catheter and abdominal drains.
4. Repeat irrigations q1h for 4 h, then q4h until returns are clear, then q8h until chemotherapy begins.
5. Change dressing at Tenckhoff catheter and abdominal drain skin sites using sterile technique once daily and prn.
6. Standard precautions must be used for all body fluids from this patient.

Heated Intraoperative Intraperitoneal Chemotherapy

After the cancer resection is complete, the Tenckhoff catheter and closed-suction drains are placed through the abdominal wall and made watertight with a purse-string suture at the peritoneum. Temperature probes are secured to the skin edge. Using a running 2-0 monofilament suture, the skin edges are secured to the limits of the self-retaining retractor. A plastic sheet is incorporated into these sutures to create an open space beneath. A slit in the plastic cover is made to allow the surgeon's double-gloved hand access to the abdomen and pelvis (Fig. 6). During the 2 hours of perfusion, all the anatomic structures within the peritoneal cavity are uniformly exposed to heat and to chemotherapy. The surgeon gently but continuously manipulates all viscera to minimize adherence of peritoneal surfaces. A roller pump forces the chemotherapy solution into the abdomen through the Tenckhoff catheter and pulls it out through the drains. A heat exchanger keeps the fluid being infused at 43° to 45°C so that the intraperitoneal fluid is 40° to 42°C. The circuit used for administration of heated intraoperative intraperitoneal chemotherapy is shown in Fig. 7. The smoke evacuator is used to pull air from beneath the plastic cover though activated charcoal, preventing any possible contamination of air in the operating room by chemotherapy.

The standard orders for heated intraoperative intraperitoneal chemotherapy are given in Table 6.

After the intraoperative perfusion is complete, the abdomen is suctioned dry of fluid and reopened, and reconstructive surgery is performed. Again, no anasto-

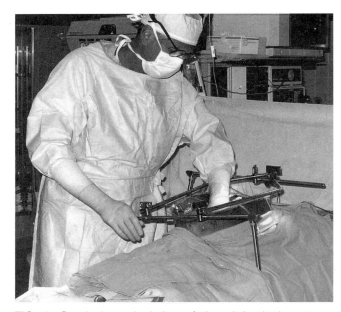

FIG. 6. Surgical manipulation of the abdominal contents after complete resection of cancer ensures uniform distribution of heat and chemotherapy.

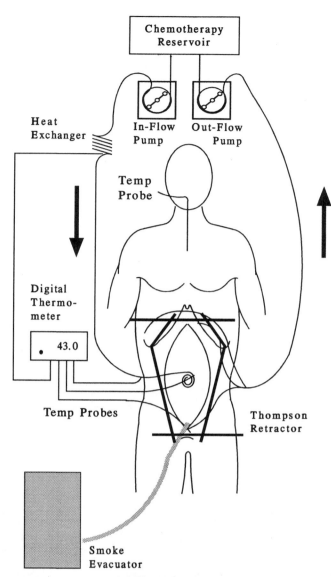

FIG. 7. Circuit for heated intraoperative intraperitoneal chemotherapy perfusion. All plastic tubes are positioned in a standard fashion, except the Tenckhoff catheter for the heated intraoperative perfusion. It is placed at the anatomic site at which the surgeon thinks there is the greatest likelihood of recurrence. This allows for a regional dose intensity of the heated chemotherapy.

moses are constructed until after the chemotherapy perfusion is complete.

Early Postoperative Intraperitoneal Chemotherapy for Adenocarcinoma

Intraperitoneal chemotherapy following complete cytoreduction in patients with appendiceal cancer, colonic cancer, rectal cancer, gastric cancer, or other gastrointestinal adenocarcinomas has used 5-fluorouracil. In pretreated ovarian cancer patients who have neurologic

TABLE 6. *Heated intraoperative intraperitoneal chemotherapy*

Mitomycin orders
1. For adenocarcinoma from appendiceal, colonic, rectal, gastric, and pancreatic cancer: add mitomycin ___ mg to 2 L 1.5% peritoneal dialysis solution.
2. Dose of mitomycin for males 12.5 mg/m², for females 10 mg/m².
3. Use a 33% dose reduction for heavy prior chemotherapy, marginal renal function, age >60, extensive intraoperative trauma to small bowel surfaces, or prior radiotherapy.
4. Send 1 L 1.5% peritoneal dialysis solution to test the perfusion circuit.
5. Send 1 L 1.5% peritoneal dialysis solution for immediate postoperative lavage.
6. Send the above to operating room ___ at ___ o'clock.

Cisplatin orders
1. For sarcoma, ovarian cancer, and mesothelioma: add cisplatin ___ mg to 2 L 1.5% peritoneal dialysis solution.
2. Dose of cisplatin 50 mg/m².
3. Use a 33% dose reduction for heavy prior chemotherapy, marginal renal function, age >60, extensive intraoperative trauma to small bowel surfaces, or prior radiotherapy.
4. Send 1 L 1.5% peritoneal dialysis solution to test the perfusion circuit.
5. Send 1 L 1.5% peritoneal dialysis solution for immediate postoperative lavage.
6. Send the above to operating room ___ at ___ o'clock.

toxicities from systemic cisplatin, no more cisplatin should be used; these patients are also treated with 5-fluorouracil. The standard orders for early postoperative administration of intraperitoneal 5-fluorouracil are shown in Table 7.

TABLE 7. *Early postoperative intraperitoneal chemotherapy with 5-fluorouracil*

Postoperative Days 1–5
1. Add to ___ mL 1.5% dextrose peritoneal dialysis solution: ___ 5-fluorouracil (650 mg/m²×___ m²) (maximal dose 1500 mg) and 50 mEq sodium bicarbonate.
2. Intraperitoneal fluid volume: 1 L for patients <1.5 m², 1.5 L for 1.5–2 m², and 2 L for >2 m².
3. Drain all fluid from the abdominal cavity before instillation, then clamp abdominal drains.
4. Run the chemotherapy solution into the abdominal cavity through the Tenckhoff catheter as rapidly as possible. Dwell for 23 hours and drain for 1 hour before next instillation.
5. Continue to drain the abdominal cavity after final dwell until the Tenckhoff catheter is removed.
6. Use 33% dose reduction for heavy prior chemotherapy, age >60, or prior radiotherapy.

TABLE 8. *Early postoperative intraperitoneal chemotherapy with Adriamycin*

Postoperative Days 1–5
1. Add to ____ mL 1.5% dextrose peritoneal dialysis solution.
2. Intraperitoneal fluid volume: 1 L for patients <1.5 m², 1.5 L for 1.5–2 m², and 2 L for >2 m².
3. Drain all fluid from the abdominal cavity before instillation, then clamp abdominal drains.
4. Run the chemotherapy solution into the abdominal cavity through the Tenckhoff catheter as rapidly as possible. Dwell for 23 hours and drain for 1 hour before next instillation.
5. Continue to drain abdominal cavity after final dwell until Tenckhoff catheter is removed.

Early Postoperative Intraperitoneal Chemotherapy with Adriamycin

In many patients who have received heated intraoperative intraperitoneal cisplatin, 5-fluorouracil does not give the necessary responses. In these patients, another drug that shows high response rates is Adriamycin. Primary ovarian cancer with pelvic or peritoneal seeding is treated after complete pelvic peritonectomy. Any ovarian cancer that has spread to the upper abdomen is cytoreduced before instituting the intraperitoneal chemotherapy. Patients with sarcomatosis are treated with early postoperative intraperitoneal Adriamycin if cytoreduction can be accomplished. Both primary and recurrent sarcomas involving the abdomen or pelvis are treated. Mesothelioma patients are treated by this regimen if complete cytoreduction can be accomplished (Table 8).

Adjuvant Intraperitoneal Chemotherapy for Adenocarcinoma and Sarcoma

Standard therapy for all patients with moderate- or high-grade cancer who are treated with intraperitoneal chemotherapy involves at least four cycles of treatment. The only patients who do not receive all four cycles of intraperitoneal chemotherapy are those in prognostic group 1 (see Table 3). These patients have grade 1 tumor and a complete cytoreduction. All other patients have at least four cycles of chemotherapy directed at both systemic and intraperitoneal sites. One of these cycles is the intraoperative and early postoperative intraperitoneal treatment. The other three cycles are on a monthly basis. Each cycle consists of five consecutive days of therapy.

The preferred method for peritoneal access for the first cycle of adjuvant chemotherapy is to have a catheter placed by paracentesis and the adequacy of chemotherapy distribution assessed radiologically (6). Most patients treated for peritoneal carcinomatosis have extensive peritoneal adhesions. To maximize distribution, chemother-apy is administered through a temporary catheter placed under radiologic control by paracentesis (8.3 French All-Purpose Drain Catheter, Meditech, Watertown, MA). Routinely, we have used a CT scan with intraperitoneal contrast to demonstrate uniform distribution of fluid within the abdomen (Fig. 8).

Access to the peritoneal cavity can be maintained using a subcutaneous infusion port and a curled Tenckhoff catheter. Access to the catheter is through the implanted port. The intraperitoneal catheter is positioned surgically in the left upper quadrant with the tip of the catheter as close as possible to the ligament of Treitz. The jejunum is a portion of the small bowel that demonstrates the most active peristalsis. Fewer catheter-related failures to infuse or drain occur if the cannula is in the mid-abdomen and surrounded by loops of small bowel.

The Tenckhoff catheter is positioned over a guide wire. The position for this wire is achieved through the drain catheter positioned by the radiologist. A tunnel for the Tenckhoff catheter and its cuff and a subcutaneous pocket for the port are created by the surgeon under local anesthesia.

The standard orders for delivery of adjuvant or induction intraperitoneal and intravenous chemotherapy for adenocarcinoma are shown in Table 9. Adjuvant or induction chemotherapy orders for sarcomatosis, ovarian cancer, or mesothelioma are shown in Table 10.

Induction Intraperitoneal and Systemic Chemotherapy

As shown in Table 9, the induction chemotherapy treatment regimen for adenocarcinomas is the same as for adjuvant intraperitoneal chemotherapy. Again, intraperi-

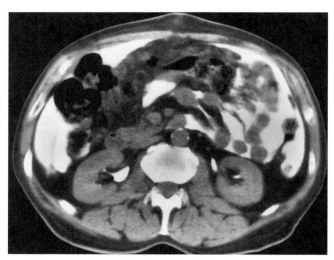

FIG. 8. CT scan of a patient who had a paracentesis for instillation of intraperitoneal chemotherapy. Intraperitoneal contrast documented wide distribution of contrast material to peritoneal surfaces.

TABLE 9. *Adjuvant or induction intraperitoneal 5-fluorouracil and intravenous mitomycin chemotherapy*

Cycle #____

1. CBC, platelets, profile A, and appropriate tumor marker before treatment; CBC and platelets 10 days after initiation of treatment.
2. 5-fluorouracil ____ mg 750 mg/m^2 (maximum dose 1600 mg) and 50 mEq sodium bicarbonate in 1,000 cc 1.5% dextrose peritoneal dialysis solution via intraperitoneal catheter each day for 5 days. Last dose ____. Dwell for 23 hours and drain for 1 hour. Continue with next administration even if no drainage obtained.
3. On Day 3 (____), 500 cc lactated Ringer's solution IV over 2 h before mitomycin infusion. Mitomycin ____ mg (10 mg/m^2×____ m^2) (maximum dose 20 mg) in 200 cc 5% dextrose and water IV over 2 h.
4. Follow routine procedure for peripheral extravasation of a vesicant if extravasation should occur.
5. Compazine 25 mg per rectum q4h prn for nausea. Outpatient only: may dose ×4 for use at home.
6. Percocet 1 tablet PO q3h prn for pain. Outpatient only: may dose ×4 for use at home.
7. Routine vital signs.
8. Out of bed at lib.
9. Diet: Regular as tolerated.
10. Daily dressing change to intraperitoneal catheter skin exit site.
11. Use 33% dose reduction for age >60 or prior radiotherapy.

TABLE 10. *Adjuvant or induction intraperitoneal cisplatin and intravenous Adriamycin chemotherapy*

Cycle #____

1. CBC, platelets, profile A, and appropriate tumor marker before treatment; CBC and platelets 10 days after initiation of treatment.
2. Cisplatin ____ mg (15 mg/m^2, maximum dose 30 mg) in 1,000 cc 1.5% dextrose peritoneal dialysis solution via intraperitoneal catheter each day for 5 days. Last dose ____. Dwell for 23 hours and drain for 1 hour. Continue with the next administration even if no drainage obtained.
3. On Day 3 (____), 500 cc lactated Ringer's solution IV over 2 h before Adriamycin infusion. Adriamycin ____ mg (30 mg/m^2, maximum dose 60 mg) in 200 cc 5% dextrose and water IV over 2 h.
4. Follow routine procedure for peripheral extravasation of a vesicant if extravasation should occur.
5. Compazine 25 mg per rectum q4h prn for nausea. Outpatient only: may dose ×4 for use at home.
6. Percocet 1 table PO q3h prn for pain. Outpatient only: may dose ×4 for use at home.
7. Routine vital signs.
8. Out of bed at lib.
9. Diet: Regular as tolerated.
10. Daily dressing change to intraperitoneal catheter skin exit site.
11. 33% dose reduction for age >60 or prior radiotherapy.

toneal chemotherapy is given only to patients with low-volume disease that is not confluent in the abdomen.

After delivering the three cycles of combined intraperitoneal and systemic chemotherapy, all treatments are discontinued for at least 2 months. If surgery follows intraperitoneal chemotherapy too quickly, an increased complication rate occurs (10–12). After the patient has recovered full activity, a complete exploratory laparotomy with meticulous cytoreduction of all residual cancer is performed. A final cycle of intraoperative and early postoperative intraperitoneal chemotherapy is then given (see Tables 6 and 7).

The standard orders for induction intraperitoneal and systemic chemotherapy for mesothelioma and sarcoma are shown in Table 10. The treatment regimen is the same as for adjuvant intraperitoneal chemotherapy. After a 2-month wait, the definitive cytoreductive surgery and a final cycle of intraoperative and early postoperative intraperitoneal chemotherapy with cisplatin and Adriamycin is given (see Tables 6 and 8).

CLINICAL RESULTS OF TREATMENT OF COLORECTAL AND APPENDICEAL PERITONEAL CARCINOMATOSIS

The disease-free survival of 155 patients with colorectal or appendiceal carcinomatosis is presented in

Table 11. Cancer of moderate or high grade by histopathology, lymph node metastases, and incomplete cytoreduction are the major poor prognostic variables. For colon cancer, the volume of cancer present as peritoneal implants is a significant prognostic variable.

TABLE 11. *Prognostic features of 155 patients with peritoneal carcinomatosis from colorectal and appendiceal cancer treated by cytoreductive surgery and intraperitoneal chemotherapy*

Prognostic feature	3-Year survivals (%)	p Value
Site		
Appendix	64	
Colon	33	.0001
Histology		
Grade I	85	
Other	29	.0001
Resection		
Complete	71	
Incomplete	20	.0001
Metastases		
Absent	63	
Present	19	.0001
Prior Chemotherapy		
Some/None	59	
Heavy	32	.0005
Volume Colon		
Moderate	62	
Large	18	.0033

MORBIDITY AND MORTALITY

The morbidity and mortality of 181 consecutive patients who had cytoreduction surgery and four cycles of combined regional and systemic chemotherapy for peritoneal carcinomatosis has been reported (13). In these 181 patients, there were three treatment-related deaths (2%). Fistula formation was a great problem in patients who had intestinal obstruction, prior radiation therapy, or prior intraperitoneal chemotherapy. Nineteen of those 72 patients (26%) developed a bowel perforation postoperatively. Only 2 of 109 (2%) patients with more normal bowel developed a fistula. Anastomotic leakage occurred in 10 of 181 patients (6%).

ALTERNATIVE APPROACHES

Peritoneal carcinomatosis was treated in the past with systemic chemotherapy. No long-term survivors have been described in the literature. Palliative surgery can give temporary relief of intestinal obstruction. However, these efforts have always been categorized as low-value surgery in that long-term survival was rarely, if ever, achieved. Other therapies—intraperitoneal immunotherapy, intraperitoneal isotopes, and intraperitoneal labeled monoclonal antibody—have not shown reproducible beneficial effects. In summary, no alternative approaches to cytoreductive surgery and intraperitoneal chemotherapy for peritoneal carcinomatosis have been reported.

PATIENT CARE CONSIDERATIONS

The major detrimental side effect of combined cytoreductive surgery and intraperitoneal chemotherapy is prolonged ileus. Patients may have a nasogastric tube in place with large volumes of secretions being aspirated for 2 to 4 weeks postoperatively. The length of time required for nasogastric suctioning seems related to the extent of the peritonectomy procedure and the extent of prior abdominal adhesions that require lysis.

The most life-threatening problem is the fistula (side wall perforation of the small bowel). Patients must be aware of the possibility of a fistula before cytoreductive surgery and intraperitoneal chemotherapy are contemplated. As mentioned above, the anastomotic leak rate is low.

After these treatments, the patient is maintained on parenteral feeding for 2 to 4 weeks. About 20% of patients, especially those who have had extensive prior procedures, need parenteral feeding when they leave the hospital.

PATIENT INFORMATION

Cytoreductive surgery and intraperitoneal chemotherapy are used in patients with peritoneal carcinomatosis. The best results are obtained when the disease treated is of low histologic grade (nonaggressive tumor) and a complete cytoreduction is possible (complete stripping of tumor from all abdominal and pelvic surfaces). If the surgery is successful, then in the operating room, the surgeon will administer chemotherapy. This chemotherapy is uniformly distributed by the surgeon's hand throughout the abdomen and pelvis. Every portion of the peritoneal surface is uniformly exposed by continuous manipulation. The drugs used intraoperatively are synergized by heat. While the abdomen is open, the fluid within the peritoneal cavity is maintained at about 42.5°C. After surgery, another drug is instilled into the abdominal cavity for 5 days in a large volume of fluid.

The most common adverse side effect is prolonged paralysis of the small bowel. Nasogastric suctioning is required for this. Also, because adequate nutrition is necessary for a full recovery, intravenous feeding (total parenteral nutrition) is started on the first postoperative day and is continued until the patient can eat normally.

In the second and third week after surgery, the most common problem revolves around small bowel fistula formation. Also, fistulae from the greater curvature of the stomach have occurred. If this does occur, reoperation is usually required. If a fistula forms, infection within the abdomen is common; this may result in prolonged hospitalization (up to 3 months).

The adverse effects of chemotherapy, other than causing a greater number of surgical complications, are few. A low white blood cell count or a low platelet count is seen in only about 10% of patients.

Despite the extensive nature of this combined treatment, the operative mortality rate remains low (2%). The likelihood of a complication remains about 25%. All these complications usually result in a complete recovery; however, the hospital stay may be prolonged.

REFERENCES

1. Jacquet P, Vidal-Jove J, Zhu BW, Sugarbaker PH. Peritoneal carcinomatosis from intra-abdominal malignancy: natural history and new prospects for management. *Acta Belgica Chirurgica* 1994;94:191–197.
2. Sugarbaker PH, Graves T, DeBruijn EA, et al. Rationale for early postoperative intraperitoneal chemotherapy (EPIC) in patients with advanced gastrointestinal cancer. *Cancer Res* 1990;50:5790–5794.
3. Sugarbaker PH, Graves T, Sweatman TW. Early postoperative intraperitoneal Adriamycin. Pharmacologic studies and a preliminary clinical report. *Reg Cancer Treat* 1991;4:127–131.
4. Sugarbaker PH, Cunliffe WJ, Belliveau JF, et al. Rationale for integrating early postoperative intraperitoneal chemotherapy (EPIC) into the surgical treatment of gastrointestinal cancer. *Sem Oncol* 1989;16: 83–97.
5. Yonemura Y, Fujimura T, Fushida S, et al. Hyperthermo-chemotherapy combined with cytoreductive surgery for the treatment of gastric cancer with peritoneal dissemination. *World J Surg* 1991;15:530–536.

6. Vidal-Jove J, Esquivel J, Buck D, Barrios P, Steves MA, Sugarbaker PH. Technical aspects of adjuvant intraperitoneal chemotherapy. *Reg Cancer Treat* 1992;4:294–297.
7. Sugarbaker PH, Steves MA, Hafner GA. Treatment of peritoneal carcinomatosis from colon or appendiceal cancer with induction chemotherapy. *Reg Cancer Treat* 1993;4:183–187.
8. Sugarbaker PH, Schellinx MET, Change D, Koslow P, Meyenfeldt M von. Peritoneal carcinomatosis from adenocarcinoma of the colon *World J Surg* 1996;20:585–592.
9. Jacquet P, Jelinek JS, Change D, Koslow P, Sugarbaker PH. Abdominal CT scan in the selection of patients with mucinous peritoneal carcinomatosis for cytoreductive surgery *J Am College Surg* 1995; 181:530–538.
10. Esquivel J, Vidal-Jove J, Steves MA, Sugarbaker PH. Morbidity and mortality of cytoreductive surgery and intraperitoneal chemotherapy. *Surgery* 1993;113:631–636.
11. Murio EJ, Sugarbaker PH. Gastrointestinal fistula following cytoreductive procedures for peritoneal carcinomatosis; incidence and outcome. *J Exp Clin Cancer Res* 1993;12:153–158.
12. Fernandez-Trigo V, Sugarbaker PH. Diagnosis and management of postoperative gastrointestinal fistulas: a kinetic analysis. *J Exp Clin Cancer Res* 1994;13:233–241.
13. Sugarbaker PH, Jablonski KA. Prognostic features of 51 colorectal and 130 appendiceal cancer patients with peritoneal carcinomatosis treated by cytoreductive surgery and intraperitoneal chemotherapy. *Ann Surg* 1995;221:124–132.

Shunting Procedures for Malignant Ascites and Pleural Effusions

H. Richard Alexander, Jr. and Douglas L. Fraker

To intervene, even briefly, between our fellow creatures and their suffering or death, is our most authentic answer to the question of our humanity.

—Howard Sackler

BACKGROUND

Extensive peritoneal carcinomatosis may result in ascites formation secondary to the exudative production of fluid directly from tumor cells or the localized inflammatory reaction of adjacent peritoneum. It is important to appreciate that less than 5% of all patients with ascites and only about two thirds of patients with cancer have ascites secondary to peritoneal carcinomatosis. However, peritoneal fluid cytology is almost always positive in patients with peritoneal carcinomatosis (1). Retroperitoneal lymph flow obstruction secondary to malignant lymphatic infiltration can also result in ascites formation, and patients with extensive liver metastases that produce either portal or hepatic venous occlusion may contract ascites on that basis.

The differential diagnosis of ascites includes cirrhosis, cardiac or pancreatic disease, nephrosis, tuberculosis, or peritoneal granulomatous disease (1,2). However, the diagnosis of malignant ascites is not usually difficult based on a previously established diagnosis of cancer in many patients. In other patients with newly diagnosed ascites who have no physical findings consistent with liver disease, the diagnosis of malignant ascites is usually apparent based on compelling clinical, radiographic, and cytologic findings.

The concept of draining peritoneal fluid into the systemic circulation was first proposed by Ruotte in 1907, when he described a technique of anastomosing the saphenous vein to the peritoneal cavity (3). LeVeen introduced the first peritoneovenous shunt in 1974, and a modification of this shunt, the Denver shunt, was introduced several years later (2) (Fig. 1).

Malignant ascites can be chylous, serous, mucinous, or bloody in nature. A serum-to-ascites albumin gradient of less than 1.1 g/dl is typically found in malignant ascites and is useful in distinguishing whether the etiology is associated with portal hypertension. The lymphocyte count is often greater than 500 cells/mm^3 (4) in malignant ascites, and tumor markers in ascites, such as carcinoembryonic antigen or CA-125, and other chemistry determinations from ascites fluid, such as fibronectin, cholesterol, interleukin-1, interleukin-6, or tumor necrosis factor levels, are nonspecific and cannot reliably distinguish between benign and malignant causes of ascites (1,5).

Malignant ascites can develop secondary to metastatic cancer of the ovary, breast, cervix, or virtually any gastrointestinal site, including gastric, pancreatic, appendiceal, or colorectal cancer. In a series of patients who presented with malignant ascites initially of unknown origin, 31 of 40 women (77%) were ultimately found to have a primary tumor of the ovary, uterus, or cervix (5). Another four (10%) were ultimately found to have a gastrointestinal primary tumor, and five (13%) had an unknown primary and were considered to have primary serous peritoneal carcinomatosis. Fourteen of 25 men (56%) who presented with malignant ascites were ultimately found to have a gastrointestinal primary, and another 9 (36%) never had a primary

H. R. Alexander, Jr.: Surgical Metabolism Section, Surgery Branch, National Cancer Institute, National Institutes of Health, Bethesda, Maryland 20892.

D. L. Fraker: Department of Surgery, University of Pennsylvania, Philadelphia, Pennsylvania 19104.

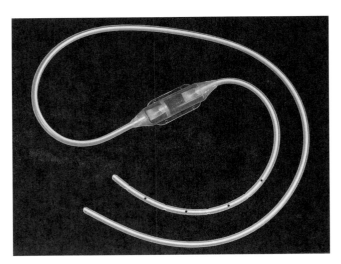

FIG. 1. Denver peritoneovenous shunt, showing the fenestrated peritoneal limb, the longer venous limb, and the pump chamber. Note the barium impregnated stripe.

site of tumor identified. Because of the potential therapeutic benefit from aggressive tumor debulking in cancers of the female reproductive organs, exploratory laparotomy has been considered appropriate for women with newly diagnosed malignant ascites, and the primary site is presumed to be ovarian. However, in men, or when an occult gastrointestinal primary tumor in a woman is suspected, then exploratory laparotomy is probably of questionable benefit.

SELECTION OF PATIENTS FOR PERITONEOVENOUS SHUNTING

Carcinomatosis with malignant ascites is usually incurable, with the exception of a subgroup of women with ovarian carcinoma. The enormous difficulty in treating this problem is reflected in the numerous innovative treatment strategies that have been used in an attempt to treat these conditions, including intraperitoneal photodynamic therapy (6), aggressive tumor debulking with peritonectomy or extensive electrocoagulation of peritoneal tumor deposits (7,8), intraperitoneal chemotherapy or biologic therapy (9–13), continuous hyperthermic peritoneal perfusion (13–15), and intraperitoneal adoptive immunotherapy (16).

The clinical course of malignant ascites is variable; however, for many patients, malignant ascites is the sole or major site of progressive and symptomatic disease for many months. Effective palliation of pain, discomfort, early satiety, or dyspnea may translate into a significant improvement in quality of life. Standard approaches have included fluid and salt restriction, diuretic therapy, and interval abdominal paracentesis. The use of diuretic therapy, usually using a combination of spironolactone and furosemide, to treat malignant ascites deserves special comment. The role of oral diuretics in controlling malignant ascites has been reported in a series of patients with either chylous malignant ascites (CMA), ascites due to peritoneal carcinomatosis (PC), or ascites secondary to massive hepatic metastases (MHM) (17). On diuretic therapy, patients in all groups lost approximately 0.5 kg/day of body weight; however, there was no change in ascites volume in patients with CMA or PC. Although there was a mean decrease in ascites volume of almost 250 ml/day in patients with ascites secondary to MHM, there was also a significant, 8% to 10%, decrease in plasma volume in patients with PC or MHM. None of the patients with MHM were symptomatic secondary to the substantial volume contraction resulting from diuretic therapy. The difficulty in mobilizing fluid in patients with PC or CMA is somewhat predictable based on the typically high concentration of albumin in malignant ascites fluid. Therefore, patients with CMA or PC do not respond to aggressive oral diuretic therapy. Patients with MHM as the etiology of their ascites have a decrease in ascites volume on oral diuretic therapy, and this occurs concomitantly with an asymptomatic reduction in plasma volume. Gough and Balderson also reported that up to 73% of patients with malignant ascites had no response to diuretic therapy (18).

Interval abdominal paracentesis has been used successfully to palliate patients with malignant ascites but has the theoretic drawbacks of depleting the patient of plasma proteins and promoting nutritional wasting (Table 1). It can result in a persistent ascites leak at the site of peritoneal puncture and can potentially cause injury to the abdominal viscera. Gough and Balderson also showed that in patients with malignant ascites treated with repeated abdominal paracentesis, serum levels of albumin are significantly lower after 1 month compared with patients treated with peritoneovenous shunting (PVS), in whom serum albumin levels were preserved (18). Repeat abdominal paracentesis may be best suited for patients with a relatively short life expectancy (ie, <2 or 3 months), for very debilitated patients in whom the risk of an operative procedure is high, and in patients with bloody, mucinous, or loculated ascites that will not be effectively drained by PVS. For patients who have a very limited life expectancy, indwelling abdominal drains to remove peritoneal fluid intermittently have been used to avoid repeat paracentesis (19,20).

TABLE 1. *General strategies to palliate malignant ascites*

Intraperitoneal chemotherapy
Intraperitoneal biologic therapy
Surgical tumor debulking
Diuretic therapy
Interval paracentesis
Peritoneovenous shunt

A paradigm outlining selection of patients for PVS has been presented by Souter et al. (21). Initially, a patient should undergo paracentesis, and the rate of reaccumulation evaluated. In general, if a patient has loculated, viscous, or bloody ascites, then a PVS will not be effective (22). If fluid reaccumulation is slow or the patient can be effectively palliated medically, then repeat interval paracentesis should be performed. Patients who have an expected survival of >1 month, preferably >3 months, and who have rapid and symptomatic reaccumulation of fluid, should be considered for a PVS.

PRETREATMENT EVALUATION

There are several clinical conditions that should be considered before placing a PVS. Because the peritoneal fluid is being reintroduced into the intravascular space, normal renal function and cardiac function is important so that the extra fluid can be excreted. The presence of peritoneal infection or elevated serum bilirubin levels are contraindications for its use. The potential adverse consequences of PVS include pulmonary edema, disseminated intravascular coagulation (DIC), and tumor dissemination from the peritoneal cavity with shortened survival.

METHODS OF PVS INSERTION

The general principles behind the use of PVS for palliation of malignant ascites are that a 15- to 20-cm pressure gradient exists between the central venous system and the abdominal cavity, favoring flow of ascites into the low-pressure central veins. The shunt is designed with a miter valve to prevent backflow of blood during periods of increased central venous pressure. The Denver shunt differs from the LeVeen shunt in that it has a small reservoir (pump chamber) that is positioned over the lower chest wall so that it can be compressed to pump fluid through the shunt and clear any cellular or fibrinous debris (Fig. 2). Hyde et al. reported that there was no difference in function between the Denver and LeVeen shunts in 26 patients who had a shunt placed primarily for palliation of ascites secondary to cirrhosis (23). However, Lund and Newkirk subsequently reported a patency rate of 90% for Denver shunts placed in 49 patients with malignant ascites or cirrhosis, which was higher than historical controls using LeVeen shunts (24). More recently, Smith et al. (25) noted that there was a trend toward better shunt patency with Denver shunts versus LeVeen shunts in patients with malignant ascites (25). In a total of 50 patients, 50% of LeVeen shunts, compared with only 26% of Denver shunts, occluded before death. The improved patency rates with the Denver shunt are explained by the ability actively to pump fluid through it and clear the high-protein fibrinous debris that may occlude LeVeen shunts. Although the mean duration of

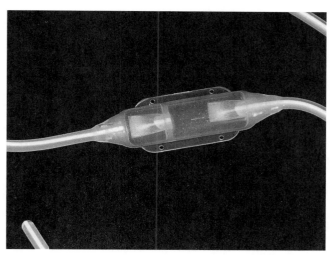

FIG. 2. Close-up of the pump chamber from a Denver PVS5. Note the dual one-way miter valve.

function was longer with Denver shunts, there was no relationship between shunt patency and survival.

A PVS can be inserted using either a local anesthetic with sedation or under a general anesthetic (26,27). The choice between the two should be based on the technical facility with which the device can be placed and the overall condition of the patient. Shunts are typically made of silicone rubber and have a barium sulfate stripe impregnated in the wall so that the shunt position can be visualized radiographically (see Fig. 1). The standard-flow Denver shunt is available with either a single- or double-miter valve in the pump chamber; these valves permit flow rates at 10 cm of water pressure from 36 to 48 ml/minute and 26 to 40 ml/minute, respectively. For most patients with malignant ascites, either type of device is suitable. The intra-abdominal portion of the drain is 27 cm in length and is fenestrated to optimize the ability to drain the ascitic fluid. The venous limb is 66 cm in length and is heparin bonded to decrease the incidence of clot formation. It is positioned in the superior vena cava through either the cephalic or, more frequently, the internal jugular vein. The shunt should be prepared for insertion by immersing it in sterile saline (the manufacturer recommends the addition of 1 million units of penicillin and 80 mg gentamicin sulfate per 500 ml of saline) and compressing the pump chamber until all air bubbles have been completely flushed from the device. The patient is positioned supine with the neck slightly extended and turned to the left. The right neck, right anterior chest wall, and abdomen are sterilely prepared and draped. A transverse cervical incision is made between the two heads of the sternocleidomastoid muscle and the internal jugular vein is exposed. Ties of 2-0 silk are passed proximally and distally around a short segment of vein and 5-0 or 6-0 pursestring using cardiovascular suture is placed. A transverse incision in the right upper quadrant is made several centimeters below the costal margin, either the external oblique or rectus abdominis fascia is exposed, and a subcutaneous pocket is bluntly made over the lower chest wall for positioning the pump chamber. The fibers of the external and internal oblique muscles or the rectus muscle are split and two concentric, pursestring, nonabsorbable sutures are placed through the posterior fascia and peritoneum to ensure a watertight closure around the catheter. A stab incision into the peritoneal cavity is made, the fenestrated limb of the shunt is placed down the right colic gutter, and the pursestring sutures are tied. To prevent fluid overload in the immediate perioperative period, approximately half of the ascitic fluid should be drained at the time of shunt insertion (28,29). After confirming flow of ascitic fluid through the venous limb of the device, it can be clamped gently to prevent continuous flow of fluid through the shunt until the venous limb is positioned. The venous limb of the catheter is tunneled subcutaneously lateral to the breast and then to the venous cutdown site. The subcutaneous tunnel is made by making several counter-incisions through the skin and using a tunneling device or a long, slender surgical clamp to pull the catheter through the subcutaneous tissue. Because most patients with malignant ascites are very asthenic, the tunnel is normally made easily along

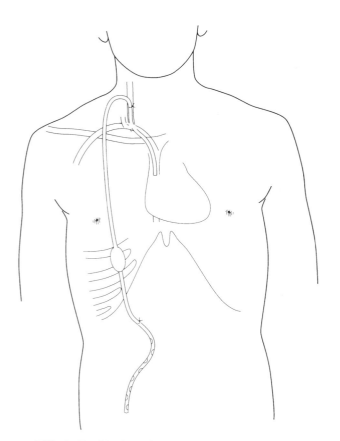

FIG. 3. Positioning of the peritoneovenous shunt.

TABLE 2. *Technical aspects of successful shunt insertion*

1. Check inflow once the catheter is positioned in the abdomen. Check fluid flow in catheter.
2. Ensure watertight peritoneal closure. Draining approximately half the fluid will help prevent leakage and facilitate postoperative management.
3. Observe strict aseptic technique.
4. Confirm placement of venous link. Check with fluoroscopy to demonstrate proper positioning in the superior vena cava and no kinking.

Modified from Hyde GL, Dillon M, Bivins BA. Peritoneal venous shunting for ascites: a 15-year perspective. *Am Surg* 1982;48:123–127.

the midaxillary line on the thoracic wall (Fig. 3). The pump chamber should be positioned over the lower thoracic wall to facilitate compression. If necessary, the venous limb of the shunt can be cut so that the tip will be positioned in the superior vena cava. After making a small venotomy in the center of the internal jugular pursestring suture, the shunt is advanced into the vein and the pursestring is tied. Fluoroscopy is used to confirm proper position of the shunt before leaving the operating room. The important technical aspects to optimize shunt function have been outlined by Hyde et al. (23) and are presented in Table 2.

CLINICAL RESULTS OF PERITONEOVENOUS SHUNTING

Numerous reports published between 1979 and 1986 outlined results and complications using the Denver or LeVeen shunt in patients with malignant ascites (2,21, 26,27,30–32). The results of these studies with respect to morbidity and mortality of the procedure and the ability to palliate malignant ascites are somewhat variable, most likely reflecting the fact that many of these reports summarized initial institutional experiences with PVS, and patient selection for shunt placement was not standard. In many of these studies, a significant percentage of patients did not survive for 30 days, and most expired within 3 months after PVS, suggesting that their advanced clinical stage may not have been ideally suited for the procedure (21,26,33–36). Straus et al. reported that 31 of 35 shunts (89%) placed in patients with malignant ascites initially functioned well and relieved symptoms of nausea, fullness, loss of appetite, and dyspnea (32). Twenty-seven of 35 (79%) functioned long-term (>3 months) or until death. The median survival in this group was only 8 weeks, and two early deaths were thought to be related to shunt placement. A transient febrile response developed in most of the patients after shunt placement, and this phenomenon has been observed by others (27,31,37). Lokich et al. reported that six of eight patients were successfully palliated with

TABLE 3. *Improvement in abdominal girth, urine output, and decreased requirement for paracenteses after peritoneovenous shunting (PVS) for malignant ascites in 40 patients*

Parameter	Before PVS[a]	After PVS[a]
Weight (kg)	61.3	58.1
	(46.3–90.4)	(42.2–81.8)
Daily urine output	1017	2333
(ml)	(510–2000)	(700–4400)
Girth (cm)	86.5	80
	(67.5–110)	(65–102.5)
Paracentesis[b]	50%	0%

[a]Mean (range).
[b]Percentage of patients requiring more than two every 3 weeks.
Modified from Qazi R, Savlov ED. Peritoneovenous shunt for palliation of malignant ascites. *Cancer* 1982;49:600–602.

TABLE 4. *Types and frequency of complications after peritoneovenous shunting for malignant ascites in 50 patients*

Complication	N (%)
Shunt occlusion	16 (32%)
Fluid overload	6 (12%)
Ascitic leak	5 (10%)
Bleeding/DIC	3 (6%)
Shunt infection	2 (4%)
IVC thrombosis	2 (4%)

DIC, disseminated intravascular coagulation; IVC, inferior vena cava.
Modified from Smith, DAP, Weaver DW, Bouwman DL. Peritoneovenous shunt (PVS) for malignant ascites: an analysis of outcome. *Am Surg* 1989;55:445–449.

PVS, but that four had transient edema after shunt placement (32). Raaf and Stroehlein reported that five patients had complete relief of tense abdominal ascites after PVS; however, four of five patients died 6 weeks or less after shunt placement (26).

In a series of 40 patients with malignant ascites refractory to medical management undergoing PVS placement, Qazi and Savlov reported that 28 (70%) were effectively palliated as evidenced by a decrease in abdominal girth, decrease in the number of paracenteses needed, and an increase in urine output (38) (Table 3). Qazi and Savlov also found that if the ascitic fluid had a high protein content (4.5 g/l) and a high number of malignant cells, the shunt did not provide good palliation. Cheung and Raaf also found that shunt failure was significantly higher in 22 patients treated with PVS when the malignant ascites was cytologically positive (36). However, the median survival was only 26 days for the 10 patients with positive cytology, compared with 80 days for the 8 patients with negative cytology, suggesting that other associated clinical conditions may have contributed to shunt failure, rather than the presence of positive cytology per se. A number of other series have reported that a positive fluid cytology is not associated with poor shunt function (22,34,37). Gough found that PVS provided good palliation of malignant ascites in 13 of 17 patients even in the face of light blood staining or positive cytology (22), and Kostroff et al. reported that positive cytology had no effect on shunt function or complication rates in 31 patients treated for malignant ascites (37). Roussel et al. reported that 21 of 36 shunts (60%) placed for control of malignant ascites functioned until death (34). The median overall survival time was 14 weeks, and shunt function was not dependent on cytology or tumor type. These reports suggest that careful patient selection for PVS is important and that a positive cytology does not preclude a patient from palliation from PVS.

Since 1989, there have been several larger series reported (18,25,39,40). Smith et al. reported that in 50 patients with malignant ascites undergoing PVS, multivariate analysis of several clinical and pathologic factors revealed that women did better than men even when "female malignancies" were excluded, leukocytosis and thrombocytopenia were associated with poor outcome, and patients with pancreatic or colon cancer had significantly shorter survival than patients with breast or gastric cancer (25). Although LeVeen shunts failed at a significantly shorter mean time interval than Denver shunts in this study and one other (30), in another recent series, this phenomenon was not observed (39). The spectrum and rate of complications observed in the series by Smith et al. is a fairly accurate reflection of those reported in other series, and these are outlined in Table 4. Clinically significant DIC was observed in only three patients. However, in patients with malignant ascites and coexisting extensive liver metastases with abnormal liver function tests, the incidence of clinically significant DIC may be higher after PVS placement (41).

Edney et al. reported that in 45 patients undergoing 55 PVS procedures, elevated coagulation parameters were actually good predictors of shunt patency (39). The

TABLE 5. *Alterations in coagulation tests after 55 peritoneovenous shunt placements in 45 patients with malignant ascites*

Parameter	Preoperative	Postoperative[a]
Platelets (10^3/mm^3)	238 ± 128	166 ± 113
Fibrinogen (mg/dl)	357 ± 168	280 ± 138
Partial thromboplastin	31.2 ± 7	
time (sec)		37.8 ± 22.8
Prothrombin time (sec)	13 ± 2	14.4 ± 4.3

[a]$P_2 < 0.05$ for all values compared with preoperative.
Modified from Edney JA, Hill A, Armstrong D. Peritoneovenous shunts palliate malignant ascites. *Am J Surg* 1989;158:598–601.

TABLE 6. *Preservation of serum albumin levels (g/dl) in patients undergoing peritoneovenous shunting versus repeat paracentesis for malignant ascites*

Serum albumin level	Peritoneovenous shunting[a]		Repeat paracentesis[b]	
	Preoperative	1 month after	Baseline	1 month after
Mean ± SD	30 ± 6.3	29.7 ± 5.7	32.5 ± 5	28 ± 5.6
Median	30	30	33	28

[a]P = 0.83, paired t-test.
[b]P < 0.001, paired t-test.
Modified from Gough IA, Balderson GA. Malignant ascites: a comparison of peritoneovenous shunting and nonoperative management. *Cancer* 1993;71:2377–2382.

typical alterations seen in various coagulation parameters are shown in Table 5. Although clinical evidence of DIC develops in up to 90% of patients undergoing PVS for ascites secondary to cirrhosis (42), only one patient with malignant ascites in Edney and colleagues' series had clinical evidence of DIC. Interestingly, all patients with a functioning shunt had fibrin split products >40 mg/dl. This finding has also been observed by Gleysteen et al., who noted that although prothrombin time and partial thromboplastin time were not altered in patients after PVS placement, fibrinogen was decreased and fibrin split products were increased maximally 1 day after shunt placement (43). Although platelets were also decreased, this correlated with a decrease in hematocrit, indicating a dilutional etiology for the thrombocytopenia. In the series reported by Edney et al., there was palliation of symptoms secondary to massive ascites in 75%, and there was considerable variation in survival depending on tumor type (39). They suggested that PVS in not indicated in most patients with pancreatic cancer.

Gough has published a report comparing the results of PVS versus nonoperative management in 85 patients with malignant ascites (18). One month after treatment, assessments of quality of life, serum creatinine, and hemoglobin levels were not different between patients treated with PVS and those treated with repeat abdominal paracentesis, although there was a slight improvement in these parameters in both groups compared with pretreatment levels. However, serum albumin levels were preserved in patients undergoing PVS (Table 6). These results suggest that in patients who are ambulatory and who would not otherwise require hospitalization or frequent clinic visits for repeat paracentesis, PVS may be preferable.

MORBIDITY AND MORTALITY

Schumacher et al. reported 30- and 60-day mortality rates of 43% and 61%, respectively, after PVS insertion in 89 patients with malignant ascites (40). Two thirds of patients had symptomatic relief and one half had complications secondary to the procedure. Shunt patency after

30 days was only about 50%. These results highlight the need for careful patient selection.

Tumor Dissemination Secondary to Peritoneovenous Shunting

Maat et al. published a case report in 1979 that was the first pathologically documented record of tumor embolization to the lungs after placement of a PVS (44). The 75-year-old patient died within 2 weeks of shunt placement, presumably due to massive tumor emboli and fluid overload. Although Smith et al. subsequently published a second case report of fatal tumor embolization after PVS in a 44-year-old patient (45), others have not been able to demonstrate clinically significant sequelae from tumor embolization or iatrogenic metastases after PVS (46–48). Tarin et al. reported that a patient who survived 27 months after PVS for palliation of ascites from ovarian cancer had no autopsy evidence of tumor dissemination outside of the peritoneal cavity, despite the fact that tumor cells from the malignant ascites were greater than 95% viable, capable of surviving for over 2 weeks in soft agar, and had clonogenic potential (46). Although the yield of malignant cells may be increased after PVS, this does not result in the development of clinically significant hematogenous metastases (49).

Souter et al. found that 5 of 12 patients (42%) undergoing autopsy after a PVS had tumor emboli and microscopic metastases scattered in the pulmonary capillaries (47). These tumors were thought to represent iatrogenic spread through the PVS, but had not been clinically significant. In a second report that included a total of 15 patients, 7 (47%) had autopsy evidence of hematogenous spread of tumor in the lungs (48). Although most of the metastases were in lung, in some patients other organs, including liver, spleen, brain, and adrenal glands, were also affected. Uniformly, these metastases were small and all patients died of progressive abdominal disease. Together, the available data suggest that even in the face of a positive cytology not all patients will have iatrogenic metastases or tumor emboli. In the approximately 45%

of patients who do, these tumors do not have any significant clinical sequelae.

Early Shunt Failure

Initial or early shunt failure presents when patients do not have any decrease in their ascites volume after PVS or, if the ascites has been drained at the time of the procedure, there is prompt reaccumulation of ascites. Overall, most shunt failures occur early after placement, and LeVeen et al. have proposed three primary mechanisms for early shunt failure: primary cardiac insufficiency, improper postoperative management, and mechanically occluded or malpositioned shunts (50). Initial clinical evaluation should eliminate the possibility of cardiac failure with chest radiography, electrocardiography, and, if possible, an assessment of central venous pressure. If occult cardiac disease is suspected, then paracentesis to reduce temporarily the volume load and treatment with bed rest, diuretics, and digitalis may improve shunt function. If cardiac disease is not suspected as the etiology of initial shunt failure, then maneuvers to optimize shunt function should be attempted. The patient should be placed flat in bed and deep inspiratory efforts with or without an abdominal binder should be tried.

If a mechanical cause of shunt failure is suspected, initial plain abdominal and chest radiography should be done to assess the position of the radiopaque shunt and determine if kinking or malposition exists. Subsequently, a superior vena cava contrast study with contrast injected into a forearm vein or into the venous limb of the shunt reveals the presence of a clot. It is safe directly to inject the shunt with contrast if a 23-gauge needle is used. If contrast is injected into the venous limb of the shunt, it should clear when the patient makes a forced inspiratory effort. If it does not, then malfunction of the valve is likely. If proper positioning and function of the venous limb can been documented, the peritoneal limb and valve may need replacement.

Late Shunt Failure

The primary causes of late shunt failure include malposition of the shunt, development of fibrin sheaths or thrombi of the venous limb, and omental fat occlusion or localized peritonitis of the peritoneal limb (50). Initially, a plain radiograph potentially reveals that the venous or peritoneal limb has become malpositioned. If the shunt is normally positioned, a contrast study through the shunt identifies a fibrin sheath or thrombus. If the venous limb does not clear with a forced inspiration, valve or peritoneal limb malfunction exists. If there is no evidence of peritonitis, attempts to clear the valve by pumping it should be made. Obviously, if there is evidence of intraperitoneal infection, pumping the shunt valve is con-

traindicated. In this situation it may be necessary to remove the device. Culture of the shunt contents should be obtained and appropriate antibiotics instituted.

PLEUROPERITONEAL SHUNTS FOR MALIGNANT PLEURAL EFFUSION

Background

There are over 100,000 new cases of malignant pleural effusion (MPE) annually in the United States, and most are secondary to lung or breast cancer (51). There are a variety of potential management options, including pleurectomy, repeat thoracentesis, and tube thoracostomy with or without sclerotherapy, intracavitary treatment, or the use of biologic response modifiers (52). The ideal patients for a pleuroperitoneal shunt (PPS) frequently include the 20% to 30% who fail sclerotherapy or those with an entrapped lung in whom full expansion is not possible. Because the 1- and 6-month mortality rates for patients with MPE are approximately 50% and 85%, respectively, selection of patients for this procedure should be carefully considered. For patients who are hospitalized and too debilitated to pump the PPS chamber, a tube thoracostomy may be the simplest palliative maneuver. Others have reported the successful outpatient management of refractory MPE using a simple drainage tube such as a Tenckhoff pigtail catheter (53,54).

The concept of PPS to palliate symptomatic refractory MPE was introduced in the early 1980s, and several reports have established its utility in controlling symptomatic MPE in selected patients (51,55,56). The standard Denver PPS is a silicone rubber device with fenestrations in both the pleural and peritoneal limbs (Fig. 4). It has a

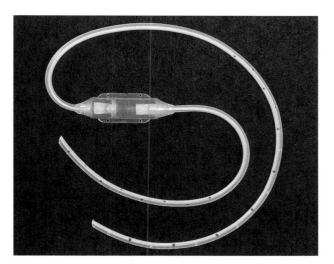

FIG. 4. A Denver pleuroperitoneal shunt with a short fenestrated pleural limb, a longer fenestrated peritoneal limb, and a dual one-way miter valve pump chamber.

one-way miter valve, similar to the PVS. The device is designed to open with a positive pressure of approximately 1 cm of water, so that theoretically there should be spontaneous flow of fluid through the device at each end expiration, when intrapleural pressure may exceed 4 cm water. Because of the different pressure dynamics between the pleural and peritoneal space compared with the peritoneal and central venous system, flow of fluid through the device is frequently assisted by repetitive compression of the pump chamber. Therefore, patients best suited for PPS are those who are alert and capable of compressing the chamber when symptoms of an enlarging pleural effusion become apparent.

Methods

The technique of PPS insertion is conceptually similar to that for PVS, and in some technical aspects is more straightforward. Although the device can be inserted using a local anesthetic with intravenous sedation, many patients undergo general anesthesia for placement. The pump chamber and peritoneal limb are inserted in a manner comparable to that for PVS. The pleural limb can be inserted into the affected hemithorax using the Seldinger technique through a 16-Fr peel-away sheath.

Clinical Results

The clinical performance of PPS in patients with MPE has been quite good. Reich et al. reported that 17 shunts placed in 13 patients over a 1-year period resulted in relief of dyspnea in all patients (57). In another series, 18 of 19 patients were relieved of symptoms after PPS placement, except for 1 who could not adequately pump the chamber (55). Complications are acceptable and include the development of a pneumothorax or wound infection. If properly managed, <25% of PPS occlude (57). A single case of massive ascites developing after placement of a PPS has been reported (58).

PATIENT INFORMATION

Peritoneovenous Shunts

A tube has been positioned in your abdominal cavity that has been designed to drain the excess fluid that has accumulated and to help relieve the symptoms of nausea, discomfort or fullness, loss of appetite, or shortness of breath that you may be experiencing. The tube has been tunneled under your skin to a large vein in the neck and is designed to allow the one-way flow of fluid from the abdominal cavity back into the vascular system. This is achieved by the presence of a one-way valve in a small compressible chamber located under your skin. Once the fluid is returned to the vascular system, it will be eliminated by the kidneys in the form of urine.

To ensure that the shunt is working properly, it will be necessary for you to compress the chamber located under your skin several times a day to prevent the buildup of any debris that may cause the shunt to clog or malfunction. The flow of fluid through the shunt is normally limited by the design of the tube, but will be increased as you take a deep breath or if you cough or bear down so that the pressure inside your abdomen exceeds that in the large vein located in your neck. After the placement of your shunt, it may be necessary for you to take a diuretic pill so that the extra fluid entering your vascular space can be adequately eliminated through the kidneys. You will be aware that the shunt is working normally if your abdominal fluid does not reaccumulate after the operation. Because the surgeon has removed some fluid from your abdominal cavity at the time of the shunt placement, your abdomen should remain smaller than it was before the procedure.

If fluid reaccumulates in your abdominal cavity, it is important that you lay flat and pump the chamber as instructed by your nurse or doctor to ensure that the flow of fluid from the abdominal cavity is adequate. It will also be necessary for you to pump the chamber on a regular basis daily to ensure that it continues to work properly. Your nurse or doctor will give you specific instructions as to how many times this should be performed. If you find that your abdominal fluid is increasing despite attempts to pump the chamber while lying flat, then you should contact your nurse or doctor and make them aware of this development.

Sometimes after the placement of the shunt patients experience shortness of breath. This is typically due to the fact that the fluid from the abdomen is flowing through the shunt more quickly than the body can eliminate it through the kidneys. When this happens, it is important to sit upright to minimize the flow of fluid through the shunt and to notify your nurse or doctor immediately. It is important not to pump the chamber if this occurs because it may make your shortness of breath worse.

In a very few patients who have shunts placed, an infection can develop. If you experience fever, abdominal pain, or chills, or there is redness or tenderness over the area of the shunt, contact your nurse or doctor immediately. This condition usually requires antibiotics administered by vein, and in rare circumstances requires that the shunt be removed to prevent the infection from worsening.

With proper care and management, your shunt should work for a long period of time and provide you with relief of your fluid buildup within the abdominal cavity. It is important to appreciate that this fluid can change the ability of your blood to clot normally or alter other laboratory values in routine blood tests. Your doctor or nurse will monitor these blood tests regularly and it is important for you to comply with the instructions regarding the intervals at which these blood tests will be performed. Although the abnormalities are frequently observed in many patients, they are often minor and have no significant consequence for your overall well-being. In fact, many believe that slight abnormalities in some blood tests are a reassurance that the shunt is functioning properly.

In summary, your shunt has been placed to improve the symptoms that you are experiencing because of the buildup of fluid in your abdominal cavity. The complications that can occur after shunt placement were described earlier, and can result from occlusion of the shunt, the too-rapid flow of fluid through the shunt, alterations in blood tests due to the effects of this fluid entering the vascular space, or shunt infection. If you have specific questions about any of these potential problems, please contact your nurse or physician.

Pleuroperitoneal Shunts

You have had a tube placed from your chest cavity into your abdominal cavity to improve the symptoms that have developed because of the accumulation of fluid in your chest cavity around your lung. Once the fluid enters the abdominal cavity, it will be absorbed into the vascular space and eliminated through the kidneys. This tube is called a shunt and has a one-way valve that prevents the flow of fluid from the abdominal cavity back into the chest cavity. It is designed to allow the spontaneous flow of fluid through the device so that with normal respiration, fluid will drain out of the chest and into the abdomen. However, to ensure that the device is functioning properly, frequent regular compressions of the pump chamber will be required. Your nurse or physician will instruct you on how to identify the pump chamber under the skin and how to compress it to push fluid through the shunt tubing.

Most patients undergo placement of a shunt to relieve symptoms of shortness of breath secondary to the buildup of fluid in the chest cavity. Because your doctor will have evacuated most of this fluid during the placement of the shunt, your symptoms should be improved by the time you are sent home. If you are experiencing shortness of breath after the shunt has been placed, it is likely fluid is accumulating in the chest cavity and should be pumped out by compressing the chamber as instructed by your physician or nurse. Also, it is helpful to sit upright to help the flow of fluid out of the chest cavity and into the abdominal cavity. If you find that your shortness of breath recurs after placement of the shunt and is not relieved by compressing the pump chamber and sitting up, then contact your nurse or physician immediately.

Rarely the shunt may become infected. If you experience fever, chills, or abdominal pain, or see redness or have tenderness over the shunt tubing, then contact your physician immediately. It is possible under these very unusual circumstances that the shunt may need to be removed and antibiotics administered to control an infection.

In summary, you have had a shunt placed to relieve the excess fluid buildup in your chest cavity. If this shunt is properly managed, the chances of it providing relief of your shortness of breath are extremely good. Please follow instructions as outlined by your nurse or physician on the care of this shunt, and remember that routine pumping of the shunt is important to maintain proper function.

REFERENCES

1. Runyon BA. Editorial: Malignancy-related ascites and ascitic fluid "humoral tests of malignancy." *J Clin Gastroenterol* 1994;18:94–98.
2. Baker AR, Weber JS. Treatment of malignant ascites. In: DeVita VT Jr, Hellman S, Rosenberg SA, eds. *Principles and practice of oncology.* Philadelphia: JB Lippincott; 1993:2255–2262.
3. Ruotte M. Abouchement de la veine saphène extrene du péritonie pour resorber les épanchements sciatiques. *Lyon Medicine* 1907;197:574–577.
4. Wang S-S, Lu C-W, Chao Y, et al. Malignancy-related ascites: a diagnostic pitfall of spontaneous bacterial peritonitis by ascitic fluid polymorphonuclear cell count. *J Hepatol* 1994;20:79–84.
5. Muggia FM, Baranda J. Management of peritoneal carcinomatosis of unknown primary tumor site. *Semin Oncol* 1993;20:268–272.
6. Sindelar WF, DeLaney TF, Tochner Z, et al. Technique of photodynamic therapy for disseminated intraperitoneal malignant neoplasms. *Arch Surg* 1991;126:318–324.
7. Esquivel J, Vidal-Jove J, Steves MA, Sugarbaker PH. Morbidity and mortality of cytoreductive surgery and intraperitoneal chemotherapy. *Surgery* 1993;113:631–636.
8. Huff T, Brand E. Pseudomyxoma peritoneii: treatment with the argon beam coagulator. *Obstet Gynecol* 1992;80:569–571.
9. Markman M. Intraperitoneal chemotherapy for malignant diseases of the gastrointestinal tract. *Surg Gynecol Obstet* 1987;164:89–93.
10. Stuart GCE, Nation JG, Snider DD, Thunberg P. Intraperitoneal interferon in the management of malignant ascites. *Cancer* 1993;71:2027–2030.
11. Dedrick RL. Theoretical and experimental bases of intraperitoneal chemotherapy. *Semin Oncol* 1985;12:1–6.
12. Hardy J, Jones A, Gore ME, Viner C, Selby P, Wiltshaw E. Treatment of advanced ovarian cancer with intraperitoneal tumour necrosis factor. *Eur J Cancer* 1990;26:771.
13. Gilly FN, Carry PY, Brachet A, et al. Treatment of malignant peritoneal effusion in digestive and ovarian cancer. *Medical Oncology and Tumor Pharmacotherapy* 1992;9:177–181.
14. Fujimoto S, Shrestha RD, Kokuban M, et al. Positive results of combined therapy of surgery and intraperitoneal hyperthermic perfusion for far-advanced gastric cancer. *Ann Surg* 1990;212:592–596.
15. Sayag AC, Gilly FN, Carry PY, et al. Intraoperative chemohyperthermia in the management of digestive cancers. *Oncology* 1993;50:333–337.
16. Eggermont AMM, Sugarbaker PH. Efficacy of intracavitary administration of cyclophosphamide, interleukin-2 and lymphokine activated killer cells against established intraperitoneal tumor. *Acta Med Austriaca* 1989;16:47–60.
17. Pockros PJ, Esrason KT, Nguyen C, Duque J, Woods S. Mobilization of malignant ascites with diuretics is dependent on ascitic fluid characteristics. *Gastroenterology* 1992;103:1302–1306.
18. Gough IA, Balderson GA. Malignant ascites: a comparison of peritoneovenous shunting and nonoperative management. *Cancer* 1993;71:2377–2382.
19. Lomas DA, Wallis PJW, Stockley RA. Palliation of malignant ascites with a Tenckhoff catheter. *Thorax* 1989;44:828.
20. Belfort MA, Stevens PJd'E, DeHaek K, Soeters R, Krige JEJ. A new approach to the management of malignant ascites: a permanently implanted abdominal drain. *Eur J Surg Oncol* 1990;16:47–53.
21. Souter RG, Tarin D, Kettlewell MGW. Peritoneovenous shunts in the management of malignant ascites. *Br J Surg* 1983;70:478–481.

22. Gough IR. Control of malignant ascites by peritoneovenous shunting. *Cancer* 1984;54:2226–2230.
23. Hyde GL, Dillon M, Bivins BA. Peritoneal venous shunting for ascites: a 15-year perspective. *Am Surg* 1982;48:123–127.
24. Lund RH, Newkirk JB. Peritoneo-venous shunting system for surgical management of ascites. *Contemp Surg* 1979;14:31–45.
25. Smith, DAP, Weaver DW, Bouwman DL. Peritoneovenous shunt (PVS) for malignant ascites: an analysis of outcome. *Am Surg* 1989;55: 445–449.
26. Raaf JH, Stroehlein JR. Palliation of malignant ascites by the LeVeen peritoneo-venous shunt. *Cancer* 1980;45:1019–1024.
27. Holman JM Jr, Albo D Jr. Peritoneovenous shunting in patients with malignant ascites. *Am J Surg* 1981;142:774–776.
28. Reinhold RB, Lokich JJ, Tomashefski J, Costello P. Management of malignant ascites with peritoneovenous shunting. *Am J Surg* 1983; 145:455–457.
29. Holm A, Halpern NB, Aldrete JS. Peritoneovenous shunt for intractable ascites of hepatic nephrogenic, and malignant causes. *Am J Surg* 1989; 158:162–166.
30. Lund RH, Moritz MW. Complications of Denver peritoneovenous shunting. *Arch Surg* 1982;117:924–928.
31. Lokich J, Reinhold R, Silverman M, Tullis J. Complications of peritoneovenous shunt for malignant acites. *Cancer Treat Rep* 1980;64: 305–309.
32. Straus AK, Roseman DL, Shapiro TM. Peritoneovenous shunting in the management of malignant ascites. *Arch Surg* 1979;114:489–491.
33. Söderlund C. Denver peritoneovenous shunting for malignant or cirrhotic ascites. *Scand J Gastroenterol* 1986;21:1161–1172.
34. Roussel JGJ, Krron BBR, Hart GAM. The Denver type for peritoneovenous shunting of malignant ascites. *Surg Gynecol Obstet* 1986; 162:235–239.
35. Sonnenfeld T, Tydéen G. Peritoneovenous shunts for malignant ascites. *Acta Chir Scand* 1986;152:117–121.
36. Cheung DK, Raaf JH. Selection of patients with malignant ascites for a peritoneovenous shunt. *Cancer* 1982;50:1204–1209.
37. Kostroff KM, Ross DW, Davis JM. Peritoneovenous shunting for cirrhotic versus malignant ascites. *Surg Gynecol Obstet* 1985;161: 204–208.
38. Qazi R, Savlov ED. Peritoneovenous shunt for palliation of malignant ascites. *Cancer* 1982;49:600–602.
39. Edney JA, Hill A, Armstrong D. Peritoneovenous shunts palliate malignant ascites. *Am J Surg* 1989;158:598–601.
40. Schumacher DL, Saclarides TJ, Staren ED. Peritoneovenous shunts for palliation of the patient with malignant ascites. *Annals of Surgical Oncology* 1994;1:378–381.
41. Tempero MA, Davis RB, Reed E, Edney, J. Thrombocytopenia and laboratory evidence of disseminated intravascular coagulation after shunmts for ascites in malignant disease. *Cancer* 1985;55: 2718–2721.
42. Ragni MV, Lewis JH, Sperio JA. Ascites-induced LeVeen shunt coagulopathy. *Ann Surg* 1983;193:91–95.
43. Gleysteen JJ, Hussey CV, Heckman MG. The cause of coagulopathy after peritoneovenous shunt for malignant ascites. *Arch Surg* 1990;125: 474–477.
44. Maat B, Oosterlee J, Spaas JAJ, White H, Lammes FB. Dissemination of tumour cells via LeVeen shunt. *Lancet* 1978;1:988.
45. Smith RRL, Sternberg SS, Paglia MA, Golbey RB. Fatal pulmonary tumor embolization following peritoneovenous shunting for malignant ascites. *J Surg Oncol* 1981;16:27–35.
46. Tarin D, Vass ACR, Kettlewell MGW, Price JE. Absence of metastatic sequelae during long-term treatment of malignant ascites by peritoneovenous shunting. *Invasion Metastasis* 1984;4:1–12.
47. Souter RG, Wells C, Tarin D, Kettlewell MGW. Surgical and pathologic complications associated with peritoneovenous shunts in management of malignant ascites. *Cancer* 1985;55:1973–1978.
48. Tarin D, Price JE, Kettlewell MGW, Souter RG, Vass ACR, Crossley B. Mechanisms of human tumor metastasis studied in patients with peritoneovenous shunts. *Cancer Res* 1984;44:3584–3592.
49. Campioni N, Lasagni RP, Vitucci C, et al. Peritoneovenous shunt and neoplastic ascites: a 5-year experience report. *J Surg Oncol* 1986;33: 31–35.
50. LeVeen HH, Vujic I, d'Ovidio NG, Hutto RB. Peritoneovenous shunt occlusions: etiology, diagnosis, therapy. *Ann Surg* 1984;200:212–223.
51. Pina E, Harvey JC, Katariya K, Beattie EJ. Malignant pleural effusions: emphasis on newer surgical treatments. *Compr Ther* 1994;20:294–299.
52. Lynch TJ Jr. Management of malignant pleural effusions. *Chest* 1993; 103:385S–389S.
53. Robinson RD, Fullerton DA, Albert JD, Sorensen J, Johnston MR. Use of pleural Tenckhoff catheter to palliate malignant pleural effusion. *Ann Thorac Surg* 1994;57:286–288.
54. Le LV, Parker LA, DeMars LR, MacKoul P, Fowler WC. Pleural effusions: outpatient management with pigtail catheter chest tubes. *Gynecol Oncol* 1994;54:215–217.
55. Lee KA, Harvey JC, Reich H, Beattie EJ. Management of malignant pleural effusions with pleuroperitoneal shunting. *J Am Coll Surg* 1994; 178:586–588.
56. Wong PS, Goldstraw P. Pleuroperitoneal shunts. *Br J Hosp Med* 1993; 50:16–21.
57. Reich H, Beattie EJ, Harvey JC. Pleuroperitoneal shunt for malignant pleural effusions: a one-year experience. *Semin Surg Oncol* 1993;9: 160–162.
58. Roukema JA, Lobach HJC, van der Werken C. Ascites after pleuroperitoneal shunting. *Cancer* 1990;66:675–676.

CHAPTER **22**

Intraoperative Radiation Therapy

William F. Sindelar and Peter A. S. Johnstone

Our Constitution is in actual operation; everything appears to promise that it will last; but in this world nothing is certain but death and taxes.

—*Benjamin Franklin (1789)*

Intraoperative radiation therapy (IORT) involves the administration of large single doses of radiation during operative procedures directly to surgically exposed tissues. IORT offers the opportunity to deliver high doses of radiation to areas of neoplastic involvement while simultaneously minimizing the risk of radiation toxicity by limiting the dose to surrounding radiosensitive normal tissues, which may be physically shielded or displaced from the radiation treatment volume. IORT was explored in various malignancies during the 1970s in Japan, with reports of benefit in both disease control and survival in selected patients with various types of malignancies (1,2).

The use of IORT spread as an investigative modality throughout Japan and to several United States institutions during the early 1980s. Selected European centers began using IORT during the late 1980s. Currently, IORT is used worldwide at more than 250 institutions, and the accumulated clinical experience exceeds 5000 patients with malignancies at various sites.

The use of IORT may increase the therapeutic ratio in several ways: first, the fraction size of radiation therapy is increased severalfold over conventional fractionated external beam radiation therapy (EBRT), with a corresponding increase in tumor cell kill for a defined radiation dose. Second, the possibility exists for complementary preoperative or postoperative EBRT to be used in

addition to IORT to cover large treatment volumes. Third, the radiation beam, typically electrons, may be modified by energy selection or by the use of surface bolus for precise dose delivery at defined depths. Fourth, the radiation dose is delivered only to the target volume and not to other mobile normal tissues that might otherwise be dose limiting and that might be excluded from the IORT portal by retraction and physical displacement. Last, nonmobile tissues in the field may be directly shielded with sterile lead sheets, thereby reducing the likelihood of toxicity.

At present, there is an accumulation of preclinical data, as well as a rapidly enlarging worldwide experience with IORT's clinical use. IORT has not yet gained universal acceptance because of the sophisticated equipment necessary, the difficulties inherent in the procedure, and the current relative lack of controlled clinical trials unequivocally illustrating superiority of IORT over conventional modes of therapy. However, increasing numbers of institutions have initiated clinical programs in IORT, and reliable, well controlled clinical trials are underway in gastric cancer, pancreatic cancer, advanced colorectal cancer, and other malignancies. The ultimate determination of IORT's utility within the oncologic armamentarium must await this evolving clinical information.

METHODS OF INTRAOPERATIVE RADIATION

The rationale for the use of IORT is the delivery of a maximum dose of radiation to regions at risk for harboring tumor or neoplastic cells while attempting to spare surrounding normal tissues from radiation exposure. IORT is delivered as a single fraction during surgery, where there are opportunities operatively to expose the tumor and physically displace or shield normal tissues from the radiation volume.

W.F. Sindelar: Surgery Branch, National Cancer Institute, National Institutes of Health, Bethesda, Maryland 20892.

P.A.S. Johnstone: Department of Radiation Oncology, University of California, Naval Medical Center, San Diego, California 92134–5000.

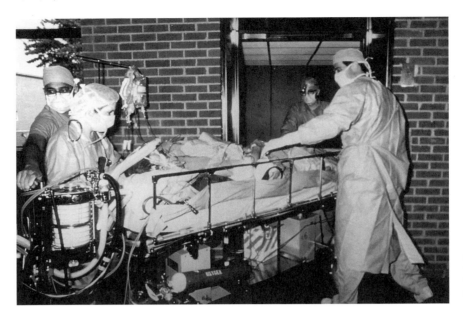

FIG. 1. Moving patient from operating room to radiation therapy suite for intraoperative radiation therapy. The patient is under anesthesia, the surgical incision is temporarily closed, and the patient is protected with layers of sterile drapes.

Most institutions performing IORT have operating theaters and radiation therapy suites that are physically separate. A patient undergoing IORT is surgically explored in the operating room, where tumor resection is carried out and the tissues at risk for harboring residual tumor are exposed. Typically, large incisions and complete mobilization of viscera are required to provide adequate exposure for IORT. After tumor resection and delineation of the regions to be irradiated, but before any necessary reconstruction of the gastrointestinal tract, the patient's incision is temporarily closed and protected with layers of sterile drapes. While maintaining anesthesia, the patient is then transferred to a mobile cart and transported to the radiation therapy treatment room (Fig. 1). The patient is then transferred to the radiation treatment table, the incision is reopened, and the radiation treatment volume is surgically re-exposed (Fig. 2). Self-retaining retractors are used in maintaining exposure of the surgical bed (Fig. 3). The treatment volume is then defined by placing a treatment applicator (usually acrylic or stainless steel cylinders of various sizes) over the tissues at risk for tumor contamination. The applicator serves primarily to collimate the IORT treatment beam and secondarily to retract mobile viscera such as intestine from the treatment volume. The applicator is then docked to the radiation treatment unit (Fig. 4). The position of the applicator is then checked with a periscopic device that allows viewing down the

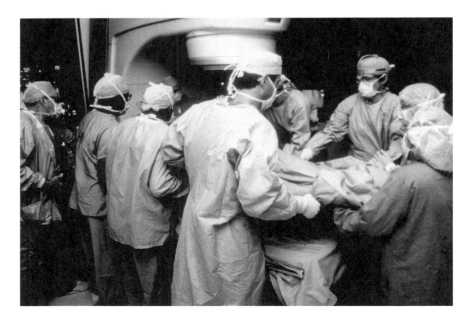

FIG. 2. Positioning patient on radiation therapy treatment table. Protective drapes are removed, the surgical sterile field is established, and the surgical incision is opened.

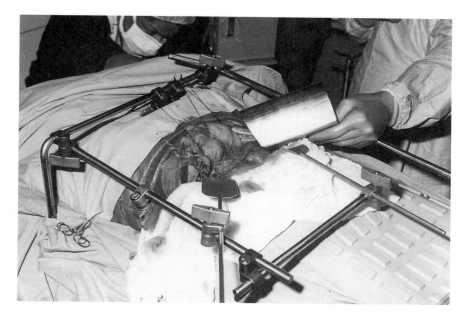

FIG. 3. Exposing the surgical field for intraoperative irradiation. Self-retaining retractors are used, and treatment applicators of various sizes are used to define the portal to be irradiated by placing the applicators over the surgically exposed tumor bed.

axis of the applicator, either by a direct optical system or closed-circuit television monitor. The patient is then irradiated, while surgical and radiation therapy treatment personnel leave the room. The patient is under continuing anesthesia and is remotely monitored electronically. After completion of radiation, the treatment applicator is removed. The surgery is then completed in the radiation treatment room, or the patient is transported back to the operating theater for completion of the operative procedure.

Some institutions have a dedicated IORT suite, a combination operating and radiation therapy room, which simplifies the logistics of IORT delivery by eliminating the need to transport patients under anesthesia between physically separated surgical and radiation therapeutic facilities (Fig. 5).

Most institutions performing IORT use electron beam radiation to limit the radiation dose deep to the treatment volume. Radiosensitive normal tissues and structures such as kidney, spinal cord, or skin may underlie regions of tumor that are irradiated. The dose to the underlying normal structures must be minimized. High-energy electron radiation from a linear accelerator has a steep fall-off in dose at tissue depths that are defined by the electron energy. X-ray and photon radiation can have deep tissue penetration and therefore may allow unacceptably high doses to be delivered to tissues deep to tumor if used intraoperatively.

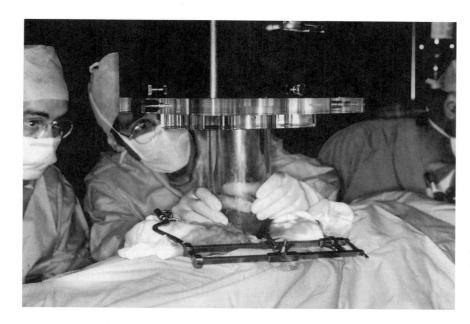

FIG. 4. Docking the treatment applicator to the linear accelerator. Movements of the treatment table and the gantry of the linear accelerator are used to join the treatment applicator to the head of the accelerator unit.

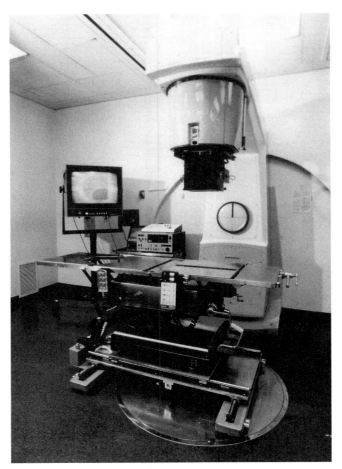

FIG. 5. Intraoperative radiation therapy unit with linear accelerator and combined surgery–radiation therapy treatment table.

EARLY CLINICAL EXPERIENCES

The clinical application of IORT to intra-abdominal tumors was investigated in the 1970s at Kyoto University by Mitsuyuki Abe and his colleagues. After developing preclinical techniques in dogs (3), Abe et al. applied IORT to patients with advanced cancers.

In 1974, Abe et al. reported using IORT in the treatment of 38 patients with gastric carcinoma (1). Using both photons from a cobalt source and electrons (8 to 20 MeV) from a betatron unit, patients received IORT to unresectable tumors, to residual tumor after attempts at resection, or to the surgical bed after resection. IORT doses ranged from 18 to 40 Gy, although most patients received 30 Gy of 8-MeV electrons. An initial group of 14 patients with metastatic disease had IORT to the unresected primary tumor with no toxicity, and a median survival of 6 months. A second group of seven patients had incomplete resections of large gastric cancers followed by IORT to the gastric bed, and two patients survived more than 5 years. A third group of 17 patients had complete resection of gross disease, and received IORT to the gas-

tric bed and regional nodal basin, showing a median survival of 20 months and a 5-year survival of 29%. Significant complications were not reported. An enlarged experience of Abe and colleagues using IORT in 43 patients with gastric cancer confirmed that the technique was feasible and could result in the long-term survival of some patients with advanced disease (4).

The early Kyoto experience with IORT prompted several Japanese institutions to explore the modality in various intra-abdominal malignancies (5). Based on reports of good local tumor control as well as occasional cures of patients with locally advanced cancers, IORT was adopted for common use throughout Japan, particularly for advanced-stage gastric cancers (6).

The Japanese experience prompted worldwide exploration of IORT, even though few controlled clinical trials were instituted in Japan. With wider application of IORT, more clinical experiences did accumulate to allow some assessments to be made of the efficacy and utility of this modality.

CLINICAL EVALUATIONS

Most of the clinical evaluations of IORT have been performed as small, single-institution series. This is expected, because until recently the capability of delivering IORT was limited to relatively few institutions that demonstrated interest in and a commitment to the modality. Collected reviews of various clinical reports examining IORT have been published (7,8).

Recently, some controlled trials of IORT compared to conventional radiation therapy or compared to no radiation treatment have been performed in some diseases. Most of these investigations involved limited numbers of selected patients, and no large-scale trials have been performed to date. The relative lack of controlled trials makes it impossible to draw definitive conclusions regarding the indications and efficacy of IORT. However, examination of selected clinical trials, which represent critical observations, can be used to draw inferences about IORT's utility. Such trials are discussed in the following sections. The important data in certain of the clinical trials cited are summarized in Table 1.

Prospective Single-Arm Trials

Gastric Cancer

The use of IORT in gastric cancer has been evaluated in several Japanese institutions. Because of the high prevalence of gastric cancer in Japan, most of the world's experience using IORT as a treatment adjunct for gastric carcinoma has been accumulated in Japanese centers (5,6). In the Japanese institutions where IORT is available, the routine use of IORT is advocated for patients in

TABLE 1. *Selected clinical trials of intraoperative radiation therapy*

Disease	Author/ institution	Treatment groups	Type of study	Treatments	No. patients	Results	Comments
Gastric	Abe et al./ Kyoto (27)	Surgery alone vs. surgery + IORT	Prospective, non-randomized	Gastrectomy alone vs. gastrectomy + IORT (28–40 Gy)	101 vs. 110	IORT improved 5-y survival stage IV ≈15%; improved ≈15% stage III+II; no difference stage I	Widely accepted by Japanese as indicating IORT rx of choice for advanced-stage gastric disease
	Sindelar et al./ NCI (28)	Surgery + EBRT vs. surgery + IORT	Prospective, randomized	Gastrectomy EBRT (50 Gy) vs. gastrectomy + IORT (20 Gy)	25 vs. 16	Median survival 25 mo IORT, 21 mo control; local recurrence 31% IORT, 80% control	Complication rates similar; EBRT used postoperatively in control stages III–IV
Pancreatic, unresectable	Shipley et al./ MGH (17)	Surgery + IORT + EBRT	Prospective, selected, phase I–II	Preoperative EBRT (10 Gy) + surgical bypass + IORT (15–25 Gy) + postoperative EBRT (50 Gy) + chemotherapy	29	Median survival 17 mo	Early study in highly selected patients, considered encouraging
	Gunderson et al./ Mayo (18)	Surgery + IORT + EBRT	Prospective, selected, phase II	Surgical bypass + IORT (18–20 Gy) + postoperative EBRT (50 Gy) + chemotherapy	52	Median survival 11 mo	No apparent benefit over historical data
	RTOG/ multi-institutional (24)	Surgery + IORT + EBRT	Prospective, phase II	Surgical bypass + IORT (15–20 Gy) + postoperative EBRT (50 Gy)	51	Median survival 9 mo	No apparent benefit over historical data
	Sindelar/ NCI (unpublished)	Surgery + EBRT vs. surgery + IORT + EBRT	Prospective, randomized	Surgical bypass + EBRT (60 Gy) + 5-FU vs. surgical bypass + IORT (25 Gy) + EBRT (50 Gy) + 5-FU	13 vs. 11	Median survival 9 mo IORT, 8 mo control	Similar complications, IORT no survival benefit
Pancreatic, resected	Hiraoka et al./ Kumamoto University (29)	Surgery alone vs. surgery + IORT	Prospective, non-randomized	Extended pancreatectomy alone vs. extended pancreatectomy + IORT (30 Gy)	9 vs. 16	5-y survival 29% IORT, 0% control	Similar complications
	Sindelar/ NCI (unpublished)	Surgery + EBRT vs. surgery + IORT	Prospective, randomized	Pancreatectomy + EBRT (50 Gy) vs. pancreatectomy + IORT (20 Gy)	13 vs. 12	Median survival 18 mo IORT, 12 mo EBRT; median time to local failure 31 mo IORT, 12 mo EBRT	Complication rates similar; EBRT used postoperatively in control stages II–IV
Colorectal, advanced	Willet et al./ MGH (21)	Surgery + IORT + EBRT	Prospective, selected, phase II	Preoperative EBRT (50 Gy) + maximal excision + IORT (10–15 Gy)	36	5-y survival 54% complete resection, 6% incomplete resection; local control 62% complete resection, 18% incomplete resection	Encouraging results in recurrent patients if surgical excision of gross tumor possible
	Gunderson et al./ Mayo Clinic (22)	Surgery + IORT + EBRT	Prospective, selected, phase II	Preoperative EBRT (50 Gy) maximal + excision + IORT (10–20 Gy)	70; 20 primary, 50 recurrent	Median survival 37 mo; local control 80% primary, 68% recurrent	32% incidence of neuropathy
Sarcoma, retroperitoneum	Sindelar et al./ NCI (30)	Surgery + EBRT vs. surgery + IORT + EBRT	Prospective, randomized	Resection + EBRT (55 Gy) vs. resection + IORT (20 Gy) + EBRT (40 Gy)	20 vs. 15	Median survival 45 mo IORT, 52 mo control; local recurrence 40% IORT, 80% control	Significant reduction in radiation enteritis and higher incidence of neuropathy in IORT group

IORT, intraoperative radiation therapy; EBRT, external beam radiation therapy; NCI, National Cancer Institute; MGH, Massachusetts General Hospital; RTOG, Radiation Therapy Oncology Group; 5-FU, 5-fluorouracil.

whom it is thought surgical resection alone would be unlikely to result in cure, including those with gross involvement of the regional perigastric or celiac lymph nodes and those with serosal involvement or extragastric extension of tumor (9). Typically, the indications for IORT include grossly resectable primary tumors in the gastric body or antrum, the absence of visceral metastatic disease, extragastric extension into the retroperitoneum, and nodal metastases that can be encompassed by a single IORT field covering the celiac axis and gastric resection bed.

Outside of Japan, the application of IORT to gastric cancer was carried out at a limited number of institutions (10). The National Cancer Institute (NCI) reported an experience of 11 patients with locally-advanced gastric cancer undergoing gastrectomy and IORT (20 Gy) to the resection bed. The actuarial 3-year disease-free survival rate was 25% in a patient population that was considered by the NCI to have little chance of salvage (11).

A comprehensive European program of evaluating IORT in various malignancies was initiated in Spain during the late 1980s at the University of Navarra under the direction of Felipe Calvo (12), an experience that accumulated one of the largest series of patients with gastric carcinoma treated with IORT outside of Japan (13). Patients with gastric cancer underwent gastrectomy and IORT to the celiac axis (typically 15 Gy with 9- to 20-MeV electrons) and usually received additional postoperative EBRT to the upper abdomen (46 Gy with 15-MeV photons in parallel opposed fields delivered over 5 weeks). Forty-three patients were treated. Acute treatment-related complications were observed in 35% of patients, including nausea and vomiting, diarrhea, dumping syndrome, pneumonia, pleural effusion, pulmonary abscess, cholangitis, suture line dehiscence, and esophageal hemorrhage. Late complications occurred in 23% of patients, including dysphagia, hepatic infarction, vertebral osteoradionecrosis, and hemorrhage from a ruptured celiac aneurysm within the IORT field. With a median follow-up of 18 months, the actuarial 3-year survival was 60%. Of the 10 patients who recurred during the observation period, only 30% progressed locally within the gastric bed or regional nodal areas.

Pancreatic Cancer

Pancreatic cancer ranks among the most challenging problems in oncology because current treatment methods are only rarely successful. Most patients present with locally-advanced unresectable disease, and even if a curative resection can be accomplished, subsequent local recurrences occur in at least half of the patients (14). IORT has been investigated in several clinical trials as a potential means of improving local control in pancreatic cancer. An early pilot series was reported by Goldson (15) in which 19 patients demonstrated the feasibility of defining IORT in pancreatic cancer. A larger Japanese experience of 108 patients with pancreatic cancer demonstrated a median survival of 6 months in patients with advanced disease (5). Many patients appeared to have pain relief after IORT, suggesting effective palliation.

The Massachusetts General Hospital (MGH) accumulated a series of 16 patients with unresectable pancreatic cancer treated with IORT in combination with 45 to 50 Gy of EBRT. These patients had an encouraging median survival of 18 months (16). More than half of the patients appeared to have local control of the primary lesion, which was given 15 to 20 Gy of IORT. Further experience in treating selected patients with IORT suggested a median survival of 17 months, considerably longer than that expected from conventional therapies for pancreatic carcinoma (17). However, subsequent experiences with increasing numbers of pancreatic cancer patients at the MGH resulted in a lowering of the median survival to approximately 12 months.

Large early experiences with IORT in unresectable pancreatic cancer were also accumulated at the Mayo Clinic (18), where the median survival was 11 months for 44 patients who had unresectable pancreatic cancers without distant metastases. Patients received 20 Gy IORT to the primary lesion and 45 to 50 Gy of fractionated EBRT. Disease progression was clinically documented in 71% of treated patients, although only 7% were considered to have progressed within the IORT field.

Colorectal Cancer

External beam radiation therapy to the pelvis at doses of 50 to 55 Gy has been shown to improve local control rates for bulky carcinomas of the rectum and rectosigmoid. Higher doses frequently lead to significant intestinal complications. In attempts to improve on local control rates in patients with locally advanced colorectal carcinoma, investigators at MGH combined IORT (10 to 15 Gy) as a boost treatment to the tumor bed after maximal resection (19). Patients also received high-dose pelvic EBRT (50 Gy) either before or after surgery. Among 16 patients with unresectable primary lesions, no local recurrences were detected. Three local recurrences developed among the four patients treated with unresectable recurrent disease. Further studies at MGH confirmed enhanced local disease control of IORT for advanced rectal cancers (20,21). Twenty patients with primary tumor receiving IORT who underwent complete surgical resection had an actuarial 5-year disease-free survival rate of 53%. Overall actuarial 5-year survival was 88%. Among 22 patients who were unable to be completely resected at the time of surgery, the actuarial 5-year local control was 60% and the 5-year disease-free survival rate was 32%. For recurrent colorectal cancer after previous resection, an actuarial 5-year local control rate of 62% was seen in 13 patients in whom gross surgical resection was possible at the time of IORT. If only partial resection was possible, the local control rate dropped to 18% for the 17 patients studied.

Investigations of IORT in colorectal carcinoma were carried out at the Mayo Clinic (22). Advanced marginally-resectable primary lesions or cancers recurrent after previous resection were treated with IORT at the time of attempted resection.

Preoperative or postoperative EBRT was given as part of the treatment strategy. For the treated group of 70 poor-prognosis patients, the median survival was 37 months. Long-term cures were seen in 30% of patients. There were no central failures within the IORT portal among 20 patients with primary cancers, and only a 10% central failure rate was seen among 50 patients with previously treated locally recurrent lesions. Local failures within the pelvis occurred in 20% of primary-lesion and 32% of recurrent-lesion patients.

Radiation Therapy Oncology Group Trials

Various phase I and II trials performed by the Radiation Therapy Oncology Group (RTOG) have evaluated the efficacy of IORT in certain malignancies. These trials demonstrated that IORT investigations may be successfully accomplished in a prospective, multigroup setting.

Patients with unresectable bile duct carcinoma were treated with IORT (14 to 22 Gy) and postoperative EBRT (45 to 50 Gy) (23). Intraoperative doses of 17 to 22 Gy were delivered to gross residual disease, whereas microscopic residual disease was treated with 14 Gy. Of 23 patients admitted to the study, 8 had completed planned protocol therapy. Of two living patients, one was free of disease at 11 months and a local recurrence developed in the other. IORT (17 to 22 Gy) was used in a phase I and II trial of locally advanced pancreatic carcinoma coordinated by the RTOG and carried out by multiple institutions (24). Postoperative EBRT (50 Gy) was delivered concomitantly with 5-fluorouracil chemotherapy. The median survival of 51 patients who received IORT according to protocol was 9 months, with a 2-year survival rate of 6%.

Recurrent, persistent, or unresectable rectal carcinomas were treated on an RTOG protocol (25). Preoperative (50 Gy) or postoperative (42 Gy) EBRT was delivered in conjunction with maximal surgical resection. IORT was delivered to doses varying with the degree of residual disease, with gross residual disease receiving 15 to 22 Gy and microscopic residual disease receiving 12 to 14 Gy. Of 40 patients receiving IORT, 60% were alive with a 43% local control at 18 months.

Twelve patients with retroperitoneal sarcomas who received IORT were investigated by the RTOG (26). The median IORT dose delivered was 16 Gy, and most patients received adjuvant postoperative EBRT to doses of 45 to 50 Gy. Absolute 1-year survival was 58%, with a 17% local failure rate. Peritoneal seeding occurred in 25% of patients.

The RTOG is currently enrolling patients in protocols investigating IORT in colorectal, gastric, and unresectable pancreatic carcinomas. Such multi-institution investigations of IORT should provide larger patient numbers than currently possible by most single institutions.

Comparative Dual-Arm Trials

Although single-arm clinical trials can establish patterns of treatment toxicity and make inferences of efficacy in selected patients, only prospective, comparative trials (preferably randomized phase III trials) can define any advantages of one therapeutic approach over another. Because of the large numbers of patients required for comparative trials and because of the substantial technical commitments required by an institution to perform IORT, few dual-arm trials have been performed using IORT. With increasing use of IORT, however, more phase III trials have been initiated or are planned to define precisely the advantages IORT may have over conventional EBRT.

Abe and colleagues conducted a prospective but non-randomized trial at Kyoto University investigating IORT in gastric carcinoma (27). One hundred ten patients underwent gastric resection alone, and 101 patients had gastric resection with IORT. The determination of which patients received IORT was based on the day of admission into the hospital. All patients had resection appropriate to the stage of disease. Patients who received IORT typically were given 28 Gy for microscopic residual and 35 Gy for gross residual disease. Patients were grouped according to stage for survival analysis. Patients with disease confined to the mucosa (stage I, 67 patients) showed no survival differences between those receiving IORT (87% 5-year survival rate) and those receiving surgery alone (93% 5-year survival rate). However, for all advanced stages, IORT showed statistically significant improvement over controls in 5-year survival rate: in lesions confined to the gastric wall (stage II, 31 patients), IORT patients showed a 5-year survival rate of 84%, whereas surgery-alone patients had a 5-year survival rate of 62%. Patients with nodal involvement (stage III, 68 patients) showed a 62% 5-year survival rate for those receiving IORT, and a 37% 5-year survival rate for those receiving surgery alone. In patients with extragastric extension (stage IV, 45 patients), the 5-year survival rate was 15% for patients receiving IORT and 0% for patients treated with surgery alone. These results suggested that adjunctive IORT improves survival when combined with resection in gastric cancer that has advanced beyond the mucosa.

A prospective, randomized trial of IORT in gastric carcinoma was conducted at the NCI (28). Patients were randomized before surgery to IORT or to control therapy, but protocol therapy was delivered only if the patient subsequently underwent complete resection of his or her lesions. Lesions confined to the gastric wall were randomized between 20 Gy IORT or no additional treatment, and locally-advanced but completely resected lesions were randomized to receive 20 Gy IORT or 50 Gy postoperative EBRT. The entire tumor bed and draining lymphatics were treated using multiple matched IORT fields and 11- to 15-MeV electrons. Misonidazole was used as a radiosensitizer in IORT patients and was delivered as a bolus intravenously 15 to 30 minutes before irradiation. Patients randomized to EBRT were treated with 1.5- to 1.8-Gy fractions daily, usually commencing within 3 o 4 weeks after surgery. Seven protocol patients died of treatment-related complications, for a 17% mortality rate. Randomized groups had equivalent morbidity. Thirty-three of 41 patients (80%) died of progressive disease. Although there were no differences in survival or recurrence rates between IORT and control groups, the patterns of recurrence did differ substantially between IORT and control patients. All 23 patients who recurred after conventional therapy experienced locoregional failures, and 20 (87%) patients recurred in the gastric bed. Recurrent disease developed in ten patients randomized to IORT; seven were locoregional failures (70%) and five were in the gastric bed (50%). The small number of patients on the study precluded valid statistical inferences. The NCI study concluded that IORT and EBRT are equivalent with respect to disease control and survival after complete resection of locally advanced gastric carcinoma.

An investigation of IORT in conjunction with pancreatic resection was performed at Kumamoto University (29). Patients with resectable pancreatic cancers were treated by resection alone or by resection with IORT to the regional nodes. All operations were extended beyond the typical boundaries of pancreatic resection to include all upper abdominal lymph node groups. Among the 16 patients receiving IORT with extended pancreatectomy, 29% survived 5 years or longer. By contrast, there were no 5-year survivors among nine patients receiving extended pancreatectomy alone.

The results of an NCI trial of IORT in retroperitoneal sarcomas have been published (30). Preoperative randomization of eligible patients was performed, but complete resection was required before protocol therapy began. Forty-eight patients were randomized and explored at the NCI. Thirteen patients were found to be ineligible at surgery for varying reasons, most commonly because of the finding of occult metastases. Patients were randomized to an experimental group receiving 20 Gy IORT, using multiple matched fields in the tumor bed, with 35 to 40 Gy EBRT postoperatively,

or randomized to a control group receiving postoperative EBRT alone (50 to 55 Gy). The delivery of EBRT used extensive treatment planning, and field-shrinking techniques were used to minimize dose to liver, spinal cord, kidney, and bowel. The resultant median survivals of 45 months (IORT + EBRT) and 52 months (EBRT alone) were not significantly different. Similar disease recurrence rates of 67% (IORT + EBRT) and 80% (EBRT) were observed. However, all failures after EBRT alone included a component of local failure, whereas significantly fewer patients failed locally in the cohort that received IORT. The IORT + EBRT group suffered more frequent neurologic toxicity, and the group receiving EBRT alone suffered more frequent acute and chronic radiation enteritis. Other treatment toxicities were equally distributed in the IORT and control groups.

Prospective, randomized trials of IORT in resectable and unresectable pancreatic cancer were completed at the NCI and are being analyzed. Twenty-six patients with completely resected adenocarcinoma of the pancreatic head were randomized to receive IORT (all experimental group patients received 20 Gy IORT) or to receive control treatment (standard control therapy was defined as 45- to 55-Gy EBRT for patients with extrapancreatic extension or nodal disease; control patients with disease confined in the pancreatic capsule received surgery alone, without postoperative EBRT). The medial survival was 18 months, with a 27% perioperative mortality. One IORT patient remains alive without evidence of disease more than 10 years after therapy. Histopathologic evidence of disease recurrence was analyzed for 12 patients who underwent autopsy and two patients who required antemortem laparotomy. Locoregional failures occurred in 47% of patients. Peritoneal seeding developed in 35% of patients, and distant metastases in 62%. There were no differences in overall or disease-free survival between IORT and control groups in this subset of patients.

COMPLICATIONS

The proper description of toxicity is of paramount importance in the realistic assessment of any therapeutic modality such as IORT. The potential benefits of a large single dose of radiation are diminished if complications from IORT are more frequent or severe than those from conventional fractionated radiation therapy. Large single doses of radiation can produce significant late toxicities compared with fractionated regimens to the same total dose. Studies from the NCI documented that histopathologic tissue responses observed in dogs subjected to experimental IORT were similar to those in human clinical subjects (31), establishing the dog as the model of choice for preclinical trials of IORT. Clinical experience has demonstrated that IORT may produce unique toxicities, in addition to many of the same complications seen with conventional fractionated EBRT.

Tepper and associates reviewed toxicity data from MGH (32). Sixteen percent (13 of 80) of patients treated with surgery alone for clinically-advanced but nonmetastatic rectal cancer extending through the bowel wall suffered severe or life-threatening complications of therapy. This was compared with a second group of patients with unresectable lesions who underwent 30- to 52-Gy preoperative EBRT to the pelvis followed by complete tumor resection, of whom 35% (8 of 23) experienced similar complications. These values were not significantly different. Selected subsequent colorectal cancer patients underwent IORT for primary tumors or recurrent disease after preoperative EBRT with 50 Gy and maximal resection. IORT doses of 10 Gy were delivered to patients with primary resectable disease and 20 Gy to patients with recurrent lesions. Severe or life-threatening complications were noted in 5 of the 24 patients (21%) treated in the primary lesion group, and in 8 of the 18 patients (47%) in the recurrent lesion group. These figures were not statistically different from those obtained from historically controlled patients at the MGH receiving conventional preoperative radiation therapy and definitive surgery for advanced colorectal malignancies.

Comparison of IORT toxicity was made with historical controls at the Latter Day Saints Hospital and the University of Utah Medical Center (33). Morbidity was 32% (9 of 28 individuals) for patients receiving surgery alone, compared with 19% (5 of 26) for those undergoing similar surgery with IORT. Mortality was 18% for surgery alone, compared with 8% for surgery IORT. The authors concluded that IORT had not added significantly to surgical morbidity.

Forty-one patients underwent pancreaticoduodenectomy and 10- to 20-Gy IORT for completely resectable carcinoma of the pancreatic head at the M. D. Anderson Cancer Center (34). All patients received 10- to 20-Gy IORT. Extended pancreatic resections were performed in these patients, and 32 of 41 patients also received EBRT with concomitant 5-fluorouracil chemotherapy. Thirteen patients (32%) suffered postoperative complications. The authors concluded that IORT under these conditions was well tolerated.

Complication rates have been made available from the RTOG pancreatic, rectal, and gastric carcinoma trials (35). The morbidity rate was 19% (42 of 220 patients) and the mortality rate was 1.8% (4 of 220 patients) among patients who received IORT for various neoplasms. There were no statistical differences in complication rates among the patients who received IORT (19% morbidity) compared with the patients who were placed on study but failed to receive IORT for a variety of reasons (17% morbidity). The mortality rate was similar for patients who received IORT (1.8%) and those who failed to received IORT (1.2%).

Cromack and colleagues reviewed toxicity data from the NCI IORT investigations (36). Four prospectively randomized trials were analyzed, comparing complications rates between patients randomized to IORT and those randomized to a control procedure (surgical resection with or without postoperative EBRT) in patients with gastric cancer, unresectable pancreatic cancer, resectable pancreatic cancer, or retroperitoneal sarcomas. Fifty-one of 66 patients (77%) who received control therapy had 138 separate complications. Forty-four of 53 patients (80%) who received IORT had 108 complications. Seven IORT-treated patients suffered treatment-related mortality (13%), compared with five patients in the control arms (8%). The only statistically significant difference between the IORT and control groups was an increased frequency of sepsis in the control cohort (non-IORT) of the patients with retroperitoneal sarcomas. However, an increased incidence (not statistically significant) of sensory-motor neuropathy was seen in IORT patients in whom the lumbosacral plexus was irradiated intraoperatively. IORT-related neuropathy has been recognized by several centers performing IORT and appears to occur with a significant incidence when large IORT treatment volumes include a major nerve plexus at doses above 15 Gy.

ASSESSMENTS

At present, IORT must be considered an experimental treatment. Available clinical information suggests that the use of IORT permits higher doses of radiation to be delivered, at least in intra-abdominal sites, than conventional fractionated techniques, with acceptable toxicity to most normal tissues. The higher total dose seems to enhance local control rates, compared with conventional radiation, particularly in advanced gastric and colorectal carcinoma. Consequently, in institutions with the capability to deliver it, IORT should be considered routinely in patients with locally-advanced gastric and colorectal carcinomas. Alternatively, in centers without the capability to deliver IORT, referral of patients with advanced gastric or colorectal cancers to IORT facilities should be contemplated.

Although some evidence suggests that IORT may enhance local control in resectable pancreatic cancer, in retroperitoneal sarcomas, and in some other locally-advanced intra-abdominal tumors, the application of IORT in these situations at present should be confined to approved trials designed to evaluate the efficacy and toxicity of IORT in specific clinical situations. Referral and inclusion of patients with advanced intra-abdominal malignancies will be important in the final assessment of IORT in cancer treatment.

REFERENCES

1. Abe M, Yabumoto E, Takahashi M, Tobi T, Mori K. Intraoperative radiotherapy of gastric cancer. *Cancer* 1974;34:2034–2041.
2. Abe M, Takahashi M, Yabumoto E, Adachi H, Yoshii M, Mori K. Clinical experiences with intraoperative radiotherapy of locally advanced cancers. *Cancer* 1980;45:40–48.
3. Abe M, Arakawa M. Fundamental studies on surgical irradiation: histological and hematological changes followed by irradiation during laparotomy of dogs. *J Jap Soc Cancer Ther* 1967;2:271–278.
4. Abe M, Takahashi M, Yabumoto E, et al.. Techniques, indications and results of intraoperative radiotherapy of advanced cancers. *Radiology* 1975;116:693–702.
5. Abe M, Takahashi M. Intraoperative radiotherapy: the Japanese experience. *Int J Radiat Oncol Biol Phys* 1981;7:863–868.
6. Tobe T, Hikasa Y, Matsuda S, Kaneko I, Mori K, Abe M. Treatment of gastric cancer with combined surgery and intraoperative radiotherapy. *World J Surg* 1979;3:715–719.
7. Abe M, Takahashi M, eds. *Intraoperative radiation therapy: proceedings of the Third International Symposium on Intraoperative Radiation Therapy.* New York: Pergamon Press; 1991.
8. Calvo FA, Santos M, Brady LW, eds. *Intraoperative radiotherapy: clinical experiences and results.* Berlin: Springer-Verlag; 1992.
9. Abe M. Intraoperative radiation therapy for gastric cancer. In Dobelbower RR, Abe M, eds. *Intraoperative radiation therapy.* Boca Raton, FL: CRC Press; 1989;165–179.
10. Abe M. Intraoperative radiation therapy for gastrointestinal malignancy. In DeCosse JJ, Sherlock P, eds. *Clinical management of gastrointestinal cancer.* Boston: Martinus Nijhoff; 1984:327–349.
11. Sindelar WF. Intraoperative radiotherapy in carcinoma of the stomach and pancreas. *Recent Results Cancer Res* 1988;110:226–243.
12. Calvo FA, Henriquez I, Santos M, et al. Intraoperative and external beam radiotherapy in advanced resectable gastric cancer: technical description and preliminary results. *Int J Radiat Oncol Biol Phys* 1989;17:183–189.
13. Calvo FA, Santos M, Pardo F, Hernández JL, Alverez-Cienfuegos J, Voltas J. Gastric cancer. In Calvo FA, Santos M, Brady LW, eds. *Intraoperative radiotherapy: clinical experiences and results.* Berlin: Springer-Verlag; 1992:51–56.
14. Tepper J, Nardi G, Suit H. Carcinoma of the pancreas—review of the MGH experiences from 1963–1973: analysis of surgical failure and implications for radiation therapy. *Cancer* 1976;37:1519–1524.
15. Goldson AL. Preliminary clinical experience with intraoperative radiotherapy. *J Natl Med Assoc* 1978;70:493–495.
16. Wood W, Shipley WU, Gunderson LL, Cohen AM, Nardi GL. Intraoperative irradiation for unresectable pancreatic carcinoma. *Cancer* 1982; 49:1272–1275.
17. Shipley WU, Wood WC, Tepper JC, et al. Intraoperative electron beam irradiation for patients with unresectable pancreatic carcinoma. *Ann Surg* 1984;200:289–296.
18. Gunderson LL, Martin JK, Kvols LK, et al. Intraoperative and external beam irradiation ± 5-FU for locally advanced pancreatic cancer. *Int J Radiat Oncol Biol Phys* 1987;13:319–329.
19. Gunderson LL, Cohen AC, Dosoretz DD, et al. Residual, unresectable, or recurrent colorectal cancer: external beam irradiation and intraoperative electron beam boost ± resection. *Int J Radiat Oncol Biol Phys* 1983;9:1597–1606.
20. Willett CG, Shellito PC, Tepper JE, Eliseo R, Convery K, Wood WC. Intraoperative electron beam radiation therapy for primary locally advanced rectal and rectosigmoid carcinoma. *J Clin Oncol* 1991;9: 843–849.
21. Willett CG, Shellito PC, Tepper JE, Eliseo R, Convery K, Wood WC. Intraoperative electron beam radiation therapy for recurrent locally advanced rectal or rectosigmoid carcinoma. *Cancer* 1991;67: 1504–1508.
22. Gunderson LL, Martenson JA, Devine RM, et al. Indications for and results of IORT with colorectal cancer. In Abe M, Takahashi M, eds. *Intraoperative radiation therapy: proceedings of the Third International Symposium on Intraoperative Radiation Therapy.* New York: Pergamon Press; 1991:299–301.
23. Wolkov H, Graves G, Won M, Sause W, Byhardt R, Hanks G. Intraoperative radiation therapy of extrahepatic biliary carcinoma: a report of RTOG-8506. In Abe M, Takahashi M, eds. *Intraoperative radiation therapy: proceedings of the Third International Symposium on Intraoperative Radiation Therapy.* New York: Pergamon Press; 1991:201–203.
24. Tepper JE, Noyes D, Krall JM, et al. Intraoperative radiation therapy of pancreatic carcinoma: a report of RTOG-8505. In Abe M, Takahashi M, eds. *Intraoperative radiation therapy: proceedings of the Third International Symposium on Intraoperative Radiation Therapy.* New York: Pergamon Press; 1991:231–233.
25. Lanciano R, Calkins A, Wolkov H, et al. A phase I,II study of intraoperative radiotherapy in advanced unresectable or recurrent carcinoma of the rectum: a Radiation Therapy Oncology Group (RTOG) study. In Abe M, Takahashi M, eds. *Intraoperative radiotherapy: proceedings of the Third International Symposium on Intraoperative Radiation Therapy.* New York: Pergamon Press; 1991:311–313.
26. Kiel KD, Won MH, Witt TR, et al. Preliminary results of protocol RTOG 85-07: phase II study of intraoperative radiation for retroperitoneal sarcomas. In Abe M, Takashashi M, eds. *Intraoperative radiation therapy: proceedings of the Third International Symposium on Intraoperative Radiation Therapy.* New York: Pergamon Press; 1991:371–372.
27. Abe M, Takahashi M, Ono K, Tobe T, Inamoto T. Japan gastric trials in intraoperative radiation therapy. *Int J Radiat Oncol Biol Phys* 1988;15: 1431–1433.
28. Sindelar WF, Kinsella TJ, Tepper JE, et al. Randomized trial of intraoperative radiotherapy in carcinoma of the stomach. *Am J Surg* 1993;165: 178–187.
29. Hiraoka T, Tashiro S, Kamimoto I, et al. Combination of intraoperative radiation with resection for cancer of the pancreas. In Abe M, Takahashi M, eds. *Intraoperative radiation therapy: proceedings of the Third International Symposium on Intraoperative Radiation Therapy.* New York: Pergamon Press; 1991:239–241.
30. Sindelar WF, Kinsella TJ, Chen PW, et al. Intraoperative radiotherapy in retroperitoneal sarcomas: final results of a prospective, randomized, clinical trial. *Arch Surg* 1993;128:402–410.
31. Sindelar WF, Hoekstra H, Restrepo C, Kinsella TJ. Pathological tissue changes following intraoperative radiotherapy. *Am J Clin Oncol* 1986; 9:504–509.
32. Tepper JE, Gunderson LL, Orlow E, et al. Complications of intraoperative radiation therapy. *Int J Radiat Oncol Biol Phys* 1984;10: 1831–1839.
33. Avizonis VN, Sause WT, Noyes RD. Morbidity and mortality associated with intraoperative radiotherapy. *J Surg Oncol* 1989;41: 240–245.
34. Evans DB, Termuhlen PM, Byrd DR, Ames FC, Ochran TG, Rich TA. Intraoperative radiation therapy following pancreaticoduodenectomy. *Ann Surg* 1993;218:54–60.
35. Noyes R, Weiss S, Krall J, et al. Surgical complications of intraoperative radiation therapy: the Radiation Therapy Oncology Group experience. In Abe M, Takahashi M, eds. *Intraoperative radiation therapy: proceedings of the Third International Symposium on Intraoperative Radiation Therapy.* New York: Pergamon Press; 1991:393–395.
36. Cromack DT, Maher MM, Hoekstra H, Kinsella TJ, Sindelar WF. Are complications in intraoperative radiation therapy more frequent than in conventional treatment? *Arch Surg* 1989;124:229–234.

CHAPTER 23

Diagnosis of Lymph Node Metastases

Richard Essner and Donald L. Morton

In respect of surgical treatment, two cardinal phenomena . . . call for emphatic notice and indicate corresponding principles of action. These are—(a) the usually insignificant dimensions of the primary lesion; (b) its tendency to rapidly infect the nearest lymph glands.

> —*Herbert L. Snow, M.D. Lond.,*
> *"Lecture on Melanotic Cancerous Disease," 1892*

MELANOMA

Background

The most common site of metastasis for cutaneous melanoma is the regional lymph nodes. However, management of the regional nodes has generated considerable debate, reflecting two different approaches. Prophylactic or elective regional lymph node dissection (ELND) is based on the theory that melanoma metastasizes in an orderly fashion, first to the regional lymph nodes and then to distant sites. Early removal of the regional nodes (ie, when they are clinically normal) should therefore improve the patient's clinical outcome (1–6). Therapeutic regional LND (TLND) assumes that the risk of distant spread is equivalent to the risk of regional disease. Therefore, regional lymph nodes should be removed only if they are clinically suspect or contain biopsy-proven metastases (7,8).

Advocates of ELND believe that surgical intervention is more effective when the tumor burden is lower. In addition, pathologic staging based on ELND specimens can identify candidates for adjuvant therapy. Opponents of ELND advocate a wait-and-watch approach, arguing that only 15% to 40% of patients will have regional metastases at the time of ELND, and thus up to 85% of patients will be subjected to an unnecessary procedure. They

claim that the potential risks of the operative procedure may outweigh its benefits. They also argue that ELND may trap metastases in transit between the primary lesion and regional lymph nodes. Some authors believe that removal of the regional nodes may promote hematogenous spread of the tumor.

History

The controversy regarding the surgical management of the regional lymph nodes began at least 100 years ago. In 1892, Herbert L. Snow in his lecture "Melanotic Cancerous Disease" advocated wide excision and ELND as a method to control lymphatic permeation of the metastases (9). In 1907, William Sampson Handley delivered two Hunterian Lectures describing the centrifugal permeation of melanoma from the primary lesion of a single cadaver (10). J. Hogarth Pringle emphasized the importance of regional lymph glands in the dissemination of melanoma and advocated in-continuity dissection of the regional lymph nodes (11). In 1945, George T. Pack demonstrated a 42% incidence of occult regional lymph node metastases and recommended in-continuity dissection for control of the primary tumor, intervening lymphatics, and regional lymph nodes (12,13). In 1965, Menhert and Heard presented data justifying the value of regional LND for deeper primary lesions (14).

Recent Literature

Support for ELND is based on a number of retrospective and nonrandomized reports that estimate an approximately 25% survival advantage for patients undergoing ELND instead of TLND (3,4,6,15–17). Most large studies have shown that patients who undergo removal of clinically negative, histologically positive nodes have a better prognosis than similar patients who undergo removal of

R. Essner and D. L. Morton: Department of Surgical Oncology, John Wayne Cancer Institute, Santa Monica, California 90404.

clinically positive nodes (3,4,6,15–18). In 1991, Morton and associates reported their experience with 1134 melanoma patients whose disease had spread to the regional nodes (3). Univariate analysis demonstrated that the number of tumor-containing nodes, the patient's gender, and the site of the primary melanoma were of prognostic importance. Removal of occult nodal metastases was associated with significantly better 5- and 10-year survival than removal of clinically positive nodes.

A large, prospective, nonrandomized study by the Sydney Melanoma Unit (SMU) demonstrated improved survival of patients undergoing ELND for intermediate-thickness melanomas (0.76 to 4.00 mm) arising on the extremities, torso, or head and neck (2). ELND was particularly beneficial in men with extremity primaries and in all patients with axial primaries. A similar study performed by SMU and the University of Alabama demonstrated a survival advantage for patients whose axial and extremity primaries were managed by wide excision plus ELND instead of wide excision alone. Although tumor thickness, presence of ulceration, and primary site were significant, only ELND was an independent predictor of improved survival (17).

Randomized Trials

Two independent, prospective, randomized trials have been performed to determine the benefit of ELND. Veronesi and the World Health Organization (WHO) studied 553 clinical stage I patients with melanoma confined to the distal two thirds of the extremity (19). After wide excision of the primary tumor, 267 patients underwent immediate LND and the remaining 286 underwent LND only in the presence of clinically positive nodes. Both groups were relatively well matched for prognostic variables. The study demonstrated no survival advantage for either group. The only patients to achieve a benefit from immediate LND (ELND) were those with Clark level IV lesions of intermediate thickness (1.0 to 1.9 mm and 3 to 3.9 mm). These patients had a 10% better survival at 5 years, and 20% at 10 years. The WHO trial was criticized for its preponderance of women: we now know that women with extremity primaries tend to have a favorable prognosis and are not likely to benefit significantly from ELND. Patients were also not stratified for thickness, Clark level, or ulceration of the primary. The WHO data were later reassessed to determine the prognostic significance of these factors (20): tumor thickness and ulceration had a negative impact on survival. Patients who underwent ELND had a greater proportion of ulcerated primaries (52% vs. 19%) than did patients treated by TLND. This discrepancy may have had a negative influence on the results of the trial.

The second prospective, randomized trial was reported in 1986 by Sim and associates from the Mayo Clinic (21).

One hundred seventy-one patients with American Joint Committee on Cancer stages I and II melanoma of the extremities were randomized to immediate LND (54 patients), delayed LND (55 patients), or no LND (62 patients). There was no significant difference in survival among the three groups. The only factors related to survival were tumor thickness and growth pattern. The authors concluded that immediate LND was of no benefit, but their results must be considered cautiously because most of the primary melanomas were low-risk, thin lesions with little risk of metastasis. Thus, both the WHO and the Mayo Clinic trials may have obscured the benefit of ELND. As discussed later, a primary melanoma's thickness, ulceration, and anatomic site provide important prognostic information that should be considered in designing a randomized trial of ELND.

Two randomized trials are in progress to determine the efficacy of ELND. The Intergroup Melanoma Trial is examining the outcome of wide excision plus ELND versus wide excision alone in patients with melanomas of intermediate thickness arising on the extremities or trunk. This trial is also comparing the outcome of 2- versus 4-cm margins of excision (22). The first interim analysis demonstrated only subset differences between the two treatment groups (22a). A second trial is being conducted by the WHO to determine the efficacy of wide excision plus ELND versus wide excision alone in patients with primary melanomas arising on the trunk. Final results of these trials will not be available for 1 to 2 years.

Patient Selection

Data from a number of retrospective and prospective, randomized trials suggest that certain patients benefit from ELND. Tumor thickness, Clark level of invasion, site of the primary, presence of ulceration or regression, histologic subtype, and gender serve as relative markers for the risk of metastatic disease (23–30).

Tumor Thickness

Balch and colleagues suggested that tumor thickness can be used as a quantitative method to determine the risk of regional and distant metastasis (5). Patients with thin (<0.76 mm) lesions have little risk for development of metastases and therefore are not likely to benefit from ELND. Patients with thick (>4 mm) primaries have up to a 60% to 70% risk of regional and distant metastases and also would probably not benefit from ELND. However, patients with intermediate (0.76 to 4 mm) primaries have about a 25% to 57% risk of regional metastases and less than a 20% chance of distant disease. Because their risk of systemic disease is low, this group of patients would most likely benefit from ELND. Similarly, patients with primaries of intermediate Clark level also have a moderate risk for regional metastases and little risk of distant disease.

Anatomic Site

The anatomic site of the primary may also be of prognostic importance in determining the need for ELND. Patients with primaries on the extremities have a more favorable prognosis than those whose primaries are on the trunk, head and neck, palms of the hands, or soles of the feet (5,28,30). In 1984, Urist and associates from the University of Alabama and SMU reviewed their experience of 534 patients with melanoma of the head and neck (28). After 5 years of follow-up, those patients who underwent wide excision plus ELND had significantly better survival than patients who underwent wide excision alone.

Pattern of Growth

The growth pattern of the primary is an important indicator of tumor aggressiveness. Tumors that demonstrate histologic features of ulceration or regression behave more aggressively and may indicate the need for immediate LND (27). Thus, patients with superficial spreading or nodular melanoma are more likely to benefit from ELND than are patients with lentigo maligna melanoma, which usually occurs on the head and neck, grows slowly, and is not aggressive. Urist and associates found that patients with lentigo maligna melanoma had higher 5-year survival rates than patients with superficial spreading or nodular melanoma (28).

Gender

Women may have a survival advantage and reduced risk for development of metastases. Randomized trials comparing wide excision plus ELND to wide excision alone suggest that women may not benefit from ELND (5,30). Because men have a higher risk for metastatic disease, ELND would be more likely to improve their long-term survival. The patient's age, general health, and other medical problems should also be used to determine the need for ELND.

Intraoperative Lymphatic Mapping and Sentinel Lymph Node Dissection: Rationale and Technique

Because of the long-standing controversy regarding the efficacy of ELND, in 1985 Morton and associates devised the technique of intraoperative lymphatic mapping and sentinel lymph node dissection (SLND) as a minimally invasive alternative to ELND in patients with clinically uninvolved lymph nodes (31). They hypothesized that the lymph that drains a cutaneous melanoma passes along dermal lymphatics to a regional lymph basin and initially into one or more sentinel nodes. These sentinel nodes should therefore be the first regional site of metastasis; if the sentinel nodes do not contain tumor cells from a primary melanoma, then there is no regional disease.

Intraoperative lymphatic mapping and SLND is preceded by preoperative cutaneous lymphoscintigraphy, during which technetium-labeled albumin colloid (Cis-US, Inc., Bedford, MA), sulfur colloid (Cis-US, Inc.), or human serum albumin (Medi-physics, Arlington Heights, IL) is injected intradermally (1 to 1.5 ml or 0.5 to 1.0 mCi) at the site of the primary melanoma. A scintillation camera is used to document the drainage pattern from the primary melanoma through the dermal lymphatics to the regional lymph nodes. The skin overlying the first (sentinel) draining node is marked. Because transit time varies with the pharmaceutical, the nuclear medicine physician performing the procedure must be careful to differentiate sentinel from nonsentinel nodes (32). In our experience, the sentinel node can be identified within 30 minutes (depending on the pharmaceutical and the distance between the primary melanoma and the regional lymph nodes) and usually can no longer be differentiated from adjacent nonsentinel nodes by 3 hours. Preoperative lymphoscintigraphy should be performed 1 day before surgery so that the isotope is excreted before intraoperative lymphatic mapping is undertaken. Because it identifies the regional lymph node basin at risk for metastases, preoperative lymphoscintigraphy is particularly helpful in sites on the head and neck or torso, which may have ambiguous lymphatic drainage patterns (18,33–36).

Intraoperative lymphatic mapping is undertaken in the operating room after induction of local or general anesthesia. Isosulfan blue vital dye (Lymphazurin; Hirsch Industries, Inc., Richmond, VA) in a volume of 0.5 to 1.0 ml is injected intradermally with a 25-gauge needle at the site of the primary melanoma (Fig. 1). If the primary lesion has already been excised, the dye is injected on either side of the scar. The previously marked skin overlying the sentinel node is incised; the incision is oriented so that a complete LND can be performed if needed. The skin flap closest to the primary melanoma is dissected free of underlying tissue and the subdermal lymphatics are observed as they stain blue (Fig. 2A). The blue dye typically reaches the regional nodes in 5 to 20 minutes; transit time can usually be predicted by preoperative lymphoscintigraphy. Injections are repeated every 20 minutes until all sentinel nodes are identified (see Fig. 2B). The sentinel node is excised and immediately sent for frozen-section evaluation. If metastases are demonstrated, complete regional LND is performed; otherwise, the regional lymphatic basin is closed without further resection. Some

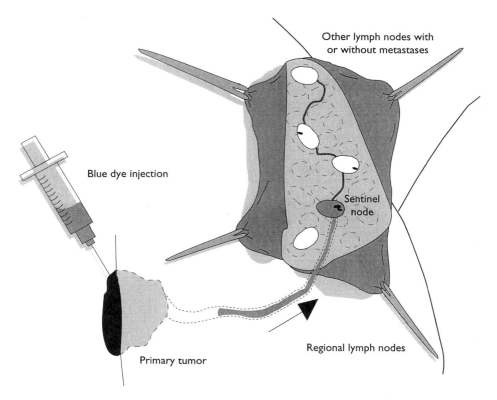

Blue dye injection

Other lymph nodes with
or without metastases

Sentinel
node

Regional lymph nodes

Primary tumor

FIG. 1. Schematic representation of intraoperative lymphatic mapping shows blue dye being injected into a primary melanoma. The dye moves along the lymphatic channel into the drainage basin. The first node to turn blue, not necessarily the proximal node, is the sentinel node. This node is removed during SLND and sent to the pathologist for immediate frozen-section or delayed permanent analysis.

surgeons prefer not to depend on frozen-section analysis of the sentinel node and will perform complete LND only as a secondary procedure, after pathologic analysis of the permanent section.

Results

In 1992, Morton and associates reported their initial experience with intraoperative lymphatic mapping and SLND (31). They were able to identify the sentinel node in 194 (82%) of 237 regional lymphatic drainage basins (Table 1). In the initial portion of the study, all patients underwent complete LND regardless of the pathology of the sentinel node. Of these specimens, 40 (21%) contained metastases in at least one lymph node. In only two (<1%) LND specimens were nonsentinel nodes the exclusive site of regional metastases, a false-negative rate of < 1%.

Occult regional metastases were identified by both standard hematoxylin and eosin staining and newer immunohistochemical techniques. Fifty-seven percent of nodal metastases were found using conventional techniques; the remainder were identified only by immunohistochemical techniques (31). Using immunohistochemical

techniques with an antiserum to S-100 protein (Dako Corp., Carpenteria, CA), Cochran and associates had previously demonstrated that 29% of lymph nodes staining negative with hematoxylin and eosin actually contained metastatic melanoma cells (37). Similarly, 14 of 100 patients who had undergone ELND had metastatic melanoma not demonstrated by conventional staining techniques (38). All specimens were stained with the melanoma-specific murine monoclonal antibody NKI/C3 (Accurate Chemical, Westbury, NY) to confirm the presence of melanoma cells. Serial sectioning rather than bivalving the nodes did not improve diagnostic accuracy. Newer molecular biology techniques looking for specific gene sequences particular to melanoma may further enhance the sensitivity of the sentinel node technique (39,40).

The accuracy of intraoperative lymphatic mapping and SLND has been verified in three studies of patients with primary melanoma draining to cervical, inguinal, or axillary regions (41–44). In a study of head and neck melanomas, the sentinel node was identified in 71 (90%) of the 79 cervical drainage basins demonstrated on preoperative lymphoscintigraphy; 15% contained metastatic disease (42). There were no regional recurrences during a mean follow-up of 27 months. In a study of melanomas on

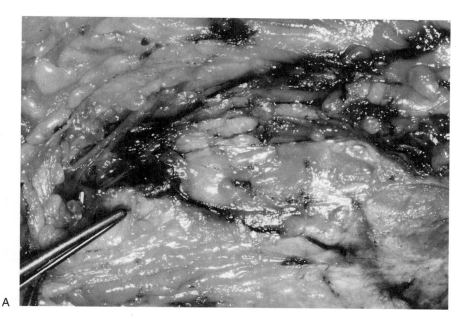

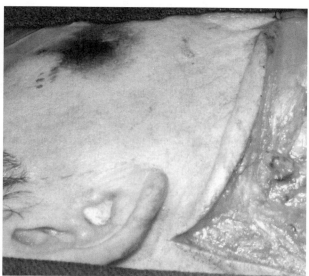

FIG. 2. A: Blue dye highlights the path of lymphatics in the inguinal basin draining a primary cutaneous melanoma on the lower back. Forceps point to the blue-staining sentinel node. (Reprinted with permission from Morton DL, Wen D-R, Wong JH, et al. Technical details of intraoperative lymphatic mapping for early stage melanoma. *Arch Surg* 1992;127:392.) **B:** Blue dye stains skin around a primary melanoma on the cheek (top left); incision over the cervical basin reveals blue-staining sentinel node (bottom right) adjacent to the superficial lobe of the parotid gland. (Reprinted with permission from Morton DL, Wen D-R, Foshag LJ, Essner R, Cochran A. Intraoperative lymphatic mapping and selective cervical lymphadenectomy for early-stage melanomas of the head and neck. *J Clin Oncol* 1993;11: 1751.) (See also Color Plate 4A,B.)

the torso or lower extremities, the sentinel node was found in > 90% of the 77 patients; 14% of the inguinal drainage basins contained metastatic disease, and the false-negative rate was 1% (45).

Thompson and SMU colleagues recently reported their experience with SLND (43). In an initial trial of 102 melanoma patients, the sentinel node was accurately demonstrated in 75% of axillary basins and 86% of cervical and inguinal basins. Twelve percent of the excised sentinel nodes contained metastases. A nonsentinel node was the exclusive site of metastasis in only one (1%) case. These results support and confirm the findings of Morton and associates.

Intraoperative lymphatic mapping with SLND is a relatively difficult procedure, but its learning curve is

steep. During his initial 58 cases, Morton and colleagues identified only 81% of sentinel nodes; however, during the next 58 cases, their rate of sentinel node identification jumped to 96%, and it now approaches 100%. The rate of sentinel node identification is highest in the inguinal region and slightly lower in the axillary and cervical basins.

Morton and colleagues at the John Wayne Cancer Institute have initiated an international multicenter trial comparing wide excision plus SLND to wide excision alone in patients with clinical stage I melanoma (localized disease) (Fig. 3). Patients with intermediate (1 to 4 mm)-thickness melanoma who have not had a wide excision (>1.5-cm margins), skin graft, or other procedures that would alter the lymphatic drainage are eligi-

TABLE 1. *Initial experience with intraoperative lymphatic mapping and selective lymph node dissection for early-stage melanoma: distribution of metastases in sentinel and nonsentinel nodes*

Total lymphadenectomies	298
237 (100%)	
Lymphadenectomies with identified sentinel nodes	194 (82%)
Lymphadenectomies with tumor in nodes	40 (21%)
Lymphadenectomies with tumor in sentinel nodes	38 (20%)
Lymphadenectomies with tumor in nonsentinel nodes (exclusively)	2 (<1%)
Total lymph nodes	3338 (100%)
Total sentinel nodes	259 (8%)
Sentinel nodes with tumor	47 (18%)
Total nonsentinel nodes	3079 (92%)
Total nonsentinel nodes with tumor (exclusively)	2 (<0.1%)

Adapted from Morton DL, Wen D-R, Wong JH, et al. Technical details of intraoperative lymphatic mapping for early

ble. Complete LND is performed only in lymphatic drainage basins containing tumor-positive sentinel nodes. The purpose of this study is to determine the benefit of early ELND without imposing the morbidity of this procedure on patients with tumor-negative sentinel nodes. The trial's organizers hope that SLND will replace blind ELND or the wait-and-watch approach as

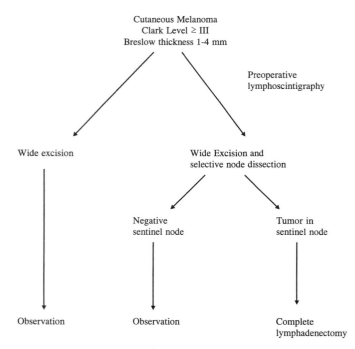

FIG. 3. Protocol for the multicenter trial of intraoperative lymphatic mapping and sentinel lymph node dissection in patients with clinical stage I melanoma.

the standard of management for patients with clinical stage I melanoma.

Morbidity and Mortality

Complications of intraoperative lymphatic mapping and SLND have been minimal (31,42). All patients report blue staining of the urine during the first 24 hours after operation, and a few patients retain dye at the injection site for a few months. The incidence of wound infection, bleeding, or seroma is less than 5%. Length of hospitalization is significantly reduced for patients undergoing SLND instead of complete LND (45).

New Approaches

In an attempt to improve the accuracy of detecting the sentinel node, especially during the learning phase and in difficult basins, Morton and associates recently modified their mapping technique by adding technetium isotope to the blue dye before it is injected (44). The blue dye is mixed by the nuclear medicine physician in a 3 : 1 ratio with 500 μCi of technetium-labeled human serum albumin (Medi-physics); a volume of 0.5 to 1.0 ml is injected at the time of surgery. A hand-held gamma counter (Neoprobe Corp., Dublin, OH) is used to follow the radioactive blue dye into the regional basin. The radioactive blue dye typically travels to the regional nodes in 5 to 20 minutes; the kinetics can be predicted by the preoperative lymphoscintigram, if the same radiopharmaceutical is used. Morton's group tested radiolymphoscintigraphic mapping in 34 lymphatic drainage basins of 30 melanoma patients. At least 1 sentinel node was identified in each basin: the blue dye identified 36 sentinel nodes, and the radiolabeled isotope found an additional 6 sentinel nodes. Overall, sentinel nodes had roughly a twofold higher radioactive count than adjacent nonsentinel nodes, and up to an eightfold higher level of radioactivity than the lymph basin or background. Although none of the sentinel nodes contained metastatic melanoma, this study demonstrated the usefulness of the hand-held gamma counter for identifying sentinel lymph nodes.

BREAST CANCER

Background

Axillary LND (ALND) for potentially curable breast cancer has been increasingly viewed as a diagnostic rather than a therapeutic procedure. Low tumor yield, potential morbidity, and expense are among the factors influencing some surgeons to limit or abandon this technique. However, no clinical characteristics, pathologic features, or genetic markers are completely accurate for demonstrating axillary lymph node metastases. Complete ALND remains the gold standard for detection.

Some surgeons now recommend limited or selective procedures for staging the axilla. These approaches have been popularized by reports suggesting no correlation between survival or distant recurrence and the number of nodes removed from the axilla (46). However, incomplete axillary dissections can increase staging errors by 2% to 45% (46).

History

Axillary LND for breast cancer was originally popularized by the French surgeon Jean Louis Petit, who noted that the axillary nodes "were the root of the cancer" and should be excised with the surrounding pectoral fascia and portions of the muscle (47). Benjamin Bell published a six-volume text that described the importance of removing axillary nodes and the associated survival advantage (47). In 1867, Charles Moore described his experience with axillary dissection and noted improved survival of those patients undergoing complete ALND (48). The controversy over axillary dissection began at this time, over 100 years ago, when James Syme and Robert Liston questioned the value of ALND in view of its limited survival data and high morbidity (49). In 1894, Halsted popularized radical mastectomy, which allowed unobstructed access to the axillary nodes. However, 23% of patients died from metastatic cancer even though Halsted found no evidence of metastases in the regional nodes. His principles of direct permeation of the tumor into the lymphatics could not explain the cause of distant failures (50).

Recent Literature

In 1987, Hayward advocated the importance of complete ALND for the treatment of early breast cancer and demonstrated decreased local recurrence rates and improved survival in patients receiving ALND in addition to radiation (51,52). However, his results are viewed with some skepticism because of the small study size and differences in management of the primary tumor. A similar study by Cabanes and associates linked ALND to a survival benefit in patients with small tumors. However, it is unclear whether the results of this study reflect the operative procedure or the adjuvant therapy (53).

Fisher and colleagues from the National Surgical Adjuvant Breast Project examined their large breast cancer database to determine differences in survival after total mastectomy, total mastectomy plus radiation to the axilla, and radical mastectomy (54). Over a 10-year follow-up, there was no difference in overall survival among the three groups. The rate of axillary recurrence was less than 5% for women who underwent either radical mastectomy or total mastectomy plus radiation. Because only about 39% of the 360 clinically negative patients in each treatment group had axillary metastases, the potential benefit of ALND could not be determined from this trial. This does not prove that axillary treatment is of no benefit, only that the number of patients was insufficient to detect a difference.

Sampling Accuracy

Although ALND remains the gold standard for determining the stage and ultimately the management of patients with breast cancer, the indications for and extent of the procedure have recently been questioned. Because of their low risk for development of axillary metastases, complete ALND is unlikely to have a benefit in breast cancer patients with pathologically negative nodes or small (<5 mm) primaries. Limited axillary dissections or axillary sampling reduces postoperative morbidity, but may prove ineffective for staging. Compared with complete ALND, dissection of level I nodes alone has a staging error of about 10% to 12%, dissection of level I and II nodes has an error of 2% to 3%, and blind sampling of the axilla produces an error of 14% to 45% (46,55).

Staging accuracy affects the rate of regional recurrences. Kjaergaard and associates demonstrated that the rate of axillary recurrence decreases as the number of excised nodes increases (56). Their rate of axillary recurrence resulting from missed or untreated disease was 12% when no nodes were excised, and only 2% when more than three lymph nodes were excised. In a similar study, Graverson and colleagues reported a 3% regional recurrence rate after removal of 5 to 10 axillary nodes (57). Mathieson and associates suggested 10 as the minimum number of nodes to be excised for adequate sampling (58).

TABLE 2. *Lymphatic mapping and selective lymph node dissection for breast cancer*

Total number of procedures	174 (100%)
Total number of positive axillary basins	62 (35.6%)
Number of procedures in which sentinel nodes were identified	114 (65.5%)
Number of sentinel nodes containing tumor	37 (32.4%)
Number of falsely negative sentinel nodes	5 (4.3%)
Number of axillary basins with concordant sentinel and nonsentinel nodes	109 (95.6%)

Adapted from Giuliano AE, Kirgan DM, Guenther JM, Morton DL. Lymphatic mapping and sentinel lymphadenectomy for breast cancer. *Ann Surg* 1994;220:391.

Intraoperative Lymphatic Mapping and Sentinel Lymph Node Dissection for Breast Cancer: Results

Because of the controversy regarding the efficacy of ALND for breast cancer, Giuliano and associates adapted the technique of intraoperative lymphatic mapping and SLND for the detection of axillary lymph node metastases (Table 2). In 1994, they reported their initial experience (59). Sentinel nodes were found in 114 (65%) of 174 procedures and accurately predicted the tumor status of the axillary basin in 109 (95%) cases. The anatomic location of the sentinel node was examined in 54 cases: in 10 cases the only site of metastasis was in level II, suggesting a high error rate for level I dissection alone.

More recently, Giuliano's group reported their continued experience with SLND (60). They compared the detection of regional metastases in 134 patients who underwent complete ALND and in 162 patients who underwent SLND before complete ALND. The rate of axillary metastases was significantly higher in the latter group (42% vs. 29%; $P < 0.03$) because SLND allowed the pathologist to focus on the nodes most likely to contain metastases. The results are likely due to the improvement in accuracy or the use of immunohistochemical staining techniques (61). The preliminary success with SLND suggests that this technique may ultimately change the management of the axilla in patients with early-stage breast cancer.

REFERENCES

1. Reitgen DS, Cox EB, McCarty KS Jr, Vollmer RT, Seigler HF. Efficacy of elective lymph node dissection in patients with intermediate thickness primary melanoma. *Ann Surg* 1983;198:379.
2. McCarthy WH, Shaw HM, Milton GW. Efficacy of elective lymph node dissection in 2,347 patients with clinical stage I malignant melanoma. *Surg Gynecol Obstet* 1985;161:575.
3. Morton DL, Wanek LA, Nizze JA, Elashoff RM, Wong JH. Improved long-term survival after lymphadenectomy of melanoma metastatic to regional nodes: analysis of prognostic factors in 1134 patients from the John Wayne Cancer Institute. *Ann Surg* 1991;214:491.
4. Das Gupta TK. Results of treatment of 269 patients with primary cutaneous melanoma: a five-year prospective study. *Ann Surg* 1977; 186: 201.
5. Balch CM, Milton GW, Cascinelli N, Sim FH. Elective lymph node dissection: pros and cons. In: Balch CM, Houghton AN, Milton GW, Sober AJ, Soong S-J, eds. *Cutaneous melanoma.* 2nd ed. Philadelphia: JB Lippincott; 1992:345.
6. McNeer G, Das Gupta TK. Prognosis in malignant melanoma. *Surgery* 1964;56:512.
7. Roses DF, Provet JA, Harris MN, et al. Prognosis of patients with pathologic stage II cutaneous melanoma. *Ann Surg* 1985;201:103.
8. Balch CM, Soong S-J, Murad TM, Ingalls AL, Maddox WA. A multifactorial analysis of melanoma: III. prognostic factors in melanoma patients with lymph node metastases (stage III). *Ann Surg* 1981; 193: 377.
9. Snow H. Melanotic cancerous disease. *Lancet* 1892;2:872.
10. Handley WS. The pathology of melanotic growths in relation to their operative treatment: lectures I & I. *Lancet* 1907;1:927:996.
11. Pringle JH. A method of operation in cases of melanotic tumours of the skin. *Edinburgh Medical Journal* 1908;23:496.
12. Pack GT, Scharnagel I, Morfit M. The principle of excision and dis-section in continuity for primary and metastatic melanoma of the skin. *Surgery* 1945;17:849.
13. Pack GT, Gerber DM, Scharnagel IM. End results in the treatment of malignant melanoma: a report of 1190 cases. *Ann Surg* 1952;131:905.
14. Menhert JH, Heard JL. Staging of malignant melanomas by depth of invasion: a proposed index to prognosis. *Am J Surg* 1965;110:168.
15. Cohen MH, Ketcham AS, Felix EL, et al. Prognostic factors in patients undergoing lymphadenectomy for malignant melanoma. *Ann Surg* 1977;186:635.
16. Callery C, Cochran AJ, Roe DJ, et al. Factors prognostic in patients with malignant melanoma spread to the regional lymph nodes. *Ann Surg* 1982;196:69.
17. Balch CM, Soong S-J, Milton GW, et al. A comparison of prognostic factors and surgical results in 1,786 patients with localized (stage I) melanoma treated in Alabama, USA and New South Wales, Australia. *Ann Surg* 1982;196:677.
18. Slingluff CL, Stidham KR, Ricci WM, Stanley WE, Seigler HF. Surgical management of regional nodes in patients with melanoma: experience with 4682 patients. *Ann Surg* 1994;219:120.
19. Veronesi U, Adamus J, Bandiera DC, et al. Inefficacy of immediate node dissection in stage I melanoma of the limbs. *N Engl J Med* 1977; 297:627.
20. Veronesi U, Adamus J, Bandiera DC, et al. Stage I melanoma of the limbs: immediate versus delayed node dissection. *Tumori* 1980;66:373.
21. Sim FH, Taylor WF, Pritchard DJ, Soule EH. Lymphadenectomy in the management of stage I malignant melanoma: a prospective randomized study. *Mayo Clin Proc* 1986;61:697.
22. Balch CM, Urist MM, Karakousis CP, et al. Efficacy of 2-cm surgical margins for intermediate-thickness melanomas (1 to 4 mm): results of a multi-institutional randomized surgical trial. *Ann Surg* 1993; 218:262.
22a. Balch CM, Soong S-J, Bartolucci A, et al. Efficacy of an elective regional lymph node dissection of 1 to 4 mm thick melanomas for patients 60 years of age or younger. *Ann Surg* 1996;224:255–266.
23. Clark WH Jr, From L, Bernardino EA, Mihm MC Jr. The histogenesis and biologic behavior of primary human malignant melanomas of the skin. *Cancer Res* 1969;29:705.
24. Breslow A. Prognostic factors in the treatment of cutaneous melanoma. *J Cutan Pathol* 1979;6:208.
25. Morton DL, Davtyan DG, Wanek LA, Foshag LJ, Cochran AJ. Multivariate analysis of the relationship between survival and the microstage of primary melanoma by Clark level and Breslow thickness. *Cancer* 1993;71:3737.
26. Balch CM, Murad TM, Soong S-J, Ingalls AL, Richards PC, Maddox WA. Tumor thickness as a guide to surgical management of clinical stage I melanoma patients. *Cancer* 1979;43:883.
27. Balch CM, Wilkerson JA, Murad TM, et al. The prognostic significance of ulceration of cutaneous melanoma. *Cancer* 1980;45:3012.
28. Urist MM, Balch CM, Soong S-J, et al. Head and neck melanoma in 534 clinical stage I patients: a prognostic factors analysis and results of surgical treatment. *Ann Surg* 1984;200:769.
29. Essner R, Wong JH, Economon JS, Morton DL. Prognostic significance of melanoma arising in the scalp. *Am J Surg* 1988;156:314.
30. Balch CM, Soong S-J, Shaw HM, Urist MM, McCarthy WH. An analysis of prognostic factors in 8500 patients with cutaneous melanoma. In: Balch CM, Houghton AN, Milton GW, Sober AJ, Soong S-J, eds. *Cutaneous melanoma.* 2nd ed. Philadelphia: JB Lippincott; 1992:165.
31. Morton DL, Wen D-R, Wong JH, et al. Technical details of intraoperative lymphatic mapping for early stage melanoma. *Arch Surg* 1992; 127:392.
32. Glass EC, Essner R, Giuliano A, Morton DL. Comparative efficacy of three lymphoscintigraphic agents. *Proceedings of the 42nd annual meeting of the Society of Nuclear Medicine* 1995;36:199p.
33. Norman J, Cruse CW, Espinosa C, et al. Redefinition of cutaneous lymphatic drainage with the use of lymphoscintigraphy for malignant melanoma. *Am J Surg* 1991;162:432.
34. Robinson DS, Sample WF, Fee HJ, et al. Regional lymphatic drainage in primary malignant melanoma of the trunk determined by colloidal gold scanning. *Surg Forum* 1977;28:147.
35. Wanebo HJ, Harpole D, Teates CD. Radionuclide lymphoscintigraphy with technetium antimony sulfide colloid to identify lymphatic drainage of cutaneous melanoma of ambiguous sites in the head and neck and trunk. *Cancer* 1985;55:1403.
36. Sappey MPC. *Injection preparation et conservation des vaisseau lym-*

phatiques. These pour le doctorate en medecine, No. 241. Paris Rignoux Imprimeur de la Faculte de Medecine, 1843.

37. Cochran AJ, Wen DR, Morton DL. Occult tumor cells in the lymph nodes of patients with pathological stage I malignant melanoma: an immunohistochemical study. *Am J Surg Pathol* 1988;12:612.

38. Cochran AJ, Wen DR, Herschman HR. Occult melanoma in lymph nodes detected by antiserum to S-100 protein. *Int J Cancer* 1984;34:159.

39. Heller R, Becker J, Wasselle J. Detection of submicroscopic lymph node metastases in patients with melanoma. *Arch Surg* 1991;126:1455.

40. Wang X, Heller R, Van Voorhis N, et al. Detection of submicroscopic lymph node metastases with polymerase chain reaction in patients with malignant melanoma. *Ann Surg* 1994;220:768.

41. Reintgen D, Cruse CW, Wells K, et al. The orderly progression of melanoma nodal metastases. *Ann Surg* 1994;220:759.

42. Morton DL, Wen D-R, Foshag LJ, Essner R, Cochran A. Intraoperative lymphatic mapping and selective cervical lymphadenectomy for early-stage melanomas of the head and neck. *J Clin Oncol* 1993;11:1751.

43. Thompson, J, McCarthy W, Robinson E, Preusse A. Sentinel lymph node biopsy in 102 patients with clinical stage I melanoma undergoing elective lymph node dissection. Presented at the Annual Meeting of the Society of Surgical Oncology, Houston, Texas, March 17–20, 1994.

44. Essner R, Foshag L, Morton DL. Intraoperative radiolymphoscintigraphy: a useful adjunct to intraoperative lymphatic mapping and selective lymphadenectomy in patients with clinical stage I melanoma. Presented at the Annual Meeting of the Society of Surgical Oncology, Houston, Texas, March 17–20, 1994.

45. Essner R, Wen DR, Cochran AJ, Morton DL, Ramming KP. Lymphatic mapping and selective lymph node biopsy: an alternative to elective lymphadenectomy for early-stage melanomas of the trunk and lower extremities. *Proceedings of the American Society of Clinical Oncology* 1993;12:391.

46. Kinne D. Controversies in primary breast cancer management. *Am J Surg* 1993;166:502.

47. Degenshein GA, Ceccarelli F. The history of breast cancer surgery: part I. Early beginnings to Halsted. *Breast* 1977;3:28.

48. Moore C: On the influence of inadequate operations on the theory of cancer. *Royal Chir Soc Lond* 1867;1:244.

49. Halsted WS. A clinical and historical study of certain adenocarcinomata of the breast. *Ann Surg* 1898;28:557.

50. Halsted WS. The results of radical operations for the cure of carcinoma of the breast. *Ann Surg* 1907;46:1.

51. Hayward JL. The Guy's Hospital trials of treatments of "early" breast cancer. *World J Surg* 1977;1:314.

52. Hayward JL, Caleffi M. The significance of local control in the primary treatment of breast cancer. *Arch Surg* 1987;122:1244.

53. Cabanes PA, Salmon RJ, Vicog JR, et al. Value of axillary dissection in addition to lumpectomy and radiotherapy in early breast cancer. *Lancet* 1992;339:1245.

54. Fisher B, Redmond C, Fisher ER, et al. Ten-year results of a randomized clinical trial comparing radical mastectomy and total mastectomy with or without radiation. *N Engl J Med* 1985;312:674.

55. Moffat F, Senofsky G, Davis K, et al. Axillary node dissection for early breast cancer: some is good, but all is better. *J Surg Oncol* 1992;51:8.

56. Kjaergaard J, Blichert-Toft M, Anderson J, et al. Probability of false negative nodal staging in conjunction with partial axillary dissection in breast cancer. *Br J Surg* 1985;72:365.

57. Graversen H, Blichert-Toft M, Andersen J, Ledeles K. Breast cancer: risk of axillary recurrence in node-negative patients following partial dissection of the axilla. *Eur J Surg Oncol* 1988;14:407.

58. Mathiesen O, Bonderup D, Panduro J. Axillary sampling and the risk of erroneous staging of breast cancer: an analysis of 960 patients. *Acta Oncol* 1990;29:721.

59. Giuliano AE, Kirgan DM, Guenther JM, Morton DL. Lymphatic mapping and sentinel lymphadenectomy for breast cancer. *Ann Surg* 1994;220:391.

60. Giuliano AE, Dale PS, Turner RR, Evans SW, Krasne DL, Morton DL. Improved axillary staging of breast cancer with sentinel lymphadenectomy. *Ann Surg* 1995;222:394.

61. Datta YH, Adams PT. Drobyski WR, et al. Sensitive detection of occult breast cancer by the reverse-transcriptase polymerase chain reaction. *J Clin Oncol* 1994;12:475.

CHAPTER 24

The Role of Lymph Node Dissection in the Treatment of Cancer

Sadiq S. Sikora and Michael T. Lotze

"Surgeons must be very careful
When they take the knife!
Underneath their fine incisions
Stirs the culprit—Life!"

—*Emily Dickinson, 1859*

The general surgical principle of wide local dissection with in-continuity removal of lymph nodes represents a basic component of the surgical management of solid tumors. En bloc dissection not only includes a margin of normal tissue around a primary solid tumor to prevent recurrence related to direct extension into the adjoining tissues, but encompasses the regional lymph nodes. Principles embodied in the Halsted radical mastectomy, with its inclusion of wide resection of the breast, overlying skin, and underlying pectoralis major muscle as well as in-continuity dissection of the axillary lymph nodes, had their logical extension to the excision of a long strip of intervening tissue from a primary melanoma to the regional draining lymph nodes, the dissection of internal mammary nodes in the setting of breast carcinoma, and the extended total pancreatectomy. Many of these procedures have been abandoned as the principles underlying the primary surgical treatment of tumors have been redefined. In addition, nonsurgical treatments for cancer, including irradiation and chemotherapy as well as immunotherapy, require a different perspective toward surgical oncologic procedures. The general use of nodal dissection as a staging procedure to determine prognosis and to place patients on clinical protocols has been firmly established. The actual role of surgical dissection with or without evidence of disease in the regional lymph nodes is the primary focus of this chapter. The ability of nodal dissections either to palliate or cure patients with solid tumors is considered. The actual dissections themselves are only briefly presented, but are well described in several operative texts (1–3).

HISTORY

It is likely that many of the "fleshy" tumors described by Hippocrates were actually nodal deposits of tumor. It was not until 1622, however, that Aselli described the lymphatic vessels in the mesentery of the dog (see Chap. 2). In 1651, Pequet described the thoracic duct, which drains the abdominal viscera and lower extremities, and its entry into the venous system. Valsalva speculated in 1704 that cancer was initially localized and then spread through the lymphatics as a subsequent manifestation of its course. This was supported by Le Dran in 1757. The father of modern surgery, John Hunter, in 1784 proposed that the lymphatic vessels were present throughout the body and served to absorb fluid. He believed that their ligation contributed to the development of edema and ascites. The concept of lymph nodes as effective barriers to the spread of cancer was suggested by Virchow in 1860, and the subsequent development of a number of radical surgical procedures, including the subtotal gastrectomy, radical mastectomy, radical prostatectomy, radical neck dissection for head and neck cancer (4), radical hysterectomy (5), and abdominal perineal resection (6), was based on the principle of the stepwise progression of cancer (7).

S. S. Sikora: Department of Surgery, Section of Surgical Oncology, University of Pittsburgh Medical Center, Pittsburgh, Pennsylvania 15213.

M. T. Lotze: University of Pittsburgh Cancer Institute, Pittsburgh, Pennsylvania 15213-2582.

DIAGNOSTIC PROCEDURES TO DETECT TUMOR WITHIN LYMPH NODES

Large tumor deposits within lymph node chains accessible to easy palpation are often discovered by the patient or during a physical examination. More difficult is the routine assessment of smaller deposits of tumor or those situated within nodes located deep within the body compartments. The recent emergence of computed tomography (CT) and magnetic resonance imaging (MRI) enables ready assessment of large deposits of disease within these sites, but this ability is usually restricted to tumor sizes of 1 cm or greater (8–10). There are a number of techniques that have been developed specifically to image lymph nodes and to confirm the diagnosis of cancer, and these are detailed in the following sections.

Lymphangiography

Modern application of lymphangiography occurred with the development by a British surgeon, J. B. Kinmonth, of a method of identifying and cannulating the lymphatics using a supravital dye (11). This dye, usually blue in color, is injected into the subcutaneous tissues and is taken up by local lymphatics. The lymphatic vessels are usually less than 1 mm in diameter and require cutdown for cannulation and successful injection. Bipedal lymphangiography is now rarely performed given the development of more modern imaging techniques. An ethiodized oil emulsion, known commercially as Ethiodol (Savage Laboratories, Melville, NY) in the United States, is most frequently used in these studies.

Complications related to lymphangiography include foreign body reactions within the nodes (12). As a matter of fact, the persistent retention of contrast material in lymph nodes was previously frequently used, especially in the treatment of lymphomas, to follow clinical responses to therapy. Other complications are rare but include pulmonary problems (13) related to blockage of pulmonary capillaries by oil, leading to decreased diffusing capacity, and very rarely to cerebral embolism. Although both upper extremity and cervical lymphangiograms have been performed, only lower extremity studies are routinely done, with cannulation of lymphatic vessels in the foot and unilateral or bipedal injection of contrast material. The use of lymphangiography is largely restricted clinically to evaluation of patients with lymphoma, but occasionally evaluations are obtained (especially in a research setting) for patients with cancer of the ovary or testes and genitourinary tumors. Unfortunately, many of the radiologic findings associated with lymphangiography are not specific to tumor (14), and may be seen in other conditions, primarily those that are inflammatory in origin. Changes associated with tumor include increases in size, filling defects, and delayed filling and obstruction. An early film obtained 2 hours after bipedal injection of contrast material is shown in Fig. 1. A different patient is presented in Fig. 2, with a 24-hour film showing excellent delineation of inguinal pelvic and abdominal lymph nodes. Unfortunately, upper pelvic and abdominal nodes are inconsistently visualized, and when absent filling is noted, conclusions regarding nodal disruption by tumor are often impossible to make. The earlier concerns that lymphangiography may cause an increase in metastases have not been borne out on further evaluation (15). Its use is limited to prospective studies evaluating the role of various diagnostic modalities for pelvic and retroperitoneal nodal disease in genitourinary tumors. Its application in the current practice is confined mainly to experimental approaches using the supravital dyes (eg, isosulfan blue to identify the sentinel node in treatment of melanomas and breast cancer; see Chap. 23).

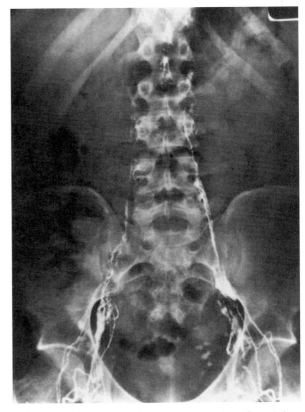

FIG. 1. Bipedal lymphangiogram (filling phase) at 2 hours. This study in a patient with ovarian carcinoma demonstrates the fine anatomy of lymphatic vessels with multiple valves. The valves in the lymphatics direct flow from the deep to the superficial system in the legs (contrary to veins) and then up through the superficial to the deep (iliac) inguinal nodal systems.

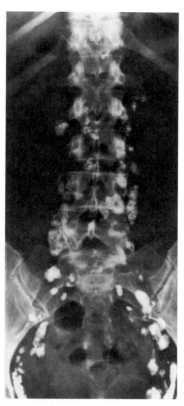

FIG. 2. Bipedal lymphangiogram (storage phase) at 24 hours. Views of the pelvis and abdomen in a patient with Hodgkin's disease confined to the neck demonstrates the long, fused Cloquet's or Rosenmiller's node at the inguinal ligament and lacunar nodes along the pelvic brim. Most of the other nodes are oval and elongated, measuring up to 2 to 4 cm normally.

Lymphoscintigraphy

The direct injection of radiolabeled substances into the skin or other organs has been carried out for many years (16). The most frequently used radionuclides include ^{131}I, ^{123}I, ^{99}Tc, and ^{111}In conjugated to albumin or other colloids. Other substances that have undergone evaluation include [193]Au, antimony sulfur colloid, stannous phytate, and [197]Hg sulfide colloid (17–22). Clinical applications of these reagents have been in the setting of diseases with frequent nodal metastases, including breast carcinoma and melanoma. Successful imaging of internal mammary nodes (which are positive in approximately 20% of patients with operable breast carcinoma) has been reported (23). This allows preoperative evaluation as well as possible subsequent radiation therapy planning.

The first reports of lymphoscintigraphy in melanoma were by Fee and colleagues (17), who used [198]Au colloid to delineate the lymph drainage in melanomas situated in ambiguous sites so that nodal dissections could be planned. Lymphoscintigraphy is used preoperatively in melanoma patients with truncal lesions to identify the nodal drainage basin as an adjunct to the sentinel node approach. Thompson et al. (24) used ^{99m}Tc-labeled antimony trisulfide colloid in melanoma patients and demonstrated that 16% of patients had more than one drainage basin (4% had three lymph node fields) and also had multiple sentinel nodes. A combination radiolymphoscintigraphic method (isosulfan blue–[99m]Tc) has been described to facilitate the identification of the sentinel node (see Chap. 23). Because the role of prophylactic nodal dissection continues to be controversial, these studies have been limited to centers performing prophylactic nodal dissections. The use of interstitial injections in patients with carcinoma of the prostate has allowed evaluation of lymphatic drainage and identification of lymph node drainage (16). The initial hope associated with the use of lymphoscintigraphy was that microscopic subclinical lymph node metastatic disease would be identified. Unfortunately, the resolution characteristics of conventional radionuclides and scanners preclude identification of very small deposits of disease. Currently, lymphoscintigraphy remains primarily a research tool, although clinical applications continue to be postulated.

Immunolymphoscintigraphy

Development of more precisely targeted radionuclides using monoclonal antibodies or polyclonal sera would supposedly identify small deposits of disease (25). Studies conducted at the National Cancer Institute (NCI) used ^{131}I-labeled specific Fab (fragment antigen-binding) fragments of monoclonal antibodies to melanoma injected subcutaneously in 10 patients (Fig. 3). Only 2 tumors were thought to have been successfully imaged, but 8 of the 10 patients had subsequently confirmed tumor (26). Four of the patients were thought to have had specific uptake by subsequent counting after axillary dissection. Use of a ^{111}In-tagged whole antibody, 9.2.27, enabled identification of lymph nodes (Fig. 4) but without convincing specific localization of tumor, presumably because of nonspecific uptake of the antibody by the reticuloendothelial system or weak staining of normal lymph node tissue by this antibody. A vast literature has accumulated on radioimmunodetection and its application in identifying primary, recurrent, and metastatic disease. Several studies have been carried out with antibodies to carcinoembryonic antigen (lung, colon) (27,28), B72.3 (colon) (29,30), HMFG1 (31) and BCD-F9 (32) (breast), CYT-356 (pelvic nodes) (33), E48 Ig (head and neck) (34), lymphoma antigens (35), and ferritin (36). Immunolymphoscintigraphy is safe, with reported sensitivity and specificity of 85% to 90% and 60% to 75%, respectively (31,37). It detects microscopic disease of up to 1 cm in size that evades the routine imaging modalities. The use of single-photon emission CT apparently improves the sensitivity (22).

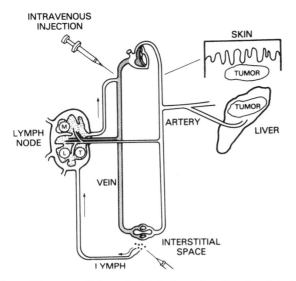

FIG. 3. Diagram of the administration of antibodies into the interstitial space or systemic circulation showing the afferent and efferent lymphatics of a lymph node. Antibodies were administered to detect nodal or systemic deposits of melanoma. M, monocytes; L, lymphocytes; T, tumor.

Computed Tomography

Frequently, a baseline CT evaluation is performed in cancer patients for assessment of the extent of local disease and to document regional spread. The CT criteria for the assessment of nodal disease are based on the size and shape of the nodes in question, presence of central necrosis, and grouping of nodes (38,39). A central low attenuation with a thick, irregular, enhancing periphery (central necrosis) is highly predictive of metastatic involvement. In general, nodes measuring more than 10 mm in the shortest diameter and of spherical shape are highly suggestive of metastatic disease. Based on these criteria, pathologic nodes can be identified with a sensitivity of 80% to 90% and specificity of 90% to 95% (38). Extracapsular nodal spread, an ominous prognostic sign, has specific CT features in the form of capsular enhancement and ill-defined nodal margins, with nearly 100% sensitivity. In head and neck malignancies, nonpalpable pathologic nodes are identified in 7% to 19% of patients (40) by critical CT evaluation. In genitourinary cancers, CT is being routinely used for the evaluation of the pelvic and para-aortic nodes. It has a high accuracy and specificity, ranging from 97% to 100%; the sensitivity varies depending on the site of nodal disease—67% for para-aortic nodes and 25% for pelvic nodes (41). In a prospective comparison of lymphangiography, CT, and abdominopel-

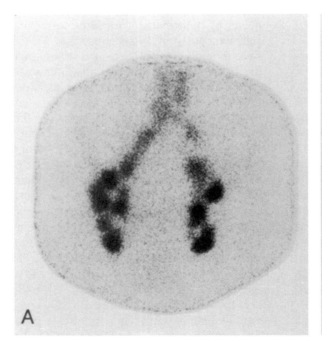
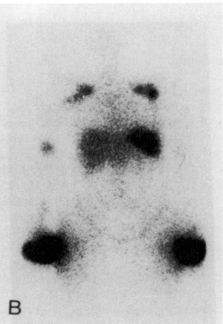

FIG. 4. A: Delineation of epitrochlear, axillary, and supraclavicular nodes in a patient injected into the web spaces of the hand with 111In-labeled monoclonal antibody 9.2.27. Uptake in the liver and spleen are also noted. **B:** A similar injection with the same antibody in the web spaces of the feet is presented, with demonstration of inguinal, iliac, and para-aortic nodes. This antibody was found to stain normal nodal tissue weakly. It was initially raised against a high–molecular-weight antigen on melanoma.

vic ultrasound in patients with carcinoma of the cervix, the sensitivity was 79%, 34%, and 19%, and the specificity was 73%, 96%, and 99%, respectively, for nodal disease (42). CT has high specificity with good negative predictive value in the assessment of metastatic nodal disease.

Magnetic Resonance Imaging

Magnetic resonance imaging is increasingly being evaluated for staging of malignant diseases. Significant differences between tumor tissues in vitro have been demonstrated, and subsequently benign and malignant tissues in vivo have been differentiated (43). Increased T1 values in tumor-bearing nodes (0.47 to 0.03 second) compared with lesser values for benign nodes (0.26 to 0.007 second) were noted in a study of breast carcinoma (44). A scan done in a patient who had previously undergone left nodal dissection is shown in Fig. 5. Delineation of small lymph nodes in the right groin was noted. These were subsequently found to be free of disease at dissection. The expected resolution of MRI techniques is approximately 0.5 to 1 cm. Very small deposits of tumor, less than 10 to 100 million cells (0.01 to 0.1 cm), are

unlikely to be detected. Technical modifications and the use of gadolinium-enhanced imaging have been proposed as measures to improve the diagnostic yield. Contrast-enhanced, fat-suppressed, T1-weighted images are the optimal sequences for evaluation, with CT-defined criteria as the basis for diagnosis of metastatic lymph nodal disease (45). On T2-weighted images, a nonhomogeneous signal intensity from within the node is suggestive of nodal metastases. In a comparative study of CT versus MRI for evaluation of cervical nodes (46), the sensitivity of identifying central necrosis was 83% to 100% by CT, versus 60% to 67% by MRI. There was disagreement in 10% to 38% of cases between CT and MRI for extracapsular disease, with MRI being less sensitive. Gadolinium enhancement did not increase the accuracy of detecting extracapsular spread. Although MRI has some advantages in the evaluation of primary head and neck and base-of-skull tumors, its efficacy in the evaluation of metastatic lymphatic disease is unclear and evolving.

Currently, CT is the preferred method of evaluation of lymph node metastases, although it is conceivable that modification in techniques and thinner (3 to 5 mm) sections in MRI may redefine the role of these imaging modalities.

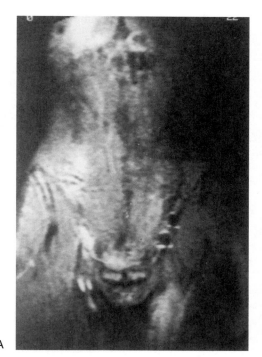 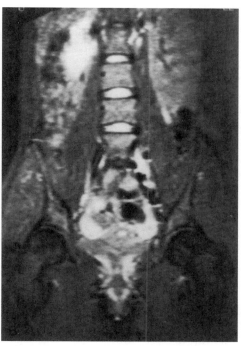

A   B

FIG. 5. Magnetic resonance imaging study in a patient with melanoma. A T1-100 study (inversion recovery time, 100 seconds) is shown in a patient who had a previous left superficial and deep nodal dissection. **A:** Three to four small lymph nodes in the superficial inguinal nodal area on the right and some lymphedema in the medial thigh on the left are noted. **B:** A deeper section from the same patient demonstrating the ovaries, iliac nodes on the right, and some clip artifact from previous dissection on the left.

Positron Emission Tomography

Positron emission tomography (PET) is a method of imaging that uses a compound labeled with a positron-emitting isotope that is incorporated into tissues during a biochemical process in the organs and tissues. PET imaging provides more of a metabolic or a functional image based on the tissue physiology, in contrast to the anatomic image obtained in a CT or MRI scan. The most widely used radiopharmaceutical for PET imaging is 2-deoxy-2-[18F] fluoro-D-glucose (FDG). FDG enters the cells, is phosphorylated, and competes with glucose for use in the tissue. Tumors have an enhanced rate of glucose metabolism and thus "light up" on a PET scan. The sensitivity and specificity of PET scanning is as high as 95% to 100% (22).

Endoscopic Ultrasonography

The advent of endoscopic ultrasonography (EUS) has revolutionized the management strategy in a number of gastrointestinal malignancies. The high resolution facilitates accurate assessment of the depth of infiltration and, with increasing familiarity, there is a distinct trend toward an accurate assessment of regional nodal disease (47–50). EUS can image a node as small as 3 mm, in contrast to the 1- to 2-cm size detectable by CT scan. A round or oval lymph node with a hypoechoic pattern and clearly demarcated boundaries is likely to harbor malignancy, in contrast to a benign node, which is bean shaped and has a hyperechoic pattern with blurred margins (51). The accuracy of EUS for staging of regional nodal disease depends not only on the site, but is influenced by a distinct learning curve. The best results have been reported in the staging of esophageal and rectal cancers (48,50). EUS also appears to be more accurate in determining the nodal status compared with CT scan (accuracy: 80% to 87% EUS vs. 57% to 72% CT) (52,53). It is now recommended as part of the preoperative staging of such patients, particularly in the setting of neoadjuvant studies. EUS has also been used in the staging of pancreatic (54), bile duct (55), and gallbladder cancers with encouraging results. Limitations to EUS are the presence of a stenosing lesion and inflammatory reactions around the site of interest. EUS has an accuracy of 70% to 80%, with a specificity ranging from 45% to 60%. The accuracy, sensitivity, and specificity of EUS in detecting metastatic nodal disease are tabulated in Table 1.

TABLE 1. *Sensitivity and specificity of endoscopic ultrasonography for nodal disease*

	Accuracy (%)	Sensitivity (%)	Specificity (%)
Esophageal tumors	82%	94%	56%
Gastric tumors	66%	86%	47%
Rectal tumors	70%	94%	55%

Compiled from references 47–53.

Fine-Needle Aspiration Biopsy

Fine-needle aspiration biopsy (FNAB) has become a widely used diagnostic tool. It is a rapid, accurate, and cost-effective method for the evaluation of mass lesions. It helps with the proper triage and planning for evaluation and therapy. In a large study of FNABs of lymph nodes on 1103 patients (56), 89% of aspirates were satisfactory for interpretation. The false-positive rate was 0.9%, with a diagnostic accuracy of 96% to 100% in solid organ malignancies, whereas the accuracy dropped to 72% in lymphomas and leukemias, accounting for the dominant share of false negatives (56,57). The major pitfalls in the accurate FNAB diagnosis are misinterpretation of reactive histiocytes as tumor, underdiagnosis of low-grade non-Hodgkin's lymphomas, and in Hodgkin's disease. Addition of flow cytometry and immunocytochemistry in the diagnosis of hematologic malignances has significantly improved the diagnostic ability (58,59). The scope of FNAB is rapidly expanding, with applications for intrathoracic and intra-abdominal lymph nodal lesions under imaging- (CT and ultrasonography), laparoscopy-, and EUS-guided approaches (47,54,60).

GENERAL PRINCIPLES

The incidence of nodal disease at presentation in various malignancies is listed in Table 2. Tumors have been

TABLE 2. *Human solid tumors with propensity to metastasize to lymph nodes*

Tumor type	Nodal disease at presentation (%)
High frequency (35%)	
Esophageal carcinoma	59
Gastric carcinoma	52
Pancreatic carcinoma	50
Lung cancer	50
Cancer of the vulva	40
Head and neck carcinoma	40
Testicular carcinoma	40
Breast carcinoma	38
Cancer of the penis	35
Moderate frequency (10%–35%)	
Colorectal carcinoma	31
Prostate carcinoma	31
Ovarian carcinoma	30
Renal carcinoma	22
Melanoma	20
Cancer of the endometrium	11
Low frequency (<10%)	
Carcinoma of the uterine cervix	8
Osteosarcoma	6
Thyroid carcinoma	5
Sarcomas, soft tissue	3
Hepatoma	1

grouped into those with a high incidence of nodal disease at presentation, those with moderate risk of nodal disease at presentation, and those with rare nodal disease at presentation.

The principles of lymphatic dissection of subcutaneous nodes and those associated with organs other than the skin include (1) gentle handling of tissue and ligation of transected tissues, (2) en bloc dissection to include adjacent structures harboring nodes, (3) adequate drainage, and (4) postoperative rehabilitation. The gentle handling of tissue and ligation of transected tissue to prevent the efflux of lymph are especially important because the consequences of lymphatic interruption include development of lymph fistulas and seromas. The lymphatics often course alongside venous or arterial vessels. En bloc dissection of veins, such as the internal jugular vein in the neck during a radical neck procedure or the femoral vein in the groin during an inguinal dissection, is frequently recommended to ensure complete nodal removal. Resection of muscle, so that identification and dissection of nodes lying below can be successfully carried out, is often included. This is recommended in the setting of axillary dissection, in which the pectoralis minor is frequently removed, and in neck dissection, in which the sternocleidomastoid and omohyoid muscles are removed. Drainage catheters are routinely inserted so that accumulated blood and lymph may be promptly evacuated and coaptation of skin and subcutaneous tissues can occur with adherence and healing. Drainage is not routinely carried out in lymph node dissections performed within the abdominal or thoracic cavities because of the normal clearance mechanisms for lymph fluid in those settings. It has, however, been recommended in pelvic lymph node dissection (61). Coverage of vessels using transposed vascularized muscle pedicles such as the sartorius muscle in the groin or dermal grafts in the neck is frequently performed. Each of four standard nodal dissections are depicted in Figs. 6 through 9.

The role of early mobilization in nodal dissection has been suggested to prevent stiffness and disuse atrophy. A randomized study evaluating early motion begun while drainage catheters were still in place was carried out at the NCI (62) in 40 patients undergoing axillary dissections for melanoma and breast carcinoma. Patients who received early motion had more total wound drainage, more days of drainage, and later postoperative days of discharge than patients who had motion started on day 7. Wound complications, including infection and small areas of skin breakdown, occurred more frequently in the early group, with no significant difference identified in the percentage of patients achieving functional range of motion. It thus appeared that the early institution of flexion and abduction exercises after axillary dissection had a deleterious effect on wound healing and drainage. This was thought likely to be the case for patients undergoing inguinal dissection as well, although this has not been formally addressed. Rehabilitation medicine consultation and initiation of physical therapy after drainage catheter removal are recommended (63,64).

Suture obliteration of the dead space (65) or injection of tetracycline into a seroma to obliterate this space have been suggested by some authors (66). In an unpublished series of patients, we have not seen a significant improvement in patients treated with tetracycline injected into the axillary space, and we have seen problems associated with subsequent restricted shoulder motion.

The incidence of complications after lymph node dissection may be related to whether a nodal dissection was prophylactic or therapeutic. A marked excess of complications in patients undergoing therapeutic nodal dissection for melanoma has been reported (67). This presumably was related to the larger amount of disease within the nodes of patients undergoing therapeutic nodal dissection as well as to long-standing lymphatic obstruction. Serum collections, infections, skin necrosis, and cellulitis occurred almost twice as frequently in patients undergoing therapeutic nodal dissection. Because only 20% of patients are found to have positive nodal disease at the time of prophylactic nodal dissection, it seems that the somewhat greater incidence of complications in the therapeutic group is outweighed by the advantages associated with the fact that 80% of patients never require therapeutic nodal dissection. Formation of lymphoceles (68) after pelvic lymphadenectomy for gynecologic or urologic procedures (originally observed in 14% to 37% of patients) is well recognized, and its incidence has been decreased by drainage of the retroperitoneum and frequent ligation of interrupted lymph vessels (61). The current reported incidence is approximately 4% to 10%. Prevention of lymphedema in extremities by emphasizing exercise, compression garments as necessary, and prevention or early treatment of infection (69) has been successful. The incidence of lymph stasis and edema after surgery for cancer of the breast has been markedly decreased since the routine use of the radical mastectomy was abandoned.

Since the mid-1960s, frequent questions have been raised as to the therapeutic role of nodal dissection. Lymph nodes were seen as serving as an effective barrier to further migration of tumor cells and as providing an important immunologic function regarding tumor antigen presentation and generation of an immunologic response. This has been difficult to demonstrate in experimental animals, and in fact in some models anergy in regional nodes has been identified when systemic tumor immunity persists (70). It is clear that immunodepression occurs after major surgery (71), but there has been no evidence from human studies that it plays an important role in subsequent manifestations of disease.

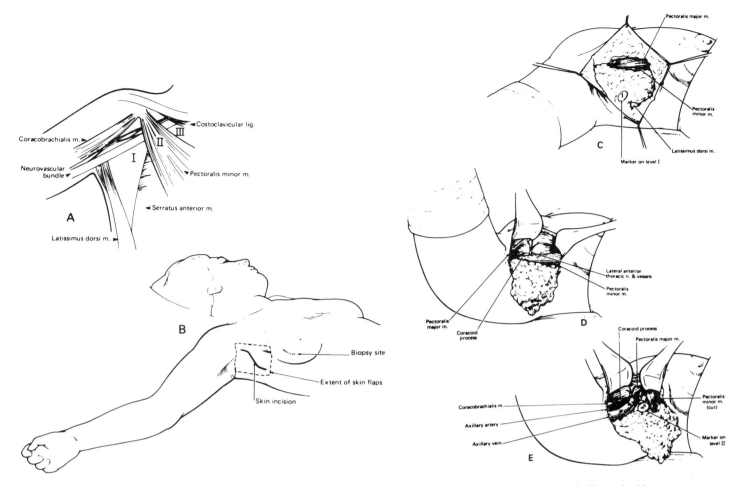

FIG. 6. Surgical procedure of complete axillary dissection. **A:** The anatomic borders are indicated with the level of node dissections indicated: I, nodes lateral to pectoralis minor; II, nodes under pectoralis minor; and III, nodes medial to pectoralis minor. **B:** The skin incision and extent of skin flaps are shown. This procedure removes the entire axillary fat pad and nodes, removes a portion of the pectoralis minor **(C)** and associated (Rotter's) nodes, divides the intercostobrachial nerve (causing some numbness of the inner upper aspect of the arm), and divides the medial pectoral nerve, which causes some flattening of the lateral pectoralis major muscle. **D:** The nerves to the serratus anterior (long thoracic nerve) and the latissimus dorsi (thoracodorsal nerve) are spared. **E:** Markers can be placed to identify level of nodes dissected. Drainage catheters are inserted routinely, and motion of the shoulder is resumed after their removal.

RANDOMIZED STUDIES EVALUATING THE ROLE OF PROPHYLACTIC NODAL DISSECTION

Most of the information reviewed in the following comes from nonrandomized, retrospective reviews of patients with procedures designed to encompass regional nodal disease. Few well conducted randomized trials have been performed to determine whether prophylactic resection of regional lymph nodes, as opposed to dissection of nodes at a time after subsequent appearance, leads to increased patient survival. The role of prophylactic nodal dissection has been supported largely by retrospective data.

The most compelling results addressing the question of prophylactic nodal dissection are from two studies: one

conducted by the World Health Organization (WHO) (72) and the other by the Mayo Clinic (73) in the setting of stage I melanoma. In these two studies, patients were randomized either to receive prophylactic nodal dissection concurrently with wide excision of the primary or to undergo dissection after nodal disease was apparent. In the WHO study, which involved 17 separate collaborating centers, a total of 553 stage I patients were analyzed. Of these, 267 patients underwent wide excision and immediate nodal dissection, and 286 had wide excision but had nodal dissection only if clinically positive nodes were detected. There was no difference in the survival curves of the two treatment groups. There was no difference in survival when sex or level (level III vs. level IV) of the

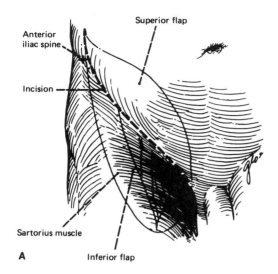

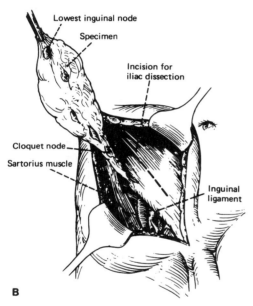

FIG. 7. Technique of superficial inguinal nodal dissection. An oblique incision is made from the anterior superior iliac spine to just lateral to the pelvic tubercle and below the inguinal crease **(A)**. Skin flaps are raised superiorly and inferiorly to include the lymph nodes lying within the femoral canal. The borders of the dissection are the sartorius laterally, the adductor magnus medially, the inguinal ligament superiorly, and a distance of approximately 15 cm inferiorly. The saphenous vein is ligated twice: once at the inferior margin and again at its confluence with the femoral vein at the fossa ovalis. The sartorius is taken off its origin from the iliac spine and transposed to cover the femoral vessels by suturing it to the inguinal ligament. This protects the exposed vessels in the event of skin flap necrosis. A deep dissection along the external iliac vessels and the obturator region may be performed if the highest (Cloquet's) node in the femoral canal is clinically positive **(B)**. This may be performed by incising the inguinal ligament and continuing the dissection superiorly. Alternatively, a separate midline incision can be performed to dissect these nodes, which leads to a lower incidence of lower extremity edema and wound complications.

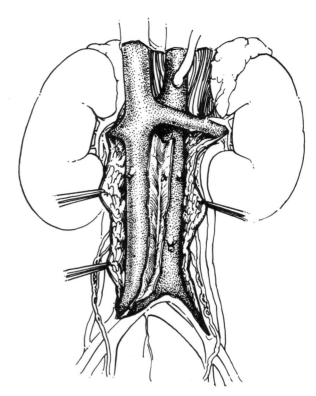

FIG. 8. Technique of retroperitoneal nodal dissection. A suprarenalhilar dissection can be performed by removing all tissue from the superior mesenteric artery (exposed by elevating the pancreas) and the crus of the diaphragm extending to both adrenals and along the renal arteries to the aorta. Infrahilar aortocaval dissection removes the anterior adventitia over the vena cava and aorta and divides the left (on the renal vein) and right (on the cava) ovarian or testicular veins as well as each lumbar vessel to facilitate en bloc removal of posterolateral nodal tissue. Adrenal arterial and venous branches entering the dissected tissue are routinely sacrificed without compromise of these highly vascular structures. The iliac extensions of this dissection proceed along the iliac vessels for several centimeters beyond the bifurcation of the hypogastric artery. Splanchnic nerves along the course of the dissection are routinely sacrificed, and all nodal tissue between both psoas muscles is removed en bloc.

primary lesion was separately analyzed in these groups. This trial is criticized for the preponderance of low-risk patients (women with extremity lesions) and the fact that these groups were not stratified for depth of infiltration and ulceration, factors that had significant impact on the survival.

The study conducted at the Mayo Clinic, with 171 patients randomized to one of three treatment arms, including follow-up only (n = 62), immediate dissection (n = 54), and dissection delayed until 30 days after removal of the primary lesion by wide local excision (n = 55), demonstrated no significant differences. The 5-year survival rate was 85% when the nodes were undissected, 85% when the nodes were removed at the time of the pri-

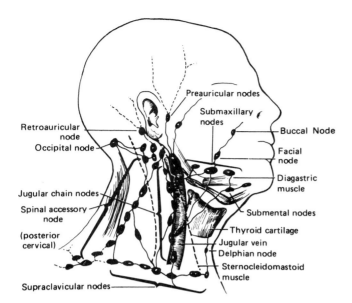

FIG. 9. Nodes encompassed in a neck dissection. A radical neck dissection may be performed through a variety of incisions that either lie in skin creases or parallel the course of the sternocleidomastoid muscle. All nodes shown are routinely removed except for the retroauricular, preauricular, facial, and buccal nodes. The spinal accessory nerve (innervating the trapezius, sternocleidomastoid, and omohyoid muscles) and the jugular vein are included with the operative specimen, but may be spared in a modified procedure. The external jugular vein, the submandibular gland, and the superficial and deep cervical fascia with their enclosed lymph nodes are routinely removed during the dissection. Great care is taken to spare the phrenic nerve, hypoglossal nerve, and vagus nerve with its associated recurrent laryngeal branch. The exposed carotid artery can be covered with a dermal graft. The superficial lobe of the parotid gland along with its nodes is often included, especially in patients with melanoma, and great care is required to protect the branches of the facial nerve, including the marginal mandibular branches that course over the mandible.

mary dissection, and 91% when operation for removal of nodes was delayed until 30 days after the initial wide local excision. They confirmed that survival and disease-free survival were related to thickness of the lesion. Thus, two well controlled studies demonstrated no advantage to prophylactic nodal dissection in melanoma. Two randomized trials, the Intergroup Melanoma Trial and the WHO trial assessing the role of prophylactic nodal dissection in patients with intermediate-thickness melanoma, have completed accrual and their results are awaited.

A similar study evaluated epidermoid carcinoma of the oral cavity and the role of elective nodal dissection (74). There appeared to be no benefit to immediate excision compared with delayed excision in a total of 75 patients evaluated. There was no difference in survival between the two groups. A total of 19 of 36 of the undissected group subsequently underwent nodal dissection for clinical node positivity. There was no difference in survival between

this group and the group undergoing immediate excision with occult positive nodes.

Radical mastectomy, which includes the pectoralis major and minor muscles as well as the axillary nodes, compared with two less extensive surgical procedures, was studied by Fisher and colleagues in the National Surgical Adjuvant Breast Project (NSABP) (75). The two other treatment groups included total (simple) mastectomy with regional irradiation (regardless of whether nodes were positive) and total mastectomy with axillary dissection performed only if nodes became positive. There were no differences in survival (38% at 10 years) in these three treatment groups, again demonstrating no apparent advantage to prophylactic nodal dissection.

A somewhat different question was asked in the study conducted by Javadpour and colleagues from the NCI (76) involving an evaluation of resection of bulky retroperitoneal nodal disease or extra-abdominal metastatic disease in the setting of testicular carcinoma. This tumor is unique in that it can be treated effectively by chemotherapy, unlike most solid tumors. This group randomized patients with bulky stage III disease to either cytoreductive surgery with chemotherapy or chemotherapy alone. It demonstrated no improvement in survival or overall response rate in individuals who underwent debulking.

Four prospective, randomized studies (77–80) comparing the extent of lymphadenectomy have been reported in the Western literature. No significant survival differences among the groups are evident in the two small series (77,78), whereas survival data are not yet mature in the two European trials. Notably, all trials document a significantly higher incidence of complications and mortality after extended resections.

Thus, for a variety of tumors (summarized in Table 3), there appears to be no benefit to prophylactic nodal dissection, and in a disease for which there is effective chemotherapy, there appears to be no role for debulking. Studies evaluating the role of nodal dissection in other diseases have yet to be performed. The following review attempts to determine the apparent benefit of either prophylactic or therapeutic nodal dissection in a number of solid tumors based primarily on retrospective reviews.

RESULTS OF NODAL DISSECTIONS IN SPECIFIC TUMORS

Cutaneous Melanoma

A number of factors with prognostic importance have been defined that relate to the outcome of patients with melanoma. Perhaps one of the most ominous findings in these patients is regional nodal disease, and this finding has prompted prophylactic nodal dissection in patients presenting without palpable nodes, with the rationale that dissection could prevent subsequent systemic spread.

TABLE 3. *Prospective, randomized studies evaluating the role of prophylactic nodal dissection and alternative therapies*

Tumor	Author	Surgical intent	No. of patients	Evidence for prophylactic nodal dissection	Comments
Melanoma, extremity	Sim et al. (73)	Early vs. late (30 days) prophylactic vs. therapeutic dissection	171	No	Three-arm study, immediate dissection, no dissection or delayed 30 days from excision of primary; no significant differences in survival
Melanoma, extremity	Veronesi et al./ WHO (72)	Prophylactic vs. therapeutic dissection	553	No	No benefit of immediate vs. delayed excision with 7–13 years of follow-up; subgroup analysis for patients (male–female; level III–level IV; <3.5 mm–3.5 mm) also without benefit of immediate node resection
Epidermoid carcinoma of oral cavity involvement	Vandenbrouck et al. (74)	Prophylactic vs. therapeutic neck dissection	75	No	50% of elective group had tumor in nodes; 14/36 of the second group of patients underwent dissection with a 47% rate; there was no difference in survival
Breast carcinoma	Fisher et al./ NSABP (75)	Radical mastectomy vs. total mastectomy plus regional irradiation vs. total mastectomy without irradiation plus subsequent dissection of nodes when clinically positive nodes	1655	No	Survival in all groups approximately 38% at 10 years; 65/365(17.8%) of patients without immmediate dissection of subsequently developed positive nodes
Gastric carcinoma	Dent et al. (77) Robertson et al. (78)	Standard lymphadenectomy D_1 vs. extended lymphadenectomy D_2/D_3	100	No	See Table 11
Lung cancer	Izbicki et al. (148)	Conventional lymphadenectomy vs. systematic mediastinal lymphadenectomy	182	No	See Table 7

WHO, World Health Organization; NSABP, National Surgical Adjuvant Breast Project.

This has been evaluated in extremity melanomas in the two randomized studies noted earlier conducted by the WHO (72) and the Mayo Clinic (73). Dissection delayed until appearance of clinically positive disease had no adverse impact on survival. The role of prophylactic nodal dissection as well as that of therapeutic nodal dissection also has been considered in a number of retrospective reviews. The estimated 5-year survival rate in patients with clinical stage II disease who undergo resection is approximately 20%, implying that some patients with nodal disease may be cured. Further follow-up of these patients, however, indicates that only 12% are alive at 10 years and 9% at 15 years (81–85). Similarly poor prognosis correlates not only with the presence of nodes but with the number of histolologically positive nodes. Balch et al. (86) in their large series demonstrated a 10-year survival of 40%, 18%, and 9% with one, two to four, and more than five nodes involved, respectively ($P <$ 0.001). Surprisingly, patients with occult primary melanomas who present with stage II disease do just as well as patients with known primaries if their nodal disease is resected (87). Nodal dissection for melanoma when clinically apparent nodes exist without evidence of systemic spread represents rational therapy. It not only offers the patient a 10% to 30% chance of 5-year survival and a 10% to 20% chance of 10-year survival, but is a significant palliative procedure that arrests the disabling effects of local tumor growth in anatomically difficult areas. The incidence of regional lymph node micrometastases varied with Clark's level in a combined series of 839 patients. Only 4% of patients with level II melanoma, 16% with level III, 35% with level IV, and 49% with level V presented with micrometastatic occult disease. Similarly, the number of patients who would have occult nodal disease can be defined by Breslow thickness. Virtually no patients have nodal metastases with a lesion <1.76 mm thick; 6% to 28% have positive nodes with lesions up to 2 mm in size; 14% to 30% have nodal positivity with lesions 2 to 3 mm; 12% to 39% have nodal metastases with lesions 3 to 4 mm; and approximately 40% to 50% of patients have nodal disease with lesions >1 mm in depth. Whether patients presented with synchronous or metachronous clinically positive nodes, the survival ranged between 30% and 40% at 5 years (88).

The role of prophylactic nodal dissection continues to be heavily debated for extremity melanoma (89–93). Proponents of prophylactic nodal dissection argue that a 15% to 20% increase in the 5-year survival can be defined for patients undergoing prophylactic nodal dissection whose lesions are in the approximate range of 2 to 4 mm. The role of prophylactic nodal dissection in patients with truncal melanoma remains unclear because no prospective trial has evaluated this group of patients, and the routes of lymphatic spread are difficult to define (94,95). Morton and colleagues (96) have demonstrated that in patients with melanoma, disease progression is in an orderly pattern—that is, the first echelon of lymph nodes, the sentinel nodes draining the primary melanoma, are the first and most likely to harbor a micrometastatic focus. The incidence of occult micrometastases in the sentinel node ranges from 18% to 20% in melanomas of >1.5 mm thickness. There is an additional 15% of micrometastases detectable by immunohistochemical staining with antibodies to S-100 and HMB-45 in specimens considered to be negative by conventional histologic techniques. The sentinel node was the only site of micrometastases in 96% of cases. If the sentinel nodes are negative, there is only a 1% possibility of a nonsentinel node harboring a malignancy (24,96). The selective node dissection based on the sentinel node status thus selects patients with occult metastatic disease who may benefit from nodal excision, and avoids nodal dissection in the node negative group. Currently, the role of selective lymph node dissection is being evaluated in a multicenter, prospective, randomized trial in the treatment of stage I and II melanomas.

Recently, alpha-interferon (alpha-IFN) has been approved by the U.S. Food and Drug Administration to be used as an adjuvant in patients with melanoma based on the evidence provided by the Eastern Cooperative Oncology Group (ECOG) 1684 study (97). The ECOG trial demonstrated a significant benefit of adjuvant alpha-IFN in the disease-free and overall survival in patients with high-risk melanoma. Most patients in this study had either recurrent regional nodal disease or clinical stage II disease (ie, palpable regional lymph nodes), and its validity for the group with micrometastatic disease needs to be determined.

Evidence to support the use of prophylactic nodal dissection in malignant melanoma of the head and neck is scant. The general consensus from multiple studies (98–103) is that finding pathologically positive nodes at either therapeutic or prophylactic nodal dissection carries a poor prognosis, and that clear benefit from elective nodal dissection at the time of occult nodal disease is difficult to demonstrate. In a series of patients reported from the New York University Medical Center by Roses and colleagues (99), systemic disease developed in 29 of 30 patients with positive nodes, most of whom had died of disease by the time of the report. Similarly, patients with histologically negative nodes did well, with 93% alive at 5 years without evidence of recurrent disease. These authors concluded that a limited dissection of nodes draining the region of the primary was sufficient. If these nodes were positive, a full nodal dissection could be considered. In a series of 100 patients reported from the Mayo Clinic (98), a 5-year survival rate of approximately 50% in patients with two or fewer positive nodes was noted. This contrasted with a 5-year survival rate of 15% in those with three or more positive nodes. A report from M. D. Anderson Hospital and Tumor Institute analyzed the results of modified neck dissection in patients with cutaneous melanoma of the head and neck (100). It estimated that only 4% of the patients would have possibly benefited from a more extensive (radical neck) dissection. Most patients in whom recurrent disease in the neck subsequently developed also had distant metastases. It appears on balance that few patients with stage I head and neck melanoma would benefit from prophylactic nodal dissection. A prospective, randomized study would be necessary to resolve this question. In patients with clinically apparent nodal disease, only a small subgroup benefits from dissection.

Cancer of the Head and Neck

Oropharyngeal Carcinoma

There are approximately 150 to 350 lymph nodes in the region above the clavicles, representing approximately one third of the total lymph nodes in the body. The risk of nodal metastasis is clearly related to the differentiation and size of the tumor, with more poorly differentiated or larger tumors metastasizing to nodes more frequently. Distant metastases are distinctly rare and occur in only approximately 10% of patients with head and neck squamous cell carcinomas. Control of regional nodal disease as well as the primary tumor is therefore of great importance. The incidence of lymph node metastases at presentation varies according to site and size of the primary tumor. Oral cavity tumors have low incidence of positive nodes (2% to 25%), whereas tumors of the nasopharynx, tonsillar fossa, base of tongue, and hypopharynx have a higher propensity for nodal metastases (60% to 90%) (104). As many as 40% of patients have demonstrable nodal disease at the time of prophylactic nodal dissection. Among patients who have no neck treatment and are initially clinically disease free, as many as one fourth to one half subsequently have nodal disease. Lesions in certain areas, such as the floor of mouth, base of tongue, soft palate, hypopharynx, and supraglottic larynx, have a high incidence of bilateral nodal metastases.

Lymph node involvement is a poor prognostic indicator, with survival decreasing by at least 50% compared with node-negative disease (105). The outcome in node-positive patients is also influenced by the number of lymph nodes involved (106), presence of extracapsular spread (107) and the level of nodal involvement (108) in the neck. The 5-year survival rate in node-negative patients is 75% and decreases proportionally to 50%, 30%, and 13% with involvement of one, two to three, and more than three nodes, respectively (109).

It is beyond the scope of this chapter to discuss the individual areas of the head and neck, the incidence of nodal metastases, and whether irradiation or surgical treatment of these nodes is more advantageous. The results and evidence of failure in the neck of irradiation, surgery, or combined treatment in a variety of head and neck tumors are presented in Table 4.

In a study of prophylactic nodal dissection in 75 patients with epidermoid carcinoma of the oral cavity, there was no benefit of early nodal dissection over procedures performed when disease in the neck became clinically apparent (74). In the treatment of N0 disease, selective neck dissections are becoming increasingly popular (eg, supraomohyoid neck dissection for oral cavity tumors or a lateral neck dissection for laryngeal and pharyngeal tumors). The role of both surgery and radiation therapy in treating clinically negative or microscopically positive neck lymph nodes continues to be defined (104). It is clear that both radiation therapy and surgery are capable of preventing neck nodal failure and are associated with a long disease-free interval or cure. In patients with N1 disease, nodal dissection that is either selective (for those patients with low-volume disease) or a modified radical neck dissection are equally effective in terms of local control and overall survival. Adjuvant radiation therapy is routinely recommended for a T3 or T4 primary tumor, more than three involved nodes, and in the presence of extracapsular spread (107,110). Combined adjuvant chemoradiation therapy in various combinations has been evaluated and has tremendous potential. In a

TABLE 4. *Failure of initial ipsilateral neck treatment[a]*

Treatment type	Failures with no treatment (%)	Failures with treatment		Failures by stage (%)				
		Partial	Complete	N1	N2A	N2B	N3A	N3B
Irradiation		15	2	15	27	27	38	34
Surgery	55 (16/29)	35	7	11	8	23	42	41
Combined		20	0	0	0	0	23	25

[a]Study of 596 patients with carcinoma of the tonsillar fossa, base of tongue, supraglottic larynx, or hypopharynx, M. D. Anderson Hospital, Houston, Texas, 1948–1967.

N1, single clinically positive homolateral node ≤3 cm in diameter; N2, single clinically positive homolateral node >6 cm in diameter; N2A, single clinically positive homolateral node >3 cm but <6 cm; N2B, multiple clinically positive homolateral nodes, none >6 cm; N3A, clinically positive homolateral nodes, one >6 cm in diameter; N3B, bilateral clinically positive nodes; N3C, contralateral positive nodes only.

Adapted from Barkely HT Jr, Fletcher GH, Jesse RH, et al.. Management of cervical lymph node metastases in squamous cell carcinoma of the tonsillar fossa, base of tongue, supraglottic larynx, and hypopharynx. *Am J Surg* 1972;124:462–467.

prospective, randomized trial (111) of chemotherapy (cisplatinum and 5-fluorouracil) and radiation in an adjuvant setting, the combined arm had a significantly better response rate (42% vs. 22%) and overall survival (median: 16.5 vs. 11.7 months). In patients with advanced locoregional disease, neoadjuvant chemoradiation therapy has been proposed to achieve reduction in tumor size to facilitate surgical excision of the tumor and eventually improve local control and prevent distant metastatic disease. Four randomized, controlled trials (112–115) for the evaluation of neoadjuvant chemoradiation followed by surgery have not demonstrated differences in the survival or local control rates compared with the standard approaches, although a consistent reduction in distant metastasis was observed in all trials.

In summary, surgery has a clearly defined role in the treatment of the patient with occult or palpable nodal disease in the neck in patients with head and neck cancers. Five-year survival rates in patients undergoing combined treatment with irradiation and surgery can often approach 60% to 70%, even in those presenting with limited nodal metastatic disease.

Thyroid Cancer

The lymphatic drainage of the thyroid accompanies the venous drainage and arterial blood supply. Drainage from the gland is into the deep cervical nodes, supraclavicular nodes, and pretracheal and prelaryngeal nodes. Nodal disease, when present in patients with papillary or papillary/follicular thyroid carcinoma, is often localized and does not necessarily portend systemic disease (116). The prognostic significance of nodal status in thyroid cancers is controversial (117). In multivariate analyses of prognostic determinants, nodal status has not been found to have any influence on long-term survival (118–121). In a retrospective, matched-pair analysis (patient groups matched for all prognostic variables except for the nodal status) to analyze the influence of nodal status on survival, there was no difference in survival between the N0 and N1 patients. In patients 45 years of age and older, however, the node-positive group had a significantly higher recurrence rate ($P = 0.008$), and in an elderly population, this difference translated into a lower survival rate at 20 years (79% vs. 90%; $P = 0.05$) (122). The adverse prognostic influence of nodal status in elderly patients has also been shown in other studies (123,124). In younger patients, nodal disease is a good prognostic factor, with surprisingly better survival in node-positive patients. Management of nodal disease, especially in the older high-risk group, by either surgical extirpation or radioiodine ablation, needs to be evaluated further in terms of benefit in local control or survival. Medullary carcinoma of the thyroid should be considered different, with approximately 40% to 50% of the patients present-

ing with nodal metastatic disease (125,126). These patients should undergo radical central neck dissection if there is clinically apparent nodal disease on palpation or biopsy and there is no evidence of systemic spread.

Breast Carcinoma

The history of nodal resection in conjunction with operative removal of a tumorous breast is representative of the changing philosophy toward the management of patients with solid malignant tumors. The initial Halstedian principles of wide, in-continuity en bloc dissection encompassing regional lymph nodes, which was applied to the treatment of carcinoma of the breast at the turn of the 20th century, was based on the belief that cancer spread in a stepwise fashion. More recently, the demonstration that comparable results could be obtained in patients subjected to nodal dissections at the time of detection of clinical nodal positivity gave credence to the belief that the appearance of nodal metastatic disease reflected the underlying biology of the host–tumor interaction and systemic spread (75). Most recently, nodal dissection has been considered to be a diagnostic and staging procedure, although controversy continues to exist about the role of complete axillary nodal dissection versus simple sampling.

The accuracy of physical examination in predicting histologic involvement of axillary nodes is fairly constant in a number of series (127). There is a 24% to 29% rate of false-positive findings and a 27% to 32% rate of false-negative findings. The incidence of nodal positivity is directly related to tumor size, and the 10-year survival rate is clearly better in patients with histologically negative nodes (72% to 76%) than in patients with histologically positive nodes (24% to 48%). Those with only one to three positive nodes can expect a 35% 10-year survival arte, compared with those with more than four positive nodes, who have an approximate 15% survival rate. Internal mammary node involvement, an area clearly not treated by standard nodal dissection, varies from 13% to 33%, depending on whether the axilla is involved and which quadrant contains the primary tumor.

Clearly, axillary dissection provides data regarding lymph nodal status that have important prognostic value and therapeutic influence. Nevertheless, the extent of nodal dissection is still controversial (ie, complete axillary dissection vs. nodal sampling). The survival rate in patients undergoing nodal dissection in NSABP-sponsored protocols was independent of the number of nodes examined (60% to 65% overall survival), as shown in Table 5, and correlated with the presence of positive nodes (128). An argument could be made that some patients were not adequately "staged," but even if this were the case, it is not clear that this affects overall survival (128,129). In a review of complete axillary dissec-

TABLE 5. *Five-year survival rate according to number of nodes examined*

Number of nodes examined	5-year survival (%)				
	All patients (N)	Negative nodes	Positive nodes	1–3 Positive nodes	>4 Positive nodes
1–5	60 (70)	74	46	44	50
6–10	162 (297)	76	44	58	27
11–15	65 (400)	77	52	68	34
16–20	61 (392)	79	44	55	32
21–25	64 (269)	81	48	68	35
26–30	65 (137)	76	56	67	46
≥30	61 (154)	81	48	76	35

Fisher B, Wolmark N, Bauer M, et al. The accuracy of clinical nodal staging and of limited axillary dissection as a determinant of histologic nodal status in carcinoma of the breast. *Surg Gynecol Obstet* 1981;152:765–772.

tion conducted at the National Institutes of Health (129), axillary levels (I, II, and III) were determined in relation to the pectoralis minor (lateral, inferior, and medial, respectively). It was apparent that there was a 29% incidence of skip metastases to levels II or III with negative nodes in level I, but only a 3% incidence of level III skip metastases (level I and II negative). An adequate staging of the axilla mandates a level I and II dissection, which clearly may not be consistently achieved with a low axillary nodal sampling.

Critical questions regarding survival after prophylactic or therapeutic nodal dissection have been addressed in the studies conducted by Fisher and colleagues in the NSABP (75). In a number of series, 30% to 40% of women with breast cancer have had occult nodal metastatic disease at presentation. If no nodes are removed, on the basis of Fisher and colleagues' studies, the axillary recurrence rate is only approximately half of this. The survival rate of patients who are initially clinically node negative but do not have axillary treatment or subsequently undergo an axillary dissection for clinically apparent nodal disease is identical to that of patients who undergo dissection at the time of presentation of their pri-

mary breast carcinoma (Table 6). The NSABP B-04 study has been criticized because about one third of patients in the total mastectomy control group had a limited axillary clearance, which may have influenced the outcome in that group (130). Although most studies (131,132) suggest no survival advantage of axillary dissection over no therapy or radiation therapy, there is a some evidence that it provides better local control in the axilla (132–134). At most institutions, patients with clinically apparent positive axillary nodes are advised to undergo axillary dissection to arrest progressive axillary growth of tumor and possibly to obtain cure. Cases of clinically apparent nodal metastases are significantly palliated by nodal dissection, and the patients are provided a 20% to 30% opportunity for long-term survival.

Only a few studies comment on the natural history of untreated nodal metastatic disease. A report by Baum and Coyle (135) from Cardiff, Wales, described 25 patients with clinically positive axillary nodes who underwent simple mastectomy, leaving the nodal disease in the axilla alone. Only half had progressive axillary disease at 2 years. In a study from Cape Town (136), 51 patients with stage I or II breast cancer underwent simple mastectomy

TABLE 6. *Results of a randomized clinical trial comparing radical mastectomy and total mastectomy with or without irradiation for breast carcinoma*

Procedure	Clinically negative nodes			Clinically positive nodes		
	Number of patients	5-year survival (%)	10-year survival (%)	Number of patients	5-year survival (%)	10-year survival (%)
Radical mastectomy	362	74.6	32.9	292	61.6	19.5
Total mastectomy and irradiation	352	75.2	30.1	294	57.4	20.4
Total mastectomy alone	365	74.0	29.0	—	—	—

Fisher B, Redmond C, Fisher ER, et al. Ten-year results of a randomized clinical trial comparing radical mastectomy and total mastectomy with or without radiation. *N Engl J Med* 1985;312:674–681.

alone. Within 3 years, axillary recurrences had developed in five patients had (10%), all of which were inoperable.

Recent data from the Early Breast Cancer Trialists Collaborative Group (137) have suggested a significant improvement in the disease-free survival rate and a marginal survival benefit of adjuvant therapy in node-negative patients. Corroboration of these data in prospective trials may necessitate a review of the philosophy of axillary dissection. Until then, level I and II axillary dissection in patients with breast cancer stratifies patients into prognostic groups (138), selects patients for adjuvant therapy or aggressive therapy (eg, in patients with more than 10 nodes) (139), and may in a select population improve local control and survival.

Lung Cancer

The incidence of nodal metastatic disease in all patients with carcinoma of the lung is approximately 50% (140,141). Overall, approximately 40% of patients have lymph node involvement at the time of resection. Seventy-seven to 96% of patients dying with lung cancer have evidence of nodal metastatic disease at autopsy. The role of surgical resection with lobectomy or pneumonectomy is controversial in the presence of established nodal metastatic disease, especially to mediastinal nodes (142). In patients who have apparent nodal metastatic disease by preoperative workup, no further surgical intervention is usually recommended. In combined series of staging mediastinoscopies, tumor is present in the lymph nodes in about one fourth of patients with squamous cell carcinoma, in approximately half of patients with adenocarcinoma or large cell carcinoma, and in about three fourths of patients with small cell carcinoma (143,144). For patients with negative nodes, resectability rates often exceed 85%. The 5-year survival rate for resectable epidermoid carcinomas is approximately 35% to 40%. In patients with nodal disease confined to the ipsilateral hilar region or parabronchial regions and with tumors smaller than 3 cm, survival approaches 60% (145,146). For patients with local nodal disease and larger tumors (up to 6 cm), survival is approximately 40% at 5 years, and for patients with disease in the mediastinal nodes and no other evidence of a poor-prognosis tumor, survival with resection is approximately 20% (145,146). Mediastinal lymphadenectomy in patients with clinically occult N2 disease (radiologically negative, mediastinoscopy negative) is associated with 3- and 5-year survival rates of 19% and 10%, respectively (147). In a prospective, controlled trial (148), 182 patients were randomized to either a conventional node sampling or a radical lymphadenectomy. The morbidity and mortality in these groups were comparable. No difference was evident in local recurrence rates (23% vs. 24%), metastatic disease (32% vs. 38%), or cancer-related deaths (32% vs. 30%; Table 7).

Hepatopancreaticobiliary Cancers

Hepatocellular Carcinoma

Although hepatocellular carcinoma is an unusual tumor in the United States, it represents the single largest killer among cancers in the world. At autopsy in 232 consecutive cases evaluated in Japan, lymphatic involvement was noted in one fourth of the patients (60 of 225 cases) (149). Nodal disease was present in the hilum, around the head of the pancreas, in the retroperitoneum, and around the aorta. In fewer than 5% of patients, disease was found in the mediastinum or neck. In contrast to these autopsy findings, only 1 of 113 patients presenting in China with hepatic resection had evidence of nodal disease (150). It seems that nodal metastases is a late consequence of tumor progression. Selby et al. (151), in a series of 105 patients undergoing liver transplantation for hepatocellular carcinoma, reported an overall 5-year survival rate of 36%. Nodal disease, bilobar involvement, and macroscopic venous invasion were poor prognostic factors. Survival after liver transplantation was no different from that after resection (5-year survival rates, 36% vs. 33%), with similar recurrence rates (43% vs. 50%), particularly in stage IVA disease (pT4N1M0) (152). Whether long-term salvage in patients with nodal metastatic disease at presentation and without other evidence of systemic spread can be obtained is not clear from the reported series.

Pancreatic Carcinoma

Lymphatic drainage is into nodes and lymphatics following the general pattern of the arterial blood supply, and is primarily to pancreaticosplenic, splenic, celiac,

TABLE 7. *Prospective, randomized trial of systematic lymphadenectomy versus conventional lymphadenectomy in patients with non-small cell lung cancer*

Type of resection	No. of patients	Morbidity	Mortality	Local recurrence	Metastasis rate	Cancer-related deaths
Systematic	82	38%	2%	23%	32%	32%
Conventional	100	47%	4%	24%	38%	30%

Izbicki JR, Thetter O, Habekost M, et al. Radical systematic mediastinal lymphadenectomy in non-small cell lung cancer: a randomized controlled trial. *Br J Surg* 1994;81:229–235.

and superior mesenteric nodes. Survival rates after a diagnosis of pancreatic carcinoma, regardless of treatment, are uniformly dismal, with overall 5-year survival rates of 5%, but in recent times a number of series have reported survival rates of 17% to 25% (153–156) in patients who can have their disease surgically extirpated. In a series of 201 patients from the Johns Hopkins Institution (156), the actuarial 5-year survival rate of 21% has been recently reported, with better survival in the group with negative nodes (36% vs. 14%). In multivariate analysis, negative lymph nodal status is a strong independent predictor of long-term survival, along with diploid DNA tumor content, tumor size <3 cm, and negative resection margins. Andersen et al. (157) have also shown a better actuarial 5-year survival in patients with negative nodes compared with those with regional node positivity (25% vs. 11%). Data from retrospective studies suggest that an extensive nodal dissection along with a total pancreatectomy may benefit patients with pancreatic cancer in terms of disease control and survival (158–160). Extended pancreatectomies, designed to include all the regional lymph nodes, as advocated by Fortner (158), have been abandoned by most surgeons. The benefits associated with a total pancreatectomy compared with a Whipple procedure (subtotal pancreaticoduodenectomy) are perhaps primarily related to the absence of a pancreatic anastomosis rather than to the inclusion of occult nodal positive disease in the operative specimen. In nonrandomized, comparative series, total pancreatectomy did not show survival benefit compared with a conventional Whipple procedure (161–163). Satake et al. (164) reported on a cumulative series of 185 patients undergoing either radical or a standard resection for small pancreatic cancers, with no difference in overall survival between the groups. The increased 1-year survival rate in patients with negative nodes was thought to be related more to the biology of the tumor than to the virtue of the operation.

Gallbladder Carcinoma

The mode of locoregional spread in gallbladder carcinoma (GBC) is complex and occurs through direct invasion and by lymphatic, portovenous, perineural, or intraductal routes. The pattern of regional lymphatic drainage was demonstrated by vital dye staining and indicated an apparently orderly spread to the cystic node, pericholedochal plexus and lymph nodes, retropancreatic nodes, and finally to the interaortocaval nodes adjacent to the right renal vein (165). Based on the pattern of spread, radical resections are designed to include the gallbladder, segments IV and V of the liver, and pericholedochal lymphatics with or without the common bile duct (166). Nodal disease is present in 50% to 55% of patients on presentation (167,168) and is an important predictor of

poor outcome in these patients (mean survival: 23.6 vs. 5.8 months in patients with node-positive disease) (168).

Radical resection with extirpation of microscopic disease (R0 resections) is the goal of surgical therapy in patients with GBC. Of 98 patients with inapparent GBC (pathologic diagnosis), in those undergoing a second surgery (completion radical resection) for pT2 cancers, the 5-year survival was significantly better compared with those patients who did not receive any further surgery (90% vs. 40%) (169). The 5-year survival rate in the node-positive patients with R0 resections was 65%, compared with 45% for patients with R1/R2 resections (170). This is substantially better than what is observed in the Western patients. Bloechle et al. (171) from Germany also demonstrated the apparent merit of radical R0 resections in patients with advanced-stage GBC. In their series of 66 patients, the mean survival for R0 resections was 25.1 (4.9) months, compared with 8.5 (1.5) months for R1 and 4.5 (0.5) months for palliative procedures. In patients with R0 resections, no difference in survival was detected between node-negative and node-positive patients (mean survival, 26.2 vs. 24.1 months). Some Japanese authors have evaluated extended radical resections to achieve an R0 resection in locoregionally advanced disease. These procedures include hepatopancreaticoduodenectomy (for the retropancreatic nodal disease) (172) or hepatoligamentectomy (for optimal pericholedochal lymphatic clearance) with vascular reconstruction (173). Unfortunately, these have been associated with very high morbidity and mortality and only a marginal benefit in outcome, and thus are not routinely recommended.

Tumors of the Gastrointestinal Tract

Carcinoma of the Thoracic Esophagus

The lymphatic drainage of the esophagus occurs through a large intercommunicating plexus between the upper and lower esophagus. Nodal involvement extending from the level of the internal jugular to the celiac artery can be noted. Regional lymph nodes are classified as being positive (N1) or without evidence of nodal involvement (N0). Most patients with esophageal carcinoma die of their disease. Even in patients who undergo resection, only 5% to 20% survive 5 years. Some increases in survival have been reported with perioperative radiation therapy or chemotherapy (174).

The incidence of lymph nodal metastasis in esophageal cancers on presentation ranges from 60% to 80%, depending on the site of involvement and depth of penetration (175–177). In a large series of Japanese patients (178) undergoing surgical treatment for carcinoma of the esophagus with extended node dissection and total thoracic and abdominal esophagectomy, an analysis of the

TABLE 8. *Distribution of nodal metastases in patients with esophageal cancer (%)*

| Site of esophageal cancer | Cervical | Mediastinal | | | Abdominal |
		Upper	Middle	Lower	
Upper	43.3	53.3	20	6.7	20
Middle	33	38	37	22	44
Lower	29.2	33	52.1	33.3	64.6
Overall	34.1	59			50

Adapted from Hennessey TPJ. Lymph node dissection. *World J Surg* 1994;18:367–372.

incidence of nodal disease and its relationship to survival was conducted. Fully 59% of patients (121/205) had positive lymph nodes at the time of dissection, and 6.4% of all resected lymph nodes (398/6258) harbored tumor. Careful anatomic studies and extensive analysis of lymph nodal dissection specimens have shown frequent metastatic involvement of cervical lymph nodes (29% to 43%) in patients with esophageal cancers regardless of the site of disease (179,180). The frequency of lymph nodal involvement in relation to the site of esophageal cancers is tabulated in Table 8. Five-year survival rate in node-positive patients ranges from 6% to 20% (171,181,182), and a worse prognosis is associated with an increasing number of lymph nodes (five or more). In node-negative patients, 45% to 83% survive for 5 years, as reported in selected series (183,184). The recurrence patterns suggest a propensity to recur in the cervicothoracic/recurrent laryngeal group of lymph nodes (185,186).

Based on the anatomic data of frequency and patterns of regional disease and recurrences, a number of authors have adopted a three-field lymphadenectomy as a procedure of choice. Three-field lymphadenectomy involves bilateral removal of lower cervical nodes, the superior, middle, and inferior mediastinal lymph nodes, and the abdominal group of nodes. In a large multi-institutional analysis of over 4500 patients from Japan, three-field lymphadenectomy had a significant survival advantage compared with a standard two-field lymphadenectomy (34% vs. 27%) (184). Similar observations have been made in a number of other retrospective comparisons (Table 9). Kato et al. (187), in the only quasirandomized

trial comparing three-field lymphadenectomy versus standard two-field lymphadenectomy, demonstrated a survival benefit in those undergoing extended resections (49% vs. 34%), although the results of this study are skewed because of the nonhomogeneous distribution of patients with regard to age and site of disease.

Three-field dissection nonetheless is a major undertaking, with increased operating time; significant morbidity (50% to 65%), primarily owing to anastomotic leakage and recurrent nerve palsy (15% to 50%); and in some series a high operative mortality (183,184,188,189). The quality of life is also significantly compromised after the extended resections (188).

It seems that lymphadenectomy may be worthwhile in stage II and III esophageal cancers, especially to stage accurately and provide prognostic information. Attention to meticulous dissection of the cervicothoracic group of lymph nodes in upper and middle thoracic lesions may provide better locoregional control and possibly prolonged survival. The significant morbidity needs to be balanced with the survival benefits in each setting.

Gastric Carcinoma

The lymphatics of the stomach drain through the various levels of the gastric wall along chains of nodes in relation to the left gastric artery, the splenic artery in the splenic hilum, and the hepatic and gastroduodenal group of nodes. Low-lying gastric carcinomas rarely have nodal involvement in the splenic hilum or along the paraesophageal region, so subtotal gastrectomy is still consid-

TABLE 9. *Comparative nonrandomized studies of standard two-field lymphadenectomy versus three-field lymphadenectomy in patients with esophageal cancers*

| Author | Standard lymphadenectomy | | | Three-field lymphadenectomy | | |
	N	Mortality (%)	5-year survival (%)	N	Mortality (%)	5-year survival (%)
Kato et al. (187)	73	12.3	34[a]	77	2.6	49
Isono et al. (184)	2800	4.6	27[a]	1800	2.8	34
Akiyama et al. (183)	392	5.9	38.3[a]	324	2.2	55
Fujita et al. (188)	65	3	36	63	2	40

[a]Statistically significant difference.

TABLE 10. *Comparative nonrandomized studies of survival after regional lymph node dissection in gastric cancer*

Author	Type of resection	No. of patients	5-year survival rate			
			Stage I	Stage II	Stage III (A/B)	Overall
Pacelli et al., Italy (205)	D_1	121	82	58	30	50
	D_{2-3}	117	86	66	40[a]	65[b]
Siewert et al., Germany (206)	D_1	558	79.5	27	35 (A) 28 (B)	—
	D_2	1096	77.5	55[c]	38[d] 18	—

[a]$P = 0.2$ (extensive versus limited node dissection).
[b]$P = 0.01$ (extensive versus limited node dissection).
[c]$P < 0.001$.
[d]$P = 0.03$ (radical versus standard dissection).

ered a regional en bloc resection (189). Blockage of nodes may, in more advanced cases, cause retrograde lymphatic flow and tumor spread to other nodal sites.

Attempts to determine whether more aggressive and radical surgical procedures could improve survival have been based largely on retrospective reviews of areas of failure (190–195). A standard subtotal or total gastrectomy along with greater omentectomy with regional node dissection has been extended to include dissections along the splenic, suprapancreatic, celiac, porta hepatis, and pancreatic duodenal lymph node regions with the intention of doing a total nodal dissection. By definition, a D1 resection removes all N1-level (along the lesser curvature and greater curvature) nodes, a D2 resection removes N1- and N2-level (long the splenic, left gastric artery, and celiac axis) nodes, and a D3 resection removes N1-, N2-, and N3-level (hepatoduodenal and root of mesentery) nodes (196). Alternatively, removal of more than 26 nodes is considered a radical lymphadenectomy (D2 resection), whereas fewer than 26 nodes would be defined as a standard lymphadenectomy (195). The factors of contamination (ie, dissection of lymph nodes outside the indicated area) and noncompliance (ie, incomplete nodal dissection) may have significant influence on the reported outcome (197). The association of the number of involved nodes and survival has been consistently documented. In patients with long follow-up, the cumulative 5-year survival rate with negative nodes is reported to be 75% to 86%, with one to three nodes, 45% to 63%, and with four or more nodes, 16% to 49% (198–201).

Retrospective data from Japan have demonstrated a survival benefit in all stages of gastric cancer after a D2 resection, with a <3% operative mortality rate (202). Among the factors influencing survival, several studies (195,203,204) have shown the extent of lymphadenectomy as an independent predictor of outcome in multivariate analysis. Two prospective, nonrandomized studies (205,206) have demonstrated at 5 years a significantly better overall survival (65% vs. 50%) in the group of patients undergoing extensive lymphadenectomy (D2 or D3) versus a standard dissection (D1), specifically in stage II (55% vs. 27%) and IIIA (38% vs. 25%) disease (Table 10).

Four prospective, randomized studies (77–80) comparing the extent of lymphadenectomy have been reported in the Western literature and are compiled in Table 11. No significant survival differences among the groups are evident in the two small series (77,78), whereas survival data are not yet mature in the two European trials. Notably, all trials document a significantly higher incidence of complications and mortality after extended resections.

Extended lymphadenectomy improves the accuracy of staging, provides radical local clearance, and perhaps prolongs survival in selected patients. Nonetheless, the

TABLE 11. *Prospective, randomized studies of survival after regional lymph node dissection in gastric cancer*

	Dent et al., South Africa (77)	Robertson et al., Hong Kong (78)	Bohenkemp et al., Netherlands (79)	Fayers et al., Great Britain (80)
N	45	55	711	400
Type of resection	D_1 vs. D_2	D_1 vs. D_3	D_1 vs. D_2	D_1 vs. D_2
Mortality (%)[a]	Nil	0 vs. 3.3	4 vs. 10	6 vs. 13
Morbidity (%)[a]	14 vs. 33	—	25 vs. 43	31 vs. 49
No. of reoperations (N)	0 vs. 4	0 vs. 3	8% vs. 18%	—
Postoperative stay (days)	9.3 vs. 13.9	8 vs. 16	18 vs. 25[b]	—
Survival	No difference	1511 vs. 992[c] d	NA	NA

[a]Significantly higher morbidity and mortality in D_{2-3} versus D_1.
[b]Total hospital stay.
[c]$P < 0.05$.

morbidity far outweighs any evident benefits, and until further data suggest significant survival advantage, its application should be limited to a controlled setting.

Carcinoma of the Colon and Rectum

The lymphatic drainage of the colon and rectum is initially into the epicolic nodes, which are directly opposed to the bowel wall. The next, more distal group is the pericolic nodes, which lie in the mesentery directly adjacent to the bowel wall. Subsequent nodal drainage and lymph flow follows the arterial blood supply rather than the portacaval system (207). The principal nodes occur around the origin of the superior mesenteric and inferior mesenteric arteries (208). These nodes further drain into the cisterna chyli (present in about 25% of patients) or other lymphatic channels, which empty into the thoracic duct. Some lymphatic drainage occurs along the portal vein and in the lower two thirds of the rectum to lateral systems and ultimately into the internal iliac nodes along the middle hemorrhoidal vessels. A third drainage area for low rectal carcinomas is through the inferior hemorrhoidal system to the superficial inguinal nodes. The lymphatic spread of tumors from carcinoma of the colon and rectum was believed initially to be to more proximal nodes and then, in a stepwise fashion, to more distal nodes. This has been challenged by an apparent finding of skip metastases bypassing earlier nodal groups in a number of series.

At presentation with colorectal carcinoma, 26% to 44% of patients have positive nodes (209). The overall incidence was 31% in a recent report of collected data on 20,515 patients. Local recurrence clearly increases in patients with nodal disease, which is also manifested by worsened survival in patients with Dukes' stage C (node-positive) carcinoma. There is a clear correlation of nodal involvement with 5-year survival in patients with carcinoma of the colon (208). In patients without nodal involvement, up to 80% survive 5 years (210). In patients with one to four positive nodes, approximately 25% survive 5 years, and in patients with five or more positive nodes, 10% or fewer survive 5 years (Table 12). Sugar-

baker and Corlew (207) have reviewed the results of extended lymph node dissections for sigmoid and rectal cancer and concluded that there is little survival advantage to be accrued from more aggressive regional nodal dissection. The French Association of Surgical Research conducted a prospective, multicenter trial (211) comparing left hemicolectomy versus left segmental colectomy for left colon cancers. The median survival was 10 years, without any significant difference between the two groups (47% vs. 54%). There was no difference among the Dukes' C patients or among patients with or without inferior mesenteric nodal involvement. The most important role of nodal dissection in patients with colon cancer is accurately to stage patients so as to select them for adjuvant therapy. Data from the North Central Cancer Treatment Group (212–214) and the pooled European study (IMPACT) (215) indicate substantial survival benefit in patients with Dukes' C cancer receiving adjuvant chemotherapy with either a combination of 5-fluorouracil and levamisole (46% vs. 60% at 6.5 years) or 5-fluorouracil and leucovorin (78% vs. 83%), compared with the surgery-alone group.

In rectal cancers, the extent of resection and nodal dissection has again not been evaluated in a controlled trial. Enker and associates (216,217) indicate that in patients with operations for rectal carcinoma, extended en bloc pelvic lymphadenectomies were of no benefit in Dukes' A or B carcinoma, but provided an approximate 20% survival benefit in patients with Dukes' C adenocarcinoma of the rectum. This conclusion must remain tentative until a randomized protocol is concluded. Cawthorn et al. (218), in a multivariate analysis of factors determining survival in rectal cancer, identified nodal metastasis, mesorectal spread, and limited surgery as adverse prognostic factors. Ng et al. (219) reported an increased incidence of local recurrence in patients with pathologic involvement of the lateral resection margin in rectal cancer. Total mesorectal excision with R0 resection has the potential to provide long-term local control and possibly prolonged survival (220–222). The most compelling evidence for total mesorectal resection comes from a long-term follow-up study in 366 patients of rectal cancer undergoing total mesorectal excision, reporting a local

TABLE 12. *Correlation of nodal involvement and 5-year survival of patients with carcinoma of the colon*

No. of nodes involved	No. of patients	Alive with no carcinoma	Alive with carcinoma	Dead with no carcinoma	Dead with carcinoma
0	584	48.5	3.0	17.6	31.9
1	112	26.8	3.5	6.2	63.5
2	68	25.0	2.9	5.9	66.2
3	40	15.0	2.5	2.5	80.0
4	24	29.1	4.2	4.2	62.5
≥5	110	9.1	0.9	4.5	85.5

Copeland EM, Miller LD, Jones RS. Prognostic factors in carcinoma of the colon and rectum. *Am J Surg* 1968;116:875.

recurrence rate of 4% for all curative resections and a 10-year disease-free survival rate of 78% (220). Postoperative adjuvant chemoradiation therapy has shown significant survival benefit in Dukes' B and C rectal cancer (56 vs. 36%) compared with surgery only in a prospective, controlled trial (223). The benefit of adjuvant therapy has also been demonstrated in several other trials (224–229), and thus, as in colon cancer, nodal dissection is used to stage these patients accurately and select for adjuvant therapy. Whether extensive nodal dissection in combination with adjuvant therapy further improves outcome is an issue that needs to be addressed in the future.

Tumors of the Urinary Tract

Renal Cell Carcinoma

The lymphatic drainage of the kidney is profuse through the retroperitoneum into lymphatics within the hilum, and extending into periaortic nodes and occasionally directly into the thoracic duct. Approximately 22% of patients with cancer of the kidney present with nodal metastatic disease, and fully one third of patients die with apparent nodal metastases (230). The benefits of regional nodal dissection are controversial because of the extensive lymphatic drainage of the kidney. Those recommending nodal dissection claim that a complete homolateral dissection from the diaphragm to the bifurcation of the aorta is required. The degree of lymphatic metastasis is related to the stage of the primary tumor, with 12% of T1 or T2, 35% of T3, and 30% to 40% of T1 to T3 V+ tumors associated with positive lymph nodes (231,232). Herrlinger et al. (233), in a comparative study of systematic lymphadenectomy versus lymph node sampling, reported a significant benefit in the 5-year (66% vs. 58%) and 10-year (56% vs. 41%) survival rates for stages I to III. Subgroup analysis of the stages demonstrated better survival rates in stage I and II, whereas in stage III the apparent benefit was lost beyond 3 years of follow-up. Similar results are reported from a number of retrospective analyses of lymphadenectomy in renal cell cancer and are presented in Table 13 (233–236). Lymphadenectomy may thus benefit a select group of patients with clinically occult nodal disease, although the available evidence is uncontrolled and controversial.

Bladder Cancer

Lymphatic spread of bladder carcinomas occurs most frequently to the obturator and external iliac nodes, followed by the common iliac, hypogastric, and perivesical nodes (237). Obturator nodal involvement without external iliac metastases is seen in 28% of patients, whereas external iliac nodal involvement without obturator metastases is observed in 19%. The incidence of pelvic node metastasis in patients undergoing cystectomy is approximately 20%, and is most frequent in patients with higher-grade tumors penetrating deeper into the bladder wall. A pelvic lymphadenectomy in this disease includes as its distal margin the lymph node of Cloquet in the femoral canal. The most proximal extent of the dissection is 1 to 2 cm above the bifurcation of the aorta. In patients with lymph node metastases, various series report a 4% to 35% 5-year survival rate, with a cumulative survival rate in 338 patients of 13% (238,239). Survival appears to vary inversely with the number of positive nodes, with 5-year survival rates of 30% to 50% for one to five positive nodes and 12% to 17% for more than six positive nodes (240–242). The current role of lymphadenectomy appears to be primarily to promote accurate staging; therapeutic benefit is confined to a select group of patients with a primary lesion confined to the bladder or with low-volume nodal disease.

Tumors of the Male Genital Tract

Prostate Carcinoma

Adenocarcinoma of the prostate is a frequent neoplasm in men, with approximately 75,000 new cases and 24,000 deaths per year. Metastatic spread occurs through both hematogenous and lymphatic routes, and it appears that prognosis is more closely related to local extension in the periprostatic space than to nodal involvement (243). Nodes that are frequently involved include the obturator nodes initially, followed by the hypogastric and then the common iliac and periaortic groups. The incidence of lymph node involvement at various sites in the pelvis is listed in Table 14 (244). Nodal metastatic disease is correlated with increasing size of the tumor in the gland and with decreasing differentiation of the tumor (27% in well

TABLE 13. *Comparative studies of survival in patients with or without lymphadenectomy for renal cell cancer*

	Peters & Brown (235)	Gilloz et al. (236)	Golimbo et al. (234)	Herrlinger et al. (233)
No. of patients	31	115	193	511
Stage	III	II + III	III	I–IV
5-Year survival (%)				
LND +	44	68	60	66
LND –	26	30	47	58

LND, Lymph node dissection.

TABLE 14. *Incidence of lymph node involvement by tumor site in adenocarcinoma of the prostate*

Lymph node group	No. of patients	Incidence of involvement	Nodes containing lymphangiogram contrast material (%)
Obturator	51	31% (16)	93
Internal iliac	63	24% (15)	95
External iliac	74	22% (16)	94
Common iliac	76	17% (13)	95
Para-aortic	74	18% (13)	93

Adapted from Pistenma DA, Bagshaw MA, Freiha FS. Extended-field radiation therapy for prostatic adenocarcinoma: status report of a limited prospective trial. In: Johnson DE, Samuels ML, eds. *Cancer of the genitourinary tract.* New York: Raven Press; 1979:229–247.

differentiated, 45% in moderately well differentiated, and 70% in poorly differentiated) (245). In well differentiated tumors, nodes are found to be positive in 2% to 5% of stage A, 5% to 31% of stage B, and 18% to 64% in stage C, whereas in poorly differentiated tumors, 27% to 80% of patients have nodal disease over all stage distributions (245,246).

Radical perineal or suprapubic prostatectomy is conducted with curative intent primarily in patients without evidence of distant or local nodal disease (247). Attempts to assess the local nodes for evidence of tumor are often recommended. Patients with evidence of local nodal involvement by either lymphangiography or pelvic nodal dissection are often refused radical prostatectomy and referred for radiation therapy. Prognosis appears to be closely correlated with nodal metastatic disease (243,248–250). A single nodal metastasis is not necessarily unfavorable (as with breast carcinoma and melanoma), with only 18% of patients showing tumor progression, as opposed to approximately 75% of patients showing progression when multiple nodes are involved (251). Follow-up of patients undergoing assessment of nodal involvement revealed that the 5-year survival rate in patients with negative pelvic nodes was 84%, compared with 34% to 66% in those with positive nodes (250,252). The role of staging lymphadenectomy is controversial. Important prognostic information may be obtained by such procedures, which therefore may be important in assessing a variety of treatments, although a 12% to 30% false-negative rate of nodal assessment is estimated after pelvic lymphadenectomy. It has been suggested that radical extirpation of regional nodes would require excision of the rectum, and consequently there is some doubt as to whether pelvic nodal dissection is ever curative. Kramer and colleagues (253) reported comparable survival rates between patients treated by radical prostatectomy and lymph node dissection and patients treated with irradiation or hormonal therapy. Occasional survivors, representing fewer than 10% of patients undergoing radical prostatectomy and lymphadenectomy, with evidence of nodal disease, can be expected at 5 years.

Cancer of the Testes

Approximately 10% to 15% of patients with seminoma have occult retroperitoneal lymph node metastases. Seminoma is a tumor of the testes that is readily curable by radiation therapy in conjunction with orchiectomy, but has more recently been demonstrated to be very effectively treated with chemotherapy alone (254). Surgical extirpation of residual retroperitoneal lymph node masses (>3 cm) after chemoradiation therapy in bulky nodal disease is probably the only indication for retroperitoneal lymph node dissection in seminomatous tumors (255).

The evolution of the treatment of nonseminomatous tumors of the testes is perhaps one of the most visible reflections of the successful development of modern chemotherapy. Chemotherapy has replaced most primary surgical procedures other than orchiectomy and retroperitoneal node dissection. In stage I disease, radical orchiectomy with retroperitoneal nodal dissection is the recommended approach. The 5-year survival rate ranges between 90% to 100%. Radical orchiectomy alone for clinical stage I disease (without evidence of retroperitoneal lymphadenopathy) cures 70% to 75% of patients and is being evaluated at some centers. Twenty to 25% have occult nodal metastatic disease or subsequently have stage II disease (positive lymph nodes in the retroperitoneum). Extensive retroperitoneal nodal dissection has been reported to be curative in patients with microscopic or low-volume (<3 cm) nodal disease (stage II) (256).

Current combination chemotherapies that include cis-platinum lead to a 70% complete response rate (254). Patients who do not respond to conventional chemotherapy with clearing of retroperitoneal lymph node metastases or metastases in other sites are considered for surgical excision. Many patients with resected, mature teratocarcinomas, however, remain free of disease. A randomized trial (76) was conducted at the NCI several years ago to evaluate the role of debulking cytoreductive surgery in patients with retroperitoneal nodal or extra-abdominal disease before chemotherapy, compared with chemotherapy alone. No significant improvement in survival was noted, and surgical debulking before chemotherapy in this setting has been abandoned. Studies of lymphangiography in this same population (257) revealed that it enabled detection of smaller deposits of disease if the results were compared with those of concurrent CT scans. In summary, some patients with clinical stage II disease with testicular carcinoma can be salvaged with retroperitoneal nodal dissections.

Carcinoma of the Penis

Carcinoma of the penis and carcinoma of the vulva metastasize frequently to the superficial and deep inguinal nodes (258). The lymphatics of the penis drain into the medial superficial inguinal nodes, and from there into the deep inguinal lymphatics along the femoral vessels, and eventually to the periaortic nodes. Occasionally, hypogastric and obturator nodes can be involved. At presentation, approximately half of patients with carcinoma of the penis have palpable nodes, but only two thirds of these contain carcinoma. This is probably related to the presence of inflammation around the primary lesion (258,259). Approximately 20% to 40% of patients without evidence of clinically palpable disease have occult deposits within the nodes, whereas 70% of N1 and 42% of N2 patients have positive nodal disease (260,261). The 5-year survival of patients with negative nodes ranges from 90% to 95%, in contrast to 30% to 40% in patients with positive nodes (262–264). Overall survival in patients undergoing lymph nodal dissection is 55% to 60%, compared with 8% to 13% in patients without lymph node dissection (260,265). Prophylactic lymphadenectomy is not recommended because the associated morbidity is prohibitive and because there is a lack of any controlled, prospective studies. Most studies indicate no significant adverse effect on survival when lymphadenectomy is delayed until clinically apparent nodal disease, although there is some evidence to the contrary (260,266). Occult node positivity is high in patients presenting with high tumor volume (T3), a high histologic grade of tumor, and invasion of the corpora, and selective lymphadenectomy may be worthwhile in this select group of patients (267,268). If unilateral disease is apparent (especially with more than two lymph nodes positive), bilateral nodal dissection is recommended because of a high rate of contralateral disease (60%).

In palpable, nonmetastatic nodal disease, the conventional recommendation is to perform a nodal dissection 4 to 6 weeks after excision of the primary, if palpable nodes persist, although some authors recommend an elective bilateral groin dissection (265,269), with improved outcome in this setting. In patients who have evidence of metachronous development of nodal disease, unilateral lymphadenectomy is considered reasonable because spread to the opposite side occurs in fewer than 10% of patients.

Tumors of the Female Genital Tract

Carcinoma of the Cervix and Endometrium

The lymphatic drainage of the cervix is through a network extending through the muscle layers to perivesical and parametrial lymphatics as well as to obturator lymph nodes, external iliac and hypogastric lymph nodes, and occasionally further to the common iliac or periaortic lymph nodes. The involvement of regional and distant nodes by carcinoma of the cervix is directly related to the local extent of the disease. Incidence of nodal metastasis is 6% in stage IB, 13% to 19% in stage II, and 20% to 30% in stages III and IV (270). The incidence of disease in pelvic nodes is clearly related to the size of the tumor, deep stromal invasion, lymphovascular invasion, and grade of tumor. Thirty-five percent of patients with tumors measuring 4 to 5 cm have associated disease in lymph nodes at presentation. Surgical procedures are limited to patients with stage I (carcinoma confined to the cervix) and stage II (carcinoma extending beyond the cervix but not onto the pelvic wall) disease (271). Radical hysterectomy and pelvic lymphadenectomy in these stages leads to 5-year survival in more than 75% of patients (272). The 5-year survival rate in patients with positive nodes is approximately 45% to 61%, and in those with negative nodes it is 82% to 94% (271,273). In a cumulative review of published series, survival data are comparable for surgical therapy (65% to 92%) and radiation therapy (53% to 92%) in stage IB/IIA cervical cancer (270).

Metastatic spread from carcinoma of the endometrium to the pelvic and periaortic nodes is associated with the local extent of the disease, the degree of differentiation of the tumor, and the depth of myometrial invasion. Of 140 patients, 11.4% were found to have pelvic nodal metastases (274). Inguinal nodal metastases are extremely rare. Patients with deep myometrial invasion have a high (50%) incidence of periaortic node metastasis. Most patients who die from endometrial carcinoma do so because of direct extension of tumor as well as distant metastatic disease. It is difficult, given the low numbers of patients with nodal metastatic disease, to determine the impact of surgery on the long-term survival of patients with either occult or clinically apparent nodes.

Carcinoma of the Ovary

Carcinoma of the ovary spreads intraperitoneally as its most frequent mode of dissemination. It may also spread through the subovarian lymphatic plexus and ascend along the ovarian blood vessels to end in nodes between the bifurcation of the aorta and renal arteries, through the broad ligaments toward the lateral and posterior pelvic wall, or rarely along the round ligaments into the external iliac and inguinal nodes (275). Nodal dissemination has been documented in as many as 15% of patients with early stage I carcinoma of the ovary. A frequent test performed earlier in ovarian carcinoma was lymphangiography (276,277), which has now been largely supplanted by CT scans (275). The incidence of positive lymphangiograms in a combined series of patients with stage I ovarian carcinoma was 14%, for stage II, 17%, stage III, 31%, and for stage IV, 64%. Because the current staging system includes patients with nodal metastatic disease in stage III along with patients with malignant extension to small bowel or omentum, it is impossible to determine the impact of nodal dissection on long-term survival from these reports. The 5-year survival rate in patients with stage III ovarian carcinoma is <5%. Although routine retroperitoneal lymphadenectomy is not recommended for carcinoma of the ovary, adequate staging, including lymph node biopsy for the purpose of chemotherapy trials, has been suggested and is routinely practiced (275).

Cancer of the Vulva

Carcinoma of the vulva is an epidermoid tumor frequently metastasizing to lymph nodes (270). Lymphatic drainage in this area is into superficial and deep inguinal and femoral nodes (270,278). It is distinctly unusual for vulva carcinoma to spread hematogenously except at advanced stages of the disease. nodal metastases develop in approximately 40% of patients with carcinoma of vulva. The incidence of deep pelvic nodes is approximately 10% and is directly related to the positivity of the highest superficial inguinal node, commonly referred to as Cloquet's node. Independent predictors of nodal disease include tumor grade, capillary space involvement, and depth of invasion. If the regional lymph nodes are negative, survival is approximately 93%. In patients with unilateral nodal disease, the 5-year survival rate is 50% to 55%, and falls to 25% to 30% with bilateral nodal involvement. Among patients with deep nodal disease, 20% survive 5 years (279,280). Surgical treatment with radical vulvectomy and bilateral nodal dissection has an overall survival rate of 80%. If the regional nodes are negative, survival is approximately 93%. In patients with stage I disease, the incidence of positive nodes ranges from 5% to 10%, and a selective superficial lymphadenectomy based on tumor location can be performed (278,281,282). In node-positive cases, ipsilateral deep nodal dissection with or without contralateral dissection is recommended. For lateral T1 lesions, contralateral node involvement is rare, and bilateral dissections may be superfluous in this group (282). For stage II disease, radical vulvectomy and bilateral groin dissection is the standard of care. In conclusion, it appears that nodal dissection has a prominent role in carcinomas of both the penis and the vulva, and is curative in a well selected group of patients.

Other Tumors

Lymphoma

With the advent of radiation therapy techniques and, more recently, the evolution of effective chemotherapy, there appears to be no substantial role for surgical excision of lymphoma. Of historical interest is the fact that in series reported before the modern era, a number of patients with head and neck lymphomas with isolated nodal disease could be cured by surgical extirpation. Claims of a 50% 5-year survival rate with an approximate 40% disease-free 5-year survival rate have been reported (283).

Among patients with gastric lymphoma, a proportion are disease free after resection of the stomach and adjacent gastric lymph nodes involved with tumor. In a series reported from Memorial Sloan-Kettering Cancer Center (284), 19 patients with nodal involvement along the lesser or greater curvature (specified as N1 disease) had an approximate 50% 5-year survival rate. Many of these patients subsequently received radiation therapy. Only 15 patients were treated by radical gastric resection alone without adjunctive radiation therapy. Five (33%) lived for an additional 5 years free of disease; two of these five had tumor that involved the perigastric lymph nodes. In stage I disease, resectional therapy with free margins is the recommended therapy, and there seems to be no additional benefit from the addition of adjuvant radiation/chemotherapy (285). In stage II disease, resection of macroscopic disease without extensive nodal dissection and adjuvant radiation therapy is optimal therapy (286–288). The use of combined chemoradiation therapy with or without surgery for treatment of stage II to IV disease has shown promise, but needs validation. Many authors still recommend combined therapy with surgical resection and irradiation.

Sarcomas of Soft Tissue and Bone

Nodal metastases from sarcomas are relatively rare and usually occur late in the course of disseminated disease. In 374 patients referred to the NCI over a 24-year period, a complete review of all nodes removed as part of surgical excisions was conducted. Only three patients had evidence of sarcoma metastatic to draining lymph nodes. The three patients with nodal disease died in less than 2 years despite surgical extirpation of their tumors. Approximately 25% of patients from collected series have nodal metastatic disease in addition to other evidence of widespread sarcomatosis at the time of autopsy. The reported incidence of nodal metastases in osteosarcoma is likewise low (289), ranging from 3.9% to 6.5%, with 31% presenting with nodal disease at autopsy. In two reviews of soft tissue sarcomas reported in literature, nodal metastases were reported in 9% to 10% of patients (290,291). In a review of 1772 patients with sarcomas from the Memorial Sloan-Kettering Cancer Center (292), the incidence of nodal involvement was 2.6%. The histologic types most frequently associated with nodal metastases were angiosarcomas, epithelioid sarcomas, and rhabdomyosarcomas (pediatric, embryonal). There was significant variation in the incidence of nodal disease in synovial sarcomas, malignant fibrous histiocytomas, and alveolar soft tissue sarcomas. Prognosis with nodal disease is poor, although resection of palpable disease may provide long-term disease control.

CONCLUSIONS

Metastatic disease to lymph nodes is a frequent occurrence in a variety of tumors. In situations in which hematogenous spread is less frequent, such as in the case of squamous cell carcinomas of the head and neck, penis, or vulva, nodal dissections clearly have a role to play and can be curative in patients with established nodal metastases. Similarly, nodal dissections for melanoma may salvage up to 20% of patients, who can be expected to survive for 5 or more years. For patients with adenocarcinomas at a number of different sites, nodal metastatic disease is most often a reflection of systemic spread. In the absence of effective chemotherapy for many of these tumors, an attempt to extirpate nodal disease surgically for both palliation and cure seems reasonable. Based on every randomized study evaluating the role of prophylactic nodal dissection, delaying dissection of nodes until their disease becomes clinically apparent appears to have no adverse effect on survival. For patients with visceral tumors, concurrent nodal dissection at the time of the primary procedure seems reasonable, given the difficulty with which subsequent nodal dissections would be performed and the 10% to 20% expected long-term survival rate in some of these patients. Surgical extirpation of nodal disease in the absence of evidence of systemic spread continues to represent rational and possibly curative treatment in many patients.

REFERENCES

1. Nora PF. *Operative surgery: principles and techniques*. 3rd ed. Philadelphia: WB Saunders; 1990.
2. Nyhus LM, Baker RJ. *Mastery of surgery*. 2nd ed. Boston: Little, Brown; 1992.
3. DeVita VT Jr, Hellman S, Rosenberg SA. *Cancer: principles and practice of oncology*. 4th ed. Philadelphia: JB Lippincott; 1993.
4. Crile G. Excision of cancer of the head and neck with special reference to the plan of dissection based on one-hundred and thirty-two operations. *JAMA* 1905;47;1780–1786.
5. Wertheim E. The extended abdominal operation for carcinoma. *Am J Obstet Gynecol* 1912;66;169–232.
6. Miles WE. A method of performing abdominoperineal excision for carcinoma of the rectum and the terminal portion of the pelvic colon. *Lancet* 1908;2;1812–1816.
7. Hill GJ III. Historic milestones in cancer surgery. *Semin Oncol* 1979; 6:409–427.
8. Jones SE, Tobias DA, Waldman RS. Complete tomographic scanning in patients with lymphoma. *Cancer* 1978;41:480–486.
9. Castellino RA, Marglin SI. Imaging of abdominal and pelvic lymph nodes: lymphography or computed tomography. *Invest Radiol* 1983; 17:433–443.
10. Best JJK, Blackledge G, Forbes WS, et al. Computed tomography of the abdomen in staging and clinical management of lymphoma. *Br Med J* 1978;2:1675–1677.
11. Kinmonth JB. Lymphangiography in man: method of outlining lymphatic trunks at operation. *Clin Sci* 1952;11:13–20.
12. Dolan PA. Lymphography: complications encountered in 522 examinations. *Radiology* 1966;86:876–880.
13. Gold WM, Youker J, Anderson S, et al. Pulmonary function abnormalities after lymphangiography. *N Engl J Med* 1965;273:519–524.
14. Ariel IM, Resnick MI. Altered lymphatic dynamics caused by cancer metastases. *Arch Surg* 1967;94:117.
15. Ujiki GT, Brand WN, O'Brien PH. Effect of lymphangiography on metastases. *Radiology* 1968;91:877–891.
16. Osborne MP, Meijer WS, Yeh SDJ, et al. Lymphoscintigraphy in the staging of solid tumors. *Surg Gynecol Obstet* 1983;156:384–391.
17. Fee HJ, Robinson DS, Sample DS, et al. The determination of lymph shed by colloidal gold scanning in patients with malignant melanoma: a preliminary study. *Surgery* 1978;84:626–632.
18. Ege GN, Warbick A. Lymphoscintigraphy: a comparison of ^{99m}Tc antimony sulphide colloid and ^{99m}Tc stannous phytate. *Br J Radiol* 1979; 52:124–219.
19. Aspegren K, Strand SE, Persson BRR. Quantitative lymphoscintigraphy for detection of metastases to the internal mammary lymph nodes: biokinetics of ^{99m}Tc-sulfur colloid uptake and correlation with microscopy. *Acta Radiol Oncol Radiat Phys Biol* 1978;17: 17–26.
20. Ege GN, Cummings BJ. Interstitial radiocolloid iliopelvic lymphoscintigraphy: technique, anatomy and clinical application. *Int J Radiat Oncol Biol Phys* 1980;6:1483–1490.
21. Jonsson PE, Strand SE, Dawiskiba S, et al. ^{99m}Tc-antimony sulfide colloid scintigraphy for identification of the lymph drainage in patients with malignancy. *Br J Surg* 1979;66:885.
22. Tempero M, Brand R, Holdeman K, Matamoros A. New imaging techniques in colorectal cancer. *Semin Oncol* 1995;5:448–471.
23. Bronskill MJ, Harauz G, Ege GN. Computerized internal mammary lymphoscintigraphy in radiation treatment planning of patients with breast cancer. *Int J Radiat Oncol Biol Phys* 1979;5:573–579.
24. Thompson JF, McCarthy WH, Bosch CMJ, et al. Sentinel lymph node status as an indicator of the presence of metastatic melanoma in regional lymph nodes. *Melanoma Res* 1995;5:255–260.
25. Weinstein JN, Parker RJ, Holton OD III, et al. Lymphatic delivery of monoclonal antibodies: potential for detection and treatment of lymph node metastases. *Cancer Invest* 1985;3:85–95.
26. Lotze MT, Carrasquillo JA, Weinstein JN, et al. Monoclonal antibody imaging of human melanoma: radioimmunodetection by subcutaneous or systemic injection. *Ann Surg* 1986;204:223–235.
27. DeLand FH, Kim EE, Goldenberg DM. Lymphoscintigraphy with radionuclide-labeled antibodies to carcinoembryonic antigen. *Cancer Res* 1980;40:2997–3000.
28. DeLand FH, Kim EE, Corgan RL, et al. Axillary lymphoscintigraphy by radioimmunodetection of carcinoembryonic antigen in breast cancer. *J Nucl Med* 1979;20:1243–1250.
29. Schneebaum S, Arnold MW, Houchens DP, et al. The significance of intraoperative periportal lymph node metastasis identification in patients with colorectal carcinoma. *Cancer* 1995;75:2809–2817.
30. Joypaul BV, Kennedy N, Hanson J, et al. Immunoscintigraphy of primary colorectal cancers with indium-111 monoclonal antibody B72.3. *J R Coll Surg Edinb* 1994;39:39–43.
31. Rosner D, Nabi H, Wild L, Ortman-Nabi J, Hreshchyshyn MM. Diagnosis of breast carcinoma with radiolabeled monoclonal antibodies (MoAbs) to carcinoembryonic antigen (CEA) and human milk fat globulin (HMFG). *Cancer Invest* 1995;13:573–582.
32. Schatten C, Barrada M, Mandeville R, et al. Combined use of ^{123}I-labeled BCD-F9 and 4C4 monoclonal antibody with dissimilar specificity for breast cancer: implication for the detection limit of

immunolymphoscintigraphy in the assessment of axillary lymph node metastases. *Nucl Med Commun* 1994;15:422–429.

33. Babaian RJ, Sayer J, Podoloff DA, Steelhammer LC, Bhadkamkar VA, Gulfo JV. Radioimmunoscintigraphy of pelvic lymph nodes with 111 indium-labeled monoclonal antibody CYT-356. *J Urol* 1994;152: 1952–1955.

34. de Bree R, Roos JC, Quak JJ, et al. Clinical imaging of head and neck cancer with technetium-99m-labeled monoclonal antibody E48 IgG or F(ab′)2. *J Nucl Med* 1994;35:775–783.

35. Keenan AM, Weinstein JN, Mulshine IL, et al. Immunolymphoscintigraphy in patients with lymphoma after subcutaneous injection of indium-111-labeled T101 monoclonal antibody. *J Nucl Med* 1987;28:42–46.

36. Order SE, Bloomer WD, Jones AG, et al. Radionuclide immunoglobulin lymphangiography: a case report. *Cancer* 1975;35:1487–1492.

37. Boilleau G, Pujol JL, Ychou M, et al. Detection of lymph node metastases in lung cancer: comparison of 13II-anti-CEA-anti-CA 19-9 immunoscintigraphy versus computed tomography. *Lung Cancer* 1994; 11:209–219.

38. Sorn PM. Detection of metastasis in cervical lymph nodes: CT and MR criteria and differential diagnosis. *AJR Am J Roentgenol* 1992;158: 961–969.

39. Van den Brekel MWM, Stel HV, Castelijns JA, et al. Cervical lymph node metastases: assessment of radiologic criteria. *Radiology* 1990; 177:379–384.

40. Reede DL, Bergeron RT. Computed tomography of cervical lymph nodes. In: Clouse ME, Wallace S, eds. *Lymphatic imaging: lymphography, computed tomography, and scintigraphy.* 2nd ed. Baltimore: Williams & Wilkins; 1985:472–495.

41. Camilien L, Gordon D, Fouchter RG, Maiman M, Boyce JG. Predictive value of CT in the presurgical evaluation of primary carcinoma of cervix. *Gynecol Oncol* 1988;30:209–215.

42. Heller PB, Maletano JH, Bundy BN, Baonhill DR, Okagaki T. Clinico-pathologic study of stage IIB, III, and IVA carcinoma of the cervix: extended evaluation for paragostic node metastasis: a Gynecologic Oncology Group Study. *Gynecol Oncol* 1990;38:425–430.

43. Hollis DP, Economou JS, Parks LC, et al. Nuclear magnetic resonance studies of several experimental and human malignant tumors. *Cancer Res* 1973;33:2156–2160.

44. Fossel ET, Brodsky G, DeLayre JL, et al. Nuclear magnetic resonance for the differentiation of benign and malignant breast tissues and axillary lymph nodes. *Ann Surg* 1983;198:541–544.

45. Van den Brekel MWM, Castelijns JA, Stel HV, et al. Detection and characterization of metastatic cervical adenopathy by MR imaging: comparison of different MR techniques. *J Comput Assist Tomogr* 1990;14:581–589.

46. Yousem DM, Som PM, Hackney DB, Schwaibold F, Hendrix RA. Central nodal necrosis and extracapsular neoplastic spread in cervical lymph nodes: MR imaging versus CT. *Radiology* 1992;182: 753–759.

47. Tio TL and Kallimanis GE. Endoscopic ultrasonography of perigastrointestinal lymph nodes. *Endoscopy* 1994;26:776–779.

48. Hildebrandt U, Schuder G, Feifel G. Preoperative staging of rectal and colonic cancer. *Endoscopy* 1994;26:810–812.

49. Akahoshi K, Misawa T, Fujishima H, Chijiiwa Y, Nawata H. Regional lymph node metastasis in gastric cancer: evaluation with endoscopic US. *Radiology* 1992;182:559–564.

50. Lightdale CJ. Endoscopic ultrasonography in the diagnosis, staging and follow up of esophageal and gastric cancer. *Endoscopy* 1992;24: 297–303.

51. Grimm H, Hamper K, Binmoeller KF, Soehendra N. Enlarged lymph nodes: malignant or not? *Endoscopy* 1992;24(Suppl 1):320–323.

52. Rifkin MD, Ehrlich SM, Marks G. Staging of rectal carcinoma: Prospective comparison of endorectal US and CT. *Radiology* 1989; 170:319–322.

53. Beynon J, Mortensen NJ McC, Foy DMA, et al. Preoperative assessment of mesorectal lymph node involvement in rectal cancer. *Br J Surg* 1989;76:276–279.

54. Tio TL, Tytgat GNJ, Houthoff JH, et al. Ampullopancreatic carcinoma: preoperative TNM classification by endosonography. *Radiology* 1990; 175:456–461.

55. Tio TL, Reeders JW, Sie LH, et al. Endosonography in the clinical staging of Klatskin tumor. *Endoscopy* 1993;25:81–85.

56. Steel BL, Schwartz MR, Ramzy I. Fine needle aspiration biopsy in the diagnosis of lymphadenopathy in 1,103 patients: role, limitations and analysis of diagnostic pitfalls. *Acta Cytol* 1995;39:76–81.

57. Gupta AL, Nayar M, Chandra M. Reliability and limitations of fine needle aspiration cytology of lymphadenopathies: an analysis of 1,261 cases. *Acta Cytol* 1991;35:777–783.

58. Sneige N, Dekmezian R, El-Naggar A, Manning J. Cytomorphologic, immunocytochemical, and nucleic acid flow cytometric study of 50 lymph nodes by fine-needle aspiration: comparison with results obtained by subsequent excisional biopsy. *Cancer* 1991;67: 1003–1007.

59. Sneige N, Dekmezian RH, Katz RL, et al. Morphologic and immunocytochemical evaluation of 220 fine needle aspirates of malignant lymphoid hyperplasia. *Acta Cytol* 1990;34:311–322.

60. Binmoeller KF, Seifert H, Soehendra N. Endoscopic ultrasonography-guided fine needle aspiration biopsy of lymph nodes. *Endoscopy* 1994; 26:780–783.

61. Ferguson JH, Maclure JG. Lymphocele following lymphadenectomy. *Am J Obstet Gynecol* 1961;83:783–792.

62. Lotze MT, Duncan MA, Gerber LH, et al. Early versus delayed shoulder motion following axillary dissection. *Ann Surg* 1981;193: 288–298.

63. Shedd DP. Rehabilitation problems of head and neck cancer patients. *J Surg Oncol* 1976;8:11–21.

64. Saunders WH, Johnson EW. Rehabilitation of the shoulder after radical neck dissection. *Ann Otol* 1975;84:812–816.

65. Aitken DR, Hunsaker R, James AG. Prevention of seromas following mastectomy and axillary dissection. *Surg Gynecol Obstet* 1984;158: 327–330.

66. Sitzmann JV, Dufresne C, Zuidema GD. The use of sclerotherapy for treatment of postmastectomy wound seromas. *Surgery* 1983;93: 345–347.

67. Ingvar C, Erichsen C, Jonsson P-E. Morbidity following prophylactic and therapeutic lymph node dissection for melanoma a comparison. *Tumori* 1984;70:529–533.

68. Kragt H, Bouma J, Aalders JG. Anticoagulants and the formation of lymphocysts after pelvic lymphadenectomy in gynecologic and oncologic operations. *Surg Gynecol Obstet* 1986;162:361–364.

69. Winick L, Robbins GF. The post-mastectomy rehabilitation group program: structure, procedure, and population demography. *Am J Surg* 1978;132:599–602.

70. Flannery GR, Chalmers PJ, Rolland JM, et al. Immune response to a syngeneic rat tumour: Development of regional node lymphocyte energy. *Br J Cancer* 1973;28:118–122.

71. Slade MS, Simmons RL, Yunis E, et al. Immunodepression after major surgery in normal patients. *Surgery* 1975;78:363–372.

72. Veronesi U, Adamus J, Bandiera DC, et al. Delayed regional lymph node dissection in stage I melanoma of the skin of the lower extremities. *Cancer* 1982;49:2420–2430.

73. Sim FH, Taylor WF, Ivins JC, et al. A prospective randomized study of the effficacy of routine elective lymphadenectomy in management of malignant melanoma. *Cancer* 1978;41:948–956.

74. Vandenbrouck C, Sancho-Gamier H, Chassagne D, et al. Elective versus therapeutic radical neck dissection in epidermoid carcinoma of the oral cavity: results of a randomized clinical trial. *Cancer* 1980;46: 386–390.

75. Fisher B, Redmond C, Fisher ER, et al. Ten-year results of a randomized clinical trial comparing radical mastectomy and total mastectomy with or without radiation. *N Engl J Med* 1985;312:674–681.

76. Javadpour N, Ozols RF, Anderson T, et al. A randomized trial of cytoreductive surgery followed by chemotherapy versus chemotherapy alone in bulky stage III testicular cancer with poor prognostic features. *Cancer* 1982;50:2004–2010.

77. Dent DM, Madden MV, Price SK. Randomized comparison of R1 and R2 gastrectomy for gastric carcinoma. *Br J Surg* 1988;75:110–112.

78. Robertson CS, Chung SCS, Woods SDS, et al. A prospective randomized trial comparing R1 subtotal gastrectomy with R3 total gastrectomy for antral cancer. *Ann Surg* 1994;220:176–182.

79. Bonenkamp JJ, Songun I, Hermans J, et al. Randomised comparison of morbidity after D1 and D2 dissection for gastric cancer in 996 Dutch patients. *Lancet* 1995;345:745–748.

80. Fayers PM, Cushieri A, Joypaul V. British Gastric Cancer Study Group: D1 versus D2 surgery for gastric cancer: morbidity and postoperative mortality in the UK MRC Randomized Trial. In: *First International Gastric Cancer Congress (Kyoto, Japan).* (Abstract P-3-1).

81. Finck SJ, Giuliano AK, Mann BD, et al. Results of ilioinguinal dissection for stage II melanoma. *Ann Surg* 1982;196:180–186.

82. Callery C, Cochran AJ, Roe DJ, et al. Factors prognostic for survival in patients with malignant melanoma spread to the regional lymph nodes. *Ann Surg* 1982;196:69–74.

83. McNeer G, DasGupta T. Prognosis in malignant melanoma. *Surgery* 1964;56:512–518.

84. Cohen MH, Ketcham AS, Felix EL, et al. Prognostic factors in patients undergoing lymphadenectomy for malignant melanoma. *Ann Surg* 1977;186:635–642.

85. Karakousis CP, Driscoll DL. Groin dissection in malignant melanoma. *Br J Surg* 1994;81:1771–1774.

86. Balch CM, Soong Sl, Muras TM, et al. A multifactorial analysis of melanoma: (III) prognostic factors in melanoma patients with lymph node metastases (stage II). *Ann Surg* 1981;193:377–388.

87. Guiliano AK, Moseley HS, Morton DL. Clinical aspects of unknown primary melanoma. *Ann Surg* 1980;191:98–104.

88. Balch CM, Houghton AN, Peters LJ. Cutaneous melanoma. In: DeVita VT, Hellman S, Rosenberg SA, eds. *Cancer: principles and practice of oncology.* 4th ed. Philadelphia: JB Lippincott; 1993: 1612–1661.

89. Balch CM, Soong Sj, Murad TM, et al. A multifactorial analysis of melanoma: II. prognostic factors in patients with stage I (localized) melanoma. *Surgery* 1979;86:343–351.

90. Balch CM, Cascinelli N, Milton GW, et al. Elective lymph node dissection: Pros and cons. In: Balch CM, Milton GW, Shaw HM, et al, eds. *Cutaneous melanoma.* Philadelphia: JB Lippincott; 1985.

91. Milton GW, Shaw HM, McCarthy WH, et al. Prophylactic lymph node dissection in clinical stage I cutaneous malignant melanoma: results of surgical treatment in 1319 patients. *Br J Surg* 1982;69:108–111.

92. Elder DE, Guerry D IV, VanHorn M, et al. The role of lymph node dissection for clinical stage I malignant melanoma of intermediate thickness (1.51–3.99 mm). *Cancer* 1985;56:413–418.

93. McCarthy WH, Shaw HM, Milton GW. Efficacy of elective lymph node dissection in 2,347 patients with clinical stage I malignant melanoma. *Surg Gynecol Obstet* 1985;161:575–580.

94. Sugarbaker EV, McBride CM. Melanoma of the trunk: the results of surgical excision and anatomic guidelines for predicting nodal metastasis. *Surgery* 1976;80:22–30.

95. Musumeci R, LaMonica G, Orefice S, et al. Lymphographic evaluation of 250 patients with malignant melanoma. *Cancer* 1976;38: 1568–1573.

96. Morton DL, Wen D-R, Wong JH, et al. Technical details of intraoperative lymphatic mapping for early stage melanoma. *Arch Surg* 1992; 127:392–399.

97. Kirkwood JM, Strawderman MH, Ernstoff MS, Smith TJ, Borden EC, Blum RH. Interferon alfa-2b adjuvant therapy of high risk resected cutaneous melanoma: the ECOG Trial EST 1684. *J Clin Oncol* 1996; 14:7–17.

98. Olson IM, Woods JE, Soule EH. Regional lymph node management and outcome in 100 patients with head and neck melanoma. *Am J Surg* 1981;142:470–473.

99. Roses DF, Harris MN, Grunberger I, et al. Selective surgical management of cutaneous melanoma of the head and neck. *Ann Surg* 1980; 192:629–632.

100. Byers RM. The role of modified neck dissection in the treatment of cutaneous melanoma of the head and neck. *Arch Surg* 1986;126: 1338–1341.

101. Eilber FR, Townsend CM, Morton DL. Results of BCG adjuvant immunotherapy for melanoma of the head and neck. *Am J Surg* 1976; 132:476–483.

102. Fitzpatrick PI, Brown TC, Reid I. Malignant melanoma of the head and neck: a clinico-pathologic study. *Can J Surg* 1972;15:90–97.

103. Simons JN. Malignant melanoma of the head and neck. *Am J Surg* 1972;124:485–493.

104. Houck JR, Medina JE. Management of cervical lymph nodes in squamous carcinomas of the head and neck. *Semin Surg Oncol* 1995;11: 228–39.

105. O Brien CJ, Smith JW, Soong SJ, et al. Neck dissection with and without radiotherapy: prognostic factors, patterns of recurrence and survival. *Am J Surg* 1986;152:456–463.

106. Leemans CR, Tiwari R, Nauta J, et al. Regional lymph node involvement and its significance in the development of distant metastases in head and neck carcinoma. *Cancer* 1993;71:452–456.

107. Johnson JT, Myers EN, Bedetti CD, Barnes EL. Cervical lymph node metastases. *Arch Otolaryngol Head Neck Surg* 1985;111:534–537.

108. Shah JP, Tollefsen HR. Epidermoid carcinoma of the supraglottic larynx. *Am J Surg* 1974;128:494–500.

109. Kalnins IK, Leonard AG, Sako K. Correlation between prognosis and degree of lymph node involvement in carcinoma of the oral cavity. *Am J Surg* 1977;134:450–455.

110. Marcial UA, Pajak TF. Radiation therapy alone or in combination with surgery in head and neck cancer. *Cancer* 1985;55:2259–2269.

111. Merlano M, Vitale V, Rosso R, et al. Treatment of advanced squamous cell carcinoma of the head and neck with alternating chemotherapy and radiotherapy. *N Engl J Med* 1992;327:1115–1121.

112. Head and Neck Contracts Program. Adjuvant chemotherapy for advanced head and neck squamous carcinoma: final report. *Cancer* 1987;60:301–311.

113. The Department of Veterans Affairs Laryngeal Cancer Study Group. Induction chemotherapy plus radiation compared with surgery plus radiation in patients with advanced laryngeal cancer. *N Engl J Med* 1991;324:1685–1690.

114. Schuller DE, Metch B, Stein DW, et al. Preoperative chemotherapy in advanced resectable head and neck cancer: final report of the Southwest Oncology Group. *Laryngoscope* 1988;98:1205–1211.

115. Paccagnella A, Orlando A, Marchiori C, et al. Phase III trial of initial chemotherapy in stage III or IV head and neck cancers: a study by the Gruppo di Studio sui Tumori della Testa e del Collo. *J Natl Cancer Inst* 1994;86:265–272.

116. McKenzie AD. The natural history of thyroid cancer: a report of 102 cases analyzed 10–15 years after diagnosis. *Arch Surg* 1971;102: 274–277.

117. Loree TR. Therapeutic implications of prognostic factors in differentiated carcinoma of the thyroid gland. *Semin Surg Oncol* 1995;11: 246–255.

118. Cunningham MP, Duda RB, Recant W, et al. Survival discriminants for differentiated thyroid cancer. *Am J Surg* 1990;160:344–347.

119. Shah JP, Loree TR, Dharker D, et al. Prognostic factors in differentiated carcinoma of the thyroid gland. *Am J Surg* 1992;164:658–661.

120. Hay ID, Taylor WF, McConahey WM. A prognostic score for predicting outcome in papillary thyroid carcinoma. *Endocrinology* 1986;119 (Suppl):1–15.

121. Cady B, Rossi RL. An expanded view of risk group definition in differentiated thyroid carcinoma. *Surgery* 1988;104:947–953.

122. Hughes CJ, Loree TR, Shah JP. Differentiated carcinoma of the thyroid gland: a matched pair analysis of cervical lymph node metastasis. Presented at the Meeting of the Society of Head and Neck Surgeons, Paris, France, May, 1994.

123. Harwood J, Clark OH, Dunphy JE. Significance of lymph node metastasis in differentiated thyroid cancer. *Am J Surg* 1978;136:107–112.

124. Sellars M, Beenken S, Blankenship A. Prognostic significance of cervical lymph node metastasis in differentiated thyroid cancer. *Am J Surg* 1992;164:578–581.

125. Chong GC, Beahrs OH, Sizemore GW, et al. Medullary carcinoma of the thyroid gland. *Cancer* 1975;35:695.

126. Corwin TR. Medullary carcinoma of the thyroid. *Surg Gynecol Obstet* 1974;138:453.

127. Fisher B, Slack NH. Number of lymph nodes examined and the prognosis of breast carcinoma. *Surg Gynecol Obstet* 1970;131:79–88.

128. Fisher B, Wolmark N, Bauer M, et al. The accuracy of clinical nodal staging and of limited axillary dissection as a determinant of histologic nodal status in carcinoma of the breast. *Surg Gynecol Obstet* 1981;152:765–772.

129. Danforth DN, Findlay PA, McDonald HD, et al. Complete axillary lymph node dissection for stage I, II carcinoma of the breast. *J Clin Oncol* 1986;4:655–662.

130. Harris JR, Osteen RT. Patients with early breast cancer benefit from effective axillary treatment. *Breast Cancer Res Treat* 1985;5:17–21.

131. Fisher B, Redmond C, Fisher E, et al. Ten-year results of a randomized clinical trial comparing radical mastectomy and total mastectomy with or without radiation. *N Engl J Med* 1985;312:674–681.

132. Cancer Research Campaign Working Party. Cancer research campaign (King's/Cambridge) trial for early breast cancer. *Lancet* 1980;2: 55–60.

133. Overgaard M, Christensen JJ, Johansen J, et al. Evaluation of radiotherapy in high-risk breast cancer patients. *Int J Radiat Oncol Biol Phys* 1990;19:1121–1124.

134. Cabanes PA, Salmon RJ, Vilcoq JR, et al. Value of axillary dissection in addition to lumpectomy and radiotherapy in early breast cancer. *Lancet* 1992;339:1245–1248.

135. Baum M, Coyle PJ. Simple mastectomy for early breast cancer and the behavior of the untreated axillary nodes. *Bull Cancer (Paris)* 1977;64:603–610.

136. Helman P, Bennett MB, Louw JH, et al. Interim report on trial of treatment for operable breast cancer. *S Afr Med J* 1972;46:1374–1375.

137. Early Breast Cancer Trialists Collaborative Group. Systemic treatment of early breast cancer by hormonal, cytotoxic, or immune therapy. *Lancet* 1992;339:1–15, 71–85.

138. Kirkland Ruffin W, Stacey-Clear A, Younger J, Hoover HC. Rationale for routine axillary dissection in carcinoma of the breast. *J Am Coll Surg* 1995;180:245–251.

139. Buzdar A, Kau S, Hortobagyi G, et al. Clinical course of patients with breast cancer with ten or more positive nodes who were treated with doxorubicin-containing adjuvant therapy. *Cancer* 1992;69:448–452.

140. Ginsberg RJ, Kins MG, Armstrong JG. Cancer of the Lung. In: DeVita VT, Hellman S, Rosenberg SA, eds. *Cancer: principles and practice of oncology*. Philadelphia: JB Lippincott; 1993:673–722.

141. Martini N, Flehinger BJ, Zaman MB, et al. Prospective study of 445 lung carcinomas with mediastinal lymph node metastases. *J Thorac Cardiovasc Surg* 1980;80:390–399.

142. Paulson DL, Reisch JS. Long-term survival after resection for bronchogenic carcinoma. *Ann Surg* 1976;184:324–332.

143. Smith RA. The importance of mediastinal lymph node invasion by pulmonary carcinoma in selection of patients for resection. *Ann Thorac Surg* 1978;25:5–11.

144. Rubinstein I, Baum GL, Kalter Y, et al. The influence of cell type and lymph node metastases on survival of patients with carcinoma of the lung undergoing thoracotomy. *American Review of Respiratory Disease* 1979;119:253–262.

145. Rubinstein I, Baum GL, Kalter Y, et al. Resectional surgery in the treatment of primary carcinoma of the lung with mediastinal lymph node metastases. *Thorax* 1979;34:33–35.

146. Martini N, Flehinger BJ, Zaman MB, et al. Results of resection in non-oat cell carcinoma of the lung with mediastinal lymph node metastases. *Ann Surg* 1983;198:386–397.

147. van Klaveren RJ, Festen J, Otten HJAM, Cox AL, de Graaf R, Lacquet LK. Prognosis of unsuspected by completely resectable N2 non-small cell lung cancer. *Ann Thorac Surg* 1993;56:300–304.

148. Izbicki JR, Thetter O, Habekost M, et al. Radical systematic mediastinal lymphadenectomy in non-small cell lung cancer: a randomized controlled trial. *Br J Surg* 1994;81:229–235.

149. Nakashima T, Okuda K, Kojiro M, et al. Pathology of hepatocellular carcinoma in Japan: 232 consecutive cases autopsied in ten years. *Cancer* 1983;51:863–877.

150. Lee C-S, Sung J-L, Hwang L-Y, et al. Surgical treatment of 109 patients with symptomatic and asymptomatic hepatocellular carcinoma. *Surgery* 1986;99:481–490.

151. Selby R, Kadry Z, Carr B, Tzakis A, Madariaga JR, Iwatsuki S. Liver transplantation for hepatocellular carcinoma. *World J Surg* 1995;19:53–58.

152. Iwatsuki S, Starzl TE. Role of liver transplantation in the treatment of hepatocellular carcinoma. *Semin Surg Oncol* 1993;9:337–340.

153. Grace PA, Pitt HA, Tompkins RK, et al. Decreased morbidity and mortality after pancreaticoduodenectomy. *Am J Surg* 1986;151:141–149.

154. Braasch JW, Deziel DJ, Rossi RL, et al. Pyloric and gastric preserving pancreatic resection: experience with 87 patients. *Ann Surg* 1986;204:411–418.

155. Trede M, Schwall G, Saeger H. Survival after pancreatico-duodenectomy: 118 consecutive resections without an operative mortality. *Ann Surg* 1990;211:447–458.

156. Yeo CJ, Cameron JL, Lillemoe KD, et al. Pancreaticoduodenectomy for cancer of the head of the pancreas. *Ann Surg* 1995;221:721–733.

157. Anderson HB, Baden H, Brahe NEB, Burcharth F. Pancreaticoduodenectomy for periampullary adenocarcinoma. *J Am Coll Surg* 1994;179:545–552.

158. Fortner JG. Regional pancreatectomy for cancer of the pancreas, ampulla, and other related sites. *Ann Surg* 1984;199:418–425.

159. Ishikawa O, Ohhigashi H, Sasaki Y, et al. Practical usefulness of lymphatic and connective tissue clearance for the carcinoma of the pancreas head. *Ann Surg* 1988;208:215–220.

160. Manabe T, Ohshio G, Baba N, et al. Radical pancreatectomy for ductal cell carcinoma of the head of the pancreas. *Cancer* 1989;64:1132–1137.

161. Connolly MM, Dawson PJ, Michelassi F, et al. Survival in 1001 patients with carcinoma of the pancreas. *Ann Surg* 1987;206:366–373.

162. Van Heerden JA. Pancreatic resection for carcinoma of pancreas: Whipple versus total pancreatectomy—an institutional perspective. *World J Surg* 1989;8:880–888.

163. Moosa AR. Pancreatic cancer: approach to diagnosis, selection of surgery and choice of operation. *Cancer* 1982;50:2689–2698.

164. Satake K, Nishiwaki H, Yokomatsu H, et al. Surgical curability and prognosis for standard versus extended resections for T1 carcinoma of the pancreas. *Surg Gynecol Obstet* 1992;175:259–265.

165. Shirai Y, Yosida K, Tsukada K, Ohtani T, Muto T. Identification of the regional lymphatic system of the gallbladder by vital staining. *Br J Surg* 1992;79:659–662.

166. Gall FP, Kockerling F, Scheele J, Schneider C, Hohenberger W. Radical operations for carcinoma of the gallbladder: present status in Germany. *World J Surg* 1991;15:328–336.

167. Onoyama H, Yamamoto M, Tseng A, Ajiki T, Saitoh Y. Extended cholecystectomy for carcinoma of the gallbladder. *World J Surg* 1995;19:758–763.

168. Pradeep R, Kaushik SP, Sikora SS, Bhattacharya BN, Pandey CM, Kapoor VK. Predictors of survival in patients with carcinoma of the gallbladder. *Cancer* 1995;76:1145–1149.

169. Shirai Y, Yoshida K, Tsukada K, Muto T. Inapparent carcinoma of the gallbladder: an appraisal of a radical second operation after simple cholecystectomy. *Ann Surg* 1992;215:326–331.

170. Shirai Y, Yoshida K, Tsukada K, Muto T, Watanabe H. Radical surgery for gallbladder carcinoma. Long-term results. *Ann Surg* 1992;216:565–568.

171. Bloechle C, Izbicki JR, Passlick B, et al. Is radical surgery in locally advanced gallbladder carcinoma justified? *Am J Gastroenterol* 1995;90:2195–2200.

172. Nakamura S, Nishiyama R, Yokoi Y, et al. Hepatopancreatoduodenectomy for advanced gallbladder carcinoma. *Arch Surg* 1994;129:625–629.

173. Mimura H, Takakura N, Kim H, Hamazaki K, Tsuge H, Ochiai Y. Block resection of the hepatoduodenal ligament for carcinoma of the bile duct and gallbladder: surgical technique and a report of 11 cases. *Hepatogastroenterology* 1991;38:561–567.

174. Herskovic A, Martz K, Al-Sarraf M, et al. Combined chemotherapy and radiotherapy compared with radiotherapy alone in patients with cancer of the esophagus. *N Engl J Med* 1992;326:1593–1598.

175. Skinner DB. En bloc resection for neoplasms of the esophagus and cardia. *J Thorac Cardiovasc Surg* 1983;85:59.

176. Akiyama H. Squamous cell carcinoma of the thoracic esophagus. In: Akiyama H, ed. *Surgery for cancer of the esophagus*. Baltimore: Williams & Wilkins; 1990:19–49.

177. Hennessy TPJ. Lymph node dissection. *World J Surg* 1994;18:367–372.

178. Akiyama H, Tsurumaru M, Kawamura T, et al. Principles of surgical treatment for carcinoma of the esophagus: analysis of lymph node involvement. *Ann Surg* 1981;194:438–446.

179. Tsurumaru M, Akiyama H, Udagawa H, Ono Y, Suzuki M, Watanabe G. Cervical-thoracic-abdominal lymph node dissection for intrathoracic esophageal carcinoma. In: Ferguson MK, Little AG, Skinner DB, eds. *Disease of the esophagus: malignant diseases*. New York: Futura; 1990:187–196.

180. Tanabe G, Baba M, Kuroshima K, et al. Clinical evaluation of esophageal lymph flow system based on the RI uptake of removed regional lymph nodes following lymphoscintigraphy. *J Jpn Surg Soc* 1986;87:315–323.

181. Siewert JR, Roder JD. Lymphadenectomy in esophageal cancer surgery. *Diseases of the Esophagus* 1992;5:91.

182. Baba M, Aikou T, Yoshinaka H, et al. Long-term results of subtotal esophagectomy with three-field lymphadenectomy for carcinoma of the thoracic esophagus. *Ann Surg* 1994;219:310–316.

183. Akiyama H, Tsurumaru M, Udagawa H, Kajiyama Y. Radical lymph node dissection for cancer of the thoracic esophagus. *Ann Surg* 1994;220:364–373.

184. Isono K, Sato H, Nakayama K. Result of a nationwide study on the three-field lymph node dissection of esophageal cancer. *Oncology* 1991;48:411.

185. Fujita H, Kakegawa T, Yamana H, et al. Lymph node metastasis and recurrence in patients with a carcinoma of the thoracic esophagus who underwent three-field dissection. *World J Surg* 1994;18:266–272,.

186. Skinner DB. Invited letter concerning: how extensive should lymph node dissection be for cancer of the thoracic esophagus? *J Thorac Cardiovasc Surg* 1994;107:1154–1174.

187. Kato H, Watanabe H, Tachmimori, Iizuka T. Evaluation of neck lymph node dissection for thoracic esophageal carcinoma. *Ann Thorac Surg* 1991;51:931.

188. Fujita H, Kakegawa T, Yamana H, et al. Mortality and morbidity rates, postoperative course, quality of life, and prognosis after extended radical lymphadenectomy for esophageal cancer: comparison of three-field lymphadenectomy with two-field lymphadenectomy. *Ann Surg* 1995;222:654–662.

189. Kato H. Lymph node dissection for thoracic esophageal carcinoma. *Ann Chir Gynaecol* 1995;84:193–199.

190. Baba H, Maehara Y, Inutsuka S, et al. Effectiveness of extended lymphadenectomy in noncurative gastrectomy. *Am J Surg* 1995;169: 261–264.

191. Lisborg P, Jatzko G, Horn M, et al. Radical surgery (R2 resection) for gastric cancer: a multivariate analysis. *Scand J Gastroenterol* 1994;29:1024–1028.

192. Stipa S. DiGiorgio A, Ferri M, Botti C. Results of curative gastrectomy for carcinoma. *J Am Coll Surg* 1994;179:567–572.

193. Bunt AM, Hermans J, Boon MC, et al. Evaluation of the extent of lymphadenectomy in a randomized trial of Western- versus Japanese-type surgery in gastric cancer. *J Clin Oncol* 1994;12:417–422. ·

194. Kim JP, Hur YS, Yang HK. Lymph node metastasis as a significant prognostic factor in early gastric cancer: analysis of 1,136 early gastric cancers. *Annals of Surgical Oncology* 1995;2:308–313.

195. Roder JD, Busch R, Stein HJ, Fink U, Siewert JR. Ratio of invaded to removed lymph nodes as a predictor of survival in squamous cell carcinoma of the oesophagus. *Br J Surg* 1994;81:410–413.

196. Japanese Research Society for Stomach Cancer. The general rules for gastric cancer study. *Jpn J Surg* 1981;16:121–123.

197. Songun I, Bonenkamp JJ, Sasako M, Bunt AMG, Hermans J, van de Velde CJH. Current results of randomized studies about the extent of lymph node dissection: quality control in lymphadenectomy for gastric cancer in a prospective randomized multicenter trial in the Netherlands. *Digestive Surgery* 1994;11:86–92.

198. Okusa T, Nakane Y, Boku T, et al. Quantitative analysis of nodal involvement with respect to survival rate after curative gastrectomy for carcinoma. *Surg Gynecol Obstet* 1990;170:488–494.

199. Isozaki H, Okajima K, Kawashima Y, et al. Prognostic value of the number of metastatic lymph nodes in gastric cancer with radical surgery. *J Surg Oncol* 1993;53:247–251.

200. Noguchi M, Miyazaki I. Prognostic significance and surgical management of lymph node metastasis in gastric cancer. *Br J Surg* 1996;83:156–161.

201. Baba H, Maehara Y, Takeuchi H, et al. Effect of lymph node dissection on the prognosis of node negative early gastric cancer. *Surgery* 1995;117:165–169.

202. Maruyama K, Okabayashi K, Kinoshita T. Progress in gastric cancer surgery in Japan and its limits of radicality. *World J Surg* 1987;11: 406–411.

203. Lee WJ, Lee WC, Houng SJ, et al. Survival after resection of gastric cancer and prognostic relevance of systematic lymph node dissection: twenty years experience in Taiwan. *World J Surg* 1995; 19:707–713.

204. Volpe CM, Koo J, Miloro SM, Driscoll DL, Nava HR, Douglass HO. The effect of extended lymphadenectomy on survival in patients with gastric adenocarcinoma. *J Am Coll Surg* 1995;181:56–64.

205. Pacelli F, Doglietto GB, Bellantone R, Alfieri S, Sgadari A, Crucitti F. Extensive versus limited lymph node dissection for gastric cancer: a comparative study of 320 patients. *Br J Surg* 1993;80:1153–1156.

206. Siewert JR, Bottcher K, Roder JD, Busch R, Hermanek P, Meyer HJ. Prognostic significance of systemic lymph node dissection in gastric carcinoma: German Gastric Carcinoma Study Group. *Br J Surg* 1993; 80:1015–1018.

207. Sugarbaker PH, Corlew S. Influence of surgical techniques on survival in patients with colorectal cancer. *Dis Colon Rectum* 1982;25: 545–557.

208. Gabriel WB, Dukes C, Bussey HJ. Lymphatic spread in cancer of the rectum. *Br J Surg* 1935;23:395–413.

209. August DA, Ottow RT, Sugarbaker PH. Clinical perspective of human colon cancer metastasis. 1984;3:303–324.

210. Dukes CE, Bussey HJR. The spread of rectal cancer and its effect on prognosis. *Br J Cancer* 1958;12:309–320.

211. The French Association for Surgical Research, Rouffet F, Hay JM, Vacher B, et al. Curative resection for left colonic carcinoma: hemicolectomy vs. segmental colectomy—a prospective, controlled, multicenter trial. *Dis Colon Rectum* 1994;37:651–659.

212. Laurie JA, Mortel CG, Fleming TR, et al. Surgical adjuvant therapy of large bowel carcinoma: an evaluation of levamisole and the combination of levamisole and fluorouracil. *J Clin Oncol* 1989;7:1447–1456.

213. Moertel C, Fleming T, MacDonald J et al. Levamisole and fluorouracil for adjuvant therapy of resected colon carcinoma. *N Engl J Med* 1990; 322:352–358.

214. Moertel CG, Fleming TR, MacDonald JS, et al. Fluorouracil plus levamisole as effective adjuvant therapy after resection of stage III colon carcinoma: a final report. *Ann Intern Med* 1995;122:321–326.

215. International Multicenter Pooled Analysis of Colon Cancer Trials (IMPACT). Efficacy of adjuvant fluorouracil and folinic acid in colon cancer. *Lancet* 1995;345:939–944.

216. Enker WE, Laffer UT, Block GE. Enhanced survival of patients with colon and rectal cancer is based upon wide anatomic resection. *Ann Surg* 1979;190:350–360.

217. Enker WE, Heilweil ML, Hertz RE, et al. En bloc pelvic lymphadenectomy and sphincter preservation in the surgical management of rectal cancer. *Ann Surg* 1986;203:426–433.

218. Cawthorne SJ, Parums DV, Gibbs NM, et al. Extent of mesorectal spread and involvement of lateral resection margin as prognostic factors after surgery for rectal cancer. *Lancet* 1990;335:1055–1059.

219. Ng IOL, Luk ISC, Yuen ST, et al. Surgical lateral clearance in resected rectal carcinomas: a multivariate analysis of clinicopathologic features. *Cancer* 1993;71:1972–1976.

220. MacFarlane JK, Ryall RDH, Heald RJ. Mesorectal excision for rectal cancer. *Lancet* 1993;341:457–460.

221. Heald RJ. Total mesorectal excision is optimal surgery for rectal cancer: a Scandinavian consensus. *Br J Surg* 1995;82:1297–1299.

222. Scott N, Jackson P, Al-Jaberi T, Dixon MF, Quirke P, Finan PJ. Total mesorectal excision and local recurrence: a study of tumour spread in the mesorectum distal to rectal cancer. *Br J Surg* 1995;82:1031–1033.

223. Gastrointestinal Tumor Study Group. Radiation therapy and fluorouracil with or without semustine for the treatment of patients with surgical adjuvant adenocarcinoma of the rectum. *J Clin Oncol* 1992; 10:549–557.

224. Fisher B, Wolmark N, Rockette H, et al. Postoperative adjuvant chemotherapy or radiation therapy for rectal cancer: results from NSABP Protocol R-01. *J Natl Cancer Inst* 1988;80:21–29.

225. Krook JE, Moertel CG, Gunderson LL, et al. Effective surgical adjuvant therapy for high-risk rectal carcinoma. *N Engl J Med* 1991;324: 709–715.

226. Gerard A, Buyse M, Nordlinger B, et al. Preoperative radiotherapy as adjuvant treatment in rectal cancer: final results of a randomized study of the European Organization for Research and Treatment of Cancer (EORTC). *Ann Surg* 1988;208:606–614.

227. Cedermark B. The Stockholm II trial on preoperative short term radiotherapy in operable rectal carcinoma: a prospective randomized trial (Abstract). *Proceedings of the American Society of Clinical Oncology* 1994;13:198.

228. Freedman GM, Coia LR. Adjuvant and neoadjuvant treatment of rectal cancer. *Semin Oncol* 1995;22:611–624.

229. Bosset JF, Horiot JC. Adjuvant treatment in the curative management of rectal cancer: a critical review of the results of clinical randomised trials. *Eur J Cancer* 1993;29A:770–774.

230. McDonald MW. Current therapy for renal cell carcinoma. *J Urol* 1982;127:211–217.

231. Giulani L, Giberti C, Martorana G, et al. Radical extensive surgery for renal cell carcinoma: long-term results and prognostic factors. *J Urol* 1990;143:468.

232. Tsukamoto T, Kumamoto Y, Miyao N, et al. Regional lymph node metastasis in renal cell carcinoma: incidence, distribution and its relation to other pathological findings. *Eur Urol* 1990;8:88.

233. Herrlinger A, Schrott KM, Sigel A. What are the benefits of extended dissection of the regional renal lymph nodes in the therapy of renal cell carcinoma? *J Urol* 1991;146:1224–1227.

234. Golimbu M, Joshi P, Sperber A, Tessler A, Al-Askari S, Morales P.

Renal cell carcinoma: survival and prognostic factors. *Urology* 1986; 27:291.

235. Peters PC, Brown GL. The role of lymphadenectomy in the management of renal cell carcinoma. *Urol Clin North Am* 1980;7:705.

236. Gilloz A, Tostain J, Rusch P. L association d une cellulo-lymphadénectomie à las nèphrectomie élargie: est-elle justifiée dans le traitement des cancers du rein? *Ann Urol* 1982;16:207.

237. Lieskovsky G, Skinner DG. Role of lymphadenectomy in the treatment of bladder cancer. *Urol Clin North Am* 1984;11:709–716.

238. Whitmore WF. Surgical management of low stage bladder cancer. *Semin Oncol* 1979;6:207–216.

239. Skinner DG. Current perspectives in the management of high-grade invasive bladder cancer. *Cancer* 1980;45:1866–1874.

240. Vieweg J, Whitmore WF, Herr HW, et al. The role of pelvic lymphadenectomy and radical cystectomy for lymph node positive bladder cancer. *Cancer* 1994;73:3020–3028.

241. Lerner SP, Skinner DG, Leiskovsky G, et al. The rationale for en bloc pelvic lymph node dissection for bladder cancer patients with nodal metastases: long-term results. *J Urol* 1993;149:758–765.

242. Fair WR, Fuks ZY, and Scher HI. Cancer of the bladder. In: DeVita VT, Hellman S, Rosenberg SA, eds. *Cancer: principles and practice of oncology.* 4th ed. Philadelphia: JB Lippincott; 1993:1052–1072.

243. Hanks GE, Myers CE, Scardino PT. Cancer of the prostate. In: DeVita VT, Hellman S, Rosenberg SA, eds. *Cancer: principles and practice of oncology.* 4th ed. Philadelphia: JB Lippincott; 1993:1073–1113.

244. Pistenma DA, Bagshaw MA, Freiha FS. Extended-field radiation therapy for prostatic adenocarcinoma: status report of a limited prospective trial. In: Johnson DE, Samuels ML, eds. *Cancer of the genitourinary tract.* New York: Raven Press; 1979:229–247.

245. Fowler JE, Jr., Whitmore, WF, et al. The incidence and extent of pelvic lymph node metastases in apparently localized prostatic cancer. *Cancer* 1981;47:2941.

246. Donahue RE, Mau JH, Whitsel JA, et al. Pelvic lymph node dissection: guide to patient management in clinically locally confined adenocarcinoma of the prostate. *Urology* 1982;20:559–565.

247. Walsh PC, Jewett HJ. Radical surgery for prostatic cancer. *Cancer* 1980;45:1906–1911.

248. Schmidt JD, McLaughlin AP III, Saltzstein SL, et al. Risk factors for the development of distant metastases in patients undergoing pelvic lymphadenectomy for prostatic cancer. *Am J Surg* 1982;144:131–135.

249. Paulson DF. The prognostic role of lymphadenectomy in adenocarcinoma of the prostate. *Urol Clin North Am* 1980;7:615–622.

250. Cline WA, Kramer SF, Farnham R, et al. Impact of pelvic lymphadenectomy in patients with prostatic adenocarcinoma. *Urology* 1981;17:129–131.

251. Prout GR Jr, Heaney JA, Grifffin P, et al. Nodal involvement as a prognostic indicator in patients with prostatic carcinoma. *J Urol* 1980; 124:226–231.

252. Hanks GE, Asbell S, Krall JM, et al. Outcome for lymph node dissection negative T-16, T-2 (A-2,B) prostate cancer treated with external beam radiation therapy in RTOG 77-06. *Int J Radiat Oncol Biol Phys* 1991;21:1099–1103.

252a. Hanks GE, Krall JM, Pilepich MV, et al. Comparison of pathologic and clinical evaluation of lymph nodes in prostate cancer: implications of RTOG data for patient management and trial design and stratification. *Int J Radiat Oncol Biol Phys* 1992;23:293–298.

253. Kramer SA, Cline WA Jr, Farnham R, et al. Prognosis of patients with stage D-1 prostatic adenocarcinoma. *J Urol* 1981;125:817–819.

254. Einhorn LH, Richie JP, Shipley WU. Cancer of the testis. In: DeVita VT, Hellman S, Rosenberg SA, eds. *Cancer: principles and practice of oncology.* 4th ed. Philadelphia: JB Lippincott; 1993:1126–1151.

255. Motzer RJ, Bosh GJ, Geller N, et al. Advanced seminoma: The role of chemotherapy and adjunctive surgery. Ann Intern Med 108:513–518, 1988.

256. Einhorn LH, Wiliams SD, Mandelbaum I, et al. Surgical resection in disseminated testicular cancer following chemotherapeutic cytoreduction. *Cancer* 48:904–908, 1981;.

257. Dunnick NR, Javodpour N. Value of CT and lymphography: distinguishing retroperitoneal metastases from nonseminomatous testicular tumors. *AJR Am J Roentgenol* 1981;136:1093–1099.

258. Fair WR, Fuks ZY, Scher HI. Cancer of the urethra and penis. In DeVita VT, Hellman S, Rosenberg SA, eds. *Cancer: principles and*

practice of oncology. 4th ed. Philadelphia: JB Lippincott; 1993: 1114–1125.

259. Cabanas R. An approach to the treatment of penile carcinoma. *Cancer* 1977;39:456.

260. Ornellas AA, Seixas ALC, Marota A, Wisnescky A, Campos F, de Moreas JR. Surgical treatment of invasive squamous cell carcinoma of the penis: retrospective analysis of 350 cases. *J Urol* 1994;151: 1244–1249.

261. Grabstald H. Controversies concerning lymph node dissection for cancer of the penis. *Urol Clin North Am* 1980;7:793. .

262. Beggs JH, Spratt JS. Epidermoid carcinoma of the penis. *J Urol* 1964;91:166–177.

263. Hardner GJ, Bhanalph T, Murphy GP, Albert DJ, Moore RH. Carcinoma penis: analysis of therapy in 100 conservative cases. *J Urol* 1972;108:428–430.

264. Dekernion JB, Tynberg P, Persky L. Carcinoma of the penis. *Cancer* 1973;32:1256–1262.

265. Johnson DE, Lo RK. Management of regional lymphnodes in penile carcinoma: Five year result following therapeutic groin dissections. *Urology* 1984;24:308–311.

266. Whitmore WF Jr, Vagaiwala MR. A technique of ilioinguinal lymph node dissection for carcinoma of the penis. *Surg Gynecol Obstet* 1984;159:573.

267. McDougal WS. Carcinoma of the penis: improved survival by early regional lymphadenectomy based on the histological grad and depth of invasion of the primary lesion. *J Urol* 1995;154:1364–1366.

268. Kulkarni JN, Kamat MR. Prophylactic bilateral groin node dissection versus prophylactic radiotherapy and surveillance in patients with N0 and N1-2A carcinoma of the penis. *Eur Urol* 1994;26:123–128.

269. Abi-Aad AS, de Kernion JB. Controversies in ilio-inguinal lymphadenectomy for cancer of the penis. *Urol Clin North Am* 1992;19: 319–324.

270. Hoskins WJ, Perez CA, Young RC. Gynecologic tumors. In: DeVita VT, Hellman S, Rosenberg SA, eds. *Cancer: principles and practice of oncology.* 4th ed. Philadelphia: JB Lippincott; 1993:1152–1225.

271. DiSaia PJ. Surgical aspects of cervical carcinoma. *Cancer* 1981;48: 548–559.

272. Hammond JA, Henson J, Freedman RS, et al. The impact of lymph node status on survival in cervical carcinoma. *Int J Radiat Oncol Biol Phys* 1981;7:1713–1718.

273. Burghardt E, Pickel H, Haas J, Lahausen M. Prognostic factors and operative treatment of stage IB to IIB cervical cancer. *Am J Obstet Gynecol* 1987;156:988–996.

274. Lewis GC, Bundy B. Surgery for endometrial cancer. *Cancer* 1981; 48:568–574.

275. Young RC, Perez CA, Hoskins WJ. Cancer of the ovary. In: DeVita VT, Hellman S, Rosenberg SA, eds. *Cancer: principles and practice of oncology.* Philadelphia: JB Lippincott; 1993:1226–1263.

276. Athey PA, Wallace S, Jing B, et al. Lymphangiography in ovarian cancer. *AJR Am J Roentgenol* 1975;123:106–113.

277. Musumeci R, DePalo G, Kenda R, et al. Retroperitoneal metastases from ovarian carcinoma: reassessment of 365 patients studies with lymphography. *AJR Am J Roentgenol* 1980;134:449–452.

278. DiSaia PJ, Creasman WT, Rich WM. An alternate approach to early cancer of the vulva. *Am J Obstet Gynecol* 1979;133:825–832.

279. Burger MPM, Hollema H, Emanuels AG, Krans M, Pras E, Bouma J. The importance of the groin node status for the survival of T1 and T2 vulval carcinoma patients. *Gynecol Oncol* 1995;57:327–334.

280. Podratz KC, Symmonds RE, Taylor WF, Williams TJ. Carcinoma of the vulva: analysis of treatment and survival. *Obstet Gynecol* 1983; 61:63–74.

281. Burke TW, Levenback C, Coleman RL, Morris M, Silva EG, Gershenson DM. Surgical therapy of T1 and T2 vulvar carcinoma: further experience with radical wide excision and selective inguinal lymphadenectomy. *Gynecol Oncol* 1995;57:215–220.

282. Andrews SJ, Williams BT, DePriest PD, et al. Therapeutic implications of lymph nodal spread in lateral T1 and T2 squamous cell carcinoma of the vulva. *Gynecol Oncol* 1994;55:41–46.

283. Catlin D. Surgery for head and neck lymphomas. *Surgery* 1966;60: 1160–1166.

284. Shiu MH, Karas M, Nisce L, et al. Management of primary gastric lymphoma. *Ann Surg* 1982;195:196–202.

285. Bozzetti F, Audisio RA, Giardini R, Gennari L. Role of surgery in

patients with primary non-Hodgkin's lymphoma of the stomach: an old problem revisited. *Br J Surg* 1993;80:1101–1106.

286. Valicenti RK, Wasserman TH, Kucik NA. Analysis of prognostic factors in localized gastric lymphoma: the importance of bulk of disease. *Int J Radiat Oncol Biol Phys* 1993;27:591–598.

287. Taal BG, Burgers JM, van Heerde P, Hart AA, Somers R. The clinical spectrum and treatment of primary non-Hodgkin's lymphoma of the stomach. *Ann Oncol* 1993;4:839–846.

288. Johnsson A, Brun E, Akerman M, Cavallin-Stahl E. Primary gastric non-Hodgkin's lymphoma: a retrospective clinico-pathological study. *Acta Oncol* 1992;31:525–531.

289. Jenkin RDT, Allt WEC, Fitzpatrick PJ. Osteosarcoma: an assessment of management with particular reference to primary irradiation and selective delayed amputation. *Cancer* 1972;30:393–399.

290. Weingrad DN, Rosenberg SA. Early lymphatic spread of osteogenic and soft tissue sarcomas. *Surgery* 1978;84:231–240.

291. Mazeron JJ and Suit HD. Lymph nodes as sites of metastases from sarcomas of soft tissue. *Cancer* 1987;60:1800–1808.

292. Fong Y, Coit DG, Woodruff JM, Brennan MF. Lymph node metastasis from soft tissue sarcoma in adults: analysis of data from a prospective database of 1772 sarcoma patients. *Ann Surg* 1993;217:72–77.

CHAPTER 25

Isolated Perfusion of Extremity Tumors

Douglas L. Fraker and Daniel G. Coit

Recently, as a result of experiences with a heart–lung apparatus in the treatment of intra-cardiac defects, it occurred to us that this extracorporeal circuit might provide a means of temporarily isolating and maintaining a tumor-bearing area while it was being perfused with maximal amounts of an alkylating agent. If vascular and lymphatic exclusion were complete, systemic toxic effects should be eliminated while the specific activity of the agents would be brought to bear only upon the tumor and its immediate environment.

—*Creech (1)*

RATIONALE AND HISTORY

It is estimated that 10% to 20% of patients who relapse after initial treatment of their melanoma present with metastatic in-transit disease clinically confined to an extremity (Fig. 1). From a biologic standpoint, the best evidence that all remaining disease is confined to the extremity in these patients comes from a review by Jaques and colleagues, looking at a historical series of major extremity amputations in the management of regionally recurrent melanoma (2). In this review, curative major amputation was associated with a 42% 5-year survival rate in 24 patients with in-transit metastasis of the extremity. Although not advocating amputation as the initial treatment of choice for these patients, the authors concluded that all clinically relevant disease was confined to the amputated extremity in those long-term survivors.

Isolation limb perfusion (ILP) emerged as a treatment modality in the management of patients with regionally confined melanoma in an effort to achieve control of the tumor without the attendant morbidity of major amputation. It is important to realize that, as implied by the review of major amputations, most of these patients have occult systemic disease that will be unaffected by regional therapy. Thus, even with a 100% durable complete response rate to ILP, long-term survival would be achieved in approximately one third of patients.

The extremities are uniquely suited to regional treatment because the arterial inflow and venous outflow can be identified and isolated with relative ease. A number of clinical trials have been reported using intra-arterial infusion chemotherapy without isolation, with or without temporary venous outflow occlusion (3–8). Clinical results of these earlier trials have been unimpressive, most likely because the extremities have no inherent capacity for first-pass drug extraction.

Isolation limb perfusion differs from infusion in that both the arterial inflow and venous outflow are cannulated, with the root of the limb controlled by tourniquet. Under these conditions, with an extracorporeal membrane oxygenator, a number of variables, including temperature, oxygen tension, and pH of the limb, can be controlled. More important, the limb can be exposed to extremely high concentrations of cytotoxic drugs while minimizing the risk of systemic toxicity. This can result in substantially increased tumor exposure to drug, as measured by the area under the time–concentration curve when compared with similar drug doses given systemically (9–11).

Isolation limb perfusion in humans was initially reported by Creech and associates in 1958, with 18 of 19 patients perfused with melphalan for advanced extremity malignancy showing a dramatic tumor response (12). The synergism of hyperthermia and high-dose chemotherapy was reported in vitro by Cavaliere et al. in 1967 (13), and subsequently in humans in the setting of ILP by Stehlin in 1969 (14). Over the ensuing 20 years, a large number of trials have been reported using this technique, primarily in patients with melanoma, and to a lesser extent in patients with regionally confined tumors such as extremity soft tissue sarcoma. Despite the volume of published data, meaningful interpretation of

D. L. Fraker: Division of Surgical Oncology, Department of Surgery, University of Pennsylvania, Philadelphia, Pennsylvania 19104.

D. G. Coit: Department of Surgery, Memorial Sloan-Kettering Cancer Center, New York, New York 10021.

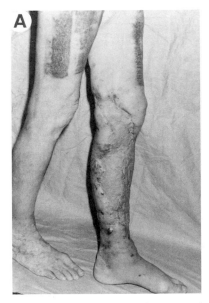 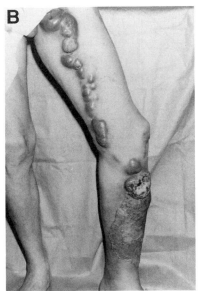 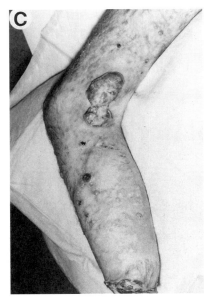

FIG. 1. Examples of three patients with regionally advanced melanoma who have failed surgical excision. **A:** Patient with a lower leg melanoma who had undergone multiple wide excisions with almost one-half of the surface of the lower leg skin grafted, now with multiple recurrences in and around the skin graft sites. **B:** Patient with an anterior calf lesion with an extensive bordering local recurrence and extension along the medial thigh. **C:** Patient with an ankle melanoma who had local recurrences treated with a below-knee amputation, and now has extensive dermal and subcutaneous in-transit lesions throughout the amputated limb.

results has been hampered by a lack of formal phase I (optimal dose, toxicity, pharmacokinetics), phase II (response rate), and phase III (efficacy) data. There has been no consistent staging system for recurrent in-transit melanoma, making comparison of results between trials and interpretation of trials using historical control patients impossible. Varying amounts of surgery are performed in association with limb perfusion, both between and within studies; the impact of perfusion in patients in whom all recurrent disease can be resected is difficult to compare to that in whom in-transit disease is unresectable. Finally, varying perfusion regimens have been reported, again both between and within studies that have evolved over extended periods of time. Perfusions may be normothermic or hyperthermic, and have used a number of drugs, either alone or in combination. The most commonly used drug in ILP is melphalan; other drugs used include nitrogen mustard, dacarbazine (DTIC), actinomycin D, cisplatinum (CDDP), and thiotepa. Although the rationale for the use of the alkylating agents is sound, the rationale for selection of other agents is less clear. DTIC, which has modest activity when given systemically, is thought to require microsomal activation in the liver for at least a portion of its antineoplastic effect, and therefore would not appear to be an ideal agent for use in a limb perfusion circuit. Finally, the optimal dose of even the most common agent, melphalan, has not been determined by formal phase I dose-escalation studies. There are number of different methods for calculating total drug dose (mg/m^2 body surface area, mg/kg body weight, or mg/l of perfused limb), and substantial variability exists in the total drug dose used, again both between and within studies.

Against this background, a number of investigators recently have been working prospectively and critically to define the role of this modality in the treatment of patients with regionally recurrent melanoma. Those results are discussed in detail later.

Indications

Indications for ILP vary widely according to the enthusiasm with which the clinician embraces this modality. There are clinicians who believe empirically that patients at risk for regionally recurrent disease, including those with intermediate or thicker primary extremity melanomas, subungual or acral lentiginous primaries, or those patients with positive regional nodes might benefit from adjuvant hyperthermic ILP to enhance locoregional control. Others believe that limb perfusion is appropriate for patients with either local recurrence or minimal in-transit disease that can be completely surgically resected—patients who are at substantial risk for further regional recurrence. Finally, there are those who think that limb perfusion should be restricted to the treatment of patients with surgically unresectable, regionally recurrent melanoma.

Although a constant visible reminder of recurrence, in-transit metastases are rarely symptomatic in the early stages. Therefore, a clear distinction needs to be made between perfusions done for relatively asymptomatic disease with curative intent, and those done for bulky, symptomatic lesions for palliative intent. In patients in whom limb perfusion is being performed with curative intent, in either the adjuvant or therapeutic setting, a very comprehensive disease evaluation is important to rule out evidence of disease outside the extremity. In patients for whom perfusion is being performed with palliative intent, minor disease outside of the field of perfusion is acceptable, as long as the extent of that disease does not preclude a reasonable survival.

Finally, patients must be suitable candidates for perfusion. In particular, for the most part, in the lower extremity disease should be confined to the leg distal to the mid-thigh, because the buttock and proximal posterior thigh are relatively poorly perfused, even with iliac cannulation. For the upper extremity, disease in the upper posterior arm is poorly perfused, even with axillary vessel cannulation. In addition, the patient should have adequate peripheral arterial circulation. Patients without palpable distal pulses are not good candidates for limb perfusion. In addition, because perfusion flow rates ultimately depend on the adequacy of venous return, patients with evidence of deep venous thrombosis are not good candidates for ILP.

DETAILED METHODOLOGY

Isolation limb perfusion consists of an initial dissection to prepare vessels for cannulation, the perfusion itself, decannulation, and closure (15,16). The first deci-

sion when performing an ILP is to select at which anatomic level the vessels are to be cannulated. The choices for lower extremity perfusion are external iliac, common femoral, or the popliteal vessels. Choices for upper extremity perfusions are axillary or brachial vessels. For patients with melanoma, the most proximal cannulation site should be selected to maximize the area of treatment of the extremity because the entire limb is at risk for in-transit metastases with this histologic type. Therefore, either external iliac or common femoral vessel cannulation for lower extremities and axillary vessel cannulation for upper extremities are the best choices for melanoma patients. Distal cannulation sites (popliteal/brachial) have the advantages of being a much shorter and simpler approach and having a lower incidence of perfusate leak. The disadvantage of these distal approaches is that the proximal half of the extremity is untreated and subject to recurrent in-transit melanoma lesions. A distal cannulation site for ILP may be selected for melanoma patients who require a second or third procedure in which a repeat vascular dissection may be difficult or hazardous. A second indication is in patients with extremity sarcoma. The natural history of sarcoma is to spread hematogenously to the lungs, and not locoregionally, as for in-transit melanoma lesions. For this reason, in sarcoma patients undergoing limb perfusion, vessels should be chosen for cannulation at the most distal site that would clearly perfuse the entire tumor mass.

The most common patient eligible for ILP is one with melanoma of the lower extremity. Therefore, the most common procedure is an external iliac ILP, and this operation is described in detail, with highlights of other types of ILP mentioned (Fig. 2). The external iliac vessels are exposed by an oblique lower abdominal incision with entry into the retroperitoneal space. The initial dissection

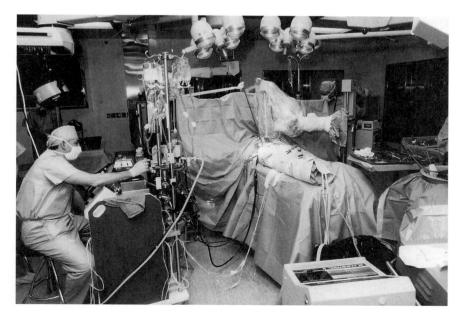

FIG. 2. A view of the overall operative setup to perform an isolation limb perfusion. This patient is being treated with a right lower extremity perfusion through the external iliac vessels. The perfusionist operating the roller pump is located on the left-hand side of the picture. Warming blankets are wrapped circumferentially around the extremity. Note the gamma counter positioned over the precordium and prepared into the field to monitor perfusate leak. Also, a Steinmann pin in the anterior superior iliac spine is connected to a pole that is secured to the anesthesia machine to maintain tourniquet tension.

circumferentially clears the external iliac artery and vein from their origin to where they become the common femoral vessels passing under the inguinal ligament, ligating all side branches. In performing this dissection, an obligatory deep inguinal lymph node sampling is necessary, and if there is any evidence of metastatic disease in this area, a formal lymph node dissection of this area is appropriate.

Proximally, the internal iliac artery is isolated such that it can be clamped during perfusion. The obturator artery is identified in the deep pelvis and ligated but not divided. The internal iliac vein has variable anatomy and may consist of a single large trunk or many moderate-sized branches directed posteriorly or laterally toward the buttocks or inferiorly toward the leg. Either the large main trunk or, preferably, specific branches that are directed toward the leg should be ligated. Control of the internal iliac vessels is important in minimizing perfusate leak in either direction through collateral vessels from the contralateral pelvis.

The final component of vascular isolation is placement of a circumferential tourniquet above the level of the tips of the cannula. For the external iliac approach, the inguinal crease secures the tourniquet medially, and laterally a Steinmann pin is placed into the anterior superior iliac spine to provide an anchor point for the tourniquet (see Fig. 2). A 4- to 6-inch–wide Esmarch tourniquet is used because it is strong enough as well as having the necessary elasticity. For additional safety, a long metal rod can be placed over the external part of the Steinmann pin to anchor it in an upright position so the pin will not become dislodged by tension from the tourniquet. The purpose of the tourniquet is to block flow through subcutaneous collaterals that are not controlled by the vascular dissection. The deep pelvic collaterals are not affected by this external tourniquet, and tourniquet placement does not replace appropriate surgical dissection.

Before placing the tourniquet, the vessels are cannulated. The external iliac vein is most posterior and it is easier to cannulate this vessel first. After the patient has been heparinized (200 U/kg), the vessel is clamped proximally and distally and a transverse venotomy is made with the cannula passed distally into the common femoral vein such that all side holes are well below the level of the tourniquet. An identical procedure is followed to place the arterial cannula through the external iliac artery. Long, straight venous cannulas are used for both the arterial and venous side of the circuit. The size range for the arterial cannula is generally between 12 and 20 Fr, and for the venous cannula between 18 and 24 Fr for an external iliac perfusion. For the more distal perfusions at the popliteal or brachial level, the appropriately smaller-sized cannulas are used.

After vessels are cannulated and the tourniquet is secured, the pump is started with the mean inflow line pressure monitored. The typical flow rate used for an external iliac perfusion varies widely depending on the patient's leg size and the isolation achieved. Target flow rates for external iliac perfusion perfusions vary between 400 ml/minute for small patients up to 900 to 1000 ml/minute for large patients, with an average rate of 600 to 700 ml/minute. The goal of the surgeon performing an ILP is to achieve the ideal situation with no communication between the perfusion circuit and the systemic circulation. Indications of leak include changes in the venous reservoir volume or signals from the radionuclide monitoring system, discussed later. Venous return is gravity-drained into a calibrated reservoir in the perfusion circuit. An increase in reservoir volume signifies a systemic-to-perfusate leak, and a decrease in reservoir volume signifies a perfusate-to-systemic leak. An equal but opposite leak would show no change in reservoir level and would be detected only by a monitoring system.

The perfusate leak monitoring system is based on continual assessment of a finite volume of systemic blood calibrated with a dose of a radioactive gamma emitter that remains in the vascular system during the perfusion (17–19). A larger amount of isotope is injected into the perfusion circuit, and any increase in counts seen on the gamma counter signifies a leak of perfusate to systemic circulation. Specifically, a thyroid counter on a movable arm is prepared in the sterile field and positioned over the precordium to monitor the systemic circulation (see Fig. 2). Twenty microcuries of ^{131}I albumin is injected systemically and allowed to distribute equally such that an increase from room background is defined for that particular patient (19). The degree of this increase depends on blood volume, chest wall size and configuration, and the precise position of the gamma counter. This calibration dose is not injected until the extremity is isolated with stable flow rates and reservoir volumes. After the increased counts detected from the calibration dose plateau, 200 µCi of ^{131}I albumin is injected into the perfusion circuit. Because the perfusion dose is 10-fold higher than the systemic calibration dose, a doubling of the initial increment signifies a 10% leak of perfusates. The reliability of this model is based on several assumptions. This model assumes a stable cardiac blood volume, no loss of ^{131}I albumin from the vascular space, and no breakdown into free iodine. Nevertheless, the ability to adapt the output from the gamma counter to a continuous readout system, such as a stripchart recorder or a digital meter, allows the surgeon to follow constantly the trend in counts detected, which very successfully identifies a perfusate leak and allows adjustments to be made to limit drug exposure.

Using these two pieces of information—the leak rate and the reservoir volume—the surgeon can manipulate the perfusion to minimize leak in either direction. Major initial leaks such as a 1% volume per minute or dramatic shifts in reservoir blood volume suggest a missed collateral vessel that needs to be ligated. Extension of the incision distally and division of the inguinal ligament almost always identifies a missed arterial or venous branch. A second possibility is malposition of the cannula such that the side holes are above the tourniquets, and this must be assessed. Minor changes or variable changes that occur during the perfusion can be managed by altering flow rate, adjusting the tourniquet, or increasing pressure in the venous outflow line. For a perfusate-to-systemic circulation leak, a decrease in the inflow rate lowers the line pressure and tends to decrease leak. Although maintaining mean perfusion pressure below mean arterial pressure may seem optimal, in certain cases the pressure relationship does not reflect the leak situation, and this guideline may be violated. Persistent perfusate leak may require turning off the pump, with adjustment of the tourniquet. For systemic-to-perfusate leaks signified by rising reservoir volume, increasing the flow in the circuit may correct the problem. A second way to decrease the systemic-to-perfusate leak is to change the venous outflow line pressure. Because this is a gravity drainage system, it may siphon off venous return that would otherwise go back to the heart, because it is positioned near the floor well below the level of the right atrium. Increasing venous line pressure by placing partial occluding clamps may rectify this problem. The clinical implication of systemic-to-perfusate leak is blood loss, and the potential problem of diluting the concentration of the perfusate drug occurs with systemic-to-perfusate leaks.

The most serious technical problem is a leak in both directions, with increasing reservoir volume but evidence of systemic exposure on the monitor system. In this situation, any adjustments made improve one situation while making the other component of the leak worse. Because the most significant toxicity to the patient arises from systemic drug exposure, efforts are made to decrease the perfusate-to-systemic leak. Again, decreasing flow rates and turning off the pump to reposition the tourniquet are potential maneuvers to improve isolation.

After the perfusion treatment period, the recirculating circuit is interrupted and the perfusate is flushed from the extremity with between 2 and 3 l of saline. The end of the wash needs to be some type of colloid (albumin, hetastarch, dextran, or blood) to maintain oncotic pressure within the vasculature during decannulation when the vessels are clamped. After the flush, the pump is turned off, the perfusion lines clamped, the tourniquet cut, and the cannula removed. The venotomy and arteriotomy are closed with vascular sutures and blood flow is re-established, first in the vein and then in the artery. A closed suction drain is placed in the deep pelvis because there may be accumulation of lymph after the lymph node dissection. The systemic heparinization may be reversed by protamine if thought necessary for hemostasis.

Mild hyperthermia is part of most limb perfusion protocols (20). Standard hyperthermia is considered to be temperatures of 41° to 42°C, with mild hyperthermia being 39° to 40°C (13). The tissue temperature in the extremity is increased in two ways. First, at the onset of the procedure, the extremity is wrapped circumferentially with one to two water jackets or warming blankets heated to 42°C (see Fig. 2). The perfusion circuit has a heat exchanger connected to a heater–cooler that warms the perfusate to 42°C. The tissue temperature is monitored by needle tip temperature probes placed subcutaneously and intramuscularly in both the leg and the thigh.

Although many of the aforementioned techniques apply to ILP at different cannulation sites, certain significant features of these other procedures should be noted. Common femoral ILP uses a tourniquet system identical to the one described for the external iliac approach. The common femoral vessels are cannulated just below the level of the inguinal ligament to perfuse both the deep and superficial femoral systems. Lateral circumflex vessels off the proximal profunda may be a source of leak and should be either clamped or ligated. A popliteal perfusion is performed through a longitudinal incision in the medial thigh to isolate the supergeniculate popliteal vessels as they exit Hunter's canal. A proximal circumferential thigh blood pressure cuff serves as a tourniquet (Fig. 3). For upper extremity perfusions, the axillary vessels are exposed by a curvilinear incision similar to that used for an axillary lymph node dissection. A small Steinmann pin is placed into the head of the humerus and an Esmarch tourniquet is wrapped around the root of the axilla. Compared to lower extremity ILP, the leak rate is usually much lower because the cross-sectional area of the root of the upper extremity is much smaller and easier to control than the similar cross-sectional area of the lower extremity. The main problem with the tourniquet is that if it is placed too tightly, the patient can suffer brachial plexus injury, and these nerves need to be protected with padding underneath the tourniquet. A brachial vessel perfusion is performed through a very small incision in the medial upper arm just proximal to the elbow. Again, the tourniquet is a blood pressure cuff above the cannulation site. For brachial and popliteal perfusions, a blood pressure cuff at 300 mm Hg provides such complete vascular isolation that minimal dissection of the vessels is needed.

SPECIAL INSTRUMENTATION OR AGENTS

The equipment needed to perform ILP consists at a minimum of the equipment used to do the perfusion, and preferably additional equipment to monitor perfusate leak and measure limb volume. The equipment used to perform the perfusion includes a pump, a heater–cooler unit, and disposable single-use perfusion packs (16). The optimal pump is a roller pump, as used for cardiopulmonary bypass in cardiac surgery. Unlike in cardiac procedures, a single-head pump is all that is required to perform ILP. The heater–cooler unit performs two functions that heat

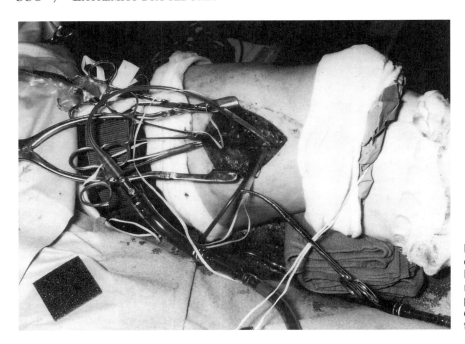

FIG. 3. A perfusion of the left lower extremity through the popliteal vessels. Note the perfusion cannula secured by the rumel tourniquet going into the proximal popliteal artery and vein. A blood pressure cuff tourniquet is used in the proximal thigh to obtain complete vascular isolation.

the tissues of the extremity. First, it heats the perfusate through the heat exchanger in the perfusion pack. Second, it connects to one or two recirculating water jackets that are wrapped circumferentially around the leg to maintain surface temperature. The disposable perfusion pack consists of tubing, a venous reservoir, and an oxygenator/heat exchanger. The typical pack used for an ILP is similar to standard, commercially available pediatric cardiac surgery packs because the lower flow rates and smaller prime volumes used in pediatric cases are more appropriate to the flow rates used in ILP. Finally, a multichannel temperature module to measure tissue temperatures at various sites throughout the limb continuously during perfusion is required.

An additional high-budget equipment item relates to monitoring of perfusate leak: a portable gamma counter with a system for continuous readout (19). Most institutions performing ILP either do not monitor leak except to follow venous reservoir volumes, or use a fluorescein injection to identify perfusate above the level of the tourniquet. Either of these approaches is inaccurate for measuring systemic exposure. The use of a precise system is mandatory with the addition of a potentially lethal dose of tumor necrosis factor (TNF) to the perfusate. Even with use of standard chemotherapeutic agents, the ability to perform ILP with low systemic exposure decreases systemic toxicity and maintains high drug levels in the perfusate. The specific equipment needed includes a gamma detector that can be positioned in the operative field over the heart—a portable thyroid scanner fulfills all of these requirements. Electronic equipment to adapt the output of disintegrations per minute (dpm) to either a digital or stripchart format completes the system.

A final piece of equipment specific for ILP is a device to measure limb volume, because many current protocols dose perfusate drugs based on the volume of the extremity treated (21). The most accurate technique is a water displacement method, in which the extremity is lowered into a calibrated cylinder filled with water. The cylinders are commercially available for upper extremities, but need to be custom made to accommodate lower extremity volumes. An alternative approach is to measure limb length and circumference at multiple points and use the mathematical formula for a cylinder to calculate an estimated limb volume.

SPECIAL PRECAUTIONS

In evaluating patients for the surgical procedure of ILP, the one specific difference from the general evaluation pertinent to any major surgical procedure is assessment of the patient's peripheral vascular system. ILP is a vascular surgical procedure and adequately sized arteries and veins are necessary to perform this operation. Evaluation of peripheral pulses and ankle–brachial index may suggest peripheral vascular disease and, if present, a formal angiogram to define the vascular anatomy is necessary. If there is unexplained leg edema, particularly in patients who had undergone a prior limb perfusion, evaluation of the venous system by ultrasound for deep venous thrombosis in the upper thigh/groin is appropriate.

RESPONSE RATES

The principal indication for performing ILP is to treat extremity melanoma, although the procedure is used to

TABLE 1. *Proportions of isolation limb perfusions done as therapeutic versus adjuvant treatments for extremity melanoma in various institutional reports*

Author	Years	No. patients	Therapeutic ILP[a]	Adjuvant ILP[b]
Bulman and Jamieson (22)	1959–79	75	29	46
Rosin and Westbury (23)	1960–79	150	80	70
Hartley and Fletcher (24)	1964–83	65	0	65
Martijn et al. (25)	1964–77	104	0	104
di Filippo et al. (26)	1969–86	116	69	57
Minor et al. (27)	NA	32	22	10
Jonsson et al. (28)	1976–81	36	15	21
Skene et al. (29)	1979–87	91	67	24
Klaase et al. (30)	1978–90	499	120	379

[a]Therapeutic ILP in which measurable macroscopic melanoma was present in perfusion field and response could be assessed.
[b]Adjuvant ILP in which patients were considered high risk for local recurrence but no visible disease was present in the perfusion field.
ILP, isolation limb perfusion; NA, not available.

treat soft tissue sarcomas of the extremity. For melanoma patients, ILP can either be considered therapeutic, in which case there is evaluable disease within the perfusion field of the limb, or as an adjuvant treatment, in which case the patients are thought to be at high risk for regional recurrence (Table 1). Treatment endpoints for therapeutic ILP include assessment of response in the measurable disease and duration of response. The only endpoint for adjuvant ILP is the disease-free intervals in the perfusion field. The most common ILP regimen used in the past two decades to treat extremity melanoma is melphalan as a single agent with mild hyperthermia (15). The use of ILP to treat extremity melanoma is discussed in four categories: therapeutic ILP with melphalan alone, adjuvant ILP with melphalan, melphalan plus other agents (particularly high-dose TNF), and ILP with other alkylating agents alone or in combination.

Therapeutic Isolation Limb Perfusion with Melphalan Alone

The data regarding response rates for therapeutic ILP with melphalan for extremity melanoma are difficult to interpret for the following reasons. First, virtually all the available data are in the form of institutional reviews in which therapeutic ILP is reported with adjuvant ILP (see Table 1) (22–30). In most series, the data on local recurrence and follow-up are combined from adjuvant and therapeutic ILP, which is difficult to interpret. Second, the precise regimen in terms of melphalan dose, time of perfusion, and level of hyperthermia is variable between institutions (Table 2). Third, the patient population treated varies widely in terms of the extent or bulk of melanoma, and with few exceptions response in terms of patient disease status is not reported. In fact, no prospective trial of ILP with objective response of tumor as the primary endpoint has been reported at this point in time.

In general, a 60-minute perfusion period is used with a melphalan dose between 1.0 and 1.5 mg/kg for lower extremity perfusions with mild hyperthermia (38°to 40°C) (see Table 2). The median complete response rate over several institutional series is between 50% and 60%, with an overall response rate of approximately 80% (Fig. 4; see Table 2). The complete response rate varies from a low of 7% (28) to a high of 82% (27) with melphalan-alone ILP. The series in which the complete response rate was only 7% consisted of only 15 patients and used the lowest dose of melphalan (28) compared with all other institutional reports, such that this is not reflective of the overall complete response rate that can be achieved. A study by Minor et al. (27) reported 18 complete responses in 22 patients (82%) with a standard dose of melphalan, and this is the highest complete response rate in the literature for melphalan-alone ILP (see Table 2). The largest study of therapeutic ILP is a recent report combining data from several Dutch groups of over 120 patients (30). The treatment regimen used in this large series was quite variable in terms of hyperthermia, with most patients having a normothermic perfusion. Nevertheless, the 54% complete response rate, 25% partial response rate, and overall objective response rate of 79% is the most accurate reflection of clinical responses that can be achieved with melphalan-alone ILP (30).

The best data for normothermic melphalan ILP come primarily from Kroon et al. in Amsterdam (31,32). One old study from St. Mary's Hospital in London reported a low overall response rate of only 48% with normothermic melphalan ILP (22). Kroon et al. reported a slightly lower complete response rate in a small number of patients (40%), but an overall response rate of 84% (31), which is again similar to that achieved with hyperthermic melphalan ILP (see Table 2). A second normothermic study by Kroon et al. was different in that it consisted of two ILP treatments 6 weeks apart, cannulating at different levels (external iliac and common femoral) (32). The complete response rate was 77% in 43 patients, which nearly equals the 82% level as the highest reported CR rate for hyperthermic melphalan ILP.

In some ways, a more important endpoint is the duration of response in the perfusion field achieved by ILP.

TABLE 2. *Perfusion characteristics and response rates for therapeutic isolation limb perfusion with melphalan for extremity melanoma*

Location	Years	Melphalan Dose LE	Melphalan Dose UE	Perfusion treatment time (min)	Target limb temperature (°C)	N	CR (%)	PR (%)	Overall response
Hyperthermic									
Westminster, London (23)	1960–79	2 mg/kg	—	50	39–40	80	21 (26%)	29 (36%)	50 (62%)
Rome (26)	1969–86	1.5 mg/kg	0.8 mg/kg	60	41.5	69	27 (39%)	30 (43%)	57 (82%)
Los Angeles (83)	1975–85	1.0 mg/kg	—	60	41–42	26	16 (62%)	5 (19%)	21 (81%)
San Francisco (27)	NA	0.8–1.5 mg/kg	0.75 mg/kg	60	39–40	22	18 (82%)	4 (18%)	22 (100%)
Lund, Sweden (28)	1976–81	0.9 mg/kg	0.45 mg/kg	120	38–40	15	1 (7%)	10 (67%)	11 (74%)
Brussels (84)	1977–82	1.3–1.5 mg/kg	75 mg	60	39–41	23	15 (65%)	6 (20%)	21 (91%)
Westminster, London (29)	1979–87	2 mg/kg	—	60	39–40	67	NA	NA	52 (74%)
Normothermic									
Netherlands (30)	1978–90	10 mg/l[a]	13 mg/l[a]	60	37–40[a]	120	65 (54%)	30 (25%)	95 (79%)
St. Mary's, London (22)	1959–79	1.5 mg/kg	1.5 mg/kg	60	37	29	NA	NA	14 (48%)
Amsterdam (31)	1978–85	10 mg/l	13 mg/l	60	37–38	18	7 (40%)	8 (44%)	15 (84%)
Amsterdam (32)	1985–90	1st: 6 mg/l[b] 2nd: 9 mg/l	—	60	37–38	43	33 (77%)	1 (2%)	34 (79%)

[a]Report is a combination of normothermic and hyperthermic perfusions from several institutions with >80% normothermic (37°) perfusion.
[b]Report of a protocol of planned sequential ILP 6 weeks apart—doses shown for first and second ILP.
LE, lower extremity; UE, upper extremity; CR, complete response; PR, partial responses; mg/l, melphalan dose as milligrams per liter of limb volume; ILP, isolation limb perfusion; N, number of patients; NA, not available.

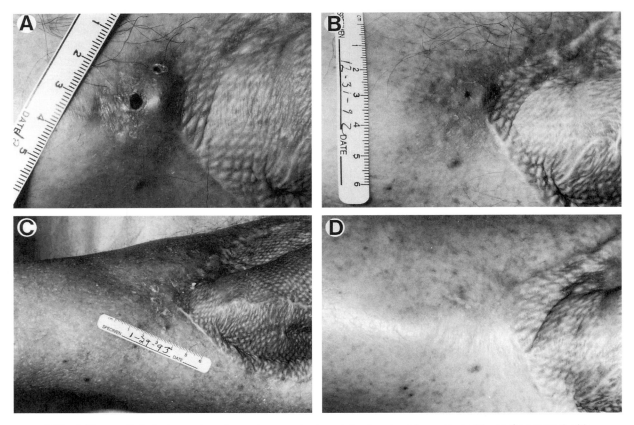

FIG. 4. Sequential photographs of a melanoma lesion at the border of previous skin grafts treated with isolation limb perfusion with melphalan. The patient had a complete response of multiple subcutaneous nodules all >1 cm in size that is ongoing 2.5 years later. **A:** Preoperatively; **B:** 2 weeks postperfusion; **C:** 6 weeks postperfusion; **D:** 4 months postperfusion.

As mentioned earlier, these data are hard to retrieve because follow-up data from therapeutic ILP is typically mixed with data from adjuvant ILP. Kroon et al. in their normothermic series reported that two of seven complete responses recurred in the perfusion field on long-term follow-up after normothermic ILP (31). Of the 33 complete responses after the double normothermic ILP, 16 recurred locally within 5 months, and the other 17 had sustained regional responses (32). The combined Netherlands report of 120 therapeutic ILPs had a median duration of complete response greater than 9 months (30).

Patients' clinical characteristics associated with an improved outcome after therapeutic ILP were evaluated by Klaase et al. (30). Factors that significantly correlated with the ability to achieve a complete response include the location of the tumor on the leg as opposed to the arm or foot, and negative regional lymph nodes. Factors positively associated with a longer duration of response included female sex, smaller number of lesions, location on the leg, recurrent lesions within 3 cm of the primary, and negative regional lymph nodes. A similar study in a smaller number of patients by di Fillipo et al. (26) agreed that small number of lesions and negative lymph nodes correlated with positive response, but found that patients with arm disease did significantly better than patients with lower extremity disease in their series.

Adjuvant Melphalan Isolation Limb Perfusion

More ILPs are performed in the adjuvant setting for high-risk patients than therapeutic ILPs in both the United States and Europe (see Table 1). However, critical evaluation of the available data indicates no survival benefit for adjuvant melphalan ILP. Two prospective, randomized trials (33,34) and two retrospective case-matched control (35) studies (36) have addressed this issue (Table 3). For patients with primary extremity melanoma, some investigators have advocated an attempt to prevent local recurrence with an adjuvant ILP for primary lesions greater than 1.5 mm in thickness (35). Ghussen et al. conducted a randomized trial of adjuvant ILP for stage I to III extremity melanoma (33). Thirty-seven patients with stage I disease were treated and randomized to excision alone versus excision plus ILP. The 5-year disease-free survival was increased from 61% with surgery alone to 95% in the ILP group (33). A retrospective study from Groningen (35) with a large number of patients showed no benefit for stage I melanoma, with equivalent disease-free survival rates and local recurrent rates (see Table 3). Finally, a retrospective study from M. D. Anderson showed no improvement in disease-free survival in all patients treated compared with case-matched controls, but in a subgroup of 25 patients from each category with lesions greater than 2.0 mm in thickness, disease-free survival was 42% for the surgery-alone group and 70% for the excision plus ILP group (36).

TABLE 3. *Adjuvant isolation limb perfusion with melphalan for extremity melanoma: results of prospective, randomized or case-matched, retrospective trials*

Stage I[a]						
Location (ref.)	Groningen, Netherlands (35)		Houston, Texas (36)		Cologne, Germany (33)	
Type of trial	Nonrandomized; case matched		Nonrandomized; case matched		Prospective, randomized	
Thickness criterion of primary melanoma	>1.5 mm		None		>1.5 mm	
Melphalan dose	1.0–1.5 mg/kg		1.5 mg/kg		1.5 mg/kg	
	Exc. Alone	Exc. + ILP	Exc. Alone	Exc. + ILP	Exc. Alone	Exc. + ILP
N	238	227	84 (>2 mm) 25	84 25	18	19
5-y DF survival	73%	77%	67% (>2 mm) 42%	78% 70%	61%	95%
LR at 10 y	13%	13%	—	—	—	—
Stage II or III[a]						
Location (ref.)			Cologne, Germany (33)		Goteborg, Sweden (34)	
Type of trial			Prospective, randomized		Prospective, randomized	
Melphalan dose			1.0–1.5 mg/kg		0.9 mg/kg	
			Exc. Alone	Exc. + ILP	Exc. Alone	Exc. + ILP
N			36	34	36	33
5-y DF survival			47%	85%	22%	28%
LR at 5 y			72%	18%	83%	70%
Deaths			22%	3%	56%	45%

[a]Stage based on M. D. Anderson staging criteria for extremity melanoma.
DF, disease free; LR, local recurrence; Exc., excision; ILP, isolation limb perfusion.

The two bits of data that suggest a potential benefit of adjuvant ILP for high-risk primaries are flawed. In the Ghussen et al. trial, only a small number of patients were treated, and the 95% disease-free 5-year survival rate in the ILP group is not reproduced by any other investigator in the field (33). The typical recurrence rates even with adjuvant ILP are four to six times higher in large populations (35). In the retrospective studies from Houston, the 42% recurrence rate in the excision-alone group for patients with >2 mm primaries is considerably higher than the natural history of this disease would predict (36). A large, multi-institutional, prospective, randomized trial in Europe has been underway for several years comparing adjuvant ILP versus observation for high-risk primary melanoma. A preliminary analysis shows a slight decrease in local recurrence after ILP but no improvement in survival, and adjuvant ILP for primary lesions is not recommended (37).

A second subgroup of patients treated with adjuvant ILP have regional recurrence in the form of satellite (stage II) or in-transit nodules (stage III) that have all been surgically resected. These patients clearly are at increased risk for further local recurrence. Both Ghussen et al. (33) and Hafström et al. (34) from Goteberg, Sweden conducted randomized trials of adjuvant melphalan ILP for patients with resected stage II or III extremity melanoma (see Table 3). Ghussen et al. reported improved 5-year disease-free survival, decreased local recurrences, and improved overall disease-specific survival after adjuvant ILP. However, the 85% disease-free survival and the 3% mortality rates at 5-year follow-up for stage II or III melanoma of the extremity are much higher than those for any other series (33). For example, for a similar group of patients, Hafström et al. reported only a 28% 5-year disease-free survival rate and a 45% mortality rate (34). Hafström et al. did show a mild to moderate decrease in local recurrence rate and improved survival, but these findings were not statistically significant in a small number of patients (see Table 3). A reasonable recommendation is that adjuvant ILP for patients with resected satellite or in-transit nodules from extremity melanoma be performed only in the setting of a clinical trial.

Melphalan Plus Tumor Necrosis Factor

Melphalan has been the predominant agent used in ILP for over 30 years (15). Other single or combination chemotherapeutic agents have been tried (38) (see below) and melphalan has been combined with other agents (39) (primarily actinomycin D) with no apparent improvement in results compared with melphalan alone, until recently. Lienard et al., working in Brussels, reported the use of high-dose TNF in ILP for extremity melanoma in 1992 (40,41). In a series of 29 patients, there was a 90% complete response rate and a 100% overall response rate (Table 4) (41). The specific regimen used included preoperative interferon-gamma, 0.2 mg subcutaneously, and a 90-minute perfusion treatment period with mild hyperthermia. Interferon-gamma 0.2 mg and TNF (4 mg lower extremity and 3 mg upper extremity) was given at time 0 and melphalan (10 mg/l for lower extremity and 13 mg/l for upper extremity) was given 30 minutes later (40). The timing and dosing of this regimen was empiric, with little or no preclinical testing. A similar study using TNF in Italy (42) reported a 64% complete response rate (7/11 patients) with a similar regimen, which is no different from the melphalan-alone ILP responses. The institution with the greatest experience outside of northern Europe with TNF limb perfusions is the National Cancer Institute (NCI) in Bethesda, Maryland (43,44). Complete response rates using the three-drug regimen of Lienard et al. are 76%, with an overall response rate of 92% (Fig. 5; see Table 2) (45). An attempt to increase the TNF dose in the perfusate to 6 mg at the NCI actually decreased the complete response rate, but this was in a small number of patients who were heavily pretreated (45). It should be noted that TNF-alone ILP has been used in six melanoma patients with only one short-lived objective response, and that as a single agent, TNF is ineffectual and not as good as melphalan alone (see Table 4) (46).

Current randomized trials of therapeutic ILP include a United States trial comparing melphalan alone versus

TABLE 4. *Use of high-dose tumor necrosis factor for therapeutic isolation limb perfusion for extremity melanoma alone or in combination with other agents*

Author	TNF Dose	Melphalan dose	Interferon-gamma dose[a]	N	CR (%)	PR (%)	Overall response (%)
Posner et al. (46)	2–4 mg	None	None	6	1 (17%)	01 (17%)	
Lienard et al. (41)	4 mg (LE) 3 mg (UE)	10 mg/l (LE) 13 mg/l (UE)	0.2 mg	29	26 (90%)	3 (10%)	29 (100%)
Hill et al. (85)	0.125–0.5 μg	1.5 mg/kg	None	4	4 (100%)	0 (100%)	
Vaglini et al. (42)	2–4 mg	10 mg/l	0.2 mg	11	7 (64%)	0 (64%)	
Fraker et al. (45)	4 mg	10 mg/l	0.2 mg	25	19 (76%)	4 (16%)	23 (92%)
Fraker et al. (45)	6 mg	10 mg/l	0.2 mg	11	4 (36%)	7 (64%)	11 (100%)

[a]Interferon-gamma given as subcutaneous injection preoperatively for 2 days and then in perfusate at the same dose.
TNF, tumor necrosis factor; CR, complete response; PR, partial response; LE, lower extremity; UE, upper extremity.

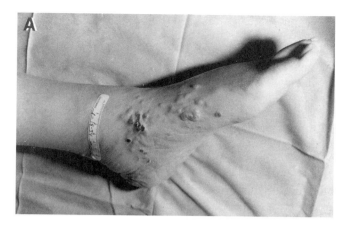

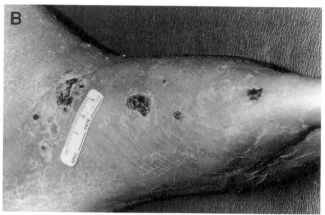

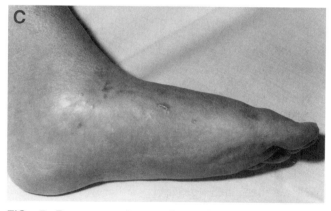

FIG. 5. Response of a patient with multiple in-transit melanoma nodules of the foot and ankle before and after an isolation limb perfusion with TNF, melphalan, and interferon-gamma. **A:** Preoperative; **B:** 4 weeks postoperative; **C:** 4 months postoperative. Note the changes after the ILP, with scabbing and crusting of the larger lesions, which are characteristic of a TNF-plus-melphalan limb perfusion.

melphalan, TNF, and interferon-gamma (44). A complementary randomized trial in Europe is comparing melphalan and TNF versus melphalan and TNF plus interferon-gamma to determine the impact of low- dose preoperative and perfusate interferon (43).

Isolation Limb Perfusion with Agents Other Than Melphalan

A variety of agents other than melphalan have been used, both alone and in combination in the ILP circuit. Of the single drugs reported, the most experience has been reported with CDDP and DTIC, and nitrogen mustard.

Imidazole carboxamide has modest activity against melanoma when administered systemically. In the mid-1980s, reports from Didolkar et al. described the clinical experience with this in an ILP circuit (47,48). Despite the fact that at least a portion of the effectiveness of this drug depends on the drug's hepatic microsomal activation, the initial reports were quite favorable. Didolkar et al. observed complete remission in 6 of 10 evaluable patients with recurrent in-transit melanoma. However, they found no 5-year survivors if all gross disease could not be completely resected, attesting to the fact that it was tumor burden and not response to perfusion that governed the ultimate outcome. Subsequent investigators have been unable to confirm these initial reports.

Shiu and colleagues reported on a series of 42 patients undergoing ILP with nitrogen mustard. Of 29 patients with measurable disease, complete response was observed in 8 and partial response in an additional 6, for an overall response rate of 48%. Predictors of response in their series included adequate dose of drug as well as adequate hyperthermia (49). Krementz and colleagues reported a poorer overall survival, 11% at 5 years, after ILP with nitrogen mustard as a single agent in 31 patients, compared with other current perfusion regimens; it was not clear from the data reported whether the survival difference was due to the drug or to other factors such as stage of disease (50).

The most experience with a single agent other than melphalan has been reported with CDDP. This drug would seem to be ideally suited for use in the ILP circuit. In melanoma, there seems to be a dose–response relationship with CDDP (51), with the primary systemic dose-limiting toxicity being nephrotoxicity and ototoxicity. In addition, the cytotoxic activity of CDDP is synergistic with that of hyperthermia (52–54). Klein and Ben-Ari reported an initial series of 15 patients with advanced melanoma of the limbs treated with hyperthermic ILP using CDDP with no locoregional toxicity at a dose of 75 mg/m² (55). Eight of 15 patients perfused had evidence of either local recurrence or in-transit disease; it is not clear from the report in how many patients complete resection of all gross disease was undertaken. Twelve of 15 patients were free of disease at follow-up ranging from 6 to 60 months.

Fletcher and colleagues have reported the largest series, 145 hyperthermic ILPs with CDDP, 70 in patients with "high-risk" melanoma (11). All of these were done in the adjuvant setting, and thus no response rate is reported. They thought that ILP with CDDP was well tolerated in doses of up to 250 mg/m² for lower extremities.

Dose-limiting toxicity included rhabdomyolysis and peripheral neuropathy.

Other investigators have encountered substantially more locoregional toxicity. Thompson and Gianoutsos reported on therapeutic ILP with CDDP in six patients with in-transit melanoma, only one of whom had a substantial response (38). Significant locoregional toxicity was encountered, including two patients who required amputation. Coit et al. reported on the experience at Memorial Sloan-Kettering Cancer Center with therapeutic CDDP perfusion (9). In their experience of 24 patients with measurable disease, an overall response rate of 80% was seen; only half of these responses were complete, and of those, only half were durable. Substantial locoregional toxicity was encountered in doses above 150 mg/m².

Finally, Hoekstra and colleagues reported on hyperthermic ILP with CDDP at a dose of 20 to 30 mg/l of perfused limb volume in seven patients with recurrent melanoma after prior hyperthermic ILP with melphalan (56). Of four patients with measurable disease left in situ, two had a complete response and a third had a partial response. Five of the seven patients recurred locoregionally after a median follow-up of only 5 months. Locoregional toxicity, most prominently peripheral neuropathy, was profound. The authors did not think that the modest response rates justified the significant toxicity.

In summary, although there is a substantial worldwide experience with hyperthermic ILP using CDDP, most of these perfusions have been done in the adjuvant setting. In those patients with measurable disease left in situ, the durable complete response rate appears to be modest, certainly no more than that reported with melphalan alone. Furthermore, although there is a significant variation in reported experience, in most centers locoregional toxicity appears to be unacceptably high, certainly worse than with melphalan. As such, limb perfusion with CDDP alone cannot be recommended as standard therapy.

Houghton and colleagues reported the significant clinical antitumor activity of the cytotoxic mouse monoclonal antibody R24 in patients with advanced metastatic melanoma. They noted that the antitumor activity may have been limited by the development of human anti-mouse antibodies (HAMA) in patients exposed to repeated doses of the murine protein (57). In an effort to limit the systemic HAMA response while exploiting the inherent cytotoxic properties of the antibody, Coit et al. performed normothermic ILP with R24 in 13 patients with measurable in-transit melanoma. Although postperfusion HAMA levels were negligible in all patients, only 1 of 13 patients had a transient partial response (58).

Multiple Agents

A number of authors have reported their experience with multiagent limb perfusion, using combinations of two or more of the aforementioned drugs. The broadest experience with multiagent ILP was reported by Krementz et al. (50). While their most common perfusion regimen is with melphalan alone, other regimens include melphalan with thiotepa, with an overall survival somewhat inferior to melphalan alone. Their best survival was observed in a cohort of patients using the combination of thiotepa, actinomycin D, and nitrogen mustard. The authors were not convinced that the survival differences observed were strictly attributable to the drug regimens used. At present, there is no compelling evidence in the literature to support the assumption that multiple drugs are superior to a single drug in the ILP circuit.

ISOLATION LIMB PERFUSION FOR SOFT TISSUE SARCOMA

The trend in treatment of patients with high-grade soft tissue sarcomas of the extremities over the past two to three decades has been development of limb salvage strategies to avoid amputation (59). Several techniques, including preoperative radiation therapy (60), postoperative radiation therapy (61), brachytherapy (62), neoadjuvant combination chemotherapy (63), and intra-arterial chemotherapy plus high-dose fractionated radiation therapy (64), have been combined with local resection to preserve extremities while maintaining acceptable local recurrence rates. Melphalan ILP had been used as a sole therapy for bulky sarcomas by Krementz et al. in 39 patients (65). They reported a complete response rate of 10% (4/39) and a partial response rate of 21% (8/39), with no long-term follow-up. Other investigators experienced with ILP for extremity melanoma have combined melphalan ILP with either immediate or delayed surgical resection (66,67), but in these small, nonrandomized series the impact of the ILP cannot be assessed.

Interest in the use of ILP to treat extremity sarcoma has been rejuvenated by the data combining TNF with melphalan (40). The three-drug regimen of melphalan, TNF, and interferon-gamma described earlier was used to treat 22 patients with extremity sarcoma for whom amputation was thought to be the only surgical option for local control (68). Fourteen of these patients had no systemic disease, and the tumors were resected 6 to 12 weeks after ILP. Evaluation of the tumor specimens showed no viable tumor in 6 of 14, for a 44% pathologic complete response rate (68). In these 23 patients, 21 had their limbs salvaged by the melphalan, TNF, and interferon ILP.

The benefits of ILP for treating sarcoma at the NCI are not as clear. Only 20% of patients with single bulky lesions had limb salvage by the use of three-drug ILP (Fraker DL, NCI, Bethesda, MD; unpublished observations). On the other hand, a subgroup of four patients with multifocal sarcoma, such as angiosarcoma or lymphangiosarcoma, had a complete response rate of 100%. The active agent for this response in these multifocal angiosarcomas may be melphalan, because Seyedi et al. reported a similar 100% response rate in five patients in 1990 using melphalan-alone ILP (69). Further assessment of patient characteristics and results needs to be obtained before determining the optional use of ILP to treat extremity sarcoma.

MORBIDITY AND MORTALITY

The morbidity of any regional perfusion technique can be classified into two categories—regional and systemic toxicity. All of the normal tissue in the area that is perfused is subjected to the same conditions (drug concentrations, temperature) as the tumor located in that area. Specifically for limb perfusions, all of the skin, subcutaneous tissue, muscle, peripheral nerve, and bone and joint tissue is subjected to hyperthermic drug perfusion, and each of these areas experiences its own characteristic side effects from melphalan ILP (70,71). Systemic toxicity due to drug exposure from ILP occurs in one of three ways. First, there may be leak of the perfusate to the systemic circulation during the treatment period. Second, after the extremity has been flushed, there may be redistribution of residual drug from the limb to the systemic circulation. Third, perfusion of the extremity may induce secondary products that can then cause systemic toxicity. This last mechanism is particularly important with the use of high-dose biologic agents such as TNF.

The most important type of morbidity from ILP is the regional side effects that may lead to long-term dysfunction in the perfused limb (72). Because the standard ILP uses high-dose melphalan, the typical toxicities associated with this agent are described in detail. Melphalan ILP causes a characteristic skin toxicity, with the appearance of erythema within 3 to 7 days after the ILP, gradually resolving into a darkened skin that fades over several weeks (71). All patients undergoing treatment have some skin toxicity of variable intensity. In some cases, areas of skin may develop blisters, particularly on the soles of the feet and the palms of the hand, characteristic of a second-degree burn. There is rarely full-thickness skin loss requiring grafting, but the discomfort may be a prominent side effect in the early postperfusion recovery period.

· Isolation limb perfusion in most cases causes some degree of dependent extremity edema that usually returns to baseline levels within 2 to 10 weeks (71). As described previously, at least a lymph node sampling if not a formal lymph node dissection is done for most ILPs performed for cutaneous melanoma. This node dissection combined with the hyperthermic drug treatment explains the postperfusion edema. Patients are managed postoperatively with extremity elevation because dependency augments this swelling in the immediate postoperative period. Use of support hose is helpful, but because of skin toxicity this may be intolerable for some patients. An alternative external support that is more acceptable for the patient is circumferential Ace wraps.

The most disturbing long-term morbidity that occurs in a small percentage of patients undergoing ILP is extremity pain due to effects on muscle or peripheral nerve (72,73). Nerve toxicity characterized by paresthesias and shooting pains usually has a later onset, occurring 2 to 3 weeks postperfusion. It is reported to occur in 25% to 40% of melphalan ILP procedures. Muscle pain occurs earlier, and ranges from a vague tight feeling to a severe discomfort. The cause of myopathy is probably related to swelling, with some degree of a compartment syndrome as well as some possible direct drug effects. Some surgeons perform four-compartment fasciotomies in the perfused leg, but this prophylactic measure is not needed in most cases. High tissue temperatures, low perfusion flow rates with tissue hypoxia and acidosis, repetitive ILP, and female sex (74) are all associated with prominent muscle toxicity, and patients in these categories must be watched closely for development of compartment syndrome. Long-term morbidity after melphalan ILP in a large population of patients includes an 11% rate of muscle atrophy or fibrosis, 8% chronic pain, and 4% chronic neuropathy, with an overall rate of long-term dysfunction of 15% (72).

Another type of regional toxicity that is not typically drug related is vascular side effects. ILP is associated with a 3% to 10% incidence of deep venous thrombosis in the perfused limb, which is likely due to thrombogenic effects of the drug and hyperthermia associated with decreased mobility of that extremity (75). Some practitioners advocate routine anticoagulation with warfarin but, again, the incidence of this complication does not seem to warrant this approach. For the arterial side, complications are most likely not due to drug effects but rather to technical problems. In the setting of atherosclerotic vessels, cannulation and perfusion of arteries may lead to macroemboli or microemboli causing distal ischemia.

Systemic toxicities from melphalan limb perfusion are limited and related to perfusate leak. If perfusate exposure is kept to less than 10% of the drug dose, then a typical 0.9 mg/kg or 10 mg melphalan/liter limb volume perfusion will deliver a systemic dose of less than 10 to 12 mg of melphalan. At this level, patients can experience some immediate postoperative nausea and vomiting and have short-lived bone marrow depression characterized by neutropenia 10 to 14 days postperfusion (75). Melphalan ILP does induce secondary inflammatory cytokines from the perfused limb, but levels are well under 1 ng/ml and would not be expected to contribute to systemic toxicities (76).

Addition of high-dose TNF to melphalan does not appear to alter the nature of the regional side effects that are due to melphalan, as described earlier. However, it clearly can increase the potential systemic morbidities. A

10% leak of a 4-mg TNF limb dose delivers 400 µg of drug, which is at or above the maximally tolerated systemic intravenous dose of TNF (77). Furthermore, exposure during ILP occurs in the setting of a major surgical procedure under general anesthesia, and this may augment the TNF toxicities (78).

The toxicity seen with TNF is related to the level of exposure and, as with other biologic agents, may be idiosyncratic or variable between patients. All patients who have a TNF limb perfusion with no perfusate leak have postoperative fever despite no direct systemic exposure. TNF ILP induces high levels of secondary mediators, particularly interleukin (IL)-6 and IL-8, and production of secondary pyrogens from the limb is likely the cause of this febrile response seen 2 to 4 hours after TNF exposure (79,80). Systemic leak rates of greater than 1% to 2% of the TNF perfusate dose typically cause hypotension 6 to 8 hours later, requiring treatment with fluids and vasopressors. This side effect is not surprising, because in phase I trials of systemic TNF, hypotension was almost universally the dose-limiting toxicity. In the initial report from Europe of TNF ILP, Lienard et al. used a Swan-Ganz pulmonary artery catheter in all patients and started prophylactic dopamine infusions preoperatively (40). Only about one third of patients in our recent series required vasopressors, and almost no patients except those with previous cardiac disease required pulmonary artery monitoring. Higher TNF exposures may lead to additional toxicities such as acute respiratory distress syndrome or renal failure, but with the use of the leak-monitoring system described previously, these high exposures should not occur (40).

ALTERNATIVE APPROACHES

Alternative treatments of in-transit melanoma of the extremity include regional approaches such as surgical excision or amputation and radiation therapy (81), and systemic treatments with chemotherapy or immunotherapy (82). Because of the nature of the spread of in-transit melanoma, regional excision in the form of berry-picking almost always fails, with nodules occurring in other adjacent areas of the involved extremity (see Fig. 1). Excision of in-transit melanoma nodules in patients not fit for ILP should be done with primary closure and not with wide excision requiring split-thickness skin grafts, because this would expose patients to significantly more morbidity with very little gain. For identical reasons, external beam radiation therapy has almost no utility in treatment of in-transit melanoma. The limited ability to achieve long-term responses as well as to deliver an effective dose of radiation therapy to the large areas of the extremity at risk limits the use of this technique. ILP treats all the macroscopic disease as well as the microscopic disease in the

TABLE 5. *Objective response rates for various forms of systemic and regional treatment of cutaneous melanoma*

Treatment (ref.)	Overall response (CR + PR)	Complete response rate
Single-agent chemotherapy (82)	20%	5%
Combination chemotherapy (82)	46%	11%
High-dose IL-2 (86)	17%	7%
TIL + IL-2 (87)	34%	6%
ILP with melphalan (30)	80%	55%
ILP with melphalan, TNF, and IFN (41,45)	90%–100%	75%–90%

CR, complete response; PR, partial response; IL-2, interleukin-2; TIL, tumor infiltrating lymphocytes; ILP, isolation limb perfusion; TNF, tumor necrosis factor; IFN, interferon-gamma.

perfusion field, and this is its primary advantage over the other regional types of surgical or radiation therapy.

The objective response rates in cutaneous and subcutaneous melanoma nodules after ILP are considerably higher than any other response rates achieved with systemic therapy (Table 5) (82). The ability of a single 60- to 90-minute perfusion treatment to achieve these response rates is remarkable and most likely due to the sustained drug delivery of high doses that can be achieved with this perfusion technique.

PATIENT ASSESSMENT

Pertinent data points after therapeutic ILP are response rates and duration of response in the perfusion field. Compared with almost all the types of cancer treatment, ILP of cutaneous melanoma is more accessible for evaluation of response because lesions are almost always on the surface of the extremity. Treated lesions can be visualized, palpated, photographed, measured directly, and sampled for biopsy at virtually any time point after treatment. Pigmented lesions that respond leave a flat spot that typically fades to a lighter blue-gray color over time. To document a response in these pigmented lesions, small areas of punch biopsies are done to confirm that there are no viable tumor cells in the specimen. For adjuvant ILP, the only meaningful endpoint is disease-free interval in the perfused extremity.

PATIENT CARE CONSIDERATIONS

A feature of patient care unique to ILP treatment is management of the regional limb toxicity. Our practice is to keep patients at strict bed rest for 1 to 2 days after the perfusion, with the leg elevated. Patients are then mobilized at a pace consistent with the level of toxicity for that individual. Examination of the limb in terms of skin changes, edema, and function, as well as the subjective symptoms of pain or discomfort from the patient provide a benchmark for progressive mobilization and ambulation. In some cases, ambulation-assist devices to limit the weight bearing on the perfused limb may be needed.

Patients are followed to assess response as well as regional toxicity in the early postoperative period. Patients treated by ILP for in-transit melanoma are at high risk for systemic disease at some time point, particularly those patients with positive regional lymph nodes. Therefore, these patients need to be followed with intermittent computed tomography scans of the chest, abdomen, and pelvis to screen for systemic recurrence.

PATIENT INFORMATION

The melanoma in the extremity (arm/leg) has grown to such an extent that operation to remove the tumor is impractical and has a very low chance of success. Other conventional treatments, such as chemotherapy by vein or radiation therapy, are not thought to be effective in prolonging life or curing this condition. A surgical technique called isolation limb perfusion allows delivery of very high concentrations of chemotherapy drugs to the extremity (arm/leg) where the tumor is located. By isolating the extremity from the rest of the body with surgical techniques, levels of the drug that are normally too toxic can be given directly to the limb with the tumor.

This technique of isolation limb perfusion is not new and has been done for advanced melanoma of the arm or leg for over 30 years. The operation to perform isolation limb perfusion is done under general anesthesia. During the operation, tubes will be inserted to the blood vessels going to the limb where the tumor is located. A machine like the one used in open heart surgery will circulate the blood and high-dose chemotherapy through the tube into the limb during the procedure. A tourniquet will be placed around the upper part of the arm or leg to keep most of the drug confined to the limb and not in the rest of the body. A solution with the medication in it may be heated during the operation to 102° to 105°F to increase its activity.

Complications of the medications and the operation in the involved limb include swelling, pain, stiffness in the joints, and reddening of the skin, with skin darkening lasting up to 4 months after the operation. A small proportion of patients may have blood clots in the operated limb that need to be treated with anticoagulation for several months. Severe complications in the limb can occur, including prolonged pain and swelling requiring medica-

tion, and may limit the long-term function of that extremity in rare instances.

REFERENCES

1. Creech O, Krementz ET, Ryan RF, Winblad JN. Chemotherapy of cancer: regional perfusion utilizing an extracorporeal circuit. *Ann Surg* 1958;148:616–632.
2. Jaques DP, Coit DG, Brennan MF. Major amputation for advanced malignant melanoma. *Surg Gynecol Obstet* 1989;169:1–6.
3. Einhorn LH, McBride CM, Luce JK. Intra-arterial infusion therapy with 5- (3,3-dimethyl-1 triazene) imidazole-4-carboxamide (NSC 45388) for malignant melanoma. *Cancer* 1973;32:749–755.
4. Savlov ED, Hall TC, Oberfield RA. Intra-arterial therapy of melanoma with dimethyl triazene imidazole carboxamide (NSC 45388). *Cancer* 1971;28:1161–1164.
5. Calvo DB, Patt YZ, Wallace S. Phase I–II trial of percutaneous intra-arterial cisdiamminedichloroplatinum (II) for regionally confined malignancy. *Cancer* 1980;45:1278–1283.
6. Bland KI, Kimura AK, Brenner DE, et al. A phase II study of the efficacy of diamminedichloroplatinum (Cisplatin) for the control of locally recurrent and intransit malignant melanoma of the extremities using tourniquet outflow-occlusion techniques. *Ann Surg* 1995;209: 73–80.
7. Calabro A, Singletary SE, Carrasco CH, Legha SS. Intraarterial infusion chemotherapy in regionally advanced malignant melanoma. *J Surg Oncol* 1990;43:239–244.
8. Frost DB, Patt YZ, Mavligit G, Chuang VP, Wallace S. Arterial infusion of dacarbazine and cisplatin for recurrent regionally confined melanoma. *Arch Surg* 1985;120:478–480.
9. Coit DG, Bajorin DF, Menendez-Botet C, et al. A phase I trial of hyperthermic isolation limb perfusion (HILP) using cisplatin (CDDP) for metastatic melanoma (meeting abstract). *Proceedings of the American Society of Clinical Oncology* 1991;10:1028.
10. Guchelaar HJ, Hoekstra HJ, de Vries EGE, Uges DRA, Oosterhuis JW, Koops HS. Cisplatin and platinum pharmacokinetics during hyperthermic isolated limb perfusion for human tumors of the extremities. *Br J Cancer* 1992;65:898–902.
11. Fletcher WS, Pommier RF, Woltering EA, Mueller CR, Ash O, Small KA. Pharmacokinetics and results of dose escalation in cisplatin hyperthermic isolation limb perfusion. *Ann Surg Oncol* 1994;1:236–243.
12. Creech O, Krementz ET, Ryan RF, Winbled JN. Chemotherapy of cancer: regional perfusion utilizing an extracorporeal circuit. *Ann Surg* 1958;148:616–632.
13. Cavaliere R, Ciogatto EC, Giovanelli BC, et al. Selective heat sensitivity of cancer cells. *Cancer* 1967;20:1351–1387.
14. Stehlin JS. Hyperthermic perfusion with chemotherapy for cancers of the extremities. *Surg Gynecol Obstet* 1969;129:305–308.
15. Cumberlin R, DeMoss E, Lassus M, Friedman M. Isolation perfusion for malignant melanoma of the extremity:a review. *J Clin Oncol* 1985;3:1022–1031.
16. Schraffordt-Koops H, Kroon BBR, Lejeune FJ. Isolated regional perfusion in the treatment of local recurrence, satellites and in-transit metastases of extremity melanoma. In: Rumke P, ed. *Therapy of advanced melanoma.* Basel: Karger; 1990:67–78.
17. Hoekstra HJ, Naujocks T, Schraffordt-Koops H, et al. Continuous leaking monitoring during hyperthermic isolated regional perfusion of the lower limb: techniques and results. *Regional Cancer Treatment* 1992; 4:301–304.
18. Alexander C, Omlor G, Berberich R, Gross G, Feifel G. Rapid measurement of blood leakage during regional chemotherapy. *Eur J Nucl Med* 1993;4:606–612.
19. Barker WC, Andrich MP, Alexander HR, Fraker DL. Continuous intraoperative external monitoring of perfusate leak using I-131 human serum albumin during isolated perfusion of the liver and limbs. *Eur J Nucl Med* 1996;22:1242–1247.
20. Stehlin JS, Giovanella BC, de Ipolyi PD, Muenz LR, Anderson RF. Results of hyperthermic perfusion for melanoma of the extremities. *Surg Gynecol Obstet* 1975;140:339–348.
21. Siddik ZH, Edwards MJ, Boddie AW. Isolated limb perfusion with chemotherapeutic agents for melanoma: a reevaluation of drug dosimetry. *Eur J Cancer Clin Oncol* 1989;25:1393–1397.

22. Bulman AS, Jamieson CW. Isolated limb perfusion with melphalan in the treatment of malignant melanoma. *Br J Surg* 1980;67:660–662.

23. Rosin RD, Westbury G. Isolated limb perfusion for malignant melanoma. *Practitioner* 1979;224:1031–1036.

24. Hartley JW, Fletcher WS. Improved survival of patients with stage II melanoma of the extremity using hyperthermic isolation perfusion with 1-phenylalanine mustard. *J Surg Oncol* 1987;36:170–174.

25. Martijn H, Oldhoff J, Koops HS. Regional perfusion in the treatment of patients with a locally metastasized malignant melanoma of the limbs. *Eur J Cancer* 1981;17:471–476.

26. di Filippo F, Calabro A, Giannarelli D, et al. Prognostic variables in recurrent limb melanoma treated with hyperthermic antiblastic perfusion. *Cancer* 1989;63:2551–2561.

27. Minor DR, Allen RE, Alberts D, et al. A clinical and pharmacokinetic study of isolated limb perfusion with heat and melphalan for melanoma. *Cancer* 1985;55:2638–2644.

28. Jonsson PE, Hafström L, Hagarder A. Results of regional hyperthermic perfusion for primary and recurrent melanomas of the extremities. *Recent Results Cancer Res* 1983;86:277–282.

29. Skene AI, Bulman AS, Williams TR, et al. Hyperthermic isolated perfusion with melphalan in the treatment of advanced malignant melanoma of the lower limb. *Br J Surg* 1990;77:765–767.

30. Klaase JM, Kroon BBR, van Geel AN, Eggermont AMM, Franklin HR, Hart AAM. Prognostic factors for tumor response and limb recurrence-free interval in patients with advanced melanoma of the limbs treated with regional isolated perfusion using melphalan. *Surgery* 1994;115:39–45.

31. Kroon BBR, van Geel AN, Benckhuijsen C, Wieberdink J. Normothermic isolation perfusion with melphalan for advanced melanoma of the limbs. *Anticancer Res* 1987;7:441–442.

32. Kroon BBR, Klaase JM, van Geel BN, Eggermont AMM, Franklin HR, van Dongen JA. Results of a double perfusion schedule with melphalan in patients with melanoma of the lower limb. *Eur J Cancer* 1993;29A:325–328.

33. Ghussen F, Kruger I, Groth W, Stutzer H. The role of regional hyperthermic cytostatic perfusion in the treatment of extremity melanoma. *Cancer* 1988;61:654–659.

34. Hafström L, Rudenstam C-M, Blomquist E, et al. Regional hyperthermic perfusion with melphalan after surgery for recurrent malignant melanoma of the extremities. *J Clin Oncol* 1991;9:2091–2094.

35. Franklin HR, Koops HS, Oldhoff J, et al. To perfuse or not to perfuse? A retrospective comparative study to evaluate the effect of adjuvant isolated regional perfusion in patients with stage I extremity melanoma with a thickness of 1. 5 mm or greater. *J Clin Oncol* 1988;6:701–708.

36. Edwards MJ, Soong S-J, Boddie AW, Balch CM, McBride CM. Isolated limb perfusion for localized melanoma of the extremity. *Arch Surg* 1990;125:317–321.

37. Lejeune FJ. A randomized trial on prophylactic isolation perfusion for stage 1 high risk (i.e. 1.5 mm thickness) malignant melanoma of the limbs: an interim report. *Melanoma Res* 1993;3(Suppl):95.

38. Thompson JF, Gianoutsos MP. Isolated limb perfusion for melanoma: effectiveness and toxicity of cisplatin compared with that of melphalan and other drugs. *World J Surg* 1992;16:227–233.

39. Martijn H, Oldhoff J, Koops HS. Hyperthermic regional perfusion with melphalan and a combination of melphalan and actinomycin D in the treatment of locally metastasized malignant melanomas of the extremities. *J Surg Oncol* 1982;20:9–13.

40. Lienard D, Ewalenko P, Delmotti JJ, Renard N, Lejeune FJ. High-dose recombinant tumor necrosis factor alpha in combination with interferon gamma and melphalan in isolation perfusion of the limbs for melanoma and sarcoma. *J Clin Oncol* 1992;10:52–60.

41. Lienard D, Lejeune F, Ewalenko I. In transit metastases of malignant melanoma treated by high dose rTNFα in combination with interferon-gamma and melphalan in isolation perfusion. *World J Surg* 1992;16:234–240.

42. Vaglini M, Belli F, Ammatuna M, et al. Treatment of primary or relapsing limb cancer by isolation perfusion with high-dose alpha-tumor necrosis factor, gamma-interferon, and melphalan. *Cancer* 1994;73:483–492.

43. Fraker DL, Alexander HR. Isolated limb perfusion with high-dose tumor necrosis factor for extremity melanoma and sarcoma. In: DeVita VT, Hellman S, Rosenberg SA, eds. *Important advances in oncology.* Philadelphia: JB Lippincott; 1994:179–192.

44. Fraker DL, Alexander HR. The use of tumour necrosis factor (TNF) in isolated perfusion: results and side effects. The NCI results. *Melanoma Res* 1994;4:27–29.

45. Fraker DL, Alexander HR, Andrich M, Rosenberg SA. Treatment of patients with melanoma of the extremity using hyperthermic isolated limb perfusion with melphalan, tumor necrosis factor, and interferon-gamma: results of a TNF dose escalation study. *J Clin Oncol* 1996;14:479–489.

46. Posner M, Lienard D, Lejeune F, Rosenfelder D, Kirkwood J. Hyperthermic isolated limb perfusion (HILP) with tumor necrosis factor (TNF) alone for metastatic intransit melanoma (Abstract). *Proceedings of the American Society of Clinical Oncology* 1994;13:396.

47. Didolkar MS, Fitzpatrick JL, Jackson AJ, Jonston GS. Toxicity and complications of vascular isolation and hyperthermic perfusion with imidazole carboxamide (DTIC) in melanoma. *Cancer* 1986;57:1961–1966.

48. Didolkar MS, Viens ML, Suter CM, Buda B. Phase II study of isolation perfusion with DTIC in stage IIa–IIIab melanoma of the extremity. *Proceedings of the American Society of Clinical Oncology* 1990;9:276.

49. Shiu MH, Knapper WH, Fortner JG, et al. Regional isolated limb perfusion of melanoma intransit metastases using mechlorethamine (nitrogen mustard). *J Clin Oncol* 1986;4:1819–1826.

50. Krementz ET, Carter RD, Sutherland CM, Muchmore JH, Ryan RF, Creech O. Regional chemotherapy for melanoma: a 35-year experience. *Ann Surg* 1994;220:520–535.

51. Chary KK, Higby DJ, Henderson ES, Swinerton KD. Phase I study of high dose cis-diamminedichloroplatinum (II) with forced diuresis. *Cancer Treat Rep* 1977;61:367–370.

52. Leong SPL, Xu MJ, Alberts DWS, et al. Chemosensitivity of human melanoma to cisplatin and heat at doses achievable by isolated hyperthermic perfusion. *Proceedings of the American Society of Clinical Oncology* 1990;9:277.

53. Fisher GA, Hahn GM. Enhancement of cis-platinum (II) diamminedichloride cytotoxicity by hyperthermia. *Monogr Natl Cancer Inst* 1982;61:255–257.

54. Kitamura K, Kuwano H, Matsuda H, Toh Y, Masuda H, Sugimachi K. Synergistic effects of intratumor administration of cis-diam minedichloroplatinum (II) combined with local hyperthermia in melanoma bearing mice. *J Surg Oncol* 1992;51:188–194.

55. Klein ES, Ben-Ari GY. Isolation perfusion with cisplatin for malignant melanoma of the limbs. *Cancer* 1987;59:1068–1071.

56. Hoekstra HJ, Koops HS, de Vries LGE, van Weerden TW, Oldhoff J. Toxicity of hyperthermic isolated limb perfusion with cisplatin for recurrent melanoma of the lower extremity after previous perfusion. *Cancer* 1993;72:1224–1229.

57. Vadhan-Raj S, Cordon-Cardo C, Carswell E, et al. Phase I trial of a mouse monoclonal antibody against GD# ganglioside in patients with melanoma: induction of an inflammatory response at tumor sites. *J Clin Oncol* 1988;6:1636.

58. Coit D, Houghton A, Cordon-Cardo C, Shiu MH, Old L. Isolation limb perfusion with monoclonal antibody R24 in patients with malignant melanoma. *Proceedings of the American Society of Clinical Oncology* 1988;7:248.

59. Williard WC, Collin C, Casper ES, Hajdu WI, Brennan MF. The changing role of amputation for soft tissue sarcoma of the extremity in adults. *Surg Gynecol Obstet* 1992;175:389–396.

60. Suit HD, Mankin HJ, Wood WC, et al. Treatment of the patient with stage M₀ soft tissue sarcoma. *J Clin Oncol* 1988;6:854–862.

61. Potter DA, Glenn J, Kinsella T, et al. Patterns of recurrence in patients with high grade soft tissue sarcomas. *J Clin Oncol* 1985;3:353–356.

62. Brennan MF, Hilaris B, Shiu MH, et al. Local recurrence in adult soft-tissue sarcoma: a randomized trial of brachytherapy. *Arch Surg* 1987;122:1289–1293.

63. Pezzi CM, Pollock RE, Evans HL, et al. Preoperative chemotherapy for soft-tissue sarcomas of the extremities. *Ann Surg* 1990;211:476–481.

64. Moseley HS. An evaluation of two methods of limb salvage in extremity soft-tissue sarcomas. *Arch Surg* 1992;127:1169–1174.

65. Krementz ET, Carter RD, Sutherland CM, Hutton I. Chemotherapy of sarcomas of the limbs by regional perfusion. *Ann Surg* 1977;185:555–564.

66. Hoekstra HJ, Koops HS, Molenaar WM, Oldhoff J. Results of isolated regional perfusion in the treatment of malignant soft tissue tumors of the extremities. *Cancer* 1987;60:1703–1707.

67. Rossi CR, Vecchiato A, Foletto M, et al. Phase II study on neoadjuvant

hyperthermic-antiblastic perfusion with doxorubicin in patients with intermediate or high grade limb sarcomas. *Cancer* 1994;73: 2140–2146.

68. Schraffordt-Koops H, Lienard D, Eggermont AM, Hoekstra HJ, VanGeel BN, Lejeune FJ. Isolated limb perfusion with high dose TNF-alpha, gamma-IFN, and melphalan in patients with irresectable soft tissue sarcomas: a highly effective limb salving procedure (Abstract). *Society of Surgical Oncology Cancer Symposium* 1993;46:1.

69. Seyedi JV, Liénard D, Bourgeois P, Lejeune F. Treatment of advanced angiosarcomas of the limbs by isolation perfusion. *Regional Cancer Treatment* 1990;3:98–102.

70. van Geel AN, Wijk JV, Wieberdink J. Functional morbidity after regional isolated perfusion of the limb for melanoma. *Cancer* 1989;63:1092–1096.

71. Wieberdink J, Benckhuysen C, Braat RP, van Slooten EA, Olthuis GAA. Dosimetry in isolation perfusion of the limbs by assessment of perfused tissue volume and grading of toxic tissue reactions. *Eur J Cancer Clin Oncol* 1982;18:905–910.

72. Vrouenraets BC, Klaase JM, Kroon BBR, van Geel VN, Eggermont AMM, Franklin HR. Long-term morbidity after regional isolated perfusion with melphalan for melanoma of the limbs. *Arch Surg* 1995;130:43–47.

73. Olieman AFT, Koops HS, Geertzen JHB, Kingma H, Hoekstra HJ, Oldhoff J. Functional morbidity of hyperthermic isolated regional perfusion of the extremities. *Annals of Surgical Oncology* 1994;1:382–388.

74. Klaase JM, Kroon BBR, van Geel BN, Eggermont AMM, Franklin HR, Hart GAM. Patient- and treatment-related factors associated with acute regional toxicity after isolated perfusion for melanoma of the extremities. *Am J Surg* 1994;167:618–620.

75. Schraffordt-Koops H, Oldhoff J, Oosterhuis JW, Beekhuis H. The role of isolated limb perfusion for regional metastases of the extremities. *Pigment Cell Res* 1985;7:146–164.

76. Quinn TD, Polk HC Jr, Edwards MJ. Hyperthermic isolated limb perfusion increases circulating levels of inflammatory cytokines. *Cancer Immunol Immunother* 1995;40:272–275.

77. Fraker DL, Alexander HR, Pass HI. Biologic therapy with TNF: systemic administration and isolation-perfusion. In: DeVita V, Hellman S, Rosenberg SA, eds. *Biologic therapy of cancer.* Philadelphia: JB Lippincott; 1995:329–345.

78. Fawcett WJ, Hill S, Sheldon J, et al. Hemodynamic changes and circulating recombinant tumor necrosis factor-α concentrations in a patient undergoing isolated limb perfusion. *Crit Care Med* 1993;21:796.

79. Thom AK, Alexander HR, Andrich MP, Barker WC, Rosenberg SA, Fraker DL. Cytokine levels and systemic toxicity in patients undergoing isolated limb perfusion (ILP) with high-dose TNF, interferon-gamma and melphalan. *J Clin Oncol* 1995;13:264–273.

80. Gérain J, Liénard D, Ewalenko P, Lejeune FJ. High serum levels of the TNF-α after its administration for isolation perfusion of the limb. *Cytokine* 1992;4:585–591.

81. Turnbull A, Shah J, Fortner J. Recurrent melanoma of an extremity treated by major amputation. *Arch Surg* 1973;106:496–498.

82. Balch CM, Houghton AN, Peters LJ. Cutaneous melanoma. In: DeVita VT, Hellman S, Rosenberg SA, eds. *Cancer: principles and practice of oncology.* Philadelphia: JB Lippincott; 1993:1612–1661.

83. Storm FK, Morton DL. Value of therapeutic hyperthermic limb perfusion in advanced recurrent melanoma of the lower extremity. *Am J Surg* 1985;150:32–35.

84. Lejeune FJ, Deloof T, Ewalenko P, et al. Objective regression of unexcised melanoma in-transit metastases after hyperthermic isolation perfusion of the limbs with melphalan. *Recent Results Cancer Res* 1983;86:268–276.

85. Hill S, Fawcett WJ, Sheldon J, Soni N, Williams T, Thomas JM. Low-dose tumour necrosis factor α and melphalan in hyperthermic isolated limb perfusion. *Br J Surg* 1993;80:995–997.

86. Rosenberg SA, Yang JC, Topalian SL, et al. Treatment of 283 consecutive patients with metastatic melanoma or renal cell cancer using high-dose bolus interleukin 2. *JAMA* 1994;271:907–913.

87. Rosenberg SA, Yannelli JR, Yang JC, et al. Treatment of patients with metastatic melanoma with autologous tumor-infiltrating lymphocytes and interleukin 2. *J Natl Cancer Inst* 1994;86:1159–1166.

CHAPTER 26

Surgical Treatment of Bone Metastases to the Axial Skeleton and Extremities

Kenneth M. Yaw and J. Scott Doyle

Those who are enslaved to their sects are not merely devoid of all sound knowledge but they will not even stop to learn. Praxiteles and Phidias...were unable to...reach and handle all portions of the material. It is not so, however with nature. Every part of a bone she makes bone, every part of the flesh, she makes flesh, and so with fat and all the rest; there is not part she has not touched, elaborated, and embellished.

—*Galen (150 A.D.)*

INCIDENCE

Metastatic carcinoma and multiple myeloma combined are over 100 times more common in the skeleton than primary malignant bone tumors. Any malignancy can spread to bone; however, over 80% of skeletal metastases are from breast, prostate, lung (bronchus), kidney, or thyroid primaries. Some others, such as melanoma, rarely metastasize to bone, but the primary tumors are so common that even though the percentages are low, the actual occurrence of such metastases is not uncommon. Still others have been dubbed "osteophobic" and rarely spread to bone, including primary carcinoma of the skin, oral cavity, esophagus, stomach, colon, and cervix (1).

Autopsy studies show an incidence of up to 85% of patients dying with carcinoma have skeletal metastases (2,3). Studies based on scintigraphic imaging and radiography show lower incidences, probably as a reflection of the sensitivity of the technique for detection. In men, over 60% of skeletal metastases are from prostate carcinoma (1). In women, over 70% of skeletal metastases are from

K. M. Yaw: Department of Orthopaedic Surgery, University of Pittsburgh School of Medicine, Division of Musculoskeletal Oncology, University of Pittsburgh Medical Center, Pittsburgh, Pennsylvania 15213.

J. S. Doyle: Department of Orthopaedic Surgery, University of Alabama Hospitals at Birmingham, Birmingham, Alabama 35233.

breast carcinoma (4). For breast carcinoma, the 5-year survival rate is reported at >80%, with 34% of those survivors at 5 years living with metastatic disease (5).

The distribution of metastases in the skeleton is only partly explained by patterns and rates of circulation. The spine is the most common site of skeletal metastasis from cancer. Up to 70% of patients who die from cancer have evidence of spinal involvement at autopsy (3). Approximately half of patients with vertebral metastases require treatment (3,6), but less than 10% require operative intervention (7–9). Hematopoietic malignancies such as lymphoma and myeloma have a proclivity for spinal involvement and should be considered in any differential diagnosis of spinal lesions. Most authors report that the thoracic spine is the most common site of involvement, followed by the lumbar and cervical spines (8,10). Certainly, the thoracic spine, with its smaller canal-to-cord ratio, is the most common site for neurologic involvement. The vertebral body, with its abundant red marrow and sinusoidal vascular system, is involved seven times more frequently than the posterior elements (the pedicles, lamina, and transverse and spinal processes) as the site of original metastatic deposit (11).

The paravertebral venous plexus provides an avenue for metastases to the spine. The sinusoidal vascular system within the vertebral body allows for easy escape, and the milieu of the marrow within the spongiosa has been shown to be congenial to seeded tumors (12,13). Breast and prostate carcinoma have unimpeded access to the spine through the communication of Batson's plexus with the azygous vein and pelvic venous plexus, respectively. Other tumors tend to occur in more generalized patterns about the skeleton, but often involve the spine.

The most common sites for skeletal metastases depend somewhat on the tumor of origin. In general, metastases distal to the knees or elbows are uncommon, and are particularly rare as solitary lesions (14). Acrometastases (metastases to the hands) are rare, but most often herald a bronchogenic primary and usually are associated with widespread visceral disease (15). The mechanisms of metastasis are still being explored, but much has been clarified in recent years (16–19).

EVALUATION

A patient who presents with a skeletal lesion needs that same thorough history and physical examination that every patient deserves. The suspicion of metastases may be very high based on age, distribution, or history of primary carcinoma. However, the clinician must cautiously avoid the pitfall of assuming metastatic carcinoma without solid clinical evidence. This is particularly important in the patient with a solitary lesion and no documented metastatic disease at other sites, because this is the patient who may unnecessarily lose life or limb if an otherwise curable sarcoma is mistreated on the assumption that it is metastatic carcinoma. Hence, every skeletal lesion must be approached as though it represents a primary malignancy until there is sufficient evidence to the contrary. Biopsy is not required for tissue diagnosis in every case, but biopsy must at least be considered if there is not sufficient other evidence to establish a definitive diagnosis.

The evaluation of advanced cancer in the skeleton involves identifying the sites of involvement, determining the structural compromise to those sites, and assessing the implications for any nearby anatomic structures (eg, spinal cord, major vessels). The most reliable test for locating skeletal lesions is the technetium bone scan. It is nonspecific as to the nature of a lesion and its structural implications, but it is very sensitive in finding most lesions. One notable exception is multiple myeloma, which may not show up on scintigraphic imaging as either increased or decreased activity (Fig. 1). For myeloma, a skeletal survey is essential to stage and follow the skeletal lesions. Another caution is that bone scans suffer from poor anatomic definition in the spine and lower pelvis unless special imaging angles and techniques are used.

The most efficient and useful study of any specific long bone lesion is a set of orthogonal plain radiographs. In any site where surgical intervention is being considered, it is essential that these films include the entire bone in question, and not be limited to just the site where a

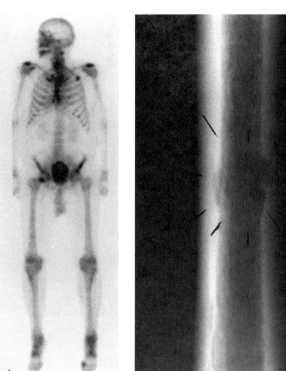
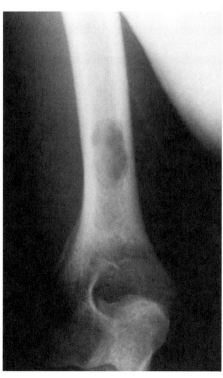

A,B rior

C

FIG. 1. A: Anterior view of a whole-body bone scan in a patient with multiple myeloma. There is abnormal uptake in the left fourth rib and right femoral neck. Skeletal survey showed multiple other lesions that do not appear on the bone scan, including the lesions shown in (B) and (C). **B:** Right distal femoral diaphyseal lesion from multiple myeloma in the patient whose bone scan is show in (A). **C:** Right distal humeral diaphyseal myeloma lesion of the patient whose bone scan is shown in (A).

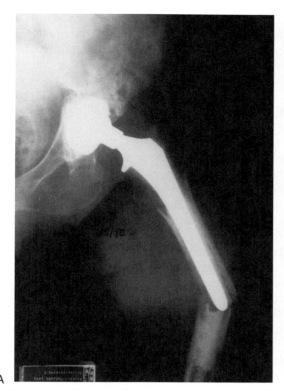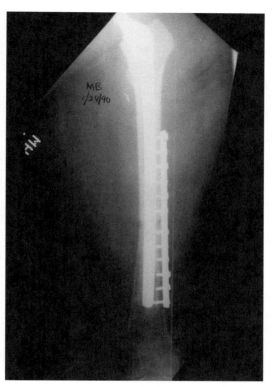

A   B

FIG. 2. A: This patient with metastatic breast carcinoma underwent total hip arthroplasty with a standard-length femoral stem. Approximately 8 weeks after surgery, she fractured through a diaphyseal femoral metastasis that was at the tip of the femoral component. **B:** She subsequently underwent revision to a long-stem component with allograft replacement of the proximal femur.

known lesion exists. Otherwise, there is a very real and significant risk of stabilizing an actual or impending pathologic fracture with hardware that ends adjacent to another undetected lesion (Fig. 2).

In the spine, magnetic resonance imaging (MRI), computed tomography (CT) scanning, and myelography may be useful adjuncts in evaluation. Thirty to 50% of the vertebral body must be destroyed before the loss is detectable on plain radiographs, and metastases may remain radiographically silent until spread occurs into the largely cortical and radiodense pedicle. The loss of pedicle markings is often the earliest radiographic clue to vertebral involvement because its cortex is often involved early and is well visualized on anteroposterior radiographs (Fig. 3).

Magnetic resonance imaging is useful in giving an accurate assessment of marrow involvement, detecting skip lesions (which may be significant if surgical intervention is being considered), and imaging the entire cord. This is an important feature of MRI because 10% of patients with cord compression have a second level of compression elsewhere in the spine (20). In most centers, MRI is supplanting myelography because it carries few risks and more completely defines the pathoanatomy. Vertebral osteomyelitis is not uncommon in debilitated

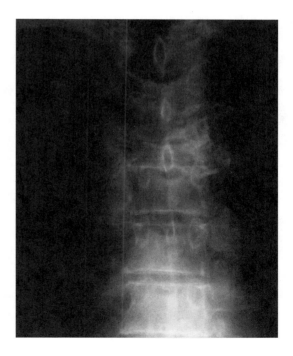

FIG. 3. Anteroposterior radiograph of the upper thoracic spine showing loss of the right pedicle of the third thoracic vertebra.

cancer patients and is reliably distinguished from tumor by MRI. The sensitivity of MRI is excellent, but its specificity suffers in the setting of a benign compression fracture. Bleeding into the marrow space and surrounding soft tissues may mimic the typical pattern of tumor on T1 imaging. If there is doubt as to the nature of the lesion, CT-guided biopsy is recommended (21). The success of CT-guided biopsy at our institution is high enough that we rarely need to perform open biopsies for diagnosis.

Computed tomography can demonstrate retropulsed bony detritus that may impinge on the cord and cause neurologic deficits. Axial thin cuts allow evaluation of the critical posterior spinal elements. Such information can help determine which approach is appropriate for decompressing or stabilizing the spine when surgery is being contemplated.

Angiography is seldom of diagnostic importance in these patients, but still serves a vital role for certain cases. A map of the local vascular anatomy can be critical in planning surgical management of these patients, particularly if surgical approach or resection will involve exposing or sacrificing major vessels. Furthermore, some lesions are so vascular that simply making a hole in them can lead to uncontrollable, life-threatening hemorrhage, and angiography allows the physician to know this preoperatively. Frequently, the radiologist can also prevent such bleeding problems by embolizing the lesion at the time of angiography (Fig. 4). If this is done as a preoperative procedure, then surgery is usually planned within 3 days of the embolization to avoid any significant revascularization effect. Although any lesion may be very vascular, ones that are notorious for being dangerously hypervascular are metastatic renal carcinoma, thyroid carcinoma, and myeloma.

FRACTURE RISK

Long-standing clinical guidelines for prophylactic internal fixation of long bone metastases include lesions greater than 2.5 cm in size or cortical destruction exceeding 50% of the circumference of the bone. These criteria were established based on retrospective review of limited numbers of cases, and have been shown to have significant false-positive and false-negative rates in predicting risk of pathologic fracture. Clinical application needs to be tempered by the surgeon's judgment and experience, with particular consideration given to high-stress areas (eg, intertrochanteric region of the femur) and to presence of pain. In general, activity- and load-related pain localized at the site of a lesion in a weight-bearing bone should be considered a sign of impending fracture regardless of the size of the lesion. New methods to provide noninvasive estimates of load-bearing capacity in affected bones apply engineering principles to the analysis of CT examinations, including defect size, defect geometry, defect location, normal bone density, and expected loading patterns (22). These methods show promise, but have yet to be validated for sites other than the spine.

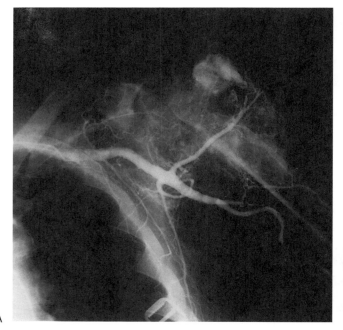

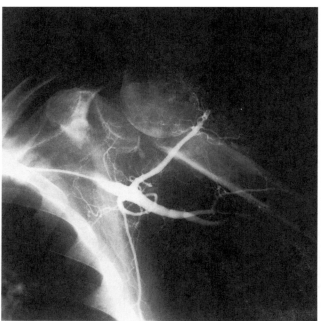

A

B

FIG. 4. A: Displaced pathologic fracture of the proximal humerus that occurred through a renal carcinoma metastasis. Preoperative angiography showed the lesion to be extremely vascular and fed primarily from the anterior humeral circumflex artery. Embolization was performed. **B:** Postembolization angiography showed dramatic decrease in blood flow to the region, and minimal bleeding was encountered at the time of surgery.

SURGICAL INDICATIONS

Reasons for operating on metastatic malignancies in the skeleton are usually one of the following:

Biopsy to establish the diagnosis
Stabilization of a pathologic fracture
Prevention of a pathologic fracture
Resection for cure

In patients with or without a past history of malignancy who do not have documented metastatic disease at any site, a biopsy is essential to prove diagnosis. This dogma may sometimes be violated in the patient with highly suspect multifocal skeletal lesions, but in doing so, the clinician must carefully balance the morbidity of the biopsy with the potential for embarking on incorrect treatment for an incorrect diagnosis. In the patient with known metastatic disease at any site, a biopsy of newly detected skeletal lesions is probably not necessary unless the lesions are suspect for some disease process other than metastatic tumor (such as infection or other primary neoplasm).

For patients in whom pathologic fracture develops, the treatment should be aggressive and directed toward rapid rehabilitation and maximal early function. In weight-bearing bones of the lower extremities, this most often requires surgical stabilization or resection and replacement of diseased segments. In the upper extremities, the morbidity of prolonged healing is less as long as reasonable pain control can be achieved by bracing and analgesics, so surgical stabilization is less often essential for reasonable quality of life.

When a pathologic fracture is considered imminent based on the imperfect criteria mentioned previously and the judgment of an experienced orthopedic surgeon, some intervention should be undertaken to prevent such fracture. Surgical decisions must be based on a comparison of the relative morbidity of the procedure to prevent fracture and the morbidity of the fracture (and its treatment) should it occur. If it is dramatically simpler to perform a procedure to prevent fracture than to deal with the fracture once it occurs, then there should be a much lower threshold for proceeding with surgical prophylaxis of the fracture. If the procedure predictably has no greater morbidity once the fracture occurs, then there should be a higher threshold for proceeding with surgery and stronger indications would be needed. This judgment depends on the location, number, and size of the lesions in predicting the most likely pattern of structural failure.

The role of predicted longevity in determining surgical indications is unsettled, and is sometimes a more emotional and socioeconomic factor than it is a firm medical issue. In the authors' opinion, unless the patient is obtunded or clearly within days of dying, longevity predictions are so unreliable that they should not be used to decide on surgical intervention. The greater the disability associated with the actual or impending fracture, the greater the acceptable risk in intervening. For a patient whose alternative to surgery is lying in bed narcotized into oblivion, even surgical mortality exceeding 50% may be acceptable if there is some reasonable chance of restoring comfort, mobility, independence, and dignity for even a few remaining months of life. Again, the decision ultimately remains with the patient and the family, but the surgeon must give compassionate guidance unbiased by fear of marring surgical statistics with potential bad outcomes.

There is a very limited role for surgical resection of metastatic lesions for cure. When exhaustive workup has failed to reveal any other sites of disease in a patient with solitary metastases from kidney or thyroid carcinoma, there have been anecdotal reports of long-term cure obtained by wide resections with negative surgical margins. Because the morbidity and functional results of such resections usually are worse than with intralesional procedures done just for management of the mechanical problems of these lesions, substantial deliberation and patient counseling must go into making a decision to proceed with such a resection. These resections and reconstructions are more in the realm of local control for isolated primary malignant bone tumors, and are not addressed in this text, but are well covered in other references (23). In anatomic sites where wide resection with negative surgical margins does not significantly alter the magnitude of the planned procedure to deal with the mechanical problems, then such a resection should be done as a matter of course in dealing with the structural problem.

SURGICAL TECHNIQUES

There are certain general principles that apply to the choice of surgical techniques in dealing with advanced diffuse skeletal metastases that are quite different from and, in some cases, diametrically opposed to the principles of managing the same fractures in trauma to otherwise healthy bones. Pathologic fractures cannot be counted on to heal. This means implants may be load bearing for the remainder of the patient's life rather than load sharing for a period of weeks or months, as expected in usual management of traumatic fractures through normal bone. For that reason, large, rigid medullary devices with high tensile strength and stiffness are preferable to plate devices.

Furthermore, metastatic lesions notoriously occur at other sites after the surgery is done (Fig. 5), meaning that any time a procedure can stabilize or strengthen an entire bone without increasing the morbidity of the operation, it is probably a good idea to do so. A common example of this would be the use of a reconstruction rod to stabilize prophylactically an impending subtrochanteric femur lesion, rather than any sort of side-plate device.

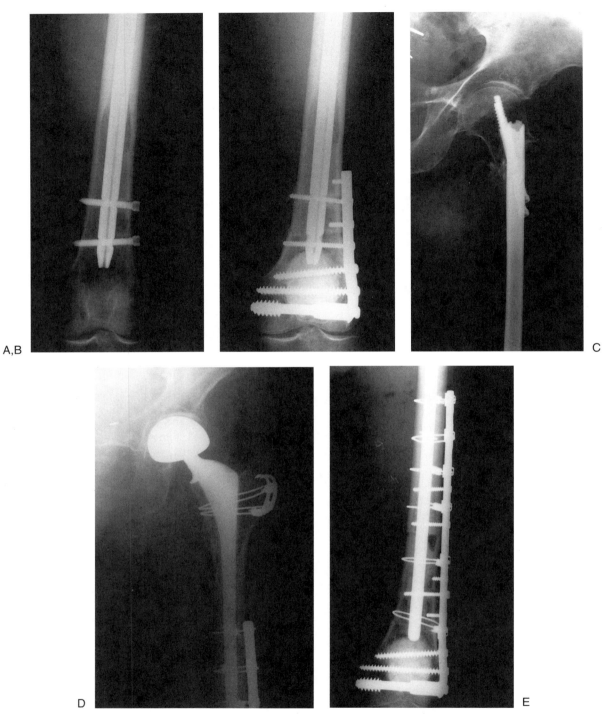

A,B

C

D

E

FIG. 5. A: This patient with metastatic thyroid carcinoma had prophylactic reconstruction rod placement for the lesion seen in his distal femoral diaphysis 2 years before the date of this radiograph. The metastatic focus at the tip of the rod in his epiphysis and metaphysis subsequently developed. **B:** The distal lesion was managed with cemented condylar screw and side plate. **C:** Approximately 1 year later, a lesion developed completely destroying the subtrochanteric region of the same femur, along with an associated pathologic avulsion fracture of his lesser trochanter. He was completely debilitated by pain and loss of function in the leg. **D,E:** He went on to have removal of the reconstruction rod and resection of the proximal two thirds of his femur with long-stem bipolar hemiarthroplasty and allograft replacement of the proximal femur. The distal screw fixation was kept intact, but the side plate was replaced with a longer plate to bridge the allograft and give sufficient overlap on the femoral stem.

In addition to implanting metal rigidly to fix fractures or bridge mechanical weak points, there is great benefit to filling defects with polymethylmethacrylate bone cement (PMMA). This gives greater mechanical integrity to the composite reconstruction. However, there are some significant caveats to using this technique. It is usually unwise to put the PMMA in before the hardware is in place, because the working time available once the PMMA is placed is in the neighborhood of 3 to 5 minutes. Instead, once the hardware is in place, the cement should be injected or pushed in around it. If such a procedure requires creating a cortical hole that further weakens the bone, serious consideration should be given to skipping the cement. If PMMA is injected, care must be given to where it may extravasate and what anatomic structures will be touched. The PMMA gets hot enough to be lethal to tissues, and a large bolus of it hardening next to a nerve or vessel can lead to disaster. Recent work has investigated the mixing of chemotherapeutic agents in the PMMA, and this technique shows some promise for the future (24).

More than in any other aspect of orthopedic surgery, the key to successful tumor surgery is contingency planning. The surgeon should prepare for failure of devices or the bone, and always think ahead of time what the options will be when it occurs. This may require having special or customized implants available. Several tumors are notorious for being hypervascular (ie, renal, thyroid, myeloma), so there should always be preparation for major blood loss. The more proximal a lesion, the more uncontrollable the situation can become, and the more thought should be given to preoperative angiography and embolization. Patient positioning on the operating table and draping of the surgical field should be done so as to allow flexibility and implementation of contingency plans as needed.

Upper Extremity

Metastases to the hand (acrometastases) are uncommon, and are especially rare in the absence of lesions elsewhere. They are more common with lung carcinoma than with other primary tumors (15). They are usually best managed with radiation therapy to symptomatic lesions, and functional bracing of actual or impending fractures. If surgery is needed, it will usually be some improvisational use of pin and PMMA fixation, or amputation (such as a highly symptomatic distal phalanx lesion).

Forearm lesions, like hand lesions, usually can be managed nonoperatively with functional bracing and radiation therapy. If surgical stabilization is done, it should be done with heavy plate fixation augmented by PMMA packing. Ordinarily, a 3.5-mm compression plate is used for its mechanical strength even if the site does not require or permit placing in compression mode. Probably

at least six cortices of fixation should be achieved on each side of the lesion if it is technically feasible.

Humeral shaft lesions can be managed operatively with medullary rod fixation supplemented with PMMA (Fig. 6). They can also be managed nonoperatively with a plastic fracture orthosis. In this non–weight-bearing bone, the decision should be based on the patient's functional demand, symptoms, expectations, and willingness to accept potential surgical morbidity. These lesions also usually lend themselves to cementation, and this is the one site where the authors frequently inject cement before final hardware insertion. When this is done, however, it is with a medullary rod which is 2 mm smaller than the reamed medullary diameter, and only after trial insertion that demonstrates the metal will fit easily and quickly over a guide wire placed down the medullary canal. Although the authors have yet to face the problem of having a rod end up cemented in an incompletely inserted position or with the guide wire cemented in place, our contingency plan for when that occurs is to use a high-speed diamond cutting disc and simply discard whatever metal remains sticking out of the bone. Humeral shaft lesions can also be operatively managed with plates and screws, but in general, large plates should be used for mechanical strength (eg, broad 4.5-mm com-

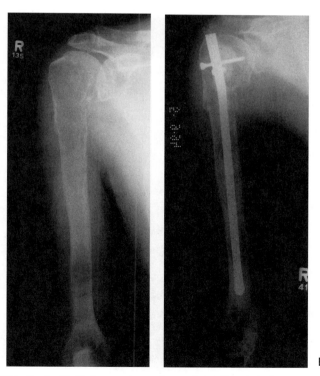

FIG. 6. **A:** Multiple myeloma throughout the right humerus with proximal diaphyseal pathologic fracture. **B:** Cemented locked medullary humeral rod.

pression plates and eight cortices of screw fixation on each side of the lesion).

Lesions about the elbow on either side of the joint seldom need surgical intervention. When radiation therapy and bracing are not sufficient, plates and PMMA packing usually are the best option. Because of the limited space available and the amount of contouring necessary to fit the irregular bony surfaces, the more pliable plates known as reconstruction plates are often the best option. In very unusual situations where destruction is massive and the patient's condition and prognosis are thought to justify the magnitude and morbidity of the procedure, joint arthroplasty may be done. This can be with custom or standard prosthetic implants, allograft transplant bone, or composites of both.

Humeral head lesions causing significant functional problems despite nonoperative treatment are usually best managed by hemiarthroplasty (Fig. 7). If there are associated humeral shaft lesions, then a long-stem implant should be used to provide fixation that bridges them. If the bone destruction is massive, then proximal humeral replacement can be done with either modular tumor prostheses or composite allograft–prosthesis reconstruction.

Scapular lesions seldom need surgery, and when they do it is usually best by resection alone. If the glenoid can be preserved, then shoulder function usually remains quite good. Even if the glenoid must be removed, the patient may be symptomatically and functionally improved with a pain-free flail shoulder and a helper hand with poor shoulder motion. Total shoulder arthroplasty is seldom needed for scapular lesions.

Lower Extremity

Foot and ankle lesions are uncommon, and usually are not a surgical problem. The structural problems are often best treated by bracing, and a patellar tendon-bearing double-upright brace can significantly unload the stress on lesions in this area. Otherwise, for the lesions that demand surgical intervention, consideration must be between PMMA-supplemented plates and ablative resection (amputation).

Tibial lesions may require surgery if large or fractured, and this can usually be done with a reamed medullary rod supplemented by cement as needed. Instead of or in addition to such surgery, a polyethylene molded tibial fracture orthosis gives a great deal of mechanical support for diaphyseal lesions.

Lesions in the knee joint are best managed with total knee arthroplasty, and the major consideration is whether patient condition and prognosis justify the surgical morbidity. Often, some symptomatic relief can be obtained

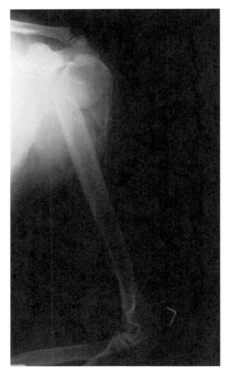
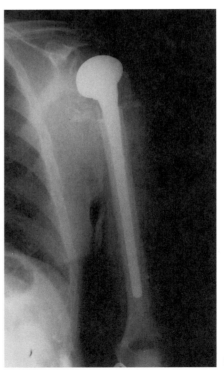

FIG. 7. A: Completely displaced proximal humerus pathologic fracture in a patient with renal carcinoma whose angiogram is shown in Fig. 4A and 4B. **B:** Cemented long-stem shoulder hemiarthroplasty with preservation of the greater tuberosity and rotator cuff.

with a hinged brace even if it does not directly support or bypass the area of the lesion.

Femoral shaft lesions should be managed according to the criteria for impending fracture discussed earlier. Because of the forces to which the femur is subjected, it is seldom appropriate to use plate fixation for diaphyseal lesions. Medullary rod is the fixation of choice, and the authors prefer a reconstruction-type rod in nearly all cases to give maximum protection to the entire bone (see Fig. 5a). In contrast to traumatic fractures through normal bone, where the trend has been toward smaller, unreamed nails, the trend in treating actual or impending pathologic fractures remains "bigger is better." Seldom should anything smaller than a 13-mm diameter rod be implanted, and bigger is preferable. A caveat for anyone unfamiliar with rodding intact bones—the canal should be over-reamed a full 2 mm to minimize the risk of fracture through a lesion during the rod insertion. Lesions that are destructive of large segments of bone are best managed by marginal resection of the involved area and replacement with prosthetic or allograft implants (see Fig. 5d,e; Fig. 8).

Lesions in the femoral head and acetabulum are best managed by total hip arthroplasty, and these sites should always be investigated and considered for such a procedure before performing a medullary rod insertion on a more distal lesion. If there are lesions in the diaphysis, a long-stem femoral implant should be used to go at least 5 cm beyond the most distal extent. In general, it can be assumed that if there is tumor in the femoral head, there is tumor in the acetabulum, so hemiarthroplasty is not usually done for metastatic disease. The best preoperative evaluation of the acetabulum is with CT scan to map the bony defect that must be filled.

Acetabular defects present a special problem for reconstruction and should be so recognized. The major factor in deciding the appropriate course of action is where the socket is deficient. If the medial wall, peripheral rim, and lateral pelvic cortex are all intact, then the defect can be filled with PMMA and a conventional cemented acetabular component can be used (Fig. 9). If the medial wall is deficient but the rim and cortex are intact, then a protrusio ring can be used to prevent medial migration, and acetabular mesh is used to contain the cement; otherwise, a conventional cemented acetabular component can be used (Fig. 10). If the acetabular rim or lateral cortex is not intact, reconstruction is done with large threaded Steinmann pins to transmit load across the deficient region of the pelvis, and the tumor void is filled with bone cement (Figs. 11 and 12). These techniques are most concisely described in the original article by Harrington reporting the technique (25). Although not unanimously agreed on by orthopedic surgeons, the general consensus and the opinion of the authors is that cement should be used on both sides of the joint in contrast to arthroplasty done for

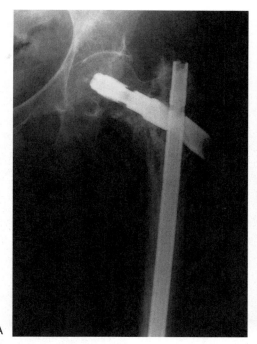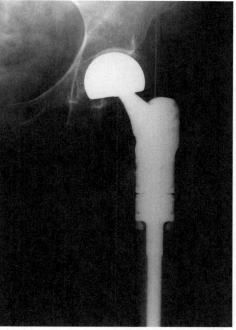

FIG. 8. A: Proximal hardware breakage through the rod connector in a reconstruction rod for pathologic intertrochanteric fracture through multiple myeloma. This cemented rod was placed 2 years before this radiograph, and the patient had been at full weight bearing with no significant pain until 1 week before this radiograph. **B:** Bipolar proximal femoral replacement hemiarthroplasty after removal of the rod and the unsalvageable portion of the proximal femur.

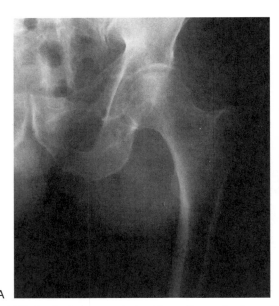

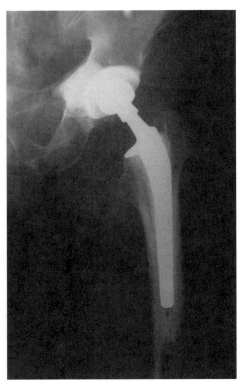

A

B

FIG. 9. A: Anteroposterior hip radiograph of a patient with multiple myeloma involving the left acetabulum, anterior column, and superior pubic ramus. **B:** Postoperative radiographs showing a cemented total hip arthroplasty including filling of the lesion with methacrylate bone cement.

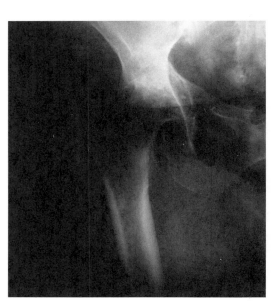

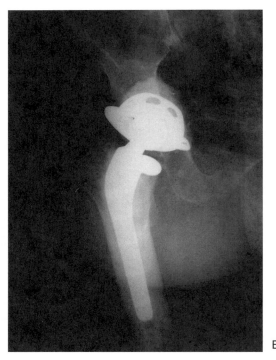

A

B

FIG. 10. A: Right hip radiograph in a patient with metastatic carcinoma of the cervix, pathologic fracture of the acetabulum with protrusio (medial migration of the femoral head), and osteonecrosis of the femoral head related to previous radiation therapy. **B:** Anteroposterior radiograph of the right hip after cemented total hip arthroplasty including use of a Harris-Oh protrusio shell to prevent migration of the components.

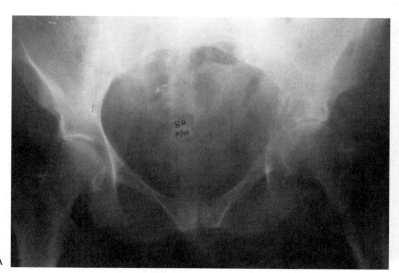

A

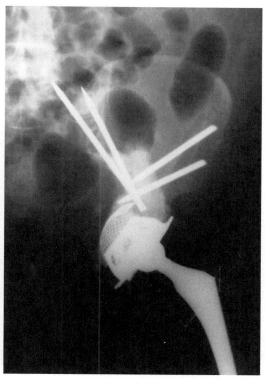

B

FIG. 11. A: Anteroposterior radiograph of the pelvis in a patient with metastatic breast carcinoma involving the left acetabulum. There is complete destruction of the anterior column and medial wall as well as superior dome and loss of the superior articular rim. **B:** Postoperative radiograph after total hip arthroplasty showing reconstruction of the medial wall with acetabular mesh, filling of the pelvic defect with methacrylate, use of a protrusio shell to prevent medial migration, and Steinmann pin fixation to allow load transfer across the cement-filled lesion.

arthritis, and that there is no role for noncemented implants in the management of metastatic disease.

Spine

Acute pathologic vertebral body fracture (in the absence of significant deformity or neurologic deficit) can usually be managed with bracing. A consensus of the indications for surgery for most authors includes:

1. To obtain tissue diagnosis
2. Symptomatic, radioresistant tumor
3. Progressive neurologic deficit during radiation therapy
4. Spinal instability or bony compression of the spinal cord

Spinal cord compression has been reported to occur in 5% to 10% of patients with spinal metastasis and usually is due to either bony fragments retropulsed into the vertebral canal or direct tumor impingement (26,27). Spinal cord dysfunction is most often related to direct compression from the anteriorly located tumor mass. As such, motor function, traveling in the anterior part of the spinal cord, is usually compromised first. Severe kyphosis may be a cause of neurologic compromise and is usually focal as a result of vertebral collapse. Intradural metastases are rare, and the dura seems to be an excellent local barrier to direct invasion (27,28). Histologic examination of spinal cords from patients who died with evidence of cord compression fails to reveal consistent patterns. The histologic changes do not strictly adhere to vascular distributions, but it has been suggested that venous congestion is the most important factor leading to neuronal degeneration (29). Parenteral steroids are widely recommended as an adjunct to other therapies, but their efficacy has never been proven in a controlled clinical trial in this setting.

Rapid onset of deficits and severe neurologic compromise are poor prognosticators of recovery regardless of the therapeutic modality. The traditional treatment for cord compression was decompressive laminectomy. Studies have shown that laminectomy offers no advantage in outcome over irradiation (30–32). Forty-four to 83% of patients with radiosensitive tumors show neurologic improvement with radiation therapy, but the average neurologic response time is 5 to 6 days, and this delay must

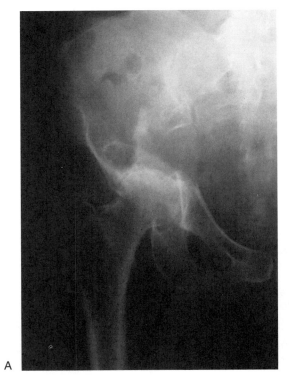

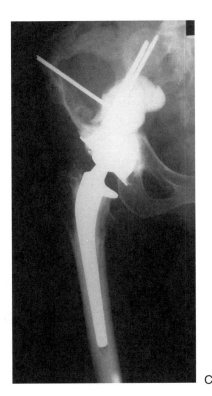

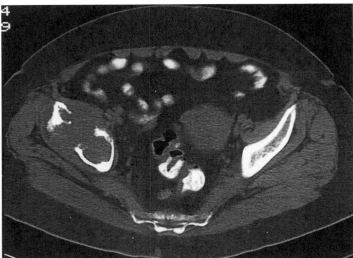

FIG. 12. A: Right hip radiograph showing destruction of the weight-bearing dome of the acetabulum and much of the right iliac wing by metastatic breast carcinoma. There is superior migration of the femoral head. **B:** Computed tomography scan through the lesion showing destruction involving anterior and posterior columns of the hip. **C:** Anteroposterior radiograph of the right hip after total hip arthroplasty using Steinmann pins and a protrusio shell.

be considered when selecting a treatment option (32). It should be emphasized that radiation therapy is likely to be effective only in the absence of retropulsed bony fragments or disk detritus. The threshold level of irradiation that interferes with bone graft incorporation and wound healing appears to be around 3000 to 3500 cGy (21). Wound complications in an irradiated patient are far more likely with posterior spinal surgery than after an anterior approach (6).

Results with laminectomy alone were poor and sometimes the procedure actually precipitated neurologic deterioration and instability (10). Laminectomy should usu-

ally be reserved for those unusual cases in which the source of compression is posterior to the cord or where multiple levels of involvement preclude anterior decompression. Laminectomy is most likely to be successful in the lumbar spine (where the cauda equina provides more room for exposure) and when the tumor mass is posteriorly located. Experimental evidence demonstrating failure of a posterior laminectomy to relieve anterior cord compression of greater than 4 mm confirms the futility of this approach (33).

Laminectomy (especially when combined with an anterior decompression) may be useful in those unusual

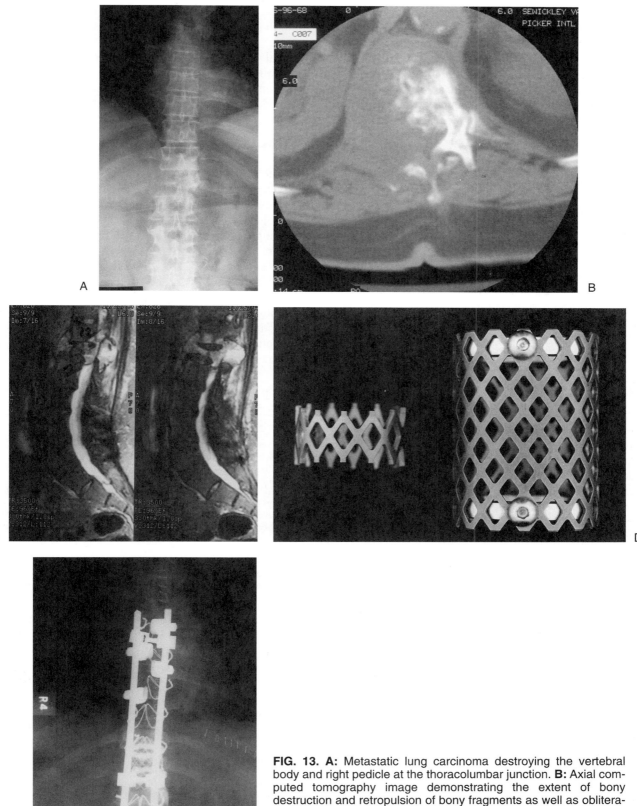

FIG. 13. A: Metastatic lung carcinoma destroying the vertebral body and right pedicle at the thoracolumbar junction. **B:** Axial computed tomography image demonstrating the extent of bony destruction and retropulsion of bony fragments as well as obliteration of epidural fat shadow. **C:** Sagittal T2-weighted magnetic resonance images showing collapse through the lesion and compression of the spinal cord by tumor as well as retropulsed bone. **D:** Metallic cage vertebral body replacement. **E:** Postoperative anteroposterior radiograph after anterior vertebral corpectomy and stabilization combined with posterior spinal instrumentation for improved stability.

cases of a "napkin ring" constriction of the cord. In cases where laminectomy is chosen, consideration should be given to instrumented stabilization because of the relatively high rate of postlaminectomy kyphosis (34). Hooks, pedicle screws, and sublaminal wires can all be used to stabilize the spinal segments above and below the involved area to the rods. The selection of specific instrumentation is often a matter of surgeons' preference and is beyond the scope of this chapter. PMMA may be used in an attempt to improve fixation to osteopenic spines, but it is less useful than in the anterior columns of the spine because of the tendency of PMMA to fail under tensile forces of the posterior spine. Bone grafting to attempt to achieve fusion is appropriate if the patient has a life expectancy of greater than 6 to 12 months; however, the risk of nonunion is probably increased from local radiation to the involved areas.

The anterior approach allows direct access to the site of neural compression and recent reports show results superior to those with laminectomy (27,35,36). This approach also allows biomechanically sound reconstruction of the anterior and middle columns of the spine, which is usually necessary after decompression. After extensive anterior decompression, often only the anterior longitudinal ligament, a shell of the far-sided cortex, and variable amounts of the pedicle remain. Because of this, it is usually necessary to reconstruct the anterior and middle columns of the spine. Structural bone grafts, PMMA–rod constructs, and metallic cage vertebral body replacements have all been used successfully to reconstruct the vertebral body (Fig. 13). The use of PMMA does not interfere with subsequent radiation therapy. If a patient's life expectancy is greater than 6 to 18 months, it is our practice to use autologous bone grafting to promote fusion. Extensive destruction, incompetent posterior elements, and a lumbar location may all militate for posterior instrumentation in addition to anterior reconstruction. In the thoracic and lumbar spine, the extent of anterior decompression possible is limited to one or two adjacent vertebral levels because of the severe instability created by a more extensive decompression.

The recovery of neurologic function depends on the rapidity of onset and degree of involvement. Regardless of treatment, if a patient progresses to a major deficit within 48 hours from the onset of symptoms, he or she has a poor prognosis for recovery. Of patients presenting with paraparesis, 35% to 65% regain their ability to ambulate, whereas only one third of patients who are frankly plegic regain ambulation. In Harrington's series, of 62 patients with major neurologic deficits, 26 recovered completely, 16 improved significantly, 20 remained unchanged, and 1 patient (without a prior deficit) deteriorated neurologically (6).

Pain associated with spinal metastases often responds to chemotherapy or local irradiation. Pathologic compression fractures not leading to significant instability can be managed with bracing. This is particularly true in the thoracic spine, where the ribs impart stability to the spine. Harrington estimates that 80% of patients with spinal metastases can be managed with nonoperative modalities. When a patient fails to respond to conservative measures, anterior decompression and stabilization provide significant relief in most patients (37).

CONCLUSION

The orthopedic management of skeletal metastases is directed to improve quality of life by relieving pain and improving function. This is accomplished by preventing pathologic fractures by prophylactic internal fixation, stabilizing fractures when they do occur, restoring destroyed joints, and decompressing sites of neurologic compression. The means used are orthotics, internal fixation fracture implants, PMMA, and the judicious use of prosthetic joint replacements and allograft bone transplants. By following the principles outlined and carefully defining realistic goals before any procedure is undertaken, a tremendous amount can be done to help the patient with advanced metastatic disease to the skeleton.

REFERENCES

1. Lane JM, Healey JH. *Diagnosis and management of pathological fractures*. New York: Raven Press; 1993.
2. Abrams HL, Sprio R, Goldstein N. Metastasis in carcinoma: analysis of 1000 autopsied cases. *Cancer* 1950;3:74.
3. Jaffe HL. *Tumors and tumorous conditions of bones and joints*. Philadelphia: Lea and Febiger; 1958.
4. Wilner D. *Radiology of bone tumors and allied disorders*. Philadelphia: WB Saunders; 1982.
5. Silverberg E. Cancer statistics: 1985. *CA Cancer J Clin* 1985;35:19.
6. Harrington KD. Anterior decompression and stabilization of the spine as a treatment for vertebral collapse and spinal cord compression from metastatic malignancy. *Clin Orthop* 1988;233:177.
7. Barron KD, Hirano A, Araki S. Experiences with metastatic neoplasms involving the spinal cord. *Neurology* 1959;9:91.
8. Black P. Spinal metastases: current status and recommended guidelines for treatment. *Neurosurgery* 1979;5:726.
9. Harrington KD. The use of methylmethacrylate for vertebral body replacement and anterior stabilization of pathologic fracture dislocations of the spine due to metastatic malignant disease. *J Bone Joint Surg [Am]* 1981;63:36.
10. Gilbert RW, et al. Epidural spinal compression from metastatic tumor: diagnosis and treatment. *Ann Neurol* 1978;3:40.
11. Harrington KD. Current concepts review: metastatic disease of the spine. *J Bone Joint Surg [Am]* 1986;68:1110.
12. Galasko CSB. The development of skeletal metastases. In: Weiss L, Gilbert HA, eds. *Bone metastases*. Boston: GK Hall Medical; 1981.
13. Powles TJ, Dowsett M, Easty GC, et al. Breast cancer osteolysis, bone metastases, and the anti-osteolytic effect of aspirin. *Lancet* 1976;1:608.
14. Leeson MC, Makley JT, Carter JR. Metastatic skeletal disease distal to the elbow and knee. *Clin Orthop* 1986;206:94.
15. Healey JH, Turnbull ADM, Miedema B, Lane JM. Acrometastases. *J Bone Joint Surg [Am]* 1986;68:743.
16. Kitazawa S, Maeda S. Development of skeletal metastases. *Clin Orthop* 1995;312:45.
17. Miyasaka M. Cancer metastasis and adhesion molecules. *Clin Orthop* 1995;312:10.
18. Mundy GR, Yoneda T. Facilitation and suppression of bone metastasis. *Clin Orthop* 1995;312:34.

19. Orr FW, Sanchez-Sweatman OH, Kostenuik P, Singh G. Tumor–bone interactions in skeletal metastasis. *Clin Orthop* 1995;312:19.
20. Harrington KD. Metastatic disease of bone. In: Chapman M, ed. *Operative orthopaedics*. Philadelphia: JB Lippincott; 1993:2567.
21. Harrington KD. Metastatic tumors of the spine: diagnosis and treatment. *Journal of the American Academy of Orthopaedic Surgeons* 1993;1:76.
22. Hipp JA, Springfield DS, Hayes WC. Predicting pathologic fracture risk in the management of metastatic bone defects. *Clin Orthop* 1995; 312:120.
23. Springfield DS, ed. Limb salvage in the treatment of musculoskeletal tumors. *Orthop Clin North Am* 1991;22:1.
24. Wang HM, Galasko CSB, Crank S, Oliver G, Ward CA. Methotrexate loaded acrylic cement in the management of skeletal metastases: biomechanical, biological, and systemic effect. *Clin Orthop* 1995;312:173.
25. Harrington KD. The management of acetabular insufficiency secondary to metastatic malignant disease. *J Bone Joint Surg [Am]* 1981; 63:653.
26. Constans JP, deDivitiis E, Donzelli R, Spaziante R, Meder JF, Hay C. Spinal metastases with neurologic manifestations: a review of 600 cases. *J Neurosurg* 1983;59:111.
27. Siegal T, Tiqva P, Siegal T. Vertebral body resection for epidural compression by malignant tumors. *J Bone Joint Surg [Am]* 1985;67:375.
28. Kostuik JP, Weinstein JN. Differential diagnosis and surgical treatment of metastatic spine tumors. In: Frymoyer JW, ed. *The adult spine: principles and practice*. New York: Raven Press; 1991:861.
29. Boland PJ, Lane JM, Sundaresan N. Metastatic disease of the spine. *Clin Orthop* 1982;169:95.
30. Cobb CA, Leavens ME, Eckles N. Indications for non-operative treatment of spinal cord compression due to breast cancer. *J Neurosurg* 1977;47:653.
31. Gilbert HA, Kagan AR, Nussbaum H, et al. Evaluation of radiation therapy for bone metastases: pain relief and quality of life. *AJR Am J Roentgenol* 1977;129:1095.
32. Young RF, Post EM, King GA. Treatment of spinal epidural metastases: a randomized prospective comparison of laminectomy and radiotherapy. *J Neurosurg* 1980;53:741.
33. Doppmann JL, Girton M. Angiographic study of the effect of laminectomy in the presence of acute anterior epidural masses. *J Neurosurg* 1976;45:195.
34. Sherman RMP, Waddell JP. Laminectomy for metastatic epidural compression by malignant tumors: results of forty-seven consecutive operative procedures. *J Bone Joint Surg [Am]* 1985;66:375.
35. Kostuik JP. Anterior spinal cord decompression for lesions of the thoracic and lumbar spine: techniques, new methods of internal fixation, results. *Spine* 1983;8:512.
36. Sundaresan N, Galich JH, Lane JM, Bains MS, McCormack P. Treatment of neoplastic epidural cord compression by vertebral body resection and stabilisation. *J Neurosurg* 1985;63: 676.
37. Fidler MW. Anterior decompression and stabilization of metastatic spinal fractures. *J Bone Joint Surg [Br]* 1986;68:83.

CHAPTER 27

Metastasectomy for Islet Carcinoma

Sally E. Carty

Even a rare disease can teach you something useful.
—*Dr. Jeffrey A. Norton*

Pancreatic islet tumors have, as a group, several unique features prompting clinicians to use metastasectomy to prolong survival. These include early presentation because of hormonal symptoms, indolent growth, a stepwise pattern of metastasis, and the availability of specific tumor markers that can signal both recurrence and response to therapy. Metastasectomy for gastrointestinal carcinoid tumors, the subject of an extensive literature that is beyond the scope of this chapter, yields results quite parallel to those of islet metastasectomy.

INCIDENCE AND NATURAL HISTORY

Islet tumors are interesting, complicated, and rare. In the United States in 1996 there were fewer than 1,430 new cases of nonthyroid endocrine cancer, associated with some 690 deaths (1). Pancreatic endocrine tumors arise from the islets of Langerhans, which normally exist interspersed with exocrine pancreatic tissue, and from the G-cells of the gastric antrum and duodenal wall. Secreted in response to a meal, the islet peptide hormones are each produced by a different cell type: alpha cells make glucagon, beta cells secrete insulin, gamma cells produce somatostatin, and gamma 2 cells elaborate vasoactive intestinal polypeptide.

Neoplasms can arise from islet tissue either sporadically or in association with inherited tumor syndromes such as multiple endocrine neoplasia type I (MEN-I) and von Hippel-Lindau syndrome. Characteristically, islet tumors cause clinical syndromes marked by specific hormonal excess. Insulinoma is the most common functional islet tumor; gastrinoma is the most com-

monly diagnosed. Islet tumor type may be confirmed immunohistochemically. Although a single tumor can secrete several hormones at once, generally one clinical syndrome predominates. In about a third of patients, islet tumors are clinically nonfunctional. Nonfunctional tumors present with abdominal pain, jaundice, or constitutional symptoms and are rising in frequency due to incidental detection on computed tomography (CT) (2). Islet tumor types, clinical syndromes, and diagnostic tests are detailed in Table 1. For a more comprehensive review, the reader is directed to three excellent articles (3–5).

Some islet tumors are malignant. As with other endocrine tumors, determination of malignant potential can be problematic because most islet tumors are histologically bland. The only recognized criteria of malignancy are involvement of another tissue and recurrence, which can occur two or three decades postoperatively. The absence of initial metastasis does not exclude the potential for future malignant behavior. Metastasis generally occurs in a stepwise pattern involving first regional nodes, then liver or direct invasion of adjacent viscera. Patients with widely metastatic disease can have lung or bone involvement. Lymph node primary tumors do occur, especially in gastrinoma (6,7).

Islet tumors grow slowly, and patients with islet carcinoma often enjoy years, even decades of long-term survival (8). On the other hand, every endocrine surgeon can recall patients who died rapidly and in their third decade of life. It is frequently taught that patients with islet metastases live "in harmony with disease" and die from other causes, but however protracted the course, most patients with malignant islet cancer do die from disease (66%–90%) (2,9,10).

Malignancy rates differ considerably by tumor type (Table 2). Tumor size is related to malignant potential, as exemplified by insulinoma which has a low malignancy rate and small size at diagnosis (often 5 mm or

S. E. Carty: Department of Surgery, University of Pittsburgh Medical Center, Pittsburgh, Pennsylvania 15261.

TABLE 1. *Islet tumor syndromes and diagnosis*

Tumor type	Clinical syndrome	Biochemical testing parameters
Gastrinoma	Zollinger-Ellison (intractable peptic ulcer disease)	Two of three criteria required for diagnosis: Fasting serum gastrin >100 pg/mL*, basal acid output >15 mEq/h (>5 mEq/h if prior gastric surgery), positive secretin test* (>200 pg/mL gastrin rise after 2U IV secretin)
Insulinoma	Whipple's triad (symptomatic fasting hypoglycemia)	Positive supervised 72-h fast: Fasting blood insulin >43 pmol/L, concurrent hypoglycemia (<39.6 mg/dL), elevated proinsulin component (>25%), negative urine sulfonurea screen
Glucagonoma	Gallstones, type II diabetes, weight loss, necrolytic migratory erythema	Fasting blood glucagon >500 pg/mL
Vasoactive intestinal polypeptide secreting tumor	Verner-Morrison (high-volume secretory diarrhea)	Plasma VIP >250 pg/mL; isoosmotic, alkaline, and hypokalemic diarrhea

*Off omeprazole ×7 days

less). Gastrinoma size is a determinant of both metastatic potential and survival (10,11). Perhaps because of subtle clinical symptoms, patients with glucagonoma characteristically have bulky disease that is already metastatic at presentation. Nonfunctional tumors have a worse prognosis (2,12). Liver involvement is a poor prognostic sign (2,9–11,13–15). In recent reports immunohistochemical detection of proliferating cell nuclear antigen, progesterone receptor activity, and MIB-1 labeling index may be useful in predicting metastatic potential or mortality in islet cancer (16–18).

Surgery is the only proven curative therapy for islet neoplasms. Two recent long-term nonrandomized series demonstrated that complete surgical resection of primary gastrinoma is associated with reduced metastasis and reduced mortality compared to unresected patients of like stage (7,10). These findings are remarkable because, in the modern era, clear evidence of a survival advantage for primary surgery is unusual in any type of solid tumor.

Now that the ulcer diathesis of gastrinoma is treated more easily with drugs than gastrectomy (19) islet metastasis is becoming recognized as the major determinant of mortality (7). How should patients with synchronous or metachronous islet metastases be managed, and can such therapy improve survival? Aggressive islet tumor metastasectomy has been advocated by several groups with experience in the field. A protocol initiated and studied at the National Cancer Institute for therapy of islet metastases is detailed here (9,13).

TREATMENT OPTIONS

Resection for Cure: Metastatic Pancreatic Endocrine Tumors

The protocol provides extirpative surgery for abdominal islet metastases to selected patients in whom, after careful radiologic staging, all identifiable tumor is considered resectable.

Indications: Determination of Resectability

In a study conducted from 1982 to 1991, 42 patients with metastatic pancreatic islet cancer were prospectively evaluated for extent of disease using CT, magnetic resonance (MR) imaging, ultrasound, angiography, and bone scan (9,13). The diagnosis was confirmed in each case using defined biochemical criteria for the type of islet tumor (see Table 1). Twenty-five patients (60%) were assessed as having inoperable disease due to diffuse liver or distant metastasis and were treated nonoperatively with chemotherapy (Table 3) and with medical therapy for hormonal symptoms (Table 4).

In 17 of the 42 patients (40%), the aggregate of radiologic information suggested that all imageable tumor could be resected. These patients underwent exploration with intent to cure. Surgery was considered extirpative if all identifiable tumor deposits were removed with pathologically negative margins. Surgery was considered pal-

TABLE 2. Islet tumor malignancy rates

Tumor type	Malignancy rate (%)
Insulinoma	10
Gastrinoma	60
Glucagonoma	70–90
Nonfunctional	85

TABLE 3. *Chemotherapy for patients with inoperable islet cancer*

Chemotherapy agents	Regimen
Streptozocin (3.0 mg/m²) Doxorubicin (40 mg/m²) 5-Fluorouracil (1,200 mg/m²)	Monthly ×1 year

TABLE 4. *Medical palliation of hormonal symptoms from islet cancer*

Tumor Type	Medical Therapy
Gastrinoma	Omeprazole, H_2 blockers
Insulinoma	Diazoxide, calcium channel blockers
Glucagonoma	Octreotide
VIPoma, carcinoid	Octreotide

liative if grossly visible metastatic or primary disease remained or if there were positive margins pathologically. Patients were examined and restaged biochemically and by imaging at 6-month intervals postoperatively. Biochemical cure was defined as the normalization of preoperatively elevated hormonal levels with concurrent negative imaging. Postoperative chemotherapy was administered to 10 of the 17 patients (see Table 3), and 4 patients with recurrent metastatic gastrinoma also received alpha-interferon (5 million units/day).

Subsequent to this study, patients are currently evaluated preoperatively using the following protocol modifications:

1. In most patients, abdominal imaging by CT and/or gadolinium-MR is both effective and cost-effective in assessing the extent of disease.
2. Equivocal cases are further assessed by angiography, octreotide scan, or both (20).
3. Chest CT is included in preoperative staging.
4. A bone scan is reserved for symptomatic patients only.

All instruments, including intraoperative ultrasound (IOUS) transducers, are in routine use at most tertiary referral centers. Nuclear octreotide scanning is now widely available as well. The safety of patients willing to undergo major surgery for islet carcinoma demands a surgical team, a facility, and a medical community with experience in the field.

Detailed Methodology

At surgery, the goal is to remove all preoperatively identified metastases as well as any additional tumor present at exploration. Patients are explored through a chevron incision extended into the right chest for right lobe hepatic resections. Examination of the entire abdominal contents includes mobilization and careful palpation of the duodenum and pancreas. IOUS with a 10-mHz transducer is performed to locate primary and multiple tumors and to visualize pancreatic duct anatomy. Open duodenotomy is performed to identify gastrinomas within the duodenal wall, which are treated with full-thickness excision. The lymph nodes around the porta hepatis, celiac axis, and pancreas are exposed and examined. The liver is bimanually palpated and examined using the 5-mHz IOUS transducer.

All gross identified disease is then resected. Enucleation of pancreatic primary tumor is avoided when possible because the tumor is already proven to have malignant spread. Stapled distal or subtotal pancreatectomy is used to treat pancreatic primary neoplasms, saving the spleen when possible. Involved viscera are resected conventionally. Suspicious or abnormal lymph nodes are excised. Bulky unilobar hepatic disease is treated with anatomic liver resection; superficial or contralateral hepatic metastases are excised by wedge resection. Postoperatively, pancreatic drains are pulled when patients are tolerating a regular diet off octreotide with drainage <10 cc/day.

Results of Surgery

Of 17 patients treated by aggressive metastasectomy, 7 were women and the mean age was 49 years (range 26–79). Twelve patients had gastrinoma, 2 had insulinoma, 2 had glucagonoma, and 1 patient's tumor secreted both ACTH and gastrin; 1 patient had MEN-I. These 17 patients underwent 20 operations for metastases, including 14 liver resections, 11 pancreatic resections, 8 viscerectomies and 12 regional lymphadenectomies. Preoperative imaging overestimated the extent of disease in two of 20 cases and underestimated the extent of disease in 13 of 20 cases, but surgery was palliative in only four cases. There was a 30% short-term morbidity rate commensurate with the extensive nature of the resections performed, and no mortality. The mean follow-up interval was 38.8 months (range 5–111).

Response Rates

Immediate biochemical cure after aggressive metastasectomy was achieved in 14 of 20 operations. All patients enjoyed a reduction in antisecretory medications. Survival in the operated group (Fig. 1**A**) was 87% at 2 years and 79% at 5 years, and did not differ by tumor type. In the 25 inoperable patients, demographics and tumor type were similar to the operated group; 2-year survival was 60% and 5-year survival was 28% (p=.0176 versus the resected group) (Fig. 1B). All study deaths were from islet cancer except for one unoperated patient with meningioma.

Two patients underwent three reoperations for recurrent metastatic islet cancer. In one man, multiple re-resections permitted survival for more than 9 years after initial metastasectomy. Four patients had a biochemical cure (14–51 months of follow-up). The median interval to radiologic recurrence was 44 months for the patients who underwent complete resection. Most recurrences were in the liver. Because no patient remained disease-free more than 7.5 years, it was concluded that most operated patients can expect durable survival in the face of recurrent metastases.

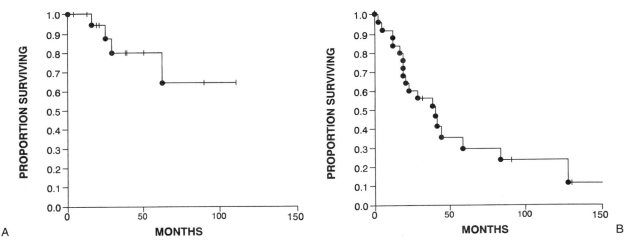

FIG. 1. A: Survival from date of operation for metastatic islet cancer. **B:** Survival from date of diagnosis of metastatic islet cancer in inoperable patients. (Carty SE, Jensen RT, Norton JA. Prospective study of aggressive resection of metastatic pancreatic endocrine tumors. *Surgery* 1992:112:1024, with permission)

Subgroup analysis was quite informative. Stratification based on the extent of surgery required to resect all metastases present at surgery yielded two directly comparable and easily identifiable groups. Nine patients had extensive disease, defined as unilobar bulky hepatic deposits requiring anatomic lobectomy (6 patients) and/or direct invasion of extrapancreatic viscera requiring viscerectomy (8 patients). Eight patients had limited metastatic disease, defined as that amenable to lymphadenectomy and hepatic wedge resection. Long-term survival was markedly improved in the group requiring limited metastasectomy (Fig. 2) compared to patients

with extensive abdominal metastases ($p<.019$). No differences were observed in time to recurrence. Although patients with resected extensive disease had survival no different than did inoperable patients (Fig. 1B), 2 of the 4 patients who enjoyed a durable biochemical cure required extensive resections to achieve that cure.

In summary, a protocol to select patients with islet carcinoma for aggressive metastasectomy demonstrated the safety, feasibility, and excellent long-term survival associated with such therapy. Half of the patients undergoing metastasectomy achieved long-term survival. Recurrence was common, and re-resection was reasonable therapy for some patients. Early islet metastasectomy conferred a clear survival advantage compared to late metastasectomy.

Review of Published Experience

Several authors have advocated islet metastasectomy to prolong survival, in both case reports (21–26) and clinical series (7–10,12,13,27,28). In an important review of 37 patients who underwent cytoreductive metastasectomy for metastatic islet and carcinoid neoplasms, hepatic metastasectomy palliated hormonal symptoms in 72% of patients (28). Danforth and colleagues obtained a median disease-free survival of 5 years after surgery for metastatic insulinoma (27). Ellison and associates determined a 62% 10-year survival in gastrinoma patients who underwent resection compared to 27% in patients incompletely resected or inoperable (29). Although analysis is limited by factors such as study design, sample size, definitions of malignancy, and inclusion of other tumor types, the preponderance of evidence strongly supports a survival advantage for islet metastasectomy (Table 5). A random-

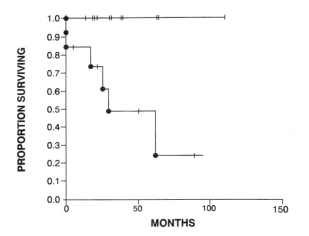

FIG. 2. Survival of aggressively resected patients with limited (*open circles*) or extensive (*closed circles*) islet metastases. (Carty SE, Jensen RT, Norton JA. Prospective study of aggressive resection of metastatic pancreatic endocrine tumors. *Surgery* 1992:112:1024, with permission)

TABLE 5. *Results of islet cancer resection and metastasectomy*

Author	Islet #	Tumor type	Extirpative rate (%)*	Resected 5-year survival (%)			Unoperated 5-y survival (%)
				Overall	Limited	Extensive	
Primary Islet Cancer							
Legaspi (30)	25	Mixed islet	†36	—	†100	—	†34
Thompson (2)	58	Mixed islet	†26	40	60	35	—
Ellison (10)	74	Gastrinoma	36	95	—	—	84
Islet Metastasectomy							
Norton (13)	5	Gastrinoma	80	†80	—	—	20
McEntee (28)	13	Mixed islet	46	77	83	71	—
Carty (9)	42	Mixed islet	80	79	100	48	28
Ellison (10)	27	Gastrinoma	†37	100	—	—	33
Danforth (27)	17	Insulinoma	†35	59	83	—	11
Evans (12)	34	Nonfunctional	—	50	72	41	38

*Frequency of complete (vs. palliative) resection performed when curative resection was the intent of surgery

† estimated

ized prospective trial to examine this issue may never take place, not only because of the rarity of the disease but also because of patient reluctance to be excluded from operative therapy.

That early metastasectomy for limited disease is demonstrably advantageous is also supported by several authors (9,12,27,28–30). Extirpative metastasectomy for extensive disease (9) and palliative cytoreductive surgery (10,27,28) do not appear to offer a significant survival advantage compared to patients with inoperable metastases (see Table 5).

Cure is possible after islet metastasectomy, with long-term cure rates remarkably similar between studies and ranging from 24% to 48%. Several recent studies have presented good evidence to support aggressive initial surgery for primary islet cancer (10,12,19,30,31). Interestingly, the long-term cure rate for primary islet carcinoma resection is comparable at 19% to 35% (2,30), and 5-year survival after primary islet resection is no different than after metastasectomy in selected patients (see Table 5). In our opinion, these data do not contradict the surgical dictum that the best time to treat a tumor is at the initial operation (5) but emphasize that the indolent nature of islet carcinoma often allows time for another try.

Postoperative Surveillance

Although cure is possible, recurrence is common after islet metastasectomy. Extirpative or palliative re-resection of metastases is frequently an issue in follow-up, and regular surveillance for recurrence is thus obligatory. To a degree perhaps not fully appreciated by those outside the field of endocrine surgery, the surveillance of patients with islet carcinoma is greatly and specifically facilitated by the ability to follow blood levels of islet hormonal peptides and tumor markers (see Table 1). Islet tumor markers detect the likelihood of recurrent disease earlier than radiologic imaging and more reliably than the known tumor markers widely used in nonendocrine cancer histologies. In patients with gastrinoma, normal fasting serum gastrin and secretin testing at 6 months, 1 year, and 2 years postoperatively predicts the 3-year disease-free interval with probabilities of 88%, 95%, and 100% respectively (32). Useful islet tumor markers not specific to islet tumor type include serum levels of pancreatic polypeptide and chromogranin A.

Palliative Resection of Metastatic Islet Carcinoma

Although resection and even multiple resection of islet metastases may prolong survival, most patients with islet cancer die of disease, often of hepatic dysfunction from liver replacement by tumor. Not only can palliative resection alleviate or improve serious tumor-related hormonal symptoms, but it can also reduce the need for medication and relieve local symptoms of obstruction, hemorrhage, or jaundice (4,5,28). The efficacy of palliative resection is difficult to evaluate critically because of varying criteria for symptom relief, but McEntee and coworkers observed a rate of symptomatic improvement of 88% independent of whether symptoms were caused by hormonal oversecretion or local mass effect (28). Thompson and colleagues observed a 51% symptomatic improvement rate with a mean duration of 39 months (2). In one retrospective series, palliative resection was reportedly associated with a survival advantage in patients with metastatic insulinoma (27). Rarely, end organ extirpation may be of benefit—for example, a patient with an ACTH-secreting islet tumor may benefit from bilateral adrenalectomy.

Other Therapeutic Options

Medical Therapy

Medical palliation may appear to be simpler than cytoreductive surgery but may be costly, ineffective, or deleterious to quality of life. For example, patients with metastatic insulinoma frequently cannot tolerate the peripheral edema that can accompany diazoxide therapy. Octreotide therapy is useful in controlled diarrhea in patients with VIPoma, can partially alleviate the characteristic rash of patients with glucagonoma, and may even provide an antitumor response in some patients (8). Octreotide therapy causes acute cholecystitis in about a third of patients with pre-existing gallstones and predisposes to the development of gallstones, so that prophylactic cholecystectomy should be performed for cholelithiasis before octreotide is started (33).

Islet carcinoma responds to systemic chemotherapy. Despite the rarity of the disease there have been several good clinical trials examining single and multiagent therapy (34–37) with possible improvement in survival (34). An effective regimen used at the National Cancer Institute employs streptozocin, doxorubicin (Adriamycin), and 5-fluorouracil with an overall 60% response rate (13). Streptozocin, a broad-spectrum antibiotic, is a potent diabetogenic agent. DTIC given as monotherapy also has produced a reasonable response rate in some patients. Interferon alpha-2b combined with continuous-infusion fluorouracil achieved a 33% response rate of mean duration 8.4 months (38). The reader is referred to two excellent reviews of this subject (4,35).

Hepatic Therapies

Prompted by slow islet tumor biology, total hepatectomy and orthotopic liver transplantation have been examined in patients with conventionally unresectable abdominal islet metastases (39,40). Early results were encouraging with 4 of 5 patients alive at median follow-up of 12 months (38). In a larger series of 14 patients undergoing abdominal cluster transplantation for islet cancer, 3-year survival was 64% (40). However, at least one patient has experienced a lethal recurrence while on immunosuppression and hepatic transplantation in this setting has not garnered the enthusiastic support of the transplant community.

Percutaneous hepatic arterial embolization with a variety of toxic agents has been used for unresectable islet cancer (8,28,35,41–43). By injuring liver tumor cells rather than the hepatic parenchyma, hepatic artery therapies are thought to decrease tumor hormone secretion and cause remission. Therapeutic agents delivered to the liver include Gelfoam particles, chemotherapeutic agents, and ethiodol. Ajani and associates noted a 60% response rate and favorable reduction in hormonal symptomatology, with projected median survival of 33.7 months from therapy (41). In patients treated with hepatic artery embolization, ligation, or both, McEntee and coworkers reported a symptomatic response of 80% to 90% and a median duration of >5 months, compared to 30% to 40% and 7 months (respectively) in patients treated with systemic chemotherapy (28). Short-term morbidity such as abdominal pain, vomiting, and fever can be considerable, so delivery of hepatic artery therapy should be limited to centers with specific experience.

In patients with bulky bilobar hepatic deposits, cirrhosis, or involvement of hepatic structures that precludes liver resection, hepatic cryotherapy may be a reasonable option. Results of cryotherapy were reported in 6 patients with metastatic neuroendocrine cancer (carcinoid, islet, and paraganglioma), and all had a complete radiologic response, with an 89% decrease in tumor markers and major morbidity in 50% (44).

PATIENT ASSESSMENT

Criteria for patients being considered for islet metastasectomy are detailed above. Published results may not reflect those encountered in daily practice, and the safety and well-being of any patient is of paramount importance.

The management of patients with islet tumors in MEN-I remains controversial (45–48). In this autosomal dominant disorder with 90% penetrance, islet microadenomas are present throughout the pancreas and coexist with parathyroid hyperplasia and adenomas of the anterior pituitary gland. Islet microadenomas can give rise to multiple islet neoplasms, both functional and nonfunctional. Duodenal gastrinomas, occurring up to 70% of the time in MEN-I (47) can also be multiple. When a patient with MEN-I develops a syndrome of islet hormonal excess, it can be difficult to localize the islet tumor responsible. Recently it was proposed that resection should be offered to MEN-I patients for symptomatic islet tumors that can be localized by invasive portal venous sampling or for imageable disease 3 cm or larger (7,48). This strategy seems inherently sensible because islet tumors associated with MEN-I are more indolent than sporadic gastrinomas (10). Nevertheless, islet cancer does occur in MEN-I (45); in our experience, about one third of MEN-I patients followed prospectively die of metastatic islet carcinoma. The goal of surgical therapy in patients with MEN-I is to alter the natural course of disease and improve survival. Problems with this strategy include a high rate (50%) of synchronous metastasis using the 3-cm cutoff (45,48), and further study is definitely required. Surgical cure of MEN-I gastrinoma is possible (26,46) but rare (45).

Every patient with an islet tumor should be evaluated for possible MEN-I. The disorder has been mapped to chromosome 11q2 (49), but as yet no direct gene test is available. Linkage analysis is an option in families with three or more affected members. Screening for MEN-I is currently done by clinical testing and careful family history. Any patient with an islet tumor should undergo fasting serum calcium and prolactin levels every 2 years until age 70. MEN-I should be suspected when the family history is significant for kidney stones, hyperparathyroidism, infertility, pancreatic tumors, or islet tumor symptomatology. In a patient with MEN-I manifested as both gastrinoma and hyperparathyroidism, it is now well established that the initial operation is parathyroidectomy. Total parathyroidectomy and autotransplantation can very nicely ameliorate the symptoms of MEN-I-associated gastrinoma, often for years (50).

REFERENCES

1. Cancer statistics, 1996. *CA Cancer J Clin* 1996;65:5.
2. Thompson GB, van Heerden JA, Grant CS, Carney JA, Ilstrup DM. Islet cell carcinomas of the pancreas: a twenty-year experience. *Surgery* 1988;104;6:1011.
3. Townsend Jr CM, Thompson JC. Neoplasms of the endocrine pancreas. In Greenfield LJ, Mullholland MW, Oldham KT, Zelenock GB, eds. *Surgery: scientific principles and practice.* Philadelphia: JB Lippincott, 1993:833.
4. Modlin IM, Lewis JJ, Ahlman H, Bilchik AJ, Kumar RR. Management of unresectable malignant endocrine tumors of the pancreas. *SGO* 1993;176:507.
5. Zogakis TG, Norton JA. Palliative operations for patients with unresectable endocrine neoplasia. *Surg Clin North Am* 1995;75:525.
6. Perrier ND, Batts KP, Thompson GB, Grant CS, Plummer TB, the Mayo Clinic Pancreatic Surgery Group. An immunohistochemical survey for neuroendocrine cells in regional pancreatic lymph nodes: a plausible explanation for primary nodal gastrinomas? *Surgery* 1995; 118:957.
7. Fraker DL, Norton JA, Alexander R, Venzon DJ, Jensen RT. Surgery in Zollinger-Ellison syndrome alters the natural history of gastrinoma. *Ann Surg* 1994;220:320.
8. Moertel CG. An odyssey in the land of small tumors. *J Clin Oncol* 1987;5:1503.
9. Carty SE, Jensen RT, Norton JA. Prospective study of aggressive resection of metastatic pancreatic endocrine tumors. *Surgery* 1992: 112:1024.
10. Ellison EC. Forty-year appraisal of gastrinoma: back to the future. *Ann Surg* 1995;222:511.
11. Weber HC, Venzon DJ, Lin J-T, et al. Determinants of metastatic rate and survival in patients with Zollinger-Ellison syndrome: a prospective long-term study. *Gastroenterology* 1995;108:1637.
12. Evans DB, Skibber JM, Lee JE, et al. Nonfunctioning islet cell carcinoma of the pancreas. *Surgery* 1993;114(6):1175–1182.
13. Norton JA, Doppman JL, Gardner JD. Aggressive resection of metastatic disease in selected patients with malignant gastrinoma. *Ann Surg* 1986;203:352.
14. Zollinger RM. Gastrinoma: factors influencing prognosis. *Surgery* 1985;97:49.
15. Mignon M, Ruszniewski P, Haffar S, et al. Current approach to the management of tumoral process in patients with gastrinoma. *World J Surg* 1986;10:703.
16. Pelosi G, Zamboni G, Doglioni C, et al. Immunodetection of proliferating cell nuclear antigen assesses the growth fraction and predicts malignancy in endocrine tumors of the pancreas. *Am J Surg Pathol* 1992;16:1215.
17. Viale G, Doglioni C, Gambacorta M, Zamboni G, Coggi G, Bordi C. Progesterone receptor immunoreactivity in pancreatic endocrine tumors. *Cancer* 1992;70:2268.
18. Clarke MR, Baker EE, Hill L. Proliferative activity in pancreatic

19. Maton PN, Gardner JD, Jensen RT. Diagnosis and management of Zollinger-Ellison syndrome. *Endocrinol Metab Clin North Am* 1989; 19:519.
20. Krenning EP, Kwekkeboom DJ, Bakker WH, et al. Somatostatin receptor scintigraphy wide [^{111}In-DTPA-D-Phe^1]- and [^{123}I-Tyr^3]-octreotide: the Rotterdam experience with more than 1000 patients. *Eur J Nucl Med* 1993;20:8.
21. Montenegro F, Lawrence GD, Macon W, Pass C. Metastatic glucagonoma: improvement after surgical debulking. *Am J Surg* 1980; 139:424.
22. Prinz RA, Badrinath K, Banerji M, Sparagana M, Dorsch TR, Lawrence AM. Operative and chemotherapeutic management of malignant glucagon-producing tumors. *Surgery* 1981;90:713.
23. Nagorney DM, Bloom SR, Polak JM, Blumgart LH. Resolution of recurrent Verner-Morrison syndrome by resection of metastatic VIPoma. *Surgery* 1983;93:348.
24. Rader DL, Martin Jr JK, Scheithauer BW. Cytoreduction surgery for metastatic glucagonoma. *Minn Med* 1984:483.
25. Goletti O, Chiarugi M, Buccianti P, et al. Resection of liver gastrinoma leading to persistent eugastrinemia. *Eur J Surg* 1992;158:55.
26. Cherner JA, Sawyers JJ. Benefit of resection of metastatic gastrinoma in multiple endocrine neoplasia type I. *Gastroenterology* 1992; 102:1049.
27. Danforth DN, Gorden P, Brennan MF. Metastatic insulin-secreting carcinoma of the pancreas: clinical course and the role of surgery. *Surgery* 1984;96:1027.
28. McEntee GP, Nagorney DM, Kvols LK, Moertel CG, Grant CS. Cytoreductive hepatic surgery for neuro-endocrine tumors. *Surgery* 1990;108:1091.
29. Ellison EC, Carey LC, Sparks J, et al. Early surgical treatment of gastrinoma. *Am J Med* 1987;82(suppl 5B):17.
30. Legaspi A, Brennan M. Management of islet cell carcinoma. *Surgery* 1988;104:1018.
31. Zollinger RM, Ellison EC, Fabri PJ, et al. Primary peptic ulcerations of the jejunum associated with islet cell tumors. *Ann Surg* 1980;192:422.
32. Fishbeyn VA, Norton JA, Benya RV, et al. Assessment and prediction of long-term cure in patients with the Zollinger-Ellison syndrome: the best approach. *Ann Intern Med* 1993;119:199.
33. Maton PN. The use of the long-acting somatostatin analogue, octreotide acetate, in patients with islet cell tumor. *Gastroenterol Clin North Am* 1989;18:897.
34. Kvols LK, Buck M. Chemotherapy of endocrine malignancies: a review. *Semin Oncol* 1987;14:343.
35. Ajani JA, Levin B, Wallace S. Systemic and regional therapy of advanced islet cell tumors. *Gastroenterol Clin North Am* 1989;18:923.
36. Moertel CG, Lefkopoulo M, Lipsitz S, Hahn RG, Klaassen D. Streptozocin-doxorubicin, streptozocin-fluorouracil, or chlorotozocin in the treatment of advanced islet cell carcinoma. *N Engl J Med* 1992; 326:519.
37. Moertel CG, Kvols L, O'Connell MJ, Rubin J. Treatment of neuroendocrine carcinomas with combined etoposide and cisplatin: evidence of major therapeutic activity in the anaplastic variants of these neoplasms. *Cancer* 1991;68:227.
38. Andreyev HJN, Scott-Mackie P, Cunningham D, et al. Phase II study of continuous infusion fluorouracil and interferon alpha-2b in the palliation of malignant neuroendocrine tumors. *J Clin Oncol* 1995; 13:1486.
39. Makakowa L, Tzakis AG, Mazzaferro V, et al. Transplantation of the liver for metastatic endocrine tumors of the intestine and pancreas. *Surg Gynecol Obstet* 1989;168:107.
40. Alessiani M, Tzakis A, Todo S, Demetris AJ, Fung JJ, Starzl TE. Assessment of five-year experience with abdominal organ cluster transplantation. *J Am Coll Surg* 1995;180:1.
41. Ajani JA, Carrasco CH, Charnsangavej C, Samaan NA, Levin B, Wallace S. Islet cell tumors metastatic to the liver: effective palliation by sequential hepatic artery embolization. *Ann Intern Med* 1988;108:340.
42. Mavligit GM, Pollock RE, Evans HL, Wallace S. Durable hepatic tumor regression after arterial chemoembolisation-infusion in patients with islet cell carcinoma of the pancreas metastatic to the liver. *Cancer* 1993;72:375.
43. Lai DTM, Kent-Man Chu, Thompson JF, et al. Islet cell carcinoma treated by induction regional chemotherapy and radical total pancreate-

ctomy with liver revascularization and small bowel autotransplantation. *Surgery* 1996;119:112.

44. Cozzi PJ, Englund R, Morris DL. Cryotherapy treatment of patients with hepatic metastases from neuroendocrine tumors. *Cancer* 1995;76:501.

45. Sheppard BC, Norton JA, Doppman JL, Maton PN, Gardner JD, Jensen RT. Management of islet cell tumors in patients with multiple endocrine neoplasia: a prospective study. *Surgery* 1989;106:1108.

46. Thompson NW, Bondeson A-G, Bondeson L, Vinik A. The surgical treatment of gastrinoma in MEN I syndrome patients. *Surgery* 1989;106:1081.

47. MacFarlane MP, Fraker DL, Alexander HR, Norton JA, Lubensky I, Jensen RT. Prospective study of surgical resection of duodenal and pancreatic gastrinomas in multiple endocrine neoplasia type I. *Surgery* 1995;118:973.

48. Fraker DL, Norton JA, Alexander HR, Venzon DJ, Jensen RT. Zollinger-Ellison syndrome: surgery should still play an important role in its management. *Gastroenterology* 1995;108:1600.

49. Larsson C, et al. Multiple endocrine neoplasia type I maps to chromosome 11 and is lost in insulinoma. *Nature* 1988;332:85.

50. Norton JA, Cornelius MJ, Doppman JL. Effect of parathyroidectomy in patients with hyperparathyroidism, Zollinger-Ellison syndrome, and multiple endocrine neoplasia type I: a prospective study. *Surgery* 1987;102:958.

CHAPTER 28

Gene Therapy of Local Tumors

Gerard J. McGarrity and Yawen L. Chiang

G. J. McGarrity and Y. L. Chiang: Genetic Therapy, Inc./Novartis, Gaithersburg, Maryland 20878.

There is a gift of being able to see at a glance the possibilities offered by the terrain.

—*Napoleon*

In the United States, clinical protocols in gene therapy, as in other specialties, must be approved by the Food and Drug Administration (FDA). In the past, these protocols have also been reviewed by the Recombinant DNA Advisory Committee (RAC) of the National Institutes of Health (NIH). Because of the RAC review, a public record is available of the numbers and types of protocols in all fields, including cancer. Approval by the NIH RAC does not necessarily mean that the FDA has also approved the protocol, or that the clinical study has been initiated. It does, however, offer an overview of the various approaches being considered in the field of cancer gene therapy.

In the first 7 years of gene therapy, from 1990 to the beginning of 1997, about 140 clinical studies in gene transfer were approved by the RAC. These numbers include both gene marking, where genes encoding resistance to an antibiotic marker have been administered, and genes having a therapeutic objective. Additional trials have been conducted in Europe. During that time, more than 1,500 patients received gene therapy worldwide, and the number continues to increase rapidly. About 70% of these patients received retroviral vector as a means of gene transfer. At this writing, no adverse effects due directly to this vector type have been published.

Table 1 lists the tumor targets that have been approved by the RAC. These represent all major tumor types. Most trials have used retroviral vector-mediated gene transfer. Other vector systems have included adenoviral vectors, encasing genes within liposomes, and the use of "naked" plasmid DNA. One trial has used a canary pox vector.

The clinical targets listed in Table 1 can be summarized according to their therapeutic objective:

Modulating immune functions
Restoring tumor suppressors
Blocking oncogene expression
Providing prodrug metabolizing enzymes
Producing genetic modification of tumor cells.

All the gene transfer protocols to date, both gene marking and gene therapy, have been phase I/II studies. The major objectives have been to determine if the gene could be transferred safely without adverse effects to the patient and to determine the level of gene transfer and expression in the target cells. Clinical efficacy was not a primary objective in these trials and has not been demonstrated, based on the absence of published results of controlled prospective studies. The focus of this chapter is to review the methodologies of gene transfer, to review the strategies used in the application of gene therapy to oncology, and to offer some reasonable projections of future developments. In such a new and emerging field, it is impossi-

TABLE 1. *Tumor targets of clinical studies in gene therapy*

Melanoma
Renal cell carcinoma
Colon/metastasis to liver
Breast
Leukemia (various types)
Ovarian
Neuroblastoma
Glioblastoma
Nonsmall cell lung carcinoma
Astrocytoma
Head and neck
Prostate
Mesothelioma
Lymphoma
Multiple myeloma
Hepatocellular carcinoma

ble to describe in detail each clinical protocol involving cancer gene therapy. Rather, relevant examples of major approaches are listed, defining some of the cytokines and methods of delivery. For more complete details, comprehensive reviews are cited. In addition, the journal *Human Gene Therapy* publishes clinical protocols that are available to the public.

GENE DELIVERY SYSTEMS

In one respect, gene therapy can be viewed as a novel method of drug delivery. Gene therapy itself can be defined as a method of transferring a gene or genes to a cell to supply a missing gene or to confer a new function to a cell. In the early trials, the genes that have typically been transferred are relatively small and subject to minimal gene regulation. For example, in the first therapeutic trial of gene therapy (which was for a metabolic disorder, severe combined immune deficiency due to adenosine deaminase [ADA] deficiency), the therapeutic goal was to restore about 10% to 15% of normal ADA blood levels; this was predicted to have therapeutic benefit (1).

In gene therapy, the genes of interest are transferred by instruments known as vectors. Vectors can be classified as either viral or nonviral. To date, the overwhelming number of trials have used viral vectors. The viral systems involve the use of certain viruses that have been rendered replication-incompetent by molecular engineering and then have had the gene or genes of choice, the transgene, inserted into the vector. In this way, the viral vector can enter the cell (transduction), thereby transferring the gene. Many viruses have the potential to serve as vectors. To date, murine retroviral vectors have accounted for about 70% of the protocols approved by the RAC. Adenoviral vectors account for about 15% and nonviral systems for an additional 12%. Most trials using adenoviral vectors have been for cystic fibrosis. Two clinical trials, both for cystic fibrosis, have proposed the use of a vector derived from adeno-associated virus (AAV).

Different vectors have special characteristics that allow them to have predilections for certain cell types (Table 2).

TABLE 2. *Characteristics of some viral vector systems*

Characteristic	Retro	Adeno	AAV
Maximum size of transgene	8.5	7.0*	4.7
Need for replicating cell	Y	N	N
Genomic integration	Y	N	Y
Generation of replication-competent form	Possible	Possible	Needs adeno or herpes
Inflammatory response possible to vector backbone	N	Y	N

*Maximum size of the trangene depends on the amount of adeno genome that is deleted.

Some of these basic characteristics are discussed below, and more information can be obtained in reviews of these vector types.

Retroviral Vectors

The retroviral vectors currently in clinical trials are derived from the Moloney strain of murine leukemia virus. Murine leukemia retroviruses contain two single-stranded RNAs that replicate through a DNA intermediate in the target cell. To construct a vector, the three structural genes of the murine leukemia virus (*gag*, *pol*, and *env*) are removed, essentially leaving only the long terminal repeats. The structural genes are replaced with the transgene(s) of interest. Often, two separate genes are introduced into a vector. The first gene is inserted 3′ to the long terminal repeat that acts as promoter. A second promoter can be inserted 3′ of the first gene and run off a second inserted promoter. Often a viral promoter—for instance, from cytomegalovirus or simian virus 40 virus—is used. Alternately, an internal ribosome entry site element derived from a virus can be used. Murine retroviral vectors can accommodate about 8.5 kilobases (kb) of sequence. The structural genes of the vector are supplied in trans by a packaging cell specifically engineered for a particular vector type. The vector contains a sequence (termed psi or packaging signal) needed to process or package the RNAs into the vector structure (2,3).

When the packaging cell has been transfected with the vector via plasmid DNA, it is termed a producer cell. The producer cell, containing the genes encoding the structural components, and the vector, containing the transgene and psi, will produce the replication-incompetent vector. The vectors are elaborated into the supernatant medium of the producer cell culture. Titers typically are in the range of 1×10^5 to 1×10^6 vectors/mL. However, effective clonal selection and downstream processing and concentration can significantly increase titers (to 1×10^9 for some vectors).

Retroviral vectors are characterized by their ability to transduce replicating but not nonreplicating cells. This selectivity makes retroviral vectors attractive for certain applications (eg, incorporation into tumor cells in the brain, but not into neighboring neural cells). The vectors are incorporated by the dividing cells and uncoated in the cytoplasm, and the transgenes are transported to the nucleus, where they integrate in a random fashion into the host genome. The integrated provirus is present for the life of the cell. However, the simple presence of the transgene (as, for example, detected by Southern analysis) does not guarantee gene expression. Gene expression must be validated by either Northern analysis or a functionality assay specific for the gene.

Theoretically, the random insertion of the retroviral vector into the host genome as a provirus might increase mutation rates. This has been reviewed, and the calculated increase is extremely low (4). Nevertheless, specific mutations are possible that could result in the activation of a cellular oncogene or the inactivation of a tumor suppressor. However, oncogenesis is a multistep process requiring a series of individual progressions.

Because of their ability to transduce replicating cells, retroviral vectors have often been used to transduce tumor cells (as well as lymphocytes, bone marrow, and skin fibroblast cells) as part of cancer gene therapy protocols (5). This transduction can be performed when the cells have been removed from the patient and propagated in the laboratory, a procedure termed ex vivo gene therapy. Alternately, the transduction can be carried out in situ or in vivo.

Retroviral vectors for clinical trials are produced under good manufacturing practices and assayed for sterility, safety, and the presence of replication-competent retroviruses (RCRs). RCRs could be generated from molecular recombinational events between the producer cells and the vector. Retroviruses and retroviral vectors can recombine at a high rate because of the presence of two identical RNA molecules in their virions. The rate of retroviral recombination depends on the degree of sequence homology. Special care is taken in the design of retroviral vectors to minimize the homology between vector and producer cell (3). Results of studies have been published in which RCRs have been deliberately inoculated into either rodents or nonhuman primates (6,7). With one notable exception, these studies have shown no ill effects, even when 20% of the blood volume of a primate was replaced with RCRs derived from a Moloney murine leukemia virus. However, in one study, three of 10 monkeys that were inoculated with high titers of non-replicating vector (10^9/mL nonreplicating vector) in the presence of 1×10^3 to 1×10^4/mL RCR developed lymphoma. These monkeys also received 500 rads of whole-body irradiation that destroyed their bone marrow. Two of these monkeys also received 5-fluorouracil (8). Lymphomas developed on days 182, 200, and 206 in the three monkeys following autologous bone marrow transplantation. The objective of this study was to study the use of retroviral vectors for gene transfer into hematopoietic stem cells. For this purpose, the authors generated a clone of retroviral producer cells that yielded high concentrations of vector (10^9/mL). The clone also produced a lower concentration of RCR. Because the available literature showed no harmful effects of RCR administration at that time, the mixture of RCR and replication-incompetent vector was administered to these severely immunosuppressed rhesus macaques.

Results of these studies underscore the urgency of efficiently assaying vector products for RCR and by design of vector/producer cell combinations that will minimize the homology between the vector and producer cell and thereby the potential for RCR generation. The studies cited above used an earlier version of vector known as N2 that was known to be recombinogenic. Later designs of vectors have significantly reduced the potential for these recombinations, and clinical-grade vectors are screened for the presence of RCR by several methods.

Patients who have received retroviral vectors have also been assayed for evidence of RCR. In ex vivo gene therapy, samples of transduced lymphocytes or bone marrow are assayed for RCR before reinfusion into the patient. To date, no reports have been published of any patient being exposed to RCR. However, a recent report described an artifactual recombinational event between the vector and the cell line of *Mus dunni* that was used as an indicator/expansion culture in RCR assays. The treatment of *Mus dunni* cells with 5-iodo-2′deoxyuridine or hydrocortisone activated a helper virus from *Mus dunni* (9).

To date, most cancer gene therapy patients have received retroviral vectors. No case of significant adverse event due directly to the vector has been reported.

Adenoviral Vectors

Most adenoviral vectors used for gene therapy have been derived from either serogroup 2 or serogroup 5 adenoviruses. Parental forms of the two serogroups are pathogenic for pediatric and adult populations, respectively. A review of the use of group C adenoviruses has been published (10). Both serogroup 2 and 5 adenoviruses have been prepared as vaccines. These vectors are genomically relatively large (36 kb). They can be propagated to high titers compared to retroviral vectors: titers of 1×10^{11} can be achieved following efficient downstream processing and concentration. Adenoviral vectors can transduce both replicating and nonreplicating cells. They have a natural tropism for several tissues, including the respiratory tract. For this reason, they have been widely used in cystic fibrosis trials.

Replication incompetence is typically achieved by partial or complete removal of early genes, particularly E1. Second- and third-generation adeno vectors have additional sequences removed, particularly E3, E4, or both. E1 regulates most of the transcriptional units, either directly or indirectly. E3 genes collectively encode proteins that enable the virus to evade host immune surveillance. Another adenoviral vector mutant has been constructed that interferes with a DNA binding protein.

Animal studies have been performed with adenoviral vectors, both for preclinical efficacy and toxicity. Cotton rats have been a favorite model for adenovirus and adeno vectors, although mice, rats, Rhesus monkeys, baboons, and macaques have also been used. In some species, notably mice, high multiplicities of infection must be used because of poor susceptibility of rodents for the human adenoviral serogroup. In humans, where a large percentage of the population has anti-adeno antibodies, potential problems can be encountered in clinical studies. An inflammatory response may be triggered even by the initial inoculation of the vector into an immune host. Also, the results of preclinical studies can be confounded by an immunologic response to the vector backbone. MHC class I restricted CD8$^+$ cytotoxic T-lymphocytes are activated in response to newly synthesized adeno antigens. This results in the destruction of the vector-infected cells and the ultimate cessation of transgene expression. These potential problems render repeat treatments difficult. To solve this problem, either the vector must be further modified to decrease this potential or some form of immunosuppression must be administered. Newer generations of vector should decrease the host immunologic response.

To date, most of the clinical applications with adenoviral vectors have been in cystic fibrosis. In preclinical cancer studies, transductions of target cells have been satisfactory and long-term tumor ablations have been reported (11,12). Various tumor types have been studied. RAC-approved adeno vector clinical trials include glioblastoma, mesothelioma, and p53 mutant lung tumors.

Adeno-Associated Virus Vectors

AAV is a double-stranded DNA virus having a genome of about 4.7 kb. It belongs to the parvovirus family. It is characterized by its parasitism, requiring the presence of an adenovirus or a herpesvirus in the same cell for replication. These helper viruses provide functions in trans for AAV genome replication and encapsidation (13,14). It has never been associated with human disease. It can infect a broad variety of cell types. The virus tends to integrate in a site-specific manner into the human genome, chromosome 19q. This integration depends on the nonstructural proteins encoded by the left half of the AAV genome. This tendency may be lost on the modification rendering the virus a vector. For definitive studies and for human trials, AAV vectors must be obtained that are free of contaminating adenovirus.

Several clinical trials are in progress with AAV vectors; these are confined to cystic fibrosis. Results of in vitro studies for other clinical indications have shown that increases of 15 and 500, respectively, have been obtained for AAV vectors for glucocerebrosidase and arylsulfatase. AAV vectors can transduce both replicating and quiescent cells. However, cells engaged in DNA synthesis are transduced at a 100-fold higher frequency.

Liposomes/Plasmid DNA

Most of the published reports of liposomal delivery of DNA have involved the use of cationic lipids. Liposomal/DNA complexes fuse with mammalian cell membranes and enter the endosomal uptake pathway. Immunogenicity and toxicity have not been reported to be a problem. This method of gene delivery has been traditionally associated with low transfection rates, and gene expression is of short duration. However, newer formulations of liposomes have improved this situation. Some problems have been encountered with manufacturing; the shelf life of liposomes is short, although this can be extended by lyophilization.

Newer approaches to liposomal construction have included targeting to specific receptors (eg, by the conjugation of folate moieties to the liposome) (15). Folate receptors are up-regulated in certain tumor cells (eg, breast and ovarian). Site-specific gene expression has been demonstrated in vivo following injection of cationic liposomes into the arterial wall (16). In clinical studies, a combination of a eukaryotic expression vector encoding for the HLA-B7 heavy chain and B2-microglobulin light chain proteins has been complexed with the cationic lipid DMRIE/DOPE (16–18). This has been investigated with melanoma.

Animal studies for efficacy and toxicity have included mice, pigs, rabbits, and nonhuman primates. No significant pathology has been reported in these studies, including one that involved the intravenous administration of liposomes into cynomolgus monkeys. Plasmid DNA typically does not integrate, although integrants can be selected for longer-term expression. Typically, gene expression is low with both liposomes and plasmid DNA (19).

Summary of Gene Delivery Systems

Much progress has been made in the last 10 years in the design, production, and preclinical and clinical testing of different gene delivery systems. Effective designs have significantly decreased both the potential and actual emergence of replication-competent forms of viral vectors. Vector formulations have been moderately scaled up for clinical studies, and several vectors have been thoroughly characterized. To date, more than 1,500 patients have been treated worldwide, with no apparent side effects due directly to the vector other than those described for adenoviral vectors. Other modifications of vectors have included the use of cell-specific or tumor-specific promoters that can help ensure that maximum gene delivery is directed to the appropriate tumor cell target. One study showed that an adenoviral vector encoding an alpha-fetoprotein (AFP) promoter upstream of the herpes simplex thymidine kinase gene killed only human hepatoma cells that produced AFP but not cells that did not produce AFP (20). This could have application in human treatments. The therapeutic gene, the herpes simplex thymidine kinase gene, would be expressed only in tumors and not in nontumor cells not containing AFP.

CLINICAL PROTOCOLS

Gene Marking Studies

Many protocols are aimed at the insertion of genes in peripheral blood or bone marrow cells, typically CD34[+] cells, for either gene marking or gene therapy. Many of these therapeutic trials intend to transduce the hematopoietic "stem cells" in marrow or peripheral blood. Although the ultimate goal of clinical trials in cancer gene therapy is clearly therapeutic, various clinical studies have been performed in gene marking. In gene marking, the intent is to determine cell trafficking or to determine the origin of gene-marked cells. In a representative procedure, lymphocytes or bone marrow cells are removed from the patient, propagated in vitro, and transduced with a vector during ex vivo propagation. The transduced cells are then returned to the patient. These studies have been performed almost exclusively with retroviral vectors (21).

Gene marking has also been frequently used in autologous bone marrow transplantation. Relapse has been the major failure in autologous bone marrow transplant in leukemias. The possibility that leukemic cells could be reinfused at the time of autologous transplant has been recognized. Gene marking offers a technique to evaluate this potential by inserting antibiotic resistance genes into the marrow cells. Studies have been performed to determine if harvested blood or marrow contains leukemogenic cells. In separate studies, gene-marked cells have been used to compare different purging techniques.

In a study to determine if the autologous transplant contained leukemogenic cells, patients with neuroblastoma or acute leukemia were evaluated using two different retroviral vectors. Both vectors encoded the gene for conferring resistance to G418, a neomycin analog. The vectors differed only in minor gene sequences. This slight difference could be distinguished by polymerase chain reaction (PCR). To determine if the marked leukemic cells in the marrow were the source of relapse, the genetic marker and a specific tumor cell marker had to be present in the same cell. This was possible in these studies. Results of several studies have been published (22,23). In the neuroblastoma and pediatric leukemia studies, 3 of 4 relapsed patients contained marked cells, indicating that the marrow was contaminated with leukemic cells. Similar results were obtained in a separate study in patients with chronic myelogenous leukemia (24).

Gene-marking studies with breast cancer and adult leukemia patients have demonstrated that gene-marked cells were not detectable in relapsed cells, suggesting the marrow was not a reservoir for tumor cells. An alternate explanation was that the level of gene marking was not high enough to mark the tumorigenic cells. Another possibility is that adult leukemia, multiple myeloma, and breast cancer patients may differ from pediatric leukemia patients.

Gene marking can also compare the relative sensitivity of purging methods in autologous bone marrow transplantation methods (Fig. 1). CD34[+] cells are divided into two portions; each is marked with a vector encoding for neomycin resistance, but they are distinguishable by PCR. The two fractions are purged by different methodologies and returned to the patient. If relapse occurs, the leukemic fractions are analyzed for the presence of each of the two vectors. The detection of one but not the other marker suggests, but is not conclusive evidence of, the relative effectiveness of the two purging procedures.

Another use of gene marking is to determine if the infused marrow contributes to short- and long-term bone marrow recovery. In limited studies, results have shown that neomycin-resistant colonies have been demonstrated in multilineage cells, including T- and B-lymphocytes (23). A later study suggested that peripheral blood stem cells may contribute more to long-term survival of gene-marked cells than marrow (25). These results also suggested that mobilized peripheral cells may in fact be more effective than bone marrow cells for gene therapy protocols, and that the progeny of mobilized peripheral blood cells can contribute to multilineages over the long term. In this study, 3 of 9 patients demonstrated long-term survival of gene-marked cells (mt>18 months). The level of marked cells averaged 5% at 12 to 18 months after transplantation. Other studies in cancer patients and patients who have received retroviral vector-mediated gene trans-

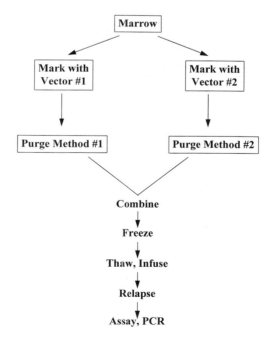

FIG. 1. Gene marking protocol to evaluate relative effectiveness of bone marrow purging techniques.

fer for severe combined immune deficiency due to ADA deficiency continued to show the presence of gene-marked cells for 2 to 5 years (1,25,26).

It is crucial to know how many stem or progenitor cells are actually being marked in these procedures. The scant information available suggests that a small number of stem or early progenitor cells are transduced. A non-cancer study that involved retroviral inoculation into CD34$^+$ cells from cord blood obtained at birth and rein-fused 3 to 4 days after birth for ADA gene therapy showed common integrants in lymphoid and myeloid cells, indicating transduction of a common precursor (26). This study reported a relatively low number of common integrants (three to five).

Another use of gene marking is to demonstrate the relative effectiveness of various cytokine cocktails on graft reconstitution. It is now possible to assess the time and efficiency of different cytokine mixtures on the relative time of marrow reconstitution. Ideally, this will allow us to identify the medium that will minimize the period of hypoplasia and immune deficiency that results from autologous bone marrow transplantation.

The results of studies from gene marking have offered important data in this emerging field. First, no evidence of an adverse event due to retroviral vector-mediated gene transfer has been reported in these patients. This has significance in its own right, demonstrating that vectors can be incorporated into the cell, as well as the genome of that cell, with no detectable toxicity to the patient. Some of the patients in these marker studies have had detectable gene markers in their lymphocytes for more than 3 years; the initial patients who received gene transfer for ADA deficiency have had gene-marked cells for more than 6 years. Second, the rate of vector transduction is low, typically <10% in most studies. This points to the need for improved vector design and type as well as an optimal and standard method for the transduction of clinically relevant target cells, whether marrow or peripheral blood. Some methods to improve transduction have been published, such as low-speed centrifugation of vectors onto target cells (27). Higher-titer vectors, as well as vectors of increased purity, should also be beneficial. A broader diversity of vector types and designs is being pursued. These include other viral systems, incorporation of specific promoters or enhancers, and alternate means of delivering vectors.

Therapeutic Trials

Immune Modulation of Tumor Cells

Various approaches have been attempted to enhance the immunogenicity of tumor cells. Results of studies in syngeneic tumor systems in animals have demonstrated the potential of this approach. However, the limitations of animal models are recognized: success in animals is no guarantee or predictor in human cancer. The general objective of modulation of the immune system is to exert an overall stimulation on the effector processing and presentation of putative tumor antigens to the immune system. This begs the question of whether there are identifiable tumor antigens in human cancer, and, if so, can they be more effectively presented through gene transfer. Gilboa and colleagues summarize some of these concepts (28). First, if tumors were immunogenic, they should have been presented by the immune system. The neoplastic state presumes that either the tumor was not immunogenic or that the patient somehow failed to mount an immune response. Somehow tumors are tolerogenic. Second, spontaneously arising tumors in rodents are typically nonimmunogenic. Does human cancer fit this model? The incidence of cancer is not significantly increased in immunocompromised patients, although Kaposi's sarcoma seems to be an exception.

On the other hand, evidence exists that tumors can down-regulate MHC class I expression or elaborate immune suppressive factors such as TGF-b. Somehow, tumors seem to have evolved mechanisms to evade a functioning, normal immune system. In one of the first reports to demonstrate this, van Pel and Boon showed that a nonimmunogenic tumor in mice could be rendered immunogenic by a small mutation (29). This demonstrated that the original tumor did in fact possess tumor antigens, but these were incapable of being presented to the immune system. Another study showed that an adjuvant, such as BCG, elicited an immune response against a previously nonimmunogenic tumor in guinea pigs (30). These and other studies clearly showed that the nonresponsiveness occurred at the level of induction of the immune response, not at the recognition step, when activated T-cells encounter their target, the tumor cell.

If immune modulation of tumor cells represents a reasonable therapeutic target, how can this modulation be exploited to the best advantage? Two possibilities exist. One is the TH1 T cell, which triggers cytotoxic T-cells and the cellular arm of immunity. Another possibility is through the interaction of the response mediated through CD4 cells. Interestingly, both approaches have advocates, based on the results of animal studies. Some papers report that TH1 responses are the primary one (28); others state that TH2 and CD4$^+$ T-cells are the major intermediary (31). As stated above, the results of animal models in cancer gene therapy must be carefully interpreted because of the nature of the cancer cell being studied, the animal strain, the conditions of the assay (especially what cytokine or other gene is being delivered), and the differences in similar studies when performed in different laboratories.

Gilboa and associates (28) argue that CD8$^+$ cytotoxic T-cells recognize antigen in the context of MHC class I molecules that are expressed on the membrane of the target cell. Interaction between the tumor cell and its cognate T-cell should be sufficient for tumor cell lysis. It should also be sufficient to reactivate memory cytotoxic T-cells. On the other hand, Lin and coworkers noted that several mouse tumors transfected with syngeneic MHC class II genes served as effective vaccines against subsequent challenge with wild-type, MHC class II-negative tumors (31). In this arm of the immune system, exogenous antigens are taken up by antigen-presenting cells and subsequently degraded by acidic proteases in acidic endosomal or lysosomal cytoplasmic compartments. The peptide fragments generated by this procedure then bind MHC class II molecules and are presented on the cell surface to CD4$^+$, MHC class II restricted T-cells. These two hypotheses are not mutually exclusive. It is difficult to generalize about the relative roles of TH1 versus TH2 in human cancer. Both are probably significant in many human tumors (32). If this is true, more than one cytokine, or a pleiotropic cytokine, may be required in antitumor therapy. The delivery and distribution of the transgene in the tumor or presentation to the immune system will be an important component of the therapeutic gene. In one study, the corequirements for CD4$^+$ T-cells and natural killer (NK) cells were demonstrated in the immune response to tumors negative for MHC class I expression. In these studies, the depletion of NK cells resulted in the selective outgrowth of tumors with downregulated MHC class I expression (33).

Transgenes Used in Tumor Vaccines

Perhaps the ambiguity described above regarding mechanistic approaches to immune recognition at least partially explains the plethora of cytokines, lymphokines, and sundry immune modulators that have been tried in cancer gene therapy trials. No universal agreement exists as to what the "magical" gene is. Perhaps no one gene will be sufficient; a mixture of two or more genes may be required. The combination of cytokines in a gene therapy trial, or the use of one transgene with a protein cytokine, will undoubtedly add a layer of complexity to clinical trials. Table 3 lists the cytokines that have received approval from the NIH RAC for gene therapy trials using various approaches to cancer vaccines.

Another question of the cancer vaccine approach is how to deliver the gene, in vivo or ex vivo. Most of the

TABLE 3. *Cytokines used as transgenes in gene therapy trials*

IL-2
IL-4
IL-7
IL-12
Interferon-gamma
GM-CSF
TNF-alpha

early approaches used the ex vivo approach, whereby the tumor cells are excised, transduced with the gene, irradiated, and then returned to the patient. Among the earliest approaches was to insert either interleukin-2 (IL-2) or tumor necrosis factor (TNF) into tumor-infiltrating lymphocytes or tumors such as melanoma or renal cell carcinoma. Gene therapy would serve as a drug delivery system, ideally producing a concentration of the cytokine in the microenvironment of the tumor high enough to be tumoricidal. The best quantitation of this approach was in the animal study reported by Dranoff and associates (34). In this study, irradiated B16 mouse melanoma cells transduced with murine granulocyte macrophage-colony stimulating factor (GM-CSF) effectively vaccinated mice against subsequent challenge with untransduced B16 cells. Seven of 10 mice were tumor-free in this study. The authors stated that elaboration on 36 ng of murine GM-CSF/1×10^6 cells/24 hours appeared to be the threshold needed to protect mice under the conditions of these experiments. The concept of local concentrations delivered by the various gene vector systems is critical to the success of these studies. This concept may explain why clinical trials using *systemic* recombinant cytokines were unsuccessful. Cytokines that are either autocrine or paracrine will probably require higher local concentrations to be effective than can be achieved by intravenous administration. Because gene delivery effectively transduces tumor cells but not adjacent normal cells, an expected advantage would be to deliver higher concentrations of drug locally while minimizing toxicity to other tissues.

A human trial was designed and conducted based on these GM-CSF animal studies. Patients with renal carcinoma (and in later trials melanoma and prostate cancer) had their tumors excised, and cell cultures were prepared from the tumor. A retroviral vector encoding GM-CSF was added, and after further ex vivo expansion, the irradiated transduced tumor cells were returned to the patient. Results have not been published, but apparently the patients tolerated the treatment well, as additional trials have been initiated. A drawback to this ex vivo approach is that it is labor-intensive. Further, not all tumors are successfully cultivated in vitro. The success will depend on the tumor type as well as the skill and experience of the cell culture laboratory. The inability to initiate a cell culture from the tumor of a particular patient will remove that patient from the study. The protocol also necessitates transport of the specimens from the clinical center to the cell-processing facility. The level of GM-CSF expressed in these trials has not been reported. Clinical success in such a protocol would be significant. Failure to effect an antitumor effect might be due to the inability of GM-CSF to elicit a response, or to the fact that the level of GM-CSF elaborated is insufficient to yield a response. The use of GM-CSF seems to influence the TH2 response to tumors also. The animal studies involving GM-CSF cited above demonstrated a significant infiltration of eosinophils and neutrophils in the area of the tumor.

Cytokines other than GM-CSF have also been used. Both IL-2 and interferon-gamma eliminated the ability of certain tumors to form tumors in syngeneic mice (35). Significantly, the animals that had been protected by these tumor vaccines also resisted subsequent challenge with wild-type tumors. This demonstrates antitumor activity as well as systemic immunity. Both IL-2 and interferon-gamma have been used in human trials involving melanoma, neuroblastoma, leukemia, and breast and brain tumors. Results of these human studies have not been published. These human studies all have used ex vivo gene therapy to transduce either the tumor or autologous fibroblasts. An IL-4 gene therapy protocol is in progress using this approach, together with recombinant IL-2.

Ex vivo gene therapy can be facilitated in several ways. Instead of establishing cell cultures from tumors, primary tumor material could be transduced without propagation in the laboratory, or freshly excised material could be irradiated, then transduced and readministered. Alternately, a universal donor cell could be identified for each particular tumor type and transduced with the gene of interest. Such a universal allogeneic donor cell would be easy to cultivate, easy to transduce, and not MHC restricted.

More recently, separate gene therapy trials using IL-7 or IL-12 have been approved by the RAC. In one proposed study, a retroviral vector encoding IL-7 will be inoculated subcutaneously into patients with malignant melanoma.

In the IL-12 trial, the study consisted of establishing autologous fibroblasts from patients with cutaneous cancer (breast, melanoma, head and neck, and cutaneous T-cell lymphoma) (36). The cultures are established and transduced with a retroviral vector encoding both IL-12 and neomycin resistance. Neomycin-resistant cultures are then assayed for IL-12 expression, expanded, and cryopreserved. Treatment consists of thawing the cultures, irradiating them with 5,000 rads, and inoculating them into the patient. This protocol could consist of up to three treatments, depending on the presence or absence of toxicity in initial patients. The targeted dose of IL-12 is 10 ng/24 hours for the first 3 patients. Depending on the absence of toxicity, this dose could be escalated to 30 ng/24 hours, then to 100, 300, 1,000, and eventually 3,000 ng/24 hours.

IL-12 has been the subject of clinical trials using the recombinant protein. Some toxicities have been reported in a phase II study in renal cell carcinoma patients who received IL-12 systemically. In 17 patients who received IL-12 in that protocol, a significant number were treated for adverse events, and 1 patient died of gastrointestinal bleeding. No toxicities were apparent when the recombinant protein was administered either intraperitoneally or subcutaneously to mice for up to 30 days. Delivery of IL-12 via gene therapy offers the potential of reducing toxicity to other organs and generating a high local concentration of the cytokine.

The biology of IL-12 shows that it apparently evokes a TH1 response. This is based on both in vitro and in vivo studies. In vivo experiments show that the administration of IL-12 to mice enhances both NK and cytotoxic T-cells and induces interferon-gamma. In an animal modeling study, IL-12 yielded a marked antitumor response even when administered as long as 28 days after injection of tumor cells into mice (37). The antitumor response consisted of inhibition of tumor growth, a decrease in the number of metastases, and increased survival time.

Prodrug Metabolizing Enzymes

An alternate method of killing tumors is through the use of "suicide" or drug sensitivity genes. This approach is designed to kill tumor cells but not neighboring normal cells. The first report of such an approach using gene transfer was by Moolten in 1986 (38). He used the gene thymidine kinase derived from herpes simplex and inserted it into a mammalian cell. The herpes simplex thymidine kinase (HsTk) gene is an effective target for the approved drug ganciclovir (GCV). HsTk phosphorylates GCV to GCV-phosphate, which is eventually converted to the triphosphate form. HsTk has a much greater affinity for GCV than the mammalian Tk isozyme. GCV is a nucleoside analog and in its triphosphate form acts as a chain terminator, interfering with DNA synthesis in replicating cells. This leads to either cell arrest or cell death.

The concept of introducing HsTk and then destroying the tumors through the use of GCV makes several assumptions. First, enough tumor cells must be cycling to be transduced by the retroviral vector. Alternately, adeno vectors or nonviral vectors would transduce not only the tumor cells, but adjacent nontumor cells as well. The transduced normal cells could be killed by the subsequent GCV treatment resulting in toxicity. Second, the transduced cells must also be cycling to be killed by the GCV treatment. One possible approach could envision the repeated infusion of retroviral particles to a tumor in situ. This would be difficult in many clinical settings. Another approach would be to introduce the mouse producer cells in vivo instead of the vectors themselves. In this way, the producer cells could be viewed as a mini-factory, generating vector particles as long as they survive in vivo and are capable of generating vectors. It is unclear how long a mouse xenograft consisting of the producer cells might last. However, in the central nervous system, a relatively privileged site, such a xenograft would theoretically be expected to last longer than in other body sites.

This approach was studied in animal models for glioblastoma (39). Fisher rats were inoculated with 4×10^4

9L gliosarcoma cells intracerebrally. Mouse producer cells that generated a retroviral vector that encoded gene for both HsTk and G418 resistance were inoculated at the same stereotactic coordinates. The animals treated with HsTk producer cells and with GCV had a significantly greater antitumor effect than untreated controls or animals that had producer cell but no GCV treatment. In a follow-up study, 10 of 12 animals (83%) had complete tumor regression 21 days after treatment with producer cell therapy (40). Producer cells were administered along with the tumor. The ratio of the tumor cells to producer cells was an important factor in the degree of tumor regression: doubling the number of producer cells roughly doubled the incidence of complete tumor regressions (38% vs 72%).

In this type of clinical study, where the producer cells are inoculated into the tumor mass, several factors can significantly affect the success of tumor regression. These include the transduction of the tumors and the ability of the GCV to kill the HsTk-transduced cells. In the studies reported by Ram and colleagues, the in vitro transduction rates ranged from 10% to 70% of the tumor cells (40). Despite this, complete tumor eradication was regularly achieved. Less than 100% transduction of the tumor cells can result in complete tumor regression. This phenomenon is due to a so-called "bystander effect," whereby the toxic metabolites of the GCV killing are transferred to adjacent cells, possibly through gap junctions. The original bystander effect in vivo with this system was demonstrated when mixtures of HsTk-transduced tumors and wild-type tumors were inoculated subcutaneously in mice and then treated with GCV. In animals bearing tumors with as few as 10% HsTk-expressing cells, complete tumor regression was demonstrated in more than 50% of the animals (40).

The bystander effect significantly amplifies the antitumor effect of this system. The two mechanisms proposed for the bystander effect include the transfer of phosphorylated GCV through direct cell-to-cell contact, presumably through gap junctions. A second theory involves the uptake of phosphorylated GCV through apoptotic vesicles between HsTk-expressing and -nonexpressing cells. However, because phosphorylated GCV transfer has been shown to occur before apoptosis has occurred, the bystander is more likely to occur via transfer of phosphorylated GCV through gap junctions. If this hypothesis is correct, one would expect better antitumor effects in tumor cells and types that express gap junctions. The expression of gap junctions is correlated with the expression of connexin genes, particularly connexin 43. Unfortunately, data are not available to correlate connexin expression or the presence of gap junctions and the effectiveness of HsTk/GCV with any specific tumor type or grade. It might be feasible to transduce the tumor cells with a vector encoding the connexin as well as the HsTk gene, although this has not been reported.

The bystander effect has been shown to occur not only between adjacent tumor cells, but also between tumor and nontumor cells, including various tumor cell types (41). Transfer between a mouse producer cell and a rat glioma cell has also been demonstrated. The ability to exhibit a bystander effect between a tumor cell and an adjacent endothelial cell could be beneficial, possibly disrupting blood supply to a tumor.

In addition to the degree of transduction and the presence of a bystander effect, the time of administration and the concentration of the GCV are critical factors. In the animal studies and in the subsequent human clinical trials, GCV was administered at a dosage similar to that safely given to patients for treatment of ocular viral infections. However, results of animal studies showed that it must be given longer—14 days compared to 7 days for ocular infections. Another factor for giving GCV for longer periods was the finding that the xenograft mouse cells could be detected for up to 14 days in nonhuman primate brain. This schedule of administration would allow the producer cells to produce vectors for 14 days after inoculation, and GCV would be administered at this time for 14 days.

The use of producer cells has particular relevance in brain tumors. In this setting, the retroviral particles should transduce tumor cells but not nondividing neurons. Endothelial cells have also been shown to be transduced in animal studies, but this could be beneficial, disrupting blood supply to a tumor. The brain is considered somewhat of an immunologically privileged site, but this is relative. Clearly, immunologic cells and reactions occur quite readily in human brain. The blood–brain barrier breaks down in glioblastoma and other brain tumors.

The RAC has approved several clinical trials that use HsTk technology, either with retroviral vectors, the producer cells, or adeno vectors. The first approved trial was for ovarian cancer using retroviral vectors. No report of that clinical study has been published. A number of other trials using HsTk producer cells to deliver HsTk to glioblastoma have been approved and conducted. These have been for glioblastoma multiforme and other tumors that have metastasized to the brain.

In the glioblastoma clinical trials, the cells are delivered in situ and GCV treatment begins 14 days later for a period of 14 days. Two methods of producer cell delivery have been used. In the first trial conducted at the NIH, producer cells were delivered stereotactically using magnetic resonance-guided coordinates. A total of 15 patients were treated in this trial, 12 of whom had primary brain tumors and 3 of whom had tumors that metastasized to the brain. The complete reports of this trial have not yet been published, but an abstract described antitumor activity as determined by reduction in the image-enhancing area on magnetic resonance scans in 5 of the first 8 patients.

In a subsequent trial exclusively for glioblastoma multiforme, the tumors were first resected, and then producer cells were inoculated into residual tumor and into the tumor margins. This trial had the option of retreatment if no tumor growth occurred. Results of this trial have not been reported. Another difference in this second trial is the use of a newer producer cell with a significantly higher titer of retroviral vector. In a comparative animal study, the newer producer cell demonstrated a 13- to 18-fold higher in vivo transduction rate (42). In addition, complete tumor ablation was achieved in mice using a 10-fold lower dose of the new producer cell, compared to the one used in the first study.

The use of retroviral vector-producer cells has application in the central nervous system, but the lability of mouse cells systemically precludes their use in other tumor applications. This lability of both mouse cells and retroviral vectors is apparently due to the presence of a 1-3 galactose-galactosyl epitope in mice and many other species (43). This epitope is due to the enzyme 1-3 galactosyl transferase, which is present in mice and most other animals. However, as reported by Galili and Swanson (43), a nonsense mutation occurred in the catarrhines, which include Old World monkeys and humans that inactivated enzymatic activity of the 1-3 galactosyl transferase. Therefore, Old World monkeys and humans do not express the epitope and contain high levels of antibodies to this epitope in their sera. Human sera quickly inactivate C-type oncoviruses from other mammals by triggering the complement cascade. In fact, this rapid inactivation may have inhibited transmission of other retroviruses from animals to humans. The retroviruses human immunodeficiency virus-1 and human T-cell leukemia virus are exceptions, being resistant to human complement. Despite these findings, the murine producer cells can apparently survive long enough in the human brain to generate sufficient retroviral vectors to exert an effect. The precise mechanism of any observed antitumor is unclear. It could be due to direct transduction of tumor or endothelial cells and hilley by GCV, the bystander effect, or some undefined immunologic response.

Suicide Gene Therapy in Allogeneic Bone Marrow Transplantation

More recently, suicide gene therapy has been applied in the area of allogeneic bone marrow transplantation (allo-BMT). Allo-BMT has emerged as an important treatment modality for patients having various hematologic malignancies: acute myelogenous leukemia, chronic myelogenous leukemia, acute lymphocytic leukemia, multiple myeloma, poor prognosis myelodysplastic syndrome, and Hodgkin's as well as non-Hodgkin's lymphoma. Originally, allo-BMT was envisioned as a method to achieve supralethal levels of myelotoxic chemoradiotherapy. It soon became apparent that an immune-mediated graft versus leukemia (GVL) is an important component in longer-term remission. It has been associated with the presence of T-lymphocytes in the donor bone marrow. A major impediment to the wider use of allo-BMT, in addition to the shortage of donors, is the development of graft-versus-host disease (GVHD). Allo-BMT has been shown to effect long-term disease-free survival. The GVHD can be either acute or chronic. Acute GVHD develops shortly after transplantation and is a major cause of early mortality. This reaction resolves in survivors. Chronic GVHD is frequently observed in survivors; it results in a greatly diminished quality of life several months after the transplant. Both reactions are mediated by host reactive lymphocytes derived from the transplant marrow. The most significant damage occurs to the skin, liver, lung, and gastrointestinal tract.

The removal of donor T-lymphocytes, the major cause of GVHD, is the most effective method of preventing GVHD. However, extensive experience has shown that T-cell depletion is associated with increased rates of graft failure and leukemia relapse and an increased incidence of Epstein-Barr virus-associated lymphomas. Therefore, donor cells are critical for the development of the engraftment of donor-derived hematopoietic stem cells as well as GVHD and GVL. Modulation of graft alloreactivity through the control of donor T-lymphocytes, administered either at the time of transplant or during later infusions, could reduce the incidence and intensity of GVHD while maintaining some GVL. The number of donor T-lymphocytes is correlated with the risk of GVHD.

To maintain the GVL while reducing or eliminating GVHD, the use of HsTk suicide technology has been proposed. It should be possible to transduce donor T-lymphocytes ex vivo, then reinfuse the transduced T-cells at the time of T-cell–depleted allo-BMT, at a predetermined time when the potential for GVHD is thought to be maximal, or when GVHD develops. Bordignon and colleagues have described a protocol based on this technology and recently published an abstract of some early results (44). All the patients treated with HsTk-transduced allolymphocytes had severe pre-existing hematologic malignancies and developed complications. After infusion of the allotransduced lymphocytes, gene-marked lymphocytes were detected by PCR, but no correlation was reported with the development of GVHD. Two patients developed GVHD. It was reported that GCV therapy eliminated the gene-marked cells and produced near-resolution of all clinical and biochemical signs of acute GVHD. This occurred apparently after a single treatment of donor T-cells and a single round of GCV administration.

Multiple administrations of HsTk vector in some applications would be problematic. In a study in AIDS patients, Riddel and coworkers reported that multiple inoculations of a vector encoding both HsTk and hygromycin-resistance gene resulted in significant antibody and cytotoxic T-cell responses to the hygromycin/Tk fusion protein (45). Typically, cancer patients receiving allo-BMT would be expected to be more immunosuppressed than the AIDS patients in that study. Also, it would be typical in an allo-BMT setting to use one, or at most two, inoculations of donor T-cells, but not multiple inoculations, as in the AIDS study. If retroviral vectors encoding the TK gene can be used successfully in an allo-BMT setting for hematologic malignancies, it could expand the population of leukemia patients who could possibly benefit from allo-BMT, including older patients as well as even more HLA-mismatched, haploidentical donors. It could expand the use of allo-BMT to other cancer types and might also allow the use of allo-BMT earlier in the disease process. In addition to the clinical trial of Bordignon that is in progress in Italy, other trials have begun at the University of Arkansas (multiple myeloma) and in France (various malignancies) using a dose-escalating schedule of increasing numbers of transduced cells per kilogram.

One report described results of preclinical studies for allo-BMT and suicide genes (46) and reported that Tk gene expression was maintained for 80 days. This could be important, as GVHD can occur late after allo-BMT. Primary lymphocytes transduced with HsTk were sensitive to GCV for 15 days after transduction. This is critical, because alloreactivity must be maintained. Results from other clinical trials that used gene therapy for ADA deficiency clearly demonstrated that gene expression continued more than 3 years after the last transduction.

Other suicide gene approaches are available besides HsTk. The most widely studied is the bacterial gene cytosine deaminase, derived from *Escherichia coli*. This enzyme converts the prodrug 5-fluorocytosine into the anti-metabolite 5-fluorouracil. Several papers have been published on in vitro and in vivo animal systems. In 1995, a clinical protocol was approved by the RAC that used an adeno vector encoding cytosine deaminase. The indication was for colon carcinoma metastasizing to the liver.

Tumor Suppressor Genes

There are many known and proposed tumor suppressor genes (47,48). Tumor suppressor genes require at least two mutational events to contribute to the development of cancer. These mutations can originate from inherited or somatic mutations. Tumor suppressor genes act by negatively affecting the transcription regulation proteins and oncogene transcription factors involved in cell division. Tumor suppressors include NF1 inactivation of G-protein GTP signal; p53 or WT1 acting as a transcription factor; p53, p21 protein and MTS1, p16 protein blocking cyclin/cyclin dependent kinase (cdk) activity as well as Rb binding and inactivating transcription factor.

Tumor suppressor genes are defined by the absence or loss of their proteins in cancer cells. The replacement of the wild-type or normal copy of the gene in a cancer cell should theoretically restore a normal phenotype and result in loss of tumorigenic potential. This would potentially be amenable to gene therapy approaches. Tumor suppressor genes often regulate the cell cycle, which is divided into four phases (G1, S, G2, M). Progression through these phases is controlled by the synthesis and degradation of cyclins, which regulate protein kinases.

When DNA in a normal cell is damaged by radiation or chemotherapy, wild-type p53 expression is increased. Increased p53 expression leads to enhanced transcription of p21 (WAF1). p21 binds to the complex of cyclin and cdk. Other proteins (eg, the retinoblastoma susceptibility gene, Rb) are not phosphorylated. This results in the failure to activate the E2F/DP1 complex. Consequently, the S-phase genes are not transcribed—so-called G1 arrest. p21 expression allows the cell to repair the DNA damage, thereby reducing the potential for mutations to occur during DNA replication.

The wild-type p53 protein has many biochemical functions. It specifically binds to DNA sequences and exhibits the characteristics of a transcription factor. p53 can up-regulate the cell cycle inhibitors p21 (WAF1/Cip1) (47,48). p21 inhibits the cell cycle-stimulating function of protein complexes, including the cyclins and cdk. p53 is mutated in many cancer types: about 56% of lung cancers and 50% of colon cancers have p53 mutations. Understanding normal p53 function is essential to understanding why mutated p53 is associated with tumor cell growth.

Protocols Involving Tumor Suppressor Genes

Results of in vitro studies have shown that reintroduction of the normal p53 gene function into cancer cells can suppress tumor growth (49,50). Clinical protocols have been designed to exploit this concept. Normal p53 gene is introduced via viral vectors into tumor cells in hopes of preventing further cell proliferation. The first p53 protocol proposed to inject a retroviral p53 vector directly or an anti k-ras retroviral vector into the tumor bed of patients with stage IV non-small cell lung cancer (51). Subsequent protocols use an adenoviral vector together with conventional cisplatin chemotherapy. Results of the preclinical studies, on which this protocol is based, have been published (52,53).

Another group proposed the use of an adeno-p53 for the treatment of hepatocellular carcinoma (52). Some concerns have been raised regarding possible contamination of wild-type p53 adenoviral preparations with mutant p53 virus. Vector preparations must be assayed for the presence of mutant p53.

The use of tumor suppressor genes and antioncogenes in gene therapy to treat cancer has technical limitations associated with the current vector systems. In using tumor suppressor genes in replacement technologies, it is necessary to correct all somatic cells containing tumor suppressor gene mutations or oncogenes for the successful treatment of cancer. This requires full transduction of all the somatic cells involved in the cancer. None of the vector systems available at this time are capable of attaining 100% transduction efficiency in vivo.

Studies in the authors' laboratory have found a high frequency of deletions in retrovirally delivered p53 genes to tumor cells in culture. As a consequence, little if any effects on growth and tumorigenicity were found. The inability to transduce a high percentage of tumor cells and the failure to maintain the intact full-length p53 transgene limit the potential efficacy of retroviral-mediated p53 cancer gene therapy (54).

Anti-Oncogenes

Oncogenes and their products are part of an intricate cell-signaling network that regulates cell division. Oncogenes can be classified into five categories (55). Generally, oncogenes behave like:

1. Growth factors that act like growth factors and stimulate growth via autocrine circuits
2. Genes that encode mutated forms of receptor tyrosine kinases that bind growth factors
3. Transducers of growth factor responses
4. Soluble cytoplasmic protein-serine kinases that regulate the cell cycle
5. Nuclear proteins that serve as transcription regulators.

Collectively, oncogenes have the characteristic of initiating a cascade of cellular events that stimulate the cell to proceed from cell quiescence to cell proliferation. Uncontrolled cell proliferation ultimately results in tumor formation. As shown by Fearon and Vogelstein, multiple events are required for carcinogenesis, using a model of colorectal cancer (56). Apparently, colorectal cancer, and perhaps other tumor types, proceed through a series of genetic alterations that include mutations in tumor suppressor genes and oncogenes. Mutations in four or five genes are required for colorectal cancer to develop. Published reports indicate that it is the accumulation of these mutations, not the sequence in which they occur, that is responsible for the tumor phenotype.

Therapeutic approaches using gene therapy approaches could theoretically involve either an antisense or ribozyme strategy that would inactivate gene expression of the oncogene involved in any specific tumor. The objective of the introduction of an antisense version of an oncogene would be to decrease and ideally to eliminate cell growth. Several gene therapy clinical trials involving oncogenes have been approved by the RAC. These include metastatic breast cancer (antisense c-fos or antisense c-myc), prostate cancer (antisense c-myc), ovarian cancer (anti-erb B2 antibody gene), and brain cancer (antisense insulin-like growth factor).

The potential for gene therapeutic approaches using wild-type tumor suppressors and antisense oncogenes is limited at present by the inability to transfer the therapeutic genes to all tumor cells. Transductions of less than all the tumor cells would not appear to be beneficial unless other factors are present. These could include some type of bystander effect, as documented in the HsTk suicide gene approach, or the combination of gene therapy with other therapies, such as radiation or chemotherapy. Alternately, vectors could be designed that would function or even replicate only in tumor cells. The combination of gene therapy with other types of conventional therapies would render the clinical trials more difficult and probably larger, as the relative contribution of each component would have to be quantitated. Published studies showed that the antitumor effects in animals of wild-type p53 persisted only as long as the other therapeutic modality was administered (53).

Genetic Modification of Tumor Cells

Nabel and colleagues have developed an alternative approach to the methods and concepts of cancer gene therapy (57). This involves the transcatheter injection of DNA liposomes directly into tumor masses. The original clinical indication was for metastatic melanoma. A DNA plasmid that encoded the histocompatibility gene HLA-B7 was encased in a cationic liposome and injected via a transcatheter into the right posterior basal pulmonary artery. No adverse events were reported with this treatment. The purpose of this study, in addition to safety, was to determine whether the introduction of a major histocompatibility gene into a tumor could induce an immunologic attack against the neoantigen. Expression of this new antigen induced a CD8[+] cytotoxic T-cell response against weak antigens in poorly immunogenic tumors (57). A report on the phase I study has been published (16). According to the authors, this study showed that no major safety concerns were identified and that some tumor shrinkage was noted. Some tumors exhibited diminished growth, and some complete regressions were observed. A second trial is being conducted. The authors also noted they are exploring the possibility of combining the HLA-B7 with a cytokine to augment antitumor responses.

Animal models of this approach have been developed (18,19). In animal studies, a poorly immunogenic B16/BL6 melanoma cell was used. This is of H-2b origin. In vivo introduction of H-2ks cDNA/liposome complexes and tumor cells before animal inoculation produced enhanced development of sensitized T-lymphocytes in draining lymph nodes. Tumors were more effectively transfected by intratumoral inoculation with naked cDNA than by lipofection. Transfection of animal tumors with allogeneic class I gene has been examined in several laboratories; results have varied. In these studies, optimal results have been observed in animals that were preimmunized to the alloantigen. In all likelihood, definitive results will come first from the clinical trials.

FUTURE APPROACHES

The clinical trials described in this report have been phase I/II studies and have focused primarily on safety and on whether and to what extent transduction/transfection has occurred. In addition, where possible, the level of gene expression has been an important study parameter. The next several years should see important data being published on the level of transgene expression as well as preliminary clinical data. Evidence of antitumor activity will heighten the urgency to refine and define the critical aspects of the human trials.

When available, clinical data reporting antitumor activity will identify not only a transgene showing activity, but what level of gene product is necessary for a specific tumor type. Even with demonstration of antitumor activity, it is likely that modifications will be needed in factors such as the method of gene delivery or the status of the patient population.

Even if antitumor activities are demonstrated, it is reasonable to project what modifications might be expected in future clinical trials. Although the present trials using various cytokines may show activity, studies with two or more cytokines delivered with vectors are likely. A variation of this technique is in progress, with one cytokine transgene and a second cytokine recombinant protein being administered. The cytokine combinations could be either those that have pleiotropic actions or those that effect both the TH1 and TH2 responses. As shown in animal studies, it will be preferable to have both antitumor activity and systemic immunity to eliminate the possibility of minimal residual disease.

In addition to combinations of transgenes, gene therapy could be combined with other antitumor modalities. This is already being performed, as noted with the combination of an adeno vector for wild-type p53 and cisplatin. The combination of p53 with radiation has also been proposed. Kim and coworkers have demonstrated that the combination of transduction with HsTk and antiviral agents such as acyclovir and GCV can increase the radiation sensitivity of tumor cells (58). The magnitude of the enhancement depends on the time and the sequence of the drug and the radiation. A possible mechanism suggested by the authors is that acyclovir (and presumably GCV) inhibits DNA polymerase b, the enzyme implicated in DNA repair of potentially lethal damage. Tumor DNA that is damaged by radiation will not have the opportunity to repair itself if it is complexed with

GCV triphosphate, which leads to chain termination. A separate study has shown that a specific gene could be activated by exposure to radiation. DNA sequences from the promoter region of Egr-1 were linked to complementary sequences that encode TNF, a radiosensitizing cytokine (59). This resulted in a radiation-inducible promoter upstream to a cDNA encoding a toxin that is transcriptionally activated within the irradiated field to enhance radiation killing. Increased animal cures were observed in the study group that received radiation and gene therapy. This could have clinical significance, as multiple radiation treatments (20 to 35) are typically given. The authors stated that a small increment in cell killing per treatment might increase the therapeutic index because the increase in tumor cell killing is magnified by an exponent equal to the number of treatments.

Another limitation is the inability to deliver a proper amount of the vector—and therefore the gene product— to either the tumor site or to antigen-presenting cells. One way to alleviate this problem is to use vectors that can express only in tumor cells, not in nontumor cells. This has been reported in several systems (20). The use of tissue-specific and tumor-specific promoters could increase the amount of transgene expressed in tumor cells while minimizing the toxicity to neighboring cells. Various tissue-specific promoters have been described for liver, prostate, breast, and other tissues as well as for certain tumors. Lymphocytes containing the gene for a tumor-specific antigen have also been used. Once the tumor cell has been targeted, it would be necessary to program a second event after the lymphocyte has attached to the tumor cell.

An alternate approach is to generate vectors that will be replication-competent in predetermined tumors (60,61). This would further increase gene delivery, although enough safety factors would have to be incorporated to ensure that the vector would not spread to either other nontumor tissues or to the public. Replication-competent viruses have been used extensively outside the area of gene therapy for years. Russell has extensively reviewed this field (62). One rationale has been that certain viruses tend to infect replicating cells. Many attempts have focused on the use of various attenuated viral vaccine preparations to kill tumor.

Obviously, the proposed use of a replicating vector would raise safety issues over and above those for replication-incompetent vectors. Such issues have been discussed by regulatory authorities for all live attenuated viral vaccines, especially regarding the potential mutability of live viruses. Russell raises several related safety concerns for any replication-competent viral vector for gene therapy:

1. Does the replicating vector have the potential either to damage normal tissue or to produce disease in the patient?

2. Can the replicating vector either mutate or recombine in the patient? If so, could this change result in increased pathogenicity for the patient or the public?

3. Could the replicating vector or its progeny spread to other individuals? If so, what are the consequences?

4. Could the recombinant virus or a derivative thereof be transmitted transplacentally, producing disease in the fetus?

Russell concludes that strong arguments exist to support laboratory studies for replicating vectors in gene therapy. Arguments will be stronger if data show that genes can be delivered efficiently with this technique and if safety data demonstrate minimal potential for these concerns.

Replication-competent herpes simplex virus-1 has been used to kill U-87MG glioma cells both in tissue culture and in nude mice and in *Aotus* monkeys (63). In safety studies, eight of eight mice survived inoculation of the herpes variant G207 compared with herpes strain F. Even more impressive, three of three *Aotus nancymai* monkeys survived, even when 1×10^7 PFU of G207 were inoculated intracerebrally (*Aotus* are known for their extreme sensitivity to herpes simplex). The G207 strain contains deletions in two beta 34.5 loci. The authors noted that strain G207 may be particularly relevant to human brain tumors because it can infiltrate along white matter tracts and can grow inside ventricles.

In addition to the use of cytokine combinations, combinations with other modalities, and tumor-specific vectors and replication-competent vectors, the method of delivering the vector is critical. As noted, ex vivo, in vivo, and in situ approaches have been attempted, and various viral and nonviral vectors have been used. Lymphocytes, CD34+ cells, autologous tumor and fibroblast cells, allogeneic cells, and mouse producer cells, among others, have been investigated. The relevant cell is clearly defined for some applications but is elusive for others. Where the objective is to present the cell containing the transgene to the proper immunologic cells, alternate means will have to be investigated. These will include subcutaneous or intradermal inoculation so that the appropriate antigens can be delivered to the Langerhans cells present in the dermis. Alternately, dendritic cells themselves could be cultivated and transduced with a cytokine or tumor antigens, which could trigger an immune cascade. In melanoma, where most of this work has been performed, human CD4+ T-cells have been identified that recognize shared melanoma-associated antigens (64). One of the shared antigens has been determined to be tyrosinase, which also has been proven to encode class I restricted epitopes that are recognized by CD8+ T-cells from melanoma patients. Recognition and identification of expressed tumor-associated antigens provide key information for cancer vaccine strategies. It is encouraging that tumor-associated antigens in one cancer type demonstrate that epitopes on these antigens have the ability to trigger both TH1 and TH2 responses.

Studies have shown that dendritic cells could initiate an immune reaction that resulted in tumor rejection (62). A study in B-cell lymphoma has further stimulated investigations into methods of exploiting dendritic cells and perhaps their precursors as vehicles for delivering appropriate genes to the immune system. These results offer exciting potential, for they showed that dendritic cells can be harvested, pulsed with antigen, and reinfused repeatedly into patients with no observable adverse effects (65). The 4 patients studied all had antitumor cellular responses, confirmed by magnetic resonance scans. Methods have been developed to isolate, characterize, and propagate dendritic cells in vitro. In view of the results in this study, additional studies will certainly be performed.

It would be premature to believe that gene therapy will miraculously transform the area of cancer therapy. Without a thorough knowledge of oncogenesis and how the immune system does or does not operate in tumor initiation and development, it will be extremely difficult to generate rational therapeutic regimens. Nevertheless, it may be possible, even in the absence of a clear knowledge of the tumor mechanisms, to design strategies that could result in significant gene therapeutics and methods of delivering them. The potential and the contribution of gene therapy toward cancer treatment will depend not only on progress in vector development and gene expression, but also on gaining additional information about the molecular events that trigger and maintain the cancer phenotype.

REFERENCES

1. Blaese RM, Culver KW, Miller AD, et al. T-lymphocyte directed gene therapy for ADA-SCID: initial trial results after 4 years. *Science* 1995; 270:475.
2. Miller AD. Retroviral packaging cells. *Hum Gene Ther* 1990;1:5.
3. Miller AD, Buttimore C. Redesign of retrovirus packaging cell lines to avoid recombination leading to helper virus production. *Mol Cell Biol* 1986;6:2895.
4. Anderson WF. What about these monkeys that got T-cell lymphoma. *Hum Gene Ther* 1993;4:1.
5. Vile R, Russell SJ. Gene transfer technologies for the gene therapy of cancer. *Gene Therapy* 1994;1:88.
6. Anderson WF, McGarrity GJ, Moen RC. Report to the NIH Recombinant DNA Advisory Committee on Murine Replication-Competent Retrovirus (RCR) Assays (Feb. 17, 1993). *Hum Gene Ther* 1993;4:311.
7. Cornetta K, Morgan RA, Anderson WF. Safety issues related to retroviral-mediated gene transfer to humans. *Hum Gene Ther* 1991;2:5.
8. Donahue RE, Kessler SW, Bodine D, et al. Helper virus induced T-cell lymphoma in nonhuman primates after retroviral medicated gene transfer. *J Exp Med* 1992;176:1125.
9. Miller AD, Bonham L, Alfano J, Kiern HP, Reynolds T, Wolgamott G. A novel retrovirus identified during testing for helper virus in human gene transfer trials. *J Virol* 1996;70:1804.
10. Shenk T. Group C adenoviruses as vectors for gene therapy. *Viral Vectors* 1995;89–107.
11. Chen SH, Shine HD, Goodman JC, Grossman RG, Woo SLC. Gene therapy for brain tumors: regression of experimental gliomas by aden-

ovirus-mediated gene transfer in vivo. *Proc Natl Acad Sci USA* 1994; 91:3054.

12. Brody SL, Jaffe HA, Han SK, Wersto RP, Crystal RG. Direct in vivo gene transfer and expression in malignant cells using adenovirus vectors. *Hum Gene Ther* 1994;5:437.

13. Fisher KJ, Gao GP, Weitzman MD, DeMatteo R, Burda JF, Wilson JM. Transduction with recombinant adeno-associated virus for gene therapy is limited by leading strand synthesis. *J Virol* 1996;70:520.

14. Flotte TR, Ifiene SA, Conrad E, et al. Stable in vivo expression of the cystic fibrosis transmembrane conductance regulator with an adeno-associated virus vector. *Proc Natl Acad Sci USA* 1993;90:10613.

15. Lee RJ, Low PS. Folate-mediated tumor cell targeting of liposome-entrapped doxorubicin in vitro. *Biochem Biophys Acta* 1995;1233:134.

16. Nabel GJ, Yang ZY, Nabel EG, et al. Direct gene transfer for treatment of human cancer. *Ann NY Acad Sci* 1995;772:227.

17. Nabel GJ, Nabel EG, Yang ZY, et al. Direct gene transfer with DNA-liposome complexes in melanoma: expression, biological activity, and lack of toxicity in humans. *Proc Natl Acad Sci USA* 1993;90:11307.

18. Plautz GE, Yang Z-Y, Wu B-Y, Gao X, Huang L, Nabel GJ. Immunotherapy of malignancy by in vivo gene transfer into tumors. *Proc Natl Acad Sci USA* 1993;90:4645.

19. Wahl WL, Strome SE, Nabel GJ, et al. Generation of therapeutic T-lymphocytes after in vivo tumor transfection with an allogeneic Class I major histocompatibility complex gene. *J Immunother* 1995;17:1.

20. Kaneko S, Hallenbeck P, Kotani T, et al. Adenovirus-mediated gene therapy of hepatocellular carcinoma using cancer specific gene expression. *Cancer Res* 1995;55:5283.

21. Dunbar CE, Emmons RVB. Gene transfer into hematopoietic progenitor and stem cells: progress and problems. *Stem Cells* 1994;12:563.

22. Brenner MK, Rill DR, Moen RC, et al. Gene-marking to trace origin of relapse after autologous bone marrow transplantation. *Lancet* 1993; 341:85.

23. Brenner MK, Rill DR, Holladay MS, et al. Gene marking to determine whether autologous marrow infusion restores long-term haemopoiesis in cancer patients. *Lancet* 1993;342:1134.

24. Deisseroth AB, Zu Z, Claxton D, et al. Genetic marking shows that Ph+ cells present in autologous transplants of chronic myelogenous leukemia (CML) contribute to relapse after autologous bone marrow transplantation. *Blood* 1995;85:3048.

25. Dunbar CE, Cottler-Fox M, O'Shaughnessy JA, et al. Retrovirally marked CD34-enriched peripheral blood and bone marrow cells contribute to long-term engraftment after autologous transplantation. *Blood* 1995;85:3048.

26. Kohn, DB, Weinberg KI, Nolta JA, et al. Engraftment of gene-modified umbilical cord blood cells in neonates with adenosine deaminase deficiency. *Nat Med* 1995;1:1017.

27. Kotani H, Newton, PB, Zhang S, et al. Improved methods of retroviral vector transduction and production for gene therapy. *Hum Gene Ther* 1994;5:19.

28. Gilboa E, Lyerly HK, Vieweg J, Saito S. Immunotherapy of cancer using cytokine gene-modified tumor vaccines. *Can Biol* 1994;5:409.

29. VanPeln A, Boon T. Protection against a nonimmunogenic mouse leukemia by an immunogenic variant obtained by mutagenesis. *Proc Natl Acad Sci USA* 1982;79:4718.

30. Key ME, Brandhorst JS, Hanna Jr MG. More on the relevance of animal tumor models: immunogenicity of transplantable leukemias of recent origin in syngeneic strain 2 guinea pigs. *J Biol Resp Modifiers* 1984;3:359.

31. Lin K, Guarnieri FG, Staveley-O'Carroll KF, et al. Treatment of established tumors with a novel vaccine that enhances major histocompatibility class II presentation of tumor antigen. *Can Res* 1996;56:21.

32. Huang AYC, Golumbek P, Ahmadzadeh M, Jaffee E, Pardoll D, Levitsky H. Role of bone marrow-derived cells in presenting MHC Class I-restricted tumor antigens. *Science* 1994;264:961.

33. Levitsky HI, Lazenby A, Hayaski RJ, Pardoll DM. In vivo primary of two distinct antitumor effecter population: the role of MHC Class I expression. *J Exp Med* 1994;179:1215.

34. Dranoff G, Jaffee E, Lazenby A, et al. Vaccination with irradiated tumor cells engineered to secrete murine granulocyte-macrophage colony-stimulating factor stimulates potent, specific and long-lasting anti-tumor immunity. *Proc Natl Acad Sci USA* 1993;90:3539.

35. Gansbacher G, Bannerji R, Daniels B, Zier K, Cronin K, Gilboa E. Retroviral vector-mediated gamma-interferon gene transfer into tumor cells generates potent and long-lasting anti-tumor immunity. *Cancer Res* 1990;50:7820.

36. Tahara H, Lotze MT, Robbins PD, Storkus WJ, Zintvogel L. IL-12 gene therapy using direct injection of tumors with genetically engineered autologous fibroblasts. *Hum Gene Ther* 1995;6:1607.

37. Brunda MJ, Luistro L, Warrier RR, et al. Antitumor and antimetastatic activity of interleukin 12 against murine tumors. *J Exp Med* 1993; 178:1223.

38. Moolten FL. Tumor chemosensitivity conferred by inserted herpes thymidine kinase genes: paradigm for a prospective cancer control strategy. *Cancer Res* 1986;46:5276.

39. Culver KW, Ram Z, Wallbridge S, Ishii H, Oldfield EH, Blaese RM. In vivo gene transfer with retroviral-producer cells for treatment of experimental brain tumors. *Science* 1992;256:1550.

40. Ram Z, Culver KA, Wallbridge S, Blaese RM, Oldfield EH. In situ retroviral mediated gene transfer for the treatment of brain tumors in rats. *Cancer Res* 1993;53:83.

41. Chen CY, Chang YN, Ryan P, Linscott M, McGarrity GJ, Chiang YL. Effect of herpes simplex virus thymidine kinase expression levels on ganciclovir-mediated cytotoxicity and the "bystander effect." *Hum Gen Ther* 1995;6:1467.

42. Lyons RM, Forry-Schaudies S, Otto E, et al. An improved retroviral vector encoding the herpes simplex virus thymidine kinase gene increases anti-tumor efficacy in vivo. *Cancer Gene Ther* 1995;2:273.

43. Galili U, Swanson K. Gene sequences suggest inactivation of X-1,3, galactosyltransferase in catarrhines after the divergence of apes from monkeys. *Proc Natl Acad Sci USA* 1991;88:740.

44. Bonini C, Verzeletti, Servida P, et al. Immunity against the transgenic product may limit efficacy of HSV-TK-transduced donor peripheral blood lymphocytes after allo-BMT. *Blood* 1995;86:628a.

45. Riddle SR, Elliott M, Lewinsohn DA, et al. T-cell mediated rejection of gene-modified HIV-specific cytotoxic T lymphocytes in HIV-infected patients. *Nat Med* 1996;2:216.

46. Tiberghegian P, Reynolds CW, Keller J, et al. Ganciclovir treatment of herpes simplex thymidine kinase-transduced primary T lymphocytes: an approach for specific in vivo donor T cell depletion after bone marrow transplantation? *Blood* 1994;84:1333.

47. Levine AJ. Tumor suppressor genes. *Sci Am* 1995:28.

48. Levine AJ. The tumor suppressor genes. *Ann Rev Biochem* 1993; 62: 623.

49. Chen Y, Chen PL, Arnaiz N, et al. Expression of wild-type p53 in human A673 cells suppresses tumorigenicity but not growth rate. *Oncogene* 1991;6:1799.

50. Takahashi T, Carbone D, Takahashi T, et al. Wild-type but not mutant p53 suppresses the growth of human lung cancer cells bearing multiple genetic lesions. *Cancer Res* 1992;52:2340.

51. Roth JA. Clinical protocol for modification of oncogene and tumor suppressor gene expression in non-small cell lung cancer. *Hum Gene Ther* 1993;4:383.

52. Fujiwara T, Grimm EA, Mukhopadhyay T, et al. Induction of chemosensitivity in human lung cancer cell in vivo by adenovirus-mediated transfer of the wild-type p53 gene. *Cancer Res* 1994;54:2287.

53. Roth JA. Clinical protocol for modified tumor suppressor gene expression and induction of apoptosis in non-small cell lung cancer (NSCLC) with an adenovirus vector expressing wild-type p53 and cisplatin. *Hum Gene Ther* 1995;6:252.

54. Venook AP, Warren RS. Gene therapy of primary and metastatic malignant tumors of the liver using ACN53 via hepatic artery infusion: a Phase I Study. *Hum Gene Ther* 1995;6:1086.

55. Hunter T. Cooperation between oncogenes. *Cell* 1991;64:249.

56. Fearon ER, Vogelstein B. A genetic model for colorectal tumorigenesis. *Cell* 1990;61:759.

57. Nabel EG, Yang Z, Muller DL, et al. Safety and toxicity of catheter gene therapy to the pulmonary vasculature in a patient with metastatic melanoma. *Hum Gene Ther* 1994;5:1089.

58. Kim JH, Kim SH, Kolozsvary A, Brown SL, Kim OB, Freytag SO. Selective enhancement of radiation response of herpes simplex virus thymidine kinase transduced by 9L gliosarcoma cells in vitro and in vivo by antiviral agents. *Int J Oncol Biol Phys* 1995;33:861.

59. Weichselbaum RR, Hallahan DE, Beckett MA, et al. Gene therapy targeted by radiation preferentially radiosensitizes tumor cells. *Can Res* 1994;54:4266.

60. Bischoff JR, Kirn DH, Williams A, et al. An adenovirus mutant that

replicates selectively in p-53 deficient human tumor cells. *Science* 1996;274:373.

61. Kucharczuk JC, Randazzo B, Chang MY, et al. Use of "replication-restricted" herpes virus to treat experimental human malignant mesothelioma. *Cancer Res* 1997;57:466.

62. Topalian SL, Rivoltini L, Mancini M, et al. Human CD4$^+$ T cells specifically recognize a shared melanoma-associated antigen encoded by the tyrosinase gene. *Proc Natl Acad Sci USA* 1994;91: 9461.

63. Hsu FJ, Benicke C, Fagnoni F, et al. Vaccination of patients with B-cell lymphoma using autologous antigen pulsed dendritic cells. *Nat Med* 1996;2:52.

CHAPTER 29

Radioimmunoguided Surgery for Recurrent and Metastatic Colorectal Cancer

Julian A. Kim and Edward W. Martin, Jr.

The difficulty lies not in new ideas, but in escaping old ones.
—*John Maynard Keynes*

HISTORY AND RATIONALE

Recurrent and metastatic colorectal cancer is a significant cause of cancer morbidity and mortality in the United States. An estimated 149,000 new cases of colorectal cancer were diagnosed in 1994, and colorectal cancer is the second leading cause of cancer mortality (1). About 25% of patients who present with primary colorectal cancer have evidence of distant metastases, and an additional 25% of patients with nonmetastatic primary colorectal cancer will develop subsequent recurrence or distant metastasis (2). Current cytotoxic chemotherapy and radiation therapy regimens have not been shown to improve overall survival in this half of the patient population.

Several lines of evidence suggest that aggressive surgical resection of recurrent or metastatic colorectal cancer can provide long-term survival in select patients. Survival rates for patients with complete surgical resection of hepatic metastases is estimated at 25% to 30%, confirming that aggressive regional treatment of metastatic disease can result in long-term survival (3,4). However, selecting patients who will have favorable outcomes from aggressive surgical resection is difficult. This selection is very important because extensive surgical procedures may carry significant associated morbidity and mortality.

Thus, a major focus of research in this area is to identify patients who have tumor biologies that would make them favorable candidates for aggressive surgical resection. Helping to identify the extent of metastatic disease at the time of surgery to aid in surgical decision making is one of the primary functions of the radioimmunoguided surgery (RIGS) system.

The RIGS system has been developed specifically for detecting cancer during surgery (5). It consists of a handheld gamma detector (the Neoprobe 1000 portable radioisotope detector, Neoprobe Corp., Columbus, OH), a tumor-specific agent tagged with a radioactive isotope, and a patented surgical method. Over the course of its 10-year clinical evolution, the RIGS system has been used in nearly 1,600 surgeries in clinical trials in the United States and Europe. The most advanced clinical experience with the RIGS system has been with colorectal cancer. Other work, in early to middle stages of development, is also ongoing to test the RIGS system for surgical detection of breast, ovarian, prostate, and neuroendocrine/endocrine cancers. The system is potentially applicable to all solid tumor types.

The RIGS system for intraoperative cancer detection is being investigated for providing the following unique benefits:

Providing immediate intraoperative staging information about the extent of disease
Assisting in intraoperative surgical decision making
Evaluating the adequacy of surgical resection bed and margins.

RIGS has the potential to give the surgeon additional information concerning the extent of disease, and this new information has potential prognostic implications that may assist intraoperative decision making.

J. A. Kim and E. W. Martin, Jr.: Department of Surgery, Division of Surgical Oncology, Arthur G. James Cancer Hospital and Research Institute, The Ohio State University College of Medicine, Columbus, Ohio 43210.

INDICATIONS

The RIGS system can be applied to any solid tumor for which an appropriate carrier substance can be developed. This chapter will review the experience in recurrent and metastatic colorectal cancer, although clinical trials in breast, ovarian, and pancreatic cancers have also been performed.

The history of surgery for recurrent colorectal cancer illustrates the controversies that surround aggressive surgery for metastatic disease. The current role of surgery in metastatic disease remains a topic of debate. The central issue appears to be that there is currently no method for predicting the biologic behavior of metastatic disease. It is clear that there is a subgroup of patients with metastatic colorectal cancer who will benefit from aggressive surgical treatment; however, selection of patients must be performed judiciously. An additional underlying theme is that to date there is no effective radiotherapy, chemotherapy, or biologic therapy that has the potential to improve patient survival in the setting of metastatic colorectal cancer. Thus, aggressive surgical resection in select patients remains a significant treatment consideration.

The RIGS system is useful for any patients who are undergoing exploratory surgery with curative intent for recurrent or metastatic disease. The selection of patients and the timing of surgery for recurrent colorectal cancer vary depending on the physician and patient. We favor close monitoring of patients by following trends in serum tumor markers such as carcinoembryonic antigen (CEA). Although CEA monitoring remains controversial, it does allow for earlier detection of colorectal cancer recurrence or metastases (6). Whether routine monitoring of CEA is cost-effective or leads to improved survival in a significant number of patients has yet to be formally tested in a randomized clinical trial. However, if aggressive surgical treatment of recurrent and metastatic colorectal cancer is to be pursued, then CEA monitoring remains an important tool.

With these points in mind, one promising indication for RIGS is for patients who are undergoing surgery for recurrent or metastatic colorectal cancer. This indication would include patients who have significant elevations of serum CEA levels but do not have measurable disease by conventional radiographic procedures. In fact, in patients undergoing "second-look" laparotomy, RIGS has been shown to increase the percentage of patients with positive findings at laparotomy from 40% to almost 80% (7).

In patients who have measurable metastatic disease who are undergoing curative resection, RIGS has provided important information at the time of surgery for patients participating in trials. For example, in patients who are undergoing hepatic resection, RIGS can help the surgeon determine whether the patient has extrahepatic disease. This information might influence the decision to perform a major hepatic resection or even place hepatic artery chemoinfusion catheters. Also, in patients who are undergoing pelvic exenteration, RIGS-provided information about the presence of extrapelvic disease may influence the nature of the resection. RIGS also provides immediate real-time information regarding resection margins and the presence or absence of residual microscopic disease.

DETAILED METHODOLOGY

Patient Selection and Preparation

The selection and preparation of a patient for RIGS surgery clinical trials is the same for any patient undergoing surgery for recurrent or metastatic or colorectal cancer. All patients must be adequately staged for extent of disease using conventional radiographic techniques such as computed tomography and magnetic resonance imaging of the abdomen, pelvis, and chest if chest radiographs show any abnormality that could represent metastases. Patients should have colonoscopy before surgery and biopsy of any suspicious areas. Antibody-based imaging studies such as OncoScint can be used at the discretion of the physician. The prior exposure of patients to murine monoclonal antibody (MAb) and the presence of human-antimurine antibodies (HAMA) has not adversely affected the efficacy of RIGS intraoperative detection in more than 100 patients studied (8).

Patients should be carefully assessed to determine risk for complications from general anesthesia as well as their ability to tolerate major surgery. They should be informed about the nature of the surgical procedure as well as the alternatives and risks, and consent should be witnessed.

Preoperative Considerations

Several unique features to the preoperative treatment of patients with RIGS deserve mention. Because RIGS intraoperative detection can be affected by blood pool background radioactivity, it is important that all radioactivity from nuclear medicine studies be adequately cleared. Some radionuclide scans may interfere with the ability of the RIGS system's gamma-detecting probe to locate the radiolabeled MAb at the time of surgery. For example, thallium-201, which is commonly used in cardiac stress tests, may have prolonged clearance from the blood and may result in a delay in the ability to perform RIGS scanning during surgery. A waiting period of 10 half-lives of any previously administered radionuclide is recommended before RIGS surgery; thus, radionuclides with long half-lives should be avoided in the preoperative period if possible.

Antibody Injection and Preoperative Monitoring

Antibody is labeled with ^{125}I using the IODO-GEN (Pierce Chemical, Rockford, IL) method (9) and is administered to the patient via a peripheral intravenous line. The dose of 1 mg antibody labeled with 2 mCi ^{125}I has shown optimal biologic activity in dose-ranging studies (10). The patient is monitored closely for any signs of adverse reaction for about 30 minutes postinjection, and external gamma counts are then performed as a baseline. Patients receive thyroid blockade by potassium iodide oral solution USP (SSKI), 130 mg/day, initiated 1 to 2 hours before antibody injection and continued daily until surgery. The SSKI saturates the thyroid and reduces uptake of the ^{125}I/antibody conjugate.

Clearance of the ^{125}I/antibody from normal tissues and the blood pool background is essential for optimal tumor localization at the time of surgery. The biologic half-life of the conjugate is about 3.5 days, and clearance consists of a rapid phase within the first 7 days followed by a more gradual decline. Precordial gamma counts are monitored weekly, with most patients exhibiting adequate clearance within 21 to 25 days.

Radioimmunoguided Surgery

Patients undergo complete bowel prep and receive antibiotic prophylaxis of choice before surgery. After induction of general anesthesia, an exploratory laparo-

tomy is performed via a midline incision. The entire peritoneal cavity and retroperitoneum are carefully inspected for any evidence of gross tumor. All adhesions from previous surgeries must be completely lysed so that the entire gastrointestinal tract can be inspected thoroughly. Systematic inspection of the abdomen includes complete mobilization of the liver and hepatic ultrasound, particularly if hepatic resection is being considered. At the completion of the traditional laparotomy, a comprehensive list of findings is documented and a surgical plan is stated based on those findings.

After the traditional exploration, a RIGS survey is performed (Fig. 1). The sound cue provided by the gamma-detecting probe is squelched on normal tissue to establish a baseline of blood background counts. Thereafter, the microprocessor in the probe's control unit gives an audible signal only when radioactivity in tissue exceeds background counts by a statistically significant amount (ie, 3 sigma). A systematic RIGS survey is performed to identify areas with increased radioactivity. RIGS-positive tissue is defined as a tissue that contains at least three standard deviations higher radioactivity than background tissue. A complete RIGS survey includes the areas listed in Table 1. Following the RIGS survey, biopsies are performed and, based on the information available to the surgeon, a revised surgical plan is established. At the completion of the surgical procedure, a detailed map of any residual gross tumor or RIGS-localized tissue that could not be resected is recorded for future data analysis.

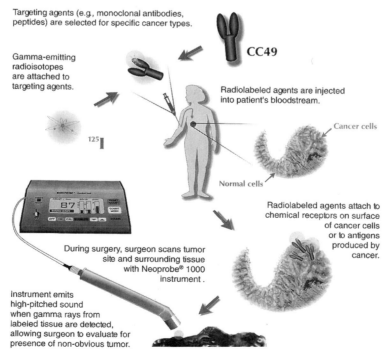

FIG. 1. The RIGS system. Patients are injected with a radiolabeled monoclonal antibody CC49 for intraoperative detection using the Neoprobe 1000. (Illustration courtesy Martin Boso)

TABLE 1. *RIGS intraoperative survey sites*

Zone	Survey sites
Zone I	Right and left lobes of liver
	Hepatoduodenal ligament
	Retropancreatic region
	Periportal and common hepatic artery regions
Zone II	Supraceliac aorta
	Celiac axis
	Stomach and duodenum
	Spleen
	Base of small bowel mesentery
	Body and tail of pancreas
Zone III	Infrapancreatic aorta
	Inferior vena cava
	Right and left kidneys
	Small and large intestines
Zone IV	Aortic bifurcation and iliac vessels
	Rectum
	Sacrum
	Bladder
	Uterus and ovaries
	Obturator foramina

Postoperatively, patients are followed throughout their hospitalization and after discharge for any evidence of toxicity or complications. Patients are followed routinely for evidence of disease recurrence and may receive additional chemotherapy or radiation therapy if deemed appropriate.

Special Agents and Instrumentation

Neoprobe 1000 Instrument

The Neoprobe 1000 is a hand-held gamma-detecting instrument that has been constructed for efficient use in the operating room. The probe is stainless steel and is gas-sterilizable (Fig. 2). It houses a cadmium/telluride crystal with sufficient sensitivity to detect low-energy radio emissions, and is connected by flexible cable to a control unit. The control unit gives a digital display of tissue radioactivity counts as well as an audible signal when statistically significant amounts of radioactivity are detected. These features provide the surgeon with real-time scanning capability and allow for probing of tissues without diverting attention from the surgical field. The protocol nurse is responsible for assisting the surgeon with immediate data collection and recording for immediate surgical decision making as well as future analysis.

The design of the probe lends itself to precise probing of tissues in isolated areas by virtue of its slender handle and angled head. The probe is an easy-to-use tool that extends the capabilities of the surgeon's hands.

Carrier Substance

The carrier substance is composed of a biologic agent that will traffic to tumor sites and be maintained in a suf-

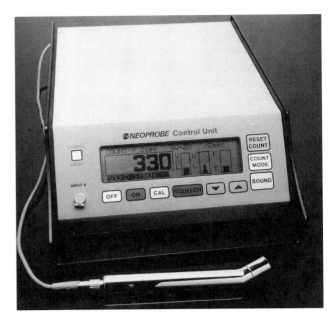

FIG. 2. The Neoprobe 1000 instrument, Neoprobe Corp., Columbus, Ohio.

ficient concentration while it is cleared from normal tissues and the blood pool. The carrier substance must also lend itself to radiolabeling and purification for use in humans. Examples of carrier substances used in the RIGS system are MAbs that bind to tumor antigens and synthetic peptides that bind to cell surface receptors. Carrier substances currently being tested in animal models include MAb fragments or chimeric humanized MAbs.

The biologic characteristics of the carrier substance, such as affinity and retention at the site of the target antigen or receptor, influence its clearance and ultimately its half-life. The half-life of the radionuclide must be suitable for each carrier substance. For example, the half-life of the radionuclide should be long enough that it does not appreciably decay during the period when the carrier substance is achieving target-specific localization. For this reason, carrier substances with short biologic half-lives are ideal, and carrier substances with longer half-lives must be labeled with a radioisotope with a long half-life (preferably five times greater than the carrier substance).

The half-life of the carrier substance determines the optimal time postinjection for RIGS surgical scanning. After the radiolabeled carrier substance is injected into the patient's peripheral vein, a high concentration of the carrier substance in the blood causes rapid distribution into the extracellular space and both normal and tumor tissues. As the carrier substance is cleared from the blood pool and concentrations of the carrier substance fall below tissue levels, secondary biodistribution results in clearance from normal tissues and retention in targeted tissues. When the ratio of the blood pool background levels of carrier substance and radioactivity are sufficiently low to provide detectable contrast to disease with concentrated levels, RIGS scanning can be performed. Thus, the biologic half-life of the carrier substance determines when RIGS can be performed after injection. For example, the biologic half-life of whole MAbs in humans is much longer than synthetic antibody fragments. Thus, despite the fact that both carrier substances may recognize similar epitopes on the same tumor antigen, their differing biologic half-lives make the timing of RIGS surgery after injection much different.

The murine MAbs used most widely with the RIGS system are the antitumor-associated (TAG)-72 antibodies. These antibodies were developed and characterized at the National Cancer Institute Laboratory of Tumor Biology and are directed against a human breast adenocarcinoma extract (11–13). The first-generation antibody, B72.3, is a murine IgG1 that shows specific binding to >85% of human adenocarcinomas, including colorectal, breast, ovarian, gastric, pancreatic, endometrial, and lung adenocarcinomas. Importantly, the antibodies do not appear to show significant nonspecific binding to normal tissues, with the exception of secretory-phase endometrium (14–16). The target TAG-72 is a high-molecular-weight glycoprotein that has the biochemical and structural characteristics of a mucin (17). The epitope recognized by the first-generation anti-TAG antibody B72.3 appears to be a carbohydrate side chain; the epitope recognized by the second-generation antibody may be a core glycoprotein (18). The affinity of CC49 for the TAG-72 antigen appears to be about eight to 10 times that of B72.3 (19). Interestingly, although TAG-72 is highly expressed on most human adenocarcinomas in vivo, its expression is down-regulated in vitro when placed in tissue culture. Both in vitro studies and human clinical trials have shown that tumor cell treatment with biologics such as interferons can up-regulate TAG-72 expression, which may provide a potential method of increasing the sensitivity of the RIGS system with CC49 (20,21).

Radioisotopes

Various radioisotopes have been evaluated using the RIGS system. The half-life of an optimal radioisotope must be significantly greater than the biologic half-life of the carrier substance. In addition, radioisotopes with low-level gamma emissions are best suited for use with the Neoprobe 1000 due to the sensitivity of the cadmium/telluride crystal in the detector, which can be placed close to tissues.

With these constraints in mind, preclinical animal models have shown ^{125}I to be ideal for use in the RIGS system (22). The half-life of 60 days enables use with MAbs, which have been shown to take about 3 to 4 weeks to clear adequately from the peripheral circulation before RIGS scanning. Alternative radioisotopes such as technetium-99m, iodine-123, and iodine-131 have been stud-

ied as well but are less suitable due to either shorter half-lives or higher energy emissions, with significant Compton scattering. However, with the advent of carrier substances with shorter biologic half-lives and differing targeting capabilities, these radionuclides may prove to be useful in the RIGS system.

CLINICAL RESULTS

RIGS human clinical studies span a period of over 10 years and consist of various completed phase I and phase II clinical trials. This section summarizes the human clinical studies published to date.

The initial phase I studies of RIGS have focused on safety issues of both the MAb and radioactive iodine as well as the dose and scheduling of these compounds to optimize RIGS detection. These studies used various MAbs to determine the feasibility of intraoperative detection. Results of a pilot study using an anti-CEA antibody in 28 patients showed that in about 68% of patients, tumor deposits were localized using the hand-held probe (23). Importantly, the RIGS surgery was found to be safe and feasible, an important step in the future development of RIGS as an intraoperative modality.

RIGS Using MAb B72.3

A continued search for MAbs directed against human colorectal cancer antigens lead to the development of the anti-TAG-72 murine MAbs. These antibodies were tested in both preclinical animal models and human clinical trials. The first-generation anti-TAG-72 antibody B72.3 was studied extensively in both phase I and phase II clinical trials. The initial cohort of patients at the Ohio State University consisted of 6 patients with primary colorectal cancer and 31 patients with recurrent disease. Fifty-seven possible intraoperative sites of radioimmunodetection were analyzed (24). Radiolabeled antibody was detected by the surgeon in 47 of the 57 possible sites, which corresponds to a RIGS localization rate of 82%. The utility of RIGS as an intraoperative detection system was confirmed due to the localization of subclinical tumor in 8 of the 31 patients with recurrent disease. The surgical procedure was altered in these patients based solely on the intraoperative RIGS findings. Additional surgical resection of RIGS-localized tumor was performed in 2 patients; in the remaining 6 patients, major surgical resection was abandoned due solely to RIGS-localized subclinical tumor. Follow-up of 66 patients confirmed intraoperative localization in 5 of 6 patients (83%) with primary colorectal cancer and 79% of those with recurrent or metastatic disease (25). These findings provided the rationale to expand to a multi-institutional study to assess the utility of RIGS.

The results of the multicenter RIGS trial were published in 1988 (26). The trial was conducted at seven medical centers, and 105 patients were enrolled over an 18-month period. RIGS localization of tumor was accomplished in 78% of patients, confirming that the single-institutional findings were reproducible. Subclinical, occult tumor was localized intraoperatively in 26 patients at 30 different sites in the pelvis, retroperitoneum, and porta hepatis. Again, a significant percentage of patients had either extended resection (23%) or abandonment of major resection (27%) based solely on RIGS detection of subclinical tumor.

The potential clinical importance of RIGS intraoperative localization and the impact on surgical decision making are illustrated in a retrospective review of 86 patients with recurrent or metastatic colorectal cancer (7). The survival of these patients was evaluated, and the results are shown in Fig. 3. Patients were assigned to one of three groups:

1. RIGS Resectable (n=40)—patients who had all gross tumor and RIGS-localized tissue resected
2. RIGS Unresectable (n=13)—all gross tumor appeared resectable but RIGS tissue was unresectable. These patients did not have resection of the gross tumor.
3. Traditional Unresectable (n=33)—patients whose gross tumor was not resectable

As evidenced by survival data, patients who were RIGS unresectable had similar survival as patients who had traditional unresectable disease. In contrast, the 5-year survival in the RIGS resectable group approached 60%, which is quite favorable compared to any previous reports on the surgical treatment of recurrent or metastatic colorectal cancer (27). These data may suggest that RIGS had an impact on patients who had gross tumor that was resectable but were spared major resection due to occult RIGS intraoperative findings. Thus, the RIGS resectable group is a highly selected group for which aggressive surgical resection can afford significant long-term survival. The study shows that RIGS appears to be a predictor of tumor biology, which may be helpful in intraoperative decision making.

RIGS Using MAbs CC49 and CC83

During the RIGS clinical trials using B72.3, a second generation of anti-TAG-72 murine MAb was developed by Jeffrey Schlom in the Laboratory of Tumor Immunology at the National Cancer Institute. The second-generation CC49 and CC83 antibodies recognize different TAG-72 epitopes than B72.3, and the resulting antibodies exhibited an approximately eightfold increase in affinity (28). A 1990 RIGS pilot study using ^{125}I CC49 evaluated 54 patients (29). Of the 30 patients with recurrent or metastatic disease, 29 (97%) showed RIGS localization of tumor, a significant improvement over the B72.3 results. As a result of this additional intraoperative information, the surgeon altered the surgical plan in 14 patients (47%) (Table 2). Specifically, 3 patients who otherwise would have undergone hepatic resection did not due to extensive occult RIGS-localized extrahepatic disease. Three additional patients had additional surgical resection of bladder, vagina, and liver based solely on occult RIGS findings. Nine patients (30%) with primary colorectal cancer

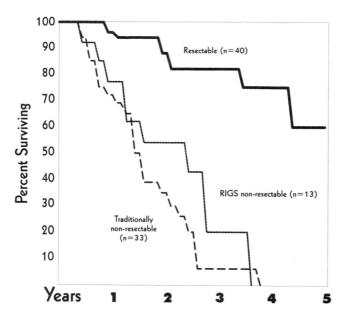

FIG. 3. Actual survival of patients with metastatic colon cancer undergoing RIGS procedures. Group 1: RIGS resectable; group 2: RIGS unresectable; group 3: traditional unresectable. (Adapted from Martin et al. [74] with permission)

TABLE 2. *RIGS-influenced operative changes*

Type of patient	Number of changes
Primary colorectal	
Rectal resection	1
Small bowel resection	2
Gastrohepatic lymph node dissection	8
Retroperitoneal lymph node dissection	4
Abandoned plans for hepatic arterial catheter	1
Total	16
Recurrent colorectal	
Added resection of intestinal anastomosis	1
Added cystectomy	1
Added vaginectomy	1
Extended planned liver resection	1
Abandoned liver resection	3
Gastrohepatic lymph node dissection	3
Added or directed brachytherapy	5
Iliac lymph node dissection	2
Total	17

were upstaged from pathologic stage I or stage II to stage III, thus making them eligible for adjuvant chemotherapy. Similar findings were observed in a pilot study using the second-generation CC83 MAb (30).

Adoptive Cellular Immunotherapy Using RIGS-Localized Lymph Nodes

Lymph nodes are a common site of RIGS localization during laparotomy. Laboratory studies of these lymph nodes show that they may be a suitable source of activated lymphocytes for adoptive cellular therapy (ACT). ACT is a form of immunotherapy in which immunologically active cells are transferred to a tumor-bearing host to effect tumor regression. Although ACT has been evaluated extensively, issues regarding the source of cells and methods of ex vivo activation remain controversial.

Immunologic Characteristics of Lymph Nodes Identified Using RIGS

In patients with metastatic colorectal cancer, the RIGS system identifies lymph nodes that appear normal grossly but that contain either foci of microscopic tumor or shed TAG-72 antigen. MAbs are distributed at the germinal centers of these RIGS-positive lymph nodes with a characteristic circular pattern, suggesting the exposure of the specific epitopes of TAG-72 on follicular dendritic cells. In the pilot study described below, RIGS-positive lymph node lymphocytes (LNLs) were characterized by a CD4$^+$ cell

pleocytosis, increased rates of expansion, and increased cytolytic activity when compared to lymphocytes from lymph nodes with macroscopic tumor, noninvolved lymph nodes, tumors, and peripheral blood. In contrast to LNLs from noninvolved lymph nodes, RIGS-positive LNLs consistently demonstrated proliferative responses to TAG-72$^+$ tumor and to soluble TAG-72$^+$ mucin (31).

We have investigated methods of short-term ex vivo activation and expansion of cells from RIGS-positive lymph nodes from patients with colorectal carcinoma. These expanded cells can be reinfused and may function in vivo as T-helper cells (32). Using anti-CD3/IL-2 and three-stage, 10-day culture in air-porous plastic bags, we have been able to effect 40- to 100-fold expansion of cells that are predominantly CD4$^+$. The cells expanded from RIGS-positive lymph nodes are noncytolytic but proliferate and, more importantly, secrete cytokines in response to autologous tumor. Technically, the expansion system is easy, highly reproducible, and expedient.

Clinical Trial of Lymph Node Lymphocytes Expanded from RIGS-Localized Lymph Nodes

A pilot study was performed to examine the clinical and biologic effects of the adoptive transfer of expanded cells from RIGS-positive lymph nodes in 12 patients with unresectable, metastatic colorectal cancer (Fig. 4). Tumor-sensitized lymphocytes were localized in all patients at laparotomy, and expanded lymph node cells were administered intravenously on postoperative day 10,

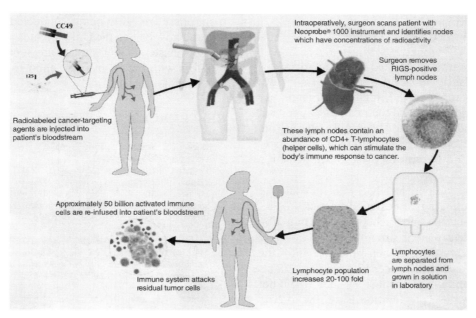

FIG. 4. Adoptive cellular therapy using lymph nodes localized during the RIGS procedure. Lymph nodes are activated ex vivo and reinfused into patients as a treatment for metastatic colon cancer. (Illustration courtesy Martin Boso)

with and without systemic IL-2 (0.1 mg/m²/d IV, days 1 to 4). Up to 4.3×10^{10} cells were expanded and infused without significant toxicity. The preliminary results of the pilot studies show significant biologic activity of the adoptively transferred cells in vivo (33). Phase II clinical trials are in progress to define further the clinical and biologic effects of this approach in patients with colorectal and pancreatic cancer.

MORBIDITY AND MORTALITY

RIGS has been performed in more than 1,600 patients in multiple medical centers. It has been used in patients with both primary and recurrent colorectal cancer. The RIGS procedure has not altered the operative mortality rate. In addition, due to the fact that many patients are spared major resection due solely to RIGS intraoperative findings, it is likely that operative morbidity for patients undergoing laparotomy for resection may actually be reduced.

Safety studies are ongoing concerning the use of murine MAbs. The results suggest that readministration of murine MAbs is safe, even in patients with circulating human antimurine antibodies at the time of reinjection (8).

Finally, there have been few documented cases of side effects from ^{125}I associated with RIGS; the side effects that have occurred are mild. Thyroid function tests have shown no evidence of hypothyroidism in patients undergoing RIGS procedures, and measurement of radioactive exposure to surgical and pathology personnel during RIGS and during pathologic evaluation of RIGS-localized tissues confirmed that levels are safe.

PATIENT INFORMATION

During cancer surgery, computed tomography, x-ray, or magnetic resonance imaging scans taken before surgery are used as references. Primarily, surgeons use their visual and tactile senses and their experience to help them find cancer and remove it. The RIGS system is an experimental tool developed to help surgeons find cancer that may not be found by any of these other detection methods.

Cancer patients taking part in RIGS clinical trials are injected with a targeting agent designed to stick to cancer-specific byproducts or cancer receptors. The targeting agent is bound to a very small amount of a radioactive chemical called iodine-125. When injected into the bloodstream, this radioactive cancer-targeting agent acts as a homing device, binding to cancer substances but not to normal cells. The dose of radiation is so low that no special precautions need to be taken, except the patient takes medication that keeps the targeting agent from accumulating in the thyroid.

A waiting period may be required between the injection and surgery to allow the targeting agent to clear from normal tissues and from the bloodstream. The waiting time varies from several hours to several weeks, depending on the cancer type and the specific agent used.

During the surgery, the surgeon scans inside the body with the highly sensitive hand-held probe. The probe can detect even very small concentrations of the radioactive targeting agent in tissues. When the probe senses the accumulated radioactive targeting agent, a control unit produces a loud sound to alert the surgeon.

In addition to cancerous tissue that is obvious to the surgeon, some tissue that looks or feels normal may cause the probe to make a sound because it contains the radioactive targeting agent. This sound alerts the surgeon to evaluate the tissue more closely because it may contain hidden cancer or other tissue involved in the disease process. If hidden cancer is found, the surgeon can use this information to help decide the best surgical or postsurgical treatment.

Patients participating in a RIGS trial must sign an informed consent form to ensure they understand possible risks and the current experimental nature of the procedure. Patients also must take a thyroid-blocking agent each day, from injection until surgery, to keep the thyroid from overaccumulating the targeting agent. Participating patients also undergo routine tests, including blood draws, before and after the RIGS procedure.

Although the RIGS system is still experimental, over 1,600 surgeries in clinical trials worldwide with various RIGS cancer-targeting agents have been performed to date, with minimal side effects and without compromising safety standards. Clinical trials are farthest along with cancer of the colon or rectum. These advanced development-phase trials are being conducted at 35 cancer centers and hospitals in the United States, Europe, and Israel. Earlier-phase, smaller studies are soon to start or are in progress with breast, ovarian, endocrine/neuroendocrine, and prostate cancers.

REFERENCES

1. Boring CC, Squires TS, Tong T, et al. Cancer statistics, 1994. *CA Cancer J Clin* 1994;44:7–26.
2. Pestana C, Reitemeyer RJ, Moertel CG, et al. The natural history of carcinoma of the colon and rectum. *Am J Surg* 1964;108:826–829.
3. Fortner JG, Silva JS, Golbey RB, et al. Multivariate analysis of a personal series of 247 consecutive patients with liver metastases from colorectal cancer. *Ann Surg* 1984;199:306–316.
4. Adson MA, van Heerden JA, Adson MH, et al. Resection of hepatic metastases from colorectal cancer. *Arch Surg* 1984;119:647–651.
5. Martin EW Jr. Introduction: the RIGS Concept. In Matin EW Jr, ed. *Radioimmunoguided surgery in the detection and treatment of colorectal cancer.* Austin: RG Landes, 1994:1–6.
6. Martin EW Jr, Minton JP, Carey LC. CEA-directed second-look surgery in the asymptomatic patient with primary resection of colorectal carcinoma. *Ann Surg* 1986;202:310–313.
7. Martin EW, Carey LC. Second-look surgery for colorectal cancer. *Ann Surg* 1991;214:321–327.
8. Ritter DC, Arnold MW, Martin EW Jr. Radioimmunolocalization in the

presence of human anti-mouse antibody (abstract). *Proc Am Soc Clin Oncol* 1995;14:423.

9. Haisma JH, Hilgers J, Zurawski V. Iodination of monoclonal antibodies for diagnosis and radiotherapy using a convenient one-vial method. *J Nucl Med* 1986;27:1890–1895.

10. Arnold MA, Schneebaum S, Berens A, et al. Intraoperative detection of colorectal cancer with radioimmunoguided surgery (RIGS) and CC49, a second-generation monoclonal. *Ann Surg* 1992;216:627–632.

11. Colcher D, Horan Hand P, Nuti M, et al. A spectrum of monoclonal antibodies reactive with human mammary tumor cells. *Proc Natl Acad Sci USA* 1981;78:3199–3203.

12. Muraro R, Kuroki M, Wunderlich D, et al. Generation and characterization of B72.3 second generation antibodies reactive with the tumor-associated glycoprotein 72 antigen. *Cancer Res* 1988;48:4588–4596.

13. Colcher DM, Milenic DE, Schlom J. Generation and characterization of monoclonal antibody B72.3: experimental and preclinical studies. In Maguire RT, Van Nostran D, eds. *Diagnosis of colorectal and ovarian carcinoma: application of immunoscintigraphic technology.* New York: Marcel Dekker, 1992:23–44.

14. Nuti M, Teramoto YA, Mariani-Constantini R, et al. Monoclonal antibody (B72.3) defines patterns of distribution of a novel tumor associated antigen in human mammary cell populations. *Int J Cancer* 1982;29:539–545.

15. Thor A, Ohuchi N, Szpak CA, et al. Distribution of oncofetal antigen tumor-associated glycoprotein-72 defined by monoclonal antibody B72.3. *Cancer Res* 1986;46:3118–3124.

16. Thor A, Viglione MJ, Muraro R, et al. Monoclonal antibody B72.3 reactivity with human endometrium: a study of normal and malignant tissues. *Int J Gynecol Pathol* 1987;6:235–247.

17. Johnson VG, Schlom J, Paterson AJ, et al. Analysis of a human tumor-associated glycoprotein (TAG-72) identified by a monoclonal antibody B72.3. *Cancer Res* 1986;246:850–857.

18. Colcher D, Minelli MF, Roselli M, et al. Radioimmunolocalization of human carcinoma xenografts with B72.3 second-generation monoclonal antibodies. *Cancer Res* 1988;48:4597–4603.

19. Molinolo A, Simpson JF, Thor A, et al. Enhanced tumor binding using immunohistochemical analyses by the second generation anti-tumor associated glycoprotein 72 monoclonal antibodies versus monoclonal antibody B72.3 in human tissue. *Cancer Res* 1990;50:1290–1298.

20. Guadnani F, Schlom J, Johnston WW, et al. Selective interferon-induced enhancement of tumor-associated antigens on a spectrum of freshly isolated human adenocarcinoma cells. *J Natl Cancer Inst* 1989; 81:502–512.

21. Greiner JW, Dansky Ullmann C, Neiroda C, et al. Improved immunotherapeutic efficacy of an anticarcinoma monoclonal antibody (^{131}I-CC49) when given in combination with gamma interferon. *Cancer Res* 1993;53:600–608.

22. Thurston MO, Kaehr JW, Martin EW Jr, et al. Radionuclide of choice for use with an intraoperative probe. *Anti Immun and Radio* 1991;4(4): 595–601.

23. Aitken DE, Hinkle GH, Thurston MO, et al. A gamma detecting probe for radioimmune detection of CEA-producing tumors. *Dis Col Rect* 1984;27:279–282.

24. Sickle-Santanello BJ, O'Dwyer PJ, Mojzisik CM, et al. Radioimmunoguided surgery using the monoclonal antibody B72.3 in colorectal tumors. *Dis Col Rect* 1987;30:761–764.

25. Martin EW Jr, Mojzisik CM, Hinkle GH, et al. Radioimmunoguided surgery: a new approach to the intraoperative detection of tumor. *Am J Surg* 1988;156:386–392.

26. Cohen AM, Martin EW, Lavery I, et al. Radioimmunoguided surgery using ^{125}I-B72.3 in patients with colorectal cancer. *Arch Surg* 1991; 126:349–351.

27. Steele G Jr, Zamcheck N, Mayer R, et al. Results of CEA-initiated second-look surgery for recurrent colon cancer. *Am J Surg* 1980;139: 544–548.

28. Arnold MW, Schneebaum S, Berens A, Mojzisik C, Hinkle G, Martin EW Jr. Radioimmunoguided surgery challenges traditional decision-making in patients with primary colorectal cancer. *Surgery* 1992;4: 624–630.

29. Arnold MA, Schneebaum S, Berens A, et al. Intraoperative detection of colorectal cancer with radioimmunoguided surgery and CC49, a second-generation monoclonal antibody. *Ann Surg* 1992;216:11–16.

30. Burak WE Jr, Schneebaum S, Kim JA, et al. Pilot study evaluating the intraoperative localization of radiolabeled monoclonal antibody CC83 in patients with metastatic colorectal carcinoma. *Surgery* 1995;118: 103–108.

31. Triozzi PL, Kim JA, Aldrich W, Young DC, Sampsel J, Martin EW Jr. Identification of tumor reacting, lymph-node lymphocytes in vivo using radiolabeled monoclonal antibody. *Cancer* 1994;73:580–588.

32. Kim JA, Martin EW, Morgan C, et al. Expansion of tumor-reactive lymph node lymphocytes from colorectal cancer patients for adoptive immunotherapy. *Cancer Biother* 1995;10:115–123.

33. Triozzi PL, Kim JA, Martin EW Jr. Adoptive immunotherapy using lymph node lymphocytes localized in vivo by radiolabeled monoclonal antibody. *J Natl Cancer Inst* 1995;87:1180–1181.

CHAPTER 30

Interventional and Ablative Procedures for Cancer Pain

Ricardo Segal and Anne Harris

Pain is a more terrible lord of mankind than even death itself.
—Albert Schweitzer

The ultimate goal of cancer treatment is not only to cure but also to palliate when cure is impossible. Improving the patient's quality of life, and especially treating cancer pain aggressively, have been the focus of clinical practice guidelines published by the Federal government (1,2). The prevalence of pain in cancer patients has been summarized by Foley (3). It is believed that about 25% of patients die without pain relief, and preventing this "tragedy of needless pain" is the challenge to all in medicine (4). Cancer pain management has advanced far beyond the first three steps on the analgesic ladder initially drawn up by the World Health Organization (5). When patients no longer attain good analgesia or are adversely affected by side effects associated with conventional pain management, many options exist to improve the situation (6–8). These patients should be referred to a specialist in pain management.

This chapter outlines options available to patients with cancer with special analgesic needs. These options should not be viewed as those of last resort, when pain is "intractable." Many tumors have patterns of neural invasion that frequently result in difficult mixed pain syndromes. In these cases, pain intractability can be anticipated by the physician. The earlier these patients are seen by a pain specialist, the more likely it is that a safe and efficacious analgesic option will be available to them.

We hope that after reading this chapter, everyone involved with the treatment of cancer will remember that the epigastric pain of pancreatic cancer, the cephalgia of head and neck tumors, the lancinating tenesmus of rectal tumors, and the pain of fractured ribs (to name just a few examples) should be an anachronism in our time.

INTERVENTIONAL PAIN TREATMENT MODALITIES

Interventional pain management modalities are classified into three categories: anatomic (corrective), augmentative (chemical/electrical stimulation), and ablative (temporary [block] or permanent [lesion: chemical, radiofrequency, section]) (9).

Anatomic modalities, being corrective by definition, are the most desirable, but unfortunately they are seldom applicable in cancer pain. Examples are an orthotic device, instrumentation for spinal instability, and resection of epidural spinal metastases for radiculopathy. Temporary ablative modalities (eg, neural blockade with local anesthetic) are used as diagnostic tests when plans include proceeding with an irreversible ablative procedure. In state-of-the-art pain control, a treatment continuum or ladder has been established in which augmentative modalities precede ablation (10). In general, when differentiating between two primary types of pain (neuropathic and nociceptive), it is important to choose the correct interventional pain control modality. Neuropathic pain responds better to electrical stimulation; nociceptive pain is more effectively controlled with implantable infusion therapy. However, in cancer patients, it is difficult to differentiate between nociceptive and neuropathic pain because they often have mixed pain syndromes (11).

NEUROSTIMULATION

Spinal Cord Stimulation

The use of spinal cord stimulation for the treatment of cancer pain has been mostly abandoned after discourag-

R. Segal: Department of Neurological Surgery, University of Pittsburgh Medical Center, Pittsburgh, Pennsylvania 15213-2582.

A. Harris: Department of Anesthesiology/Critical Care Medicine, University of Pittsburgh Medical Center and Department of Veterans Affairs Medical Center, Pittsburgh, Pennsylvania 15213-2582.

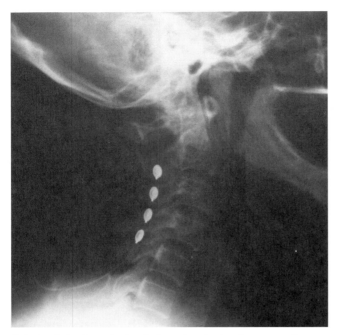

FIG. 1. Spinal cord stimulation. Cervical spine x-ray demonstrating implanted dorsal epidural stimulating electrode.

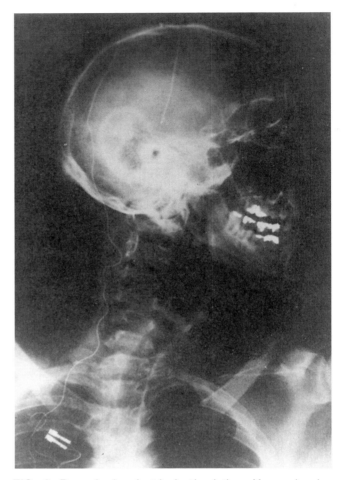

FIG. 2. Deep brain electrical stimulation. X-ray showing stimulator lead in the periventricular gray matter with wire connection to subcutaneous receiver (not shown). (Richardson DE, Akil H. Pain reduction by electrical brain stimulation in man. *J Neurosurg* 1977;47:185, with permission)

ing reports (12,13). Still, malignancy-induced plexus lesion pain syndromes may respond to spinal cord stimulation (14). The predominance of the neuropathic type of pain in these syndromes may be the rationale, and we have obtained good pain control with spinal cord stimulation in very selected patients with Pancoast syndrome (Segal, unpublished observation) (Fig. 1). Spinal cord stimulators can be implanted percutaneously under local anesthesia. The procedure does not mutilate and is reversible. The main disadvantages are the potential risk of a foreign body implant and the cost of hardware. Cost-effectiveness may be estimated according to expected survival. Although there are no studies specifically for chronic intractable cancer pain, spinal cord stimulation appears to be cost-effective when compared to alternative therapies that cost $20,000 per year or more, with 78% or lower efficacy (15).

Deep Brain Electrical Stimulation

The usefulness of brain stimulation for relief of cancer pain has been debated since Richardson and Akil reported in 1977 that chronic periventricular gray region electrical stimulation resulted in pain reduction in 2 cancer patients (Fig. 2) (16). Hosobuchi and associates' finding of increased endorphin release in the cerebrospinal fluid supported the hypothesis that deep brain stimulation provides endogenous opiate-mediated analgesia (17). In Hosobuchi's series of 122 patients who underwent electrode implantation for intractable pain, five successes and

two failures in seven cases of cancer pain treated with stimulation of the periaqueductal gray (PAG) region were reported (18). He also reported 14 complications, including one death, corresponding to the entire series; the complications for the small subgroup of cancer pain were not separately indicated. Young and colleagues remarked that adding four uncounted complications, Hosobuchi's rate of complication was close to 15% (19). Young reported in 1985 three excellent, three partial, and two poor results with PAG stimulation in cancer pain with a 19% complication rate. By 1994, Young and Rinaldi accrued 30 cancer patients for a total of 178 pain patients treated with brain stimulation (20). They reported 70% long-term pain relief in the group with the nociceptive type of pain, compared to 50% in the neuropathic type group, but they did not break down cancer versus non-cancer patients in this grouping. They had a 21% complication rate, 4% permanent (20).

In summary, deep brain stimulation is expensive and carries a significant risk, and its efficacy remains controversial.

IMPLANTABLE PROGRAMMABLE INFUSION SYSTEMS

Intraspinal

The demonstration in 1979 of the analgesic effects in cancer pain of the epidural and intrathecal administration of small doses of morphine, together with the development of implantable infusion systems, has revolutionized patient management (21–23). When pain is not controlled satisfactorily with oral or parenteral opiates or is complicated by unacceptable side effects, a trial of intraspinal opiate administration may be indicated. A cost-analysis study has demonstrated that the cost of treating a patient with an exteriorized intraspinal catheter connected to an external pump is equal to the cost of a totally implantable pump until the third month. After 1 year, the cost of treating a patient with an exteriorized system escalates to three times the cost of a totally implantable pump (24). Decisions to undertake such treatment are based on an analgesic trial with a temporary catheter. We favor the percutaneous insertion of either an epidural or intrathecal catheter, with administration of a 10-mg or 1-mg bolus of preservative-free morphine, respectively, repeating the dose once the effect wears off (usually 12 to 24 hours later) through the course of a 48-hour period. If there are doubts about the effectiveness of the pain relief, the analgesic trial is continued.

Once a satisfactory trial is achieved, patients with a life expectancy of >3 months receive an implantable pump connected to an internalized lumbar intrathecal catheter. Patients with a life expectancy of <3 months are infused via an externalized epidural catheter (25). Epidural catheter tips must be positioned close to the dermatomes subserving the pain distribution. Long-term use of epidural catheters has been associated with fibrosis (26). They must be replaced due to malfunctioning, even multi-orifice catheters, more frequently than those implanted intrathecally, and complications include epidural injectate encapsulation (27,28).

However, excellent cancer pain control with this modality is evident from a large series of reports. Onofrio and Yaksh reported 23 cancer patients implanted with an infusion pump with 65% good or excellent pain relief, and with a dose escalation of 2.5 at an average survival time of 4 months (29). Muller and associates reported 41 cancer patients implanted with a infusion pump (18 epidural, 23 intrathecal) who had good to excellent pain control with an average survival of 205 days; the average initial morphine requirement was 3.6 mg/24 hours and the final requirement was 8.3 mg/24 hours (26). Krames and colleagues implanted infusion pumps in 17 cancer patients (6 epidural catheters, 11 intrathecal) (27). Four of the epidural catheters had to be converted to intrathecal within 2 to 6 months because of failure. Fifteen patients had good to excellent pain relief, but there was very significant development of tolerance to morphine with an average 6-month study duration. The side effects included urinary retention (9 patients), constipation (17), pruritus (1), and leg myoclonic spasms (2). Penn and Paice reported 35 cancer patients infused intrathecally with pumps for an average of 5.4 months; 80% attained good to excellent pain relief, with few side effects (30). Dose escalation averaged two times the initial dose. One case required performance of a percutaneous cordotomy, after which the patient responded to the pump. Hassenbusch and coworkers entered 69 patients in an epidural catheter trial; 41 (59.4%) were selected and implanted with pumps and epidural catheters (31). With an average duration of 7 months follow-up, satisfactory pain relief with morphine (a 30% or greater decrease in pain analog values) persisted in about 81.2% of the cases at 6 months. There were few side effects, and dose escalation was about twice the initial dose after 9 months. They concluded that epidural administration is an acceptable alternative to the intrathecal route.

Intraventricular

Since first reported by Leavens in 1982, several series have been reported of the administration of microdoses (0.1 to 0.2 mg) of morphine through a subcutaneous reservoir attached to a intraventricular catheter (32–36). Continuous intraventricular administration of morphine via an implanted pump was reported in 1987 by Weigl and colleagues (37) and Brazenor (38) and later by Dennis and DeWitty (39) and Alesch (40). An implantable patient-controlled manual pump for intermittent intraventricular administration was reported by Lu and associates in 1991 (41). In 52 patients implanted with an Ommaya reservoir for intraventricular morphine administration, Cramond and Stuart (35) documented that dose escalation had occurred in 13 patients by the time of death; 29 patients had maintained a plateau, and 6 had decreased dosage requirements. Schultheiss and coworkers (42), using a manual drug delivery system for intraventricular morphine in 12 patients with an initial daily dose of 0.2 mg/day, found that 5 remained stable between 0.3 and 0.9 mg/day and 7 required a continuous increase up to 6 mg/day. In a patient with ear cancer pain, we implanted an intraventricular reservoir and pump (Fig. 3) (Segal, unpublished observation). He required gradual increases of his initial daily microdose of 0.2 mg until he reached a plateau at 0.9 mg/day in 4 weeks, remaining stable until he died from cancer progression 2 months later.

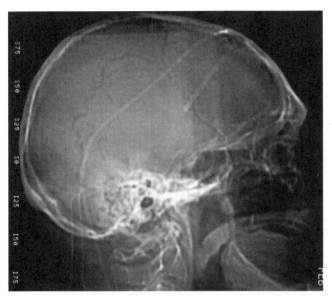
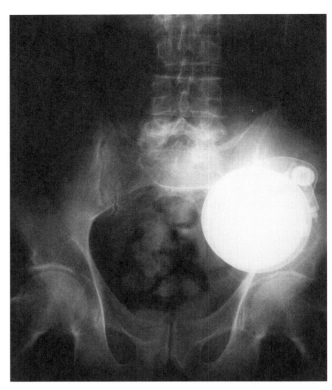

FIG. 3. Intraventricular administration of morphine. **A**: CT scout film demonstrating intraventricular catheter, Selkar subcutaneous reservoir, and connecting tubing. **B**: Abdominal x-ray demonstrating connecting tubing and subcutaneous implanted programmable infusion pump.

Increased dose requirements in patients receiving intrathecal morphine seem to be more indicative of cancer progress than development of tolerance, but the causative mechanisms in intraventricular administration remain unclear (42). Gourlay and associates (43) reported a significantly greater degree of intraspinal dose escalation in patients receiving continuous infusion compared to patients receiving repeated bolus doses. No difference was found between the epidural and intrathecal route. Still, the intraventricular route of opiate administration is being used infrequently, we believe in part because it remains unknown or feared by many physicians. The other reason may be that the Food and Drug Administration has specified that the commercially available implantable infusion pumps are for intraspinal administration only. Authors do not discuss if their patients signed informed consents. Compassionate basis may be invoked, but this could be questionable if intrathecal trials with documented failure were not performed. As shown by Anderson and colleagues, intrathecal morphine may also be effective in relieving head and neck cancer pain (44).

NEUROABLATIVE PROCEDURES

With the introduction of improved pharmacologic agents and the use of neuraxis for infusion, there are fewer indications for neuroablative procedures. Nonetheless, in patients with cancer pain, neurolysis is often the most direct route to analgesia when life expectancy is short. In addition, in this age of medical cost-benefit analysis, neurolysis may become more attractive. Current techniques for neuroablation in cancer pain are summarized here. Useful reviews with further information include those of Sundaresan, Bonica, Arbit, Jain, Patt, Lamer, and Tasker and their coworkers (45–51).

Plexus and Nerve Root Procedures

Percutaneous Peripheral Somatic Neurolysis

Peripheral somatic neurolysis is not commonly used in pain of malignant origin due to the multiple nociceptive pathways stimulated by most tumors. When it may be indicated, it must always be preceded by a diagnostic block with local anesthetics, for two reasons. The first is that the patient must be allowed to experience the sense of numbness that is anticipated to replace pain. The second is to allow time for a pain reevaluation in the presence of conduction blockade to rule out the emergence of pain that previously had been suppressed.

If a favorable response is attained, several differences between the diagnostic and neurolytic block then must be

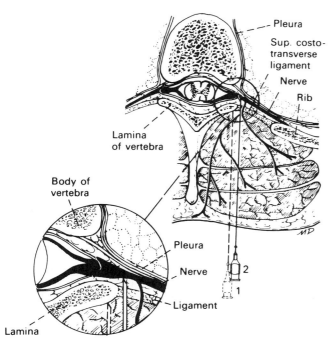

FIG. 4. Thoracic paravertebral somatic nerve block. (Bonica JJ. Regional analgesia with local anesthesia. In Bonica JJ, ed. *The management of pain*, 2d ed. Philadelphia: Lea & Febiger, 1990:1913, with permission)

made clear to the patient (49). Qualitatively, the density of analgesia attained by the neurolytic block is often less than that of the block with local anesthetics. Especially with thicker nerves, the neurolysis may need to be repeated to attain a dense block. Additionally, neurolysis is only semi-permanent: neural regeneration must be anticipated. Risks are also different. Sensory dysesthesia postinjection is problematic, and in mixed function nerves, motor or autonomic function cannot be guaranteed. Lastly, injury to adjacent nonneural tissue or its vascular supply can occur.

In clinical practice, probably the most common use of percutaneous somatic neurolysis is in patients with metastatic rib pain. Intercostal nerve blockade is extremely useful in these patients due to the limited innervation of the ribs and the unsatisfactory analgesia these patients experience despite escalations in the dosage of conventional analgesics. Unlike the approach used at the angle of the rib in conventional rib blocks with local anesthetics, the paravertebral approach is used when the intent is neurolysis (Fig. 4) (46).

Other instances of peripheral percutaneous somatic neurolysis may be indicated on a case-by-case basis. More commonly, however, somatic neurolysis is undertaken along the neuraxis for more extensive tissue involvement.

Percutaneous Neuroaxial Neurolysis

Percutaneous neuroaxial neurolysis facilitates somatic nociceptive pathway disruption at a proximal location. Use of both the epidural and intrathecal spaces for this purpose has been described in detail by numerous authors (52–66). Conceptually, the goal of both techniques is to produce selective destruction of the posterior spinal rootlets (fila radicularia) that transmit nociceptive information while sparing the motor fibers in the anterior rootlets. This is done by manipulating the position of the patient and choosing neurolytic agents with different properties.

Routine contraindications for all regional anesthetics take on special importance in the frail cancer patient. Coagulation disorders and thrombocytopenia are common and must be corrected. Skin integrity must be inspected and must be intact. Immunosuppression may lead to undetected bacteremia secondary to the inability to mount a febrile response, and must be considered. Unique to neuroaxial blockade are concerns about undetected metastatic lesions, either locally at the site of the proposed intervention (with the risk of hematoma formation) or intracranially (with the potential for elevated intracranial pressures and the risk of herniation).

Intrathecal Neurolysis

Intrathecal neurolysis is accomplished by using either dehydrated ethanol or phenol. The former is hypobaric relative to the cerebrospinal fluid and floats to the highest point; the latter, admixed with glycerine to prevent dispersion, sinks. These properties, when combined with creative positioning, can target specific areas of the spinal cord. Positioning includes not only accentuating the lumbar or thoracic curvature, but also tilting 45° laterally to tip the rootlets up or down, depending on the agent used (Fig. 5).

Further precision in the targeting of the nerves to be lysed is accomplished by use of very small volumes of neurolytic agent. When large distributions of nerves are to be lysed, use of multiple access points is recommended rather than increasing the volume of injectate (56). Neuroaxial neurolysis is done one side at a time, so treatment of bilateral pain requires that neurolysis be undertaken in two steps.

The choice of neurolytic agent varies. Both agents have their advantages and disadvantages. With alcohol, the disadvantages include its greater sensitivity to positional changes, and pain on injection. Its most notable advantage is that the patient can be positioned with the painful side up. With phenol, the painful side must be down, which is often intolerable for the patient. Phenol's hyperbaricity, nonetheless, is an advantage with positioning for sacral neurolysis. Phenol also has little of the unpleasant burning on injection experienced with alcohol.

Epidural Neurolysis

The epidural space, a potential space surrounding the intrathecal sac, contains little other than fat, veins, and

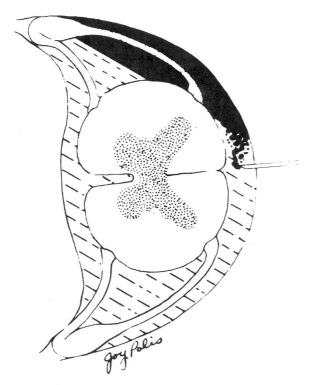

FIG. 5. Intrathecal neurolysis with alcohol. Lateral/prone positioning favors selective contact with the posterior rootlets. (Bonica JJ. Regional analgesia with local anesthesia. In Bonica JJ, ed. *The management of pain*, 2d ed. Philadelphia: Lea & Febiger, 1990:2207, with permission)

nerve roots. These properties have long made it the most widely used site for regional anesthesia and analgesia. The development of new catheters that remain chemically inert in the presence of neurolytic agents and that also can be positioned accurately with fluoroscopy has increased the use of the epidural space for neurolytic procedures as well (64).

Phenol and alcohol have been used for epidural neurolysis (55,64–66). Advantages of the technique include those inherent in avoiding dural puncture (eg, no meningeal irritation or postdural puncture headache). Other relative technical advantages and disadvantages will require more time to evaluate. One interesting study mapped the spread of epidural 5% phenol in glycerin admixed with Tc99 via scintigram (67). The findings suggest that epidural phenol can spread further and more bilaterally than suspected. In 15 patients with pain of malignant origin referable to dermatomes as cephalad as C8 in some and as low as the sacral roots in others, 13 of 15 patients had good pain relief, 1 had fair, and 1 had poor. Technical considerations included catheter migration and the decreasing spread of signal with repeated injections.

Results

No meta-analysis summarizing the safety and efficacy data for neuroaxial neurolysis techniques has been published. Bonica and associates summarized the experience of four authors using alcohol and four authors using phenol in the treatment of cancer pain (68). In these 1,872 patients, permanent complications included bladder paresis (0.1% to 4%), bowel paresis (0.1% to 2%), and muscle weakness (0.1% to 6%). Analgesic responses were reported by more authors. In a summary of 11 different authors treating 1,634 patients with alcohol, the analgesic responses were 61% good relief, 24% intermediate, and 14% little or no relief. Bonica relates that as his technique of intrathecal neurolysis evolved over time from a one-needle approach to a multiple-needle approach, the incidence of complications dropped with no change in analgesic response. In a 1978 review (69), four authors were found who treated pain of malignant origin with 5% phenol in glycerine and included complete data for analgesic response. In a total of 253 patients, satisfactory analgesia ranged from 45% to 79%; data on incomplete analgesic responses were unavailable.

Percutaneous neuroaxial neurolysis has many uses in the relief of pain of malignant origin when conventional analgesic regimens produce intolerable side effects or fail to provide adequate analgesia. The technique used must be tailored to each patient's needs. Special considerations unique to the neuraxis require imaging of the spine to rule out occult metastatic lesions.

Percutaneous Sympathetic Ganglion Neurolysis

Visceral afferent nerve fibers conduct nociceptive information to the brain via anatomic pathways shared with the sympathetic nervous system. In visceral pain, the major sympathetic ganglia therefore serve as ideal targets for disruption of the visceral afferents that travel through them. As Loeser and associates point out, sympatholysis for visceral pain is analogous to peripheral neurectomy or dorsal rhizotomy for somatic pain (70).

Sympathetic nervous system cell bodies are located in the intermediolateral column from spinal cord segments T1 to L2. Distribution of fibers to the periphery is via a ventral root to small paravertebral ganglia. There are three major locations where the fiber tracts coalesce into richly innervated fused ganglia or more midline plexi. The sympathetic outflow to the head, neck, and upper extremity passes through the most cephalad of these structures, the stellate ganglia. The abdomen and pelvis are served by the celiac and superior hypogastric plexi, respectively (71).

Whereas local anesthetics are routinely used to produce temporary conduction blockade of the stellate ganglia in a number of painful syndromes, percutaneous neurolysis of the stellate ganglia has remained uncommon and controversial. Concerns include permanent injury to adjacent neural structures that are often blocked with this technique (eg, the recurrent laryngeal and phrenic nerves), as well as the potentially catastrophic complications of inaccurate needle placement. Nonetheless, a series of 100 successful stellate ganglion neurolysis procedures was reported by Racz and Holubec (72). In these patients, fluoroscopy guidance and a modified technique were used, and no serious side effects were reported.

Celiac Plexus Neurolysis

Pain arising from tumor infiltration of the upper abdominal viscera often responds incompletely to conventional analgesic treatment. Ablation of the sympathetic innervation to the upper abdominal viscera can often relieve epigastric pain with referred patterns to the back.

The greater (T5–9), lesser (T10,11), and least (T12) splanchnic nerves descend paravertebrally, piercing the diaphragm discretely, and then dissociate into a highly irregular reticulum deep within the retroperitoneum, usually anterior to the L1 vertebral body and posterior to the celiac artery branch point from the aorta. Recent anatomic studies of the celiac plexus reveal that the plexus more often fuses into one midline structure rather than remaining discrete bilateral ganglia (73).

Percutaneous Celiac Neurolysis

Blockade of the sympathetic innervation to the abdominal viscera can be done as either bilateral splanchnic nerve blocks or the classic celiac plexus block. The splanchnic nerves are blocked retrocrurally with a bilateral paravertebral approach. The celiac plexus itself is blocked with an antecrural needle placement from either a posterior or anterior approach (Fig. 6). In both cases, imaging technologies have markedly reduced the risk of complications of incorrect needle placement. Imaging techniques include conventional as well as flow Doppler ultrasound, fluoroscopy, and computed tomographic (CT) guidance. After needle placement, a contrast dye admixed with local anesthetic is used to confirm spread and to test for analgesic response. If the response is favorable, then lysis is undertaken. Lysis is done with dehydrated ethyl alcohol. This product, admixed with local anesthetic to prevent burning on contact, is absorbed systemically and results in a variable level of intoxication. The immediate expected response to sympatholysis includes analgesia, hypotension, and diarrhea, as well as development of a blood alcohol level. Hypotension is offset by prehydra-

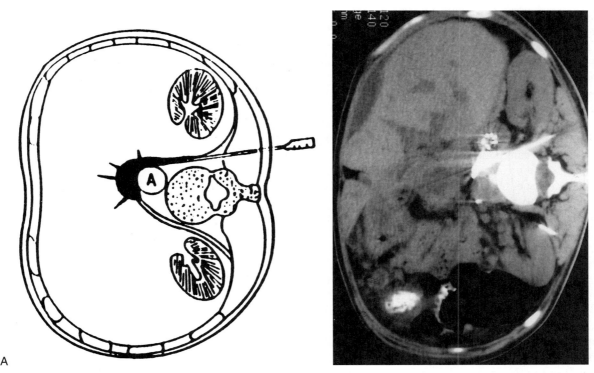

FIG. 6. A: Antecrural celiac plexus block with posterior approach, highlighting dye spread. (Hilgier M, Rykowski JJ. One-needle transcrural celiac plexus block. *Reg Anesth* 1994;19:281, with permission) **B:** Note that the inferior vena cava is highlighted by transvenous umbrella.

tion. Diarrhea, in clinical experience, usually resolves within 72 hours.

Since the original description of the percutaneous celiac plexus block by Kappis in 1914 (74), many conclusions have been drawn about its role in the management of pain of malignant origin (75–101). In a recent meta-analysis of the neurolytic celiac plexus block for the treatment of cancer pain, 24 English language reports were reviewed to assess its safety and efficacy (102). Two studies were randomized controlled trials, one was prospective, and 21 were uncontrolled retrospective studies. Most studied tumors of the pancreas. Results of efficacy were divided into short-term (<2 weeks) and long-term (2 weeks to death) time frames. Findings showed that both short- and long-term outcomes were similar for patients with tumors of the pancreas and with other abdominal tumor types. In merged data, 73% to 92% of patients had partial to complete relief when death occurred within or beyond 3 months. The need for a repeat block due to lack of effect with the first block was 7%. The three most common effects included local pain (96%), diarrhea (44%), and hypotension (38%). The more severe side effects included 1% neurologic side effects and 1% other effects, such as hematuria, diaphragmatic irritation, and pneumothorax.

Open Intraoperative Celiac Neurolysis

An underused but highly effective technique of intraoperative phenol celiac neurolysis has been employed to prevent the development of pain in patients undergoing surgical exploration of pancreatic tumor. In the approach described by Flanigan and Kraft (103), the aorta is visualized by incision of the pars flaccida of the lesser omentum and the subsequent retraction of the liver and stomach. Six percent phenol is then injected slightly lateral, posterior, and cephalad to the origin of the celiac artery between the celiac ganglia. Intermittent aspiration is necessary to rule out intravascular injection. A total volume of 15 to 20 cc is used. Of the 32 patients undergoing this procedure, 4 had no pain relief, 3 had partial relief, and 25 had complete relief. Mean duration of analgesia was 4.3 months, mean survival 5 months. Eighty-four percent of patients had no recurrence of pain before death. In a subsequent modification of this technique, bilateral injections of alcohol mixed with local anesthetic were given into the area of the plexus (104). Similar results were reported for 12 patients; no complications were reported.

Blockade of the sympathetic innervation to the upper abdominal viscera is effective for the relief of cancer pain. Percutaneous neurolysis should not be reserved for patients with intractable pain and for whom it represents the last resort, and patients who achieve inadequate relief of pain secondary to visceral tumor should be considered

appropriate candidates for celiac plexus neurolysis. Preemptive, open, intraoperative neurolysis of the celiac plexus also provides effective palliation of pain in patients with pancreatic tumors.

Percutaneous Superior Hypogastric Plexus Neurolysis

The anatomic considerations of the superior hypogastric plexus are similar to those of the celiac plexus. Once again, a diffuse reticulum of fibers forms in a prevertebral location within the retroperitoneum. In this case, the plexus derives innervation from the lumbar sympathetic chain (L2–L3) and is located anterior to the L4–5 vertebral bodies just below the aortic bifurcation (105).

Blockade of the superior hypogastric plexus, previously termed a presacral neurectomy, is accomplished using a bilateral paravertebral approach (Fig. 7). Imaging technologies are used to guide needle placement to the anterolateral face of the L5 vertebral body. If a diagnostic block with local anesthetic produces a favorable analgesic response, neurolysis is completed with phenol (Fig. 8).

The analgesic utility of percutaneous superior hypogastric plexus neurolysis was recently reported by two groups (106,107). In the former, 28 patients were treated, in the latter 26. Both series studied pain arising in the pelvis secondary to malignant causes, and in both series the patients blocked had either failed to achieve analgesia with conventional therapy or had experienced unwanted side effects.

In the first study of analgesic efficacy, the mean reduction in pain was reported as 70%. Patients without complete analgesia were thought to have pain referable to somatically innervated structures. In the second study, 3 of 26 patients were offered a second neurolysis secondary

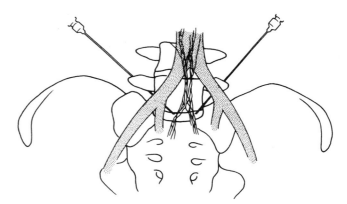

FIG. 7. Superior hypogastric plexus block. Anterior view of pelvis illustrating location of hypogastric plexus and correct bilateral needle placement. (Plancarte R. Superior hypogastric plexus block for pelvic cancer pain. *Anesthesiology* 1990;73:236, with permission)

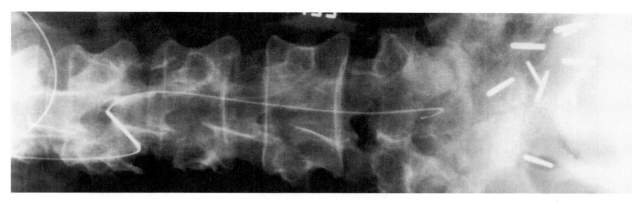

FIG. 8. Phenol epidural neurolysis, with catheter in situ.

to incomplete analgesia, with subsequent improved analgesia. These patients all had extensive documented retroperitoneal tumor spread. Thus, satisfactory pain relief was reported as 69% overall and 27% in patients with extensive retroperitoneal tumor spread. Follow-up at 6 months documented stable reports of residual pain and stable doses of opioids.

The incidence of block-related complications was reported in the second study. One of the 26 patients experienced a burning sensation in the pelvis for 48 hours. Otherwise, no bladder puncture, hematoma formation, or atherosclerotic plaque embolization to the lower extremity was reported.

This author and others (108) feel that the utility of the sympathetic plexus neurolysis may be greater for tumors of the abdomen than of the pelvis. Perhaps because the bony pelvis offers little room for expansion, the pain rapidly takes on mixed somatic, visceral, and neuropathic characteristics, subsequently necessitating further treatment. Nonetheless, superior hypogastric plexus neurolysis offers a useful, safe technique for the treatment of many patients with less extensive disease.

Percutaneous Radiofrequency Rhizotomy

The radiofrequency probe, which also serves as a stimulating electrode, is introduced into the intervertebral foramen using a percutaneous needle under C-arm fluoroscopy (Fig. 9). This procedure is performed under local anesthesia but requires an experienced anesthesiologist for the administration of short-acting intravenous sedatives such as methohexital (Brevital) and propofol (Diprivan). The patient must be fully awake and cooperative soon after each lesion is made to test for the development of hypesthesia or weakness and to ensure that the threshold to electrical stimulation of the lesioned root has been increased (109) Up to 76% pain relief has been reported with this technique (110).

We consider this technique useful for cancer pain referred in the distribution of a few adjacent nerve roots, most commonly lumbosacral and sometimes thoracic, specifically in patients with a life expectancy <3 months. The tumor must be located distal to the intervertebral foramina to allow placement of the radiofrequency electrode. Cervical percutaneous rhizotomy is technically more difficult, morbidity is higher, and it is not recommended for brachial plexus involvement (110).

Spinal Cord Procedures

Commissural Myelotomy

Commissural myelotomy consists of longitudinal splitting of about 40 to 55 mm of the thoracolumbar spinal cord into two halves, extending two or three segments rostral to the pain level. It requires a three-level laminectomy (Fig. 10). It was introduced in 1926, but its popularity has waxed and waned. Pain relief was originally thought to result from the section of the spinothalamic fibers decussating in the anterior commissure; Sourek (115) proposed that the lesion of the most medial fast conducting fibers of the dorsal funiculi may also play a role. Gildenberg and Hirshberg reported satisfactory results with a limited single-segment commissural myelotomy based in an hypothetical extralemniscal pathway in the vicinity of the central canal (111). This procedure is indicated in bilateral lower limb and midline pelvic pain most commonly seen in colorectal and urogenital cancer which it is often refractory to intraspinal opiates. Commissural myelotomy has an advantage over cordotomy in that with a single procedure, bilateral analgesia is obtained. It is also safer in continent and deambulating patients. Satisfactory pain control is obtained in 60% to 90% of patients; ataxia and dysesthesia are common but transient (111–115).

In modern series, mortality has been 0%, except for two publications reporting 3% to 8% mortality. The rate

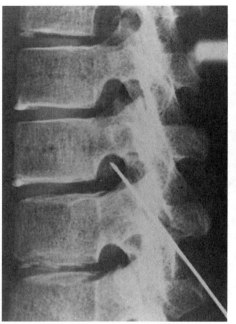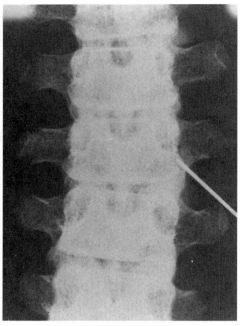

A   B

FIG. 9. Percutaneous radiofrequency rhizotomy, thoracic spine. **(A)** Lateral and **(B)** anteroposterior x-rays. The needle is introduced percutaneously under C-arm fluoroscopy into the intervertebral foramen, through which the radiofrequency probe, which also serves as a stimulating electrode, is inserted. (Uematsu S. Percutaneous electrothermocoagulation of spinal nerve trunk, ganglion and rootlets. In Schmidek HH, Sweet WH, eds. *Operative neurosurgical techniques, indications, methods, and results.* Orlando: Grune & Stratton, 1988:1207, with permission)

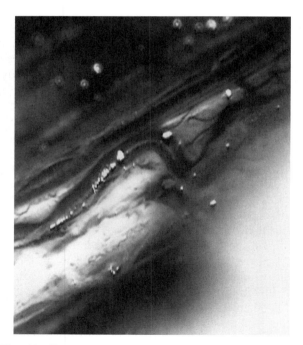

FIG. 10. Commissural myelotomy. Intraoperative photograph obtained through the operating microscope demonstrating longitudinal medial splitting of three segments of the thoracolumbar spinal cord. (See also Color Plate 5.)

of sphincter disturbances ranges from 0% to 10%. Leg weakness is usually transient and mild, but the reported incidence greatly varies between series (0% to 60%) (116). In a series of 6 patients in which microneurosurgical techniques and intraoperative neurophysiologic monitoring were used, postoperative morbidity consisted of transient ataxia (1 to 2 weeks) and in some cases a more permanent partial proprioception deficit (Segal, unpublished observation).

Percutaneous Cordotomy

Since Mullan and associates (118) performed the first percutaneous cordotomy in 1963 using a strontium-90 needle, the procedure has been periodically improved by the application of new technologies. After the introduction by Rosomoff and coworkers (119) of radiofrequency percutaneous cervical cordotomy, the high rate of satisfactory pain relief (93% Tasker [51], 90% Rosomoff) and low mortality (0.5% Tasker) in large series left no reason for performing open cordotomies (other than shortage of equipment or unfamiliarity with the technique) (Fig. 11). (117,118) The series also included nonmalignancy patients, and the long-term results have been reported in review publications.

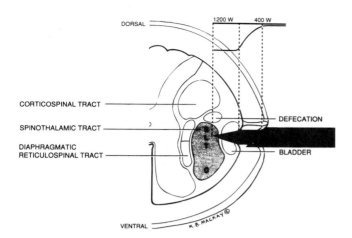

FIG. 11. Percutaneous cordotomy by lateral high cervical technique. Impedance changes from cerebrospinal fluid to cord impalation, the homuncular arrangement of the spinothalamic tract, and the locations of important pathways are shown. (Tasker RR. Neurosurgical and neuroaugmentative intervention. In Patt RB, ed. *Cancer pain.* Philadelphia: JB Lippincott, 1993:485, with permission)

Percutaneous cordotomy is indicated in cancer patients refractory to morphine with limited life expectancy (1 year) and pain below the upper extremities, because the level of analgesia ascends with time. Some patients prefer to undergo a cordotomy instead of being implanted with a morphine pump because they do not have the socioeconomic support for refilling.

The high initial success rate of both percutaneous and open cordotomy (90% to 97%) tends to fall with the life span but still remains satisfactory in 80% of patients 1 year later and in more than 60% of the patients who survive >2 years (51,119,120). Although percutaneous techniques made cordotomy much safer (mortality 0.03% to 0.5%, sphincter dysfunction in 2% to 2.9%, paresis in 0.5% to 3%, and sleep-induced apnea in 1%), the major deterrent to performing it is probably the fear, especially for cancer patients, of having to perform a contralateral cordotomy later. This occurred in 35% of Rosomoff's cancer cases. Bilateral cordotomy is associated with sphincter dysfunction (18% to 21%), paraparesis (1.6% to 3%), and sleep-induced apnea (3%) and a significant increase in mortality (1.6% to 2%) (51,122).

CT guidance, described by Kanpolat and colleagues in 1989, allows selective percutaneous radiofrequency cordotomy to be performed (123). The procedure is carried out in the CT radiology suite under local anesthesia and conscious sedation. Iohexol is injected into the lumbar subarachnoidal space for contrast imaging by CT of the cervical spinal cord silhouette. Using a technique similar to a C1–C2 lateral puncture for cervical myelography, the spinal needle is directed toward the anterolat-

eral quadrant, more anterior for upper body pain and more posterior for lower body pain. This takes advantage of the somatotopic arrangement of most nociceptive fibers in the spinothalamic tract, with the sacral fibers ascending posterolaterally, closer to the spinal cord surface at the level of the dentate ligament, and the lumbar, thoracic, and cervical fibers coursing relatively more and more anterior and, medially, deeper. A specially designed temperature-monitoring radiofrequency electrode (0.25 mm in diameter, bared 2.0 mm at the tip) is introduced through the needle and calibrated to impale the cord to the desired depth (Fig. 12). Electrical stimulation is then used to ascertain that the desired target has been approached before making the radiofrequency lesions.

Kanpolat reported the results of 54 cases of cancer pain. He achieved an initial success rate of pain control of 94%, no mortality, and only transient complications (one case of ataxia and one of hemiparesis, resolving in 1 week). The success in obtaining selective analgesia in the painful region follows a learning curve: 2 of 11 patients in 1988, 8 of 14 in 1989, 7 of 12 in 1990, and 16 of 17 in 1991–92 (124). Because this new technique is highly successful in obtaining selective cordotomy, it may allow the performance of bilateral selective cordotomy without the prohibitive risks of conventional percutaneous cordotomy techniques.

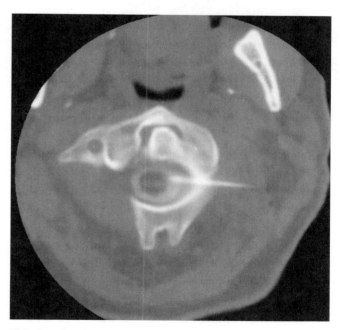

FIG. 12. C1–C2 CT-guided selective percutaneous radiofrequency cordotomy. Placement of the 0.25-mm in diameter cordotomy electrode into the anterolateral spinothalamic tract target.

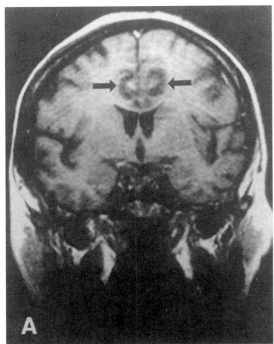

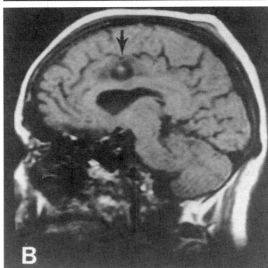

FIG. 13. Stereotactic cingulotomy. Postoperative coronal **(A)** and right hemisphere sagittal **(B)** T1 (TR, 600 ms; TE, 30 ms) MR scans without contrast enhancement. The location of the lesions *(arrows)* corresponded closely with the stereotactic targets (center of each hemisphere's cingulate gyrus). Mild apparent surrounding edema was noted but had no clinical effects. (Hassenbusch SJ, Pillay PK, Barnett GH. Radiofrequency cingulotomy for intractable cancer pain using stereotaxis guided by magnetic resonance imaging. *Neurosurgery* 1990;27:222, with permission)

Intracranial Procedures

Stereotactic Cingulotomy

Stereotactic cingulotomy requires bilateral cingulate gyrus lesions. They are obtained stereotactically with radiofrequency electrodes and are performed through 3-mm twist drill holes, with no mortality and low morbidity. Ballantine and Giriunas reported satisfactory pain relief in 57% of 35 cancer patients, but only 20% of those who survived >3 months (125). Hassenbusch and associates introduced the technique of magnetic resonance (MR) guidance for radiofrequency cingulotomy, reporting dramatic short-term pain relief in 4 cancer patients (Fig. 13) (126).

In 1980, Steiner and colleagues reported the usefulness of radiosurgery in pain control, although he performed thalamotomy as opposed to cingulotomy in 52 cancer patients (127). Currently, the feasibility of combining MR stereotactic guidance and radiosurgery to perform noninvasive intracranial lesions such as cingulotomy may lead to the popularization of this procedure (128).

Stereotactic Mesencephalotomy

This procedure is mostly indicated for cancer pain because it seems to be more effective in nociceptive pain than in neuropathic pain. Appropriate cases are head, neck, and upper body cancer pain, when cordotomy is not an option and a morphine pump is not accepted by the patient. The lesions are obtained by stereotactically placing a radiofrequency electrode in the rostral mesencephalic spinothalamic tract, usually contralaterally in

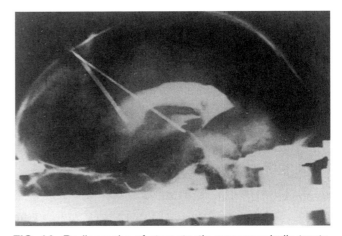

FIG. 14. Radiographs of stereotactic mesencephalic tractotomy. The electrode (thinner) is centered on the target. The thick catheter in the frontal horn was placed to perform the ventriculography. (Frank F, Fabrizzi AP, Gaist G. Stereotactic mesencephalic tractotomy in the treatment of chronic cancer pain. *Acta Neurochir (Wien)* 1989;99:38, with permission)

unilateral pain, but occasionally also bilaterally in bilateral pain (Fig. 14). Several series in cancer pain report good to "spectacular" pain relief (57% to 100%). Mortality rates differ considerably between series (0.5% to 8.8%), but there is good agreement that complications are common (oculomotor disturbances, 12% to 20%; contralateral dysesthesia, 6% to 15%) (129–132).

REFERENCES

1. Schipper H. Quality of life. Meaning and measurement. In Foley KM, ed. *Advances in pain research and therapy.* New York: Raven Press, 1990.
2. *Management of cancer pain.* Clinical Practice Guideline #9, United States Department of Health and Human Services, Agency for Health Care Policy and Research. March 1994.
3. Foley KM. The treatment of cancer pain. *N Engl J Med* 1985;313:84.
4. Melzack R. The tragedy of needless pain: a call for social action. In Dubner R, Gebhart GF, Bond MR, eds. *Pain research and clinical management:* proceedings of the 5th World Congress on Pain. Amsterdam: Elsevier, 1988:1.
5. World Health Organization. *Cancer pain relief and palliative care.* Report of WHO expert committee. WHO Technical Report Series 804. Geneva, Switzerland: WHO 1990:1.
6. Hill CS Jr, Fields WS, Thorpe DM. A call to action to improve relief of cancer pain. In Hill CS Jr, Fields WS, eds. *Advances in pain research and therapy.* New York: Raven Press, 1989:353.
7. MacDonald N. The role of medical oncology in cancer pain control. In Hill CS Jr, Fields WS, eds. *Advances in pain research and therapy.* New York: Raven Press, 1989:123.
8. Cherny NI, Portnoy RK. Cancer pain management: current strategy. *Cancer* 1993;72:11.
9. North RB. Neurosurgical procedures for chronic pain. *Clin Neurosurg* 1992;40:182.
10. North RB, Levy RM. Consensus conference on the neurosurgical management of pain. *Neurosurgery* 1994;34:756.
11. Meyerson BA. Electrical stimulation of the spinal cord and brain. In Bonica JJ, ed. *The management of pain.* Philadelphia/London: Lea & Febiger, 1990:1862.
12. Richardson RR, Siqueira EB, Cerullo LJ. Spinal epidural neurostimulation for treatment of acute and chronic intractable pain: initial and long-term results. *Neurosurgery* 1979;5:344.
13. Meglio M, Cioni B, Rossi GF. Spinal cord stimulation in management of chronic pain. A 9-year experience. *J Neurosurg* 1989;70:519.
14. Hood TW, Siegfried J. Epidural vs. thalamic stimulation for the management of brachial plexus lesion pain. *Acta Neurochir* (Suppl) 1984;33:451.
15. *Spinal cord (dorsal column) stimulation for chronic intractable pain.* ERCI Health Technology Assessment Report, Plymouth Meeting, PA, October 1993.
16. Richardson DE, Akil H. Pain reduction by electrical brain stimulation in man. Part 2: Chronic self-administration in the periventricular gray matter. *J Neurosurg* 1977;47:184.
17. Hosobuchi Y, Rossier J, Bloom FE, et al. Stimulation of human periaqueductal gray for pain relief increases immunoreactivity in ventricular fluid. *Science* 1979;203:279.
18. Hosobuchi Y. Brain stimulation for intractable pain. *J Neurosurg* 1986; 64:545.
19. Young RF, Kroening R, Fulton W, Feldman RA, Chambi I. Electrical stimulation of the brain in treatment of chronic pain. Experience over 5 years. *J Neurosurg* 1985;62:389.
20. Young RF, Rinaldi PC. Brain stimulation for relief of chronic pain. In Wall PD, Melzack R, eds. *Textbook of pain,* 3d ed. Edinburgh: Churchill-Livingstone, 1994:1225.
21. Behar M, Magora F, Olshwang D, Davidson JT. Epidural morphine in treatment of pain. *Lancet* 1979;1:527.
22. Poletti CE, Cohen AM, Todd DP, et al. Cancer pain relieved by long-term epidural morphine with permanent indwelling systems for self-administration. *J Neurosurg* 1981;55:581.
23. Wang JK, Nauss LA, Thomas JE. Pain relief by intrathecally applied morphine in man. *Anesthesiology* 1979;50:149.
24. Bedder MD, Burchiel K, Larson A. Cost analysis of two implantable narcotic delivery systems. *J Pain Symptom Manag* 1991;6:368–373.
25. Krames ES. Intrathecal infusional therapies for intractable pain: patient management guidelines. *J Pain Symptom Manag* 1993;8:36.
26. Muller H, Luben V, Zierskyi J, Hempelman G. Long-term spinal opiate treatment. *Acta Anaesthesiol Belg* (Suppl. 2) 1988;39:83.
27. Krames ES, Gershow J, Glassberg A, et al. Continuous infusion of spinally administered narcotics for the relief of pain due to malignant disorders. *Cancer* 1985;56:696.
28. Cherry DA, Gourlay GK. CT contrast evidence of injectate encapsulation after long-term epidural administration [comment]. *Pain* 1993; 53:241.
29. Onofrio BM, Yaksh TL. Long-term pain relief produced by intrathecal morphine infusion in 53 patients. *J Neurosurg* 1990;72:200.
30. Penn RD, Paice JA. Chronic intrathecal morphine for intractable pain. *J Neurosurg* 1987;67:182.
31. Hassenbusch SJ, Pillay PK, Magdinec M, et al. Constant infusion of morphine for intractable cancer pain using an implanted pump. *J Neurosurg* 1990;73:405.
32. Nurchi G. Use of intraventricular and intrathecal morphine in intractable pain associated with cancer. *Neurosurgery* 1984;15:801.
33. Lenzi A, Galli G, Gandolfini M, Marini G. Intraventricular morphine in paraneoplastic painful syndrome of the cervicofacial region: experience in 38 cases. *Neurosurgery* 1985;17:6.
34. Roquefeuil B, Benezech J, Blanchet P, Batier C, Frerebeau P, Gros C. Intraventricular administration of morphine in patients with neoplastic intractable pain. *Surg Neurol* 1984;21:155.
35. Cramond T, Stuart G. Intraventricular morphine for intractable pain of advanced cancer. *J Pain Symptom Manag* 1993;8:465.
36. Lazorthes Y, Verdie JC, Bastide R, Lavados A, Descouens D. Spinal versus intraventricular chronic opiate administration with implantable drug delivery devices for cancer pain. *Appl Neurophysiol* 1985;48:234.
37. Weigl K, Mundinger F, Chrubasik J. Continuous intraventricular morphine or peptide infusion for intractable cancer pain. *Acta Neurochir* (Suppl) 1987;39:163.
38. Brazenor GA. Long-term intrathecal administration of morphine: a comparison of bolus injection via reservoir with continuous infusion by implanted pump. *Neurosurgery* 1987;21:484.
39. Dennis GC, DeWitty RL. Long-term intraventricular infusion of morphine for intractable pain in cancer of the head and neck. *Neurosurgery* 1990;26:404.
40. Alesch F. Intraventricular morphine application in intractable pain. In Kepplinger B, Pernak JM, Ray AL, eds. *Pain: clinical aspects and therapeutic issues.* Part II. Linz: Edition Selva Verlag, 1993:1.
41. Lu S, Wang J, Weng R, Wang Q. Clinical application of a patient-controlled apparatus for intraventricular administration of morphine in intractable pain: report of 28 cases. *Neurosurgery* 1991;29:73.
42. Schultheiss R, Schramm J, Neidhardt J, Penn RD, Dennis GD. Dose changes in long- and medium-term intrathecal morphine therapy of cancer pain. *Neurosurgery* 1992;31:4.
43. Gourlay GK, Plummer JL, Cherry DA, et al. Comparison of intermittent bolus with continuous infusion of epidural morphine in the treatment of severe pain. *Pain* 1991;47:135.
44. Andersen PE, Cohen JI, Everts EC, Bedder MD, Burchiel KJ. Intrathecal narcotics for relief of pain from head and neck cancer. *Arch Otolaryngol Head Neck Surg* 1991;117:1277.
45. Sundaresan N, DiGiacinto GV, Hughes JO. Neurosurgery in the treatment of cancer pain. *Cancer* 1989;63:2365.
46. Bonica JJ, Buckley FP. Regional analgesia with local anesthesia. In Bonica JJ, ed. *The management of pain,* 2d ed. Philadelphia: Lea & Febiger, 1990:1913.
47. Arbit E. Neurosurgical management of cancer pain. In Foley KM, Bonica JJ, Ventafridda V, eds. Second International Congress on Cancer Pain. *Advances in pain research and therapy,* vol. 16. New York: Raven Press, 1990:289.
48. Jain S. *Current strategies of neurolytic procedures in cancer pain management: current concepts in cancer and acute pain management syllabus.* Postgraduate Course at Memorial Sloan-Kettering Cancer Center, 12/1992.
49. Patt RB. Peripheral neurolysis and the management of cancer pain. In Patt RB, ed. *Cancer pain.* Philadelphia: JB Lippincott, 1993:360.

50. Lamer TJ. Treatment of cancer-related pain when orally administered medications fail. *Mayo Clin Proc* 1994;69:473.

51. Tasker RR. Neurosurgical and neuroaugmentative intervention. In Patt RB, ed. *Cancer pain.* Philadelphia: JB Lippincott, 1994:471.

52. Superville-Sovak B, Rasminnsky M, Finlayson MH. Complications of phenol neurolysis. *Arch Neurol* 1975;32:226.

53. Swerdlow M. Intrathecal neurolysis. *Anaesthesia* 1978;33:733.

54. Ferrer-Brechner T. Epidural and intrathecal phenol neurolysis for cancer pain. *Anesthesiol Rev* 1981;8:14.

55. Colpitts MR, Levy DA, Lawrence M. *Treatment of cancer-related pain with phenol epidural block.* Presented at the 2d World Congress on Pain, Montreal, 1978.

56. Bonica JJ. Neurolytic blockade and hypophysectomy. In Bonica JJ, ed. *The management of pain,* 2d ed. Philadelphia: Lea & Febiger, 1990:1980.

57. Stovner J, Endresen R. Intrathecal phenol for cancer pain. *Acta Anaesthesiol Scand* 1972;16:17.

58. Ischia S, Luzzani A, Ischia A, et al. Subarachnoid neurolytic block (L5–S1) and unilateral percutaneous cervical cordotomy in the treatment of pain secondary to pelvic malignant disease. *Pain* 1984;20:139.

59. Lifshitz S, Debacker LJ, Buchsbaum HJ, et al. Subarachnoid phenol block for pain relief in gynecologic malignancy. *Obstet Gynecol* 1976;48:316.

60. Swerdlow M. Spinal and peripheral neurolysis for managing Pancoast syndrome. In Bonica JJ, Ventafridda V, Pagni CA, eds. *Advances in pain research and therapy,* vol. 4. New York: Raven Press, 1982:135.

61. Papo I, Visca A. Phenol subarachnoid rhizotomy for the treatment of cancer pain. In Bonica JJ, Ventafridda V, Pagni CA, eds. *Advances in pain research and therapy,* vol. 2. New York: Raven Press, 1979:339.

62. Gerbershagen HU. Neurolysis: subarachnoid neurolytic blockade. *Acta Anaesthesiol Belg* 1981;1:45.

63. Swerdlow M. Intrathecal and extradural block in pain relief. In Swerdlow M, Charlton JE, eds. *Relief of intractable pain,* 4th ed. Amsterdam: Elsevier, 1989:223.

64. Racz GB, Sabonghy M, Gintautus J. Intractable pain therapy using a new epidural catheter. *JAMA* 1982;248:646.

65. Jain S, Foley K, Thomas J, et al. Factors influencing efficacy of epidural neurolysis therapy for intractable cancer pain. In Dubner R, Gebhart GF, Bond MR. *Pain research and clinical management,* vol. 3. Proceedings of the 5th World Congress I.A.S.P. Amsterdam: Elsevier, 1987.

66. Korevaar WC, Kline MT, Donelly CVC. Thoracic epidural neurolysis using alcohol. In Dubner R, Gebhart GF, Bond MR. *Pain research and clinical management,* vol. 3. Proceedings of the 5th World Congress on Pain. Amsterdam: Elsevier, 1987:S133.

67. Salmon JB, Finch PM, Lovegrove FT, Warwick A. Mapping the spread of epidural phenol in cancer pain patients by radionuclide admixture and epidural scintigraphy. *Clin J Pain* 1992;8:18.

68. Bonica JJ, Buckley FP, Moricca G, Murphy TM. Neurolytic blockade and hypophysectomy. In Bonica JJ, ed. *The management of pain,* 2d ed. Philadelphia: Lea & Febiger, 1990:2007.

69. Wood KW. The use of phenol as a neurolytic agent: a review. *Pain* 1978; 5:205.

70. Loeser JD, Sweet WH, Tew JM, Van Loveren H, Bonica JJ. Neurosurgical operations involving peripheral nerves. In Bonica JJ, ed. *The management of pain,* 2d ed. Philadelphia: Lea & Febiger, 1990:2057.

71. Thompson GE, Moore DC. Celiac plexus, intercostal and minor peripheral blockade. In Cousins MJ, Bridenbaugh PO, eds. *Neural blockade,* 2d ed. Philadelphia: JB Lippincott, 1988:503.

72. Racz GB, Holubec JI. Stellate ganglion phenol neurolysis. In Racz GB, ed. *Techniques of neurolysis.* Boston: Kluwer Academic, 1989:133.

73. Hilgier M, Rykowski JJ. One-needle transcrural celiac plexus block. *Reg Anesth* 1994;19:227.

74. Kappis M. Erfahrungen mit lokalanesthesie bei bauchoperationen. Verhandlung der Deutschen Gesellschaft fur Cir, 1914;43:87.

75. Lieberman RP, Waldman SD. Celiac plexus neurolysis with the modified transaortic approach. *Radiology* 1990;175:274.

76. Ischia S, Luzzani A, Ischia A, Faggion S. A new approach to the neurolytic block of the coeliac plexus: the transaortic technique. *Pain* 1983; 16:333.

77. Gorbitz C, Leavens ME. Alcohol block of the celiac plexus for control of upper abdominal pain caused by cancer and pancreatitis. *Neurosurgery* 1972;34:575.

78. Thompson GE, Moore DC, Bridenbaugh LD, Artin RY. Abdominal pain and alcohol celiac plexus nerve block. *Anesth Analg* 1977;56:1.

79. Owitz S, Koppolu S. Celiac plexus block: an overview. *Mt Sinai J Med* 1983;50:486.

80. Brown DL, Bully CK, Quiel EL. Neurolytic celiac plexus block for pancreatic cancer pain. *Anesth Analg* 1987;66:869.

81. Leung JWC, Bowenwright M, Aveling W, et al. Coeliac plexus block for pain in pancreatic cancer and chronic pancreatitis. *Br J Surg* 1983;70:730.

82. Jones J. Coeliac plexus block with alcohol for relief of upper abdominal pain due to cancer. *Ann R Coll Surg Engl* 1977;59:46.

83. Moore DC, Bush WH, Burnett LL. Celiac plexus block: a roentgenographic, anatomic study of technique and spread of solution in patients and corpses. *Anesth Analg* 1981;60:369.

84. Sharp K, Stevens EJ. Improving palliation in pancreatic cancer: intraoperative celiac plexus block for pain relief. *South Med J* 1991;84:469.

85. Matamala AM, Lopez FV, Sanchez JL, Bach LD. Percutaneous anterior approach to the coeliac plexus using ultrasound. *Br J Anesth* 1989; 62:637.

86. Moore DC. Celiac (splanchnic) plexus block with alcohol for cancer pain of the upper intra-abdominal viscera. In *International symposium on pain of advanced cancer.* New York: Raven Press, 1979:357.

87. Ischia S, Ischia A, Polati E, Finco G. Three posterior percutaneous celiac plexus block techniques. *Anesthesiology* 1992;76:534.

88. Brown DL. A retrospective analysis of neurolytic celiac plexus block for non-pancreatic intra-abdominal cancer pain. *Reg Anesth* 1989; 14:63.

89. Squier R, Morrow JS, Roman R. Pain therapy for pancreatic carcinoma with neurolytic celiac plexus block. *Conn Med* 1989;53:269.

90. Ventafridda GC, Caraceni AT, Sbanotto AM, et al. Pain treatment in cancer of the pancreas. *Eur J Surg Oncol* 1990;16:1.

91. Herpels V, Kurdziel JC, Dondelinger RF. Percutaneous CT-guided nerve block of the coeliac plexus and splanchnic nerves. *Ann Radiol* 1988;31:291.

92. Filshie J, Golding S, Robbie DS, Husband JE. Unilateral computerized tomography guided celiac plexus block: a technique for pain relief. *Anesthesia* 1983;38:498.

93. Hupert C, Zeig N, Sieglen-Fortunato L, Ciolino RC. Celiac plexus blocks provides pain relief for malignant and benign visceral pain. *NJ Med* 1987;84:573.

94. Black A, Dwyer B. Coeliac plexus block. *Anaesth Intensive Care* 1973; 1:315.

95. Hegedus V. Relief of pancreatic pain by radiography-guided block. *Am J Radiol* 1979;133:1101.

96. Buy JN, Moss AA, Singler RC. CT-guided celiac plexus and splanchnic nerve neurolysis. *J Comput Assist Tomogr* 1982;6:315.

97. Bridenbaugh LD, Moore DC, Campbell DD. Management of upper abdominal cancer pain. *JAMA* 1964;190:877.

98. Mercadante S. Celiac plexus block versus analgesics in pancreatic cancer pain. *Pain* 1993;52:187.

99. Lebovitz AH, Lefkowitz M. Pain management of pancreatic carcinoma. *Pain* 1989;36:1.

100. Sharfman WH, Walsh TD. Has the analgesic efficacy of neurolytic celiac plexus block been demonstrated in pancreatic cancer pain? *Pain* 1990;41:267.

101. Romanelli DF, Beckmann CF, Heiss FW. Celiac plexus block: efficacy and safety of the anterior approach. *Am J Roentgenol* 1993;160:479.

102. Ersenberg E, Carr DB, Chalmers TC. Neurolytic celiac plexus block for the treatment of cancer pain: a meta-analysis. *Anesth Analg* 1995; 80:290.

103. Flanigan DP, Kraft R. Continuing experience with palliative chemical splanchnicectomy. *Arch Surg* 1978;113:509.

104. Sharp KW, Stevens EJ. Improving palliation in pancreatic cancer: intraoperative celiac plexus block for pain relief. *South Med J* 1991; 84:469.

105. Bonica JJ. General considerations of pain in the pelvis and perineum. In Bonica JJ, ed. *The management of pain,* 2d ed. Philadelphia: Lea & Febiger, 1990:1290.

106. Plancarte R, Amescua C, Patt R, Aldrete A. Superior hypogastric plexus block for pelvic cancer pain. *Anesthesiology* 1990;73:236.

107. Leon-Casasola OA, Kent E, Lema M. Neurolytic superior hypogastric plexus block for chronic pelvic pain associated with cancer. *Pain* 1993;54:145.

108. Orlandini G. Selection of patients undergoing neurolytic superior hypogastric plexus block [comment]. *Pain* 1993;56:121.

109. Uematsu S. Percutaneous electrothermocoagulation of spinal nerve trunk, ganglion, and rootlets. In Schmidek HH, Sweet WH, eds. *Operative neurosurgical techniques: indications, methods, and results.* New York: Grune & Stratton, 1988:1207.

110. Pagura JR. Percutaneous radiofrequency spinal rhizotomy. *Appl Neurophysiol* 1983;46:138.

111. Gildenberg PL, Hirshberg RM. Limited myelotomy for the treatment of intractable cancer pain. *J Neurol Neurosurg Psych* 1984:47;94.

112. Lippert RG, Hosobuchi Y, Nielson SL. Spinal commissurotomy. *Surg Neurol* 1974;2:373.

113. Cook AW, Kawakami Y. Commissural myelotomy. *J Neurosurg* 1977; 47:1.

114. Broager B. Commissural myelotomy. *Surg Neurol* 1974;2:71.

115. Sourek K. Commissural myelotomy. *J Neurosurg* 1969;31:524.

116. King RB. Anterior commissurotomy for intractable pain. *J Neurosurg* 1977;47:7.

117. Sweet HW, Poletti CE, Gybels JM. Operations in the brain stem and spinal canal, with an appendix on the relationship of open to percutaneous cordotomy. In Wall PD, Melzack R, eds. *Textbook of pain*, 3d ed. Edinburgh: Churchill-Livingstone, 1994:1225.

118. Mullan S, Harper PV, Hekmatpanah J, Torres H, Dobbin G. Percutaneous interruption of spinal-pain tracts by means of a strontium needle. *J Neurosurg* 1963:20;931.

119. Rosomoff HL, Carroll F, Brown J, Sheptak P. Percutaneous radiofrequency cervical cordotomy: technique. *J Neurosurg* 1965:23:639.

120. Rosomoff HL. Percutaneous spinothalamic cordotomy. In Wilkins RH, Rengachari SS, eds. *Neurosurgery.* New York: McGraw-Hill, 1985:2446.

121. Hitchcock E. Spinal and pontine tractotomies and nucleotomies. In Lunsford LD, ed. *Modern stereotactic neurosurgery.* Boston: Martinus Nijhoff Publishing, 1988:279.

122. Rosomoff HL, Papo I, Loeser JD. Neurosurgical operations on the spinal cord. In Bonica JJ. *The management of pain*, 2d ed. Philadelphia: Lea & Febiger, 1990:2067.

123. Kanpolat Y, Deda H, Akyar S, Bilgic S. CT-guided percutaneous cordotomy. *Acta Neurochir (Wien)* 1989;91:151.

124. Kanpolat Y, Akyar S, Caglar S, Unlu A, Bilgic S. CT-guided percutaneous selective cordotomy. *Acta Neurochir (Wien)* 1993;123:92.

125. Ballantine HT, Giriunas IE. Treatment of intractable psychiatric illness and chronic pain by stereotactic cingulotomy. In Schmidek HH, Sweet WH, eds. *Operative neurosurgical techniques: indications, methods, and results*, 2d ed. Orlando: Grune & Stratton, 1988:1069.

126. Hassenbusch SJ, Pillay PK, Barnett GH. Radiofrequency cingulotomy for intractable cancer pain using stereotaxis guided by magnetic resonance imaging. *Neurosurgery* 1990;27:220.

127. Steiner L, Forster D, Leksell L, Meyerson BA, Boethius J. Gammathalamotomy in intractable pain. *Acta Neurochir* 1980;52:173.

128. Kondziolka D, Lunsford LDL. Functional radiosurgery: current and future applications. In Gildenberg P, Tasker RR, eds. *Textbook of stereotactic and functional neurosurgery.* New York: McGraw Hill (in press).

129. Bosch DA. Stereotactic rostral mesencephalotomy in cancer pain and deafferentation pain: a series of 40 cases with follow-up results. *J Neurosurg* 1991;75:747.

130. Frank F, Fabrizzi AP, Gaist G. Stereotactic mesencephalic tractotomy in the treatment of chronic cancer pain. *Acta Neurochir* 1989;99:38.

131. Beauvillain de Montreuil C, Lajat Y, Resche F, Boutet JJ, Legent F. Use of stereotaxis neurosurgery in the treatment of pain in cervicofacial cancers. *Annales d'Oto-laryngologie et de Chirurgie Cervicofaciale* 1983:100:81.

132. Whisler WW, Voris HC. Mesencephalotomy for intractable pain due to malignant disease. *Appl Neurophysiol* 1978;41:52.

CHAPTER 31

Intraoperative Ultrasound in the Oncologic Setting: An Overview

Howard A. Zaren, Jeffrey H. Schwartz, Bernard Sigel, and Junji Machi

Every day try to help uplift, as you would help yourself or your family, whoever in your environment may be physically, mentally, or spiritually sick. Then no matter what your part is on the stage of life, you will know that you have been playing it rightly, directed by The Stage Manager Of All Destinies.

—Paramahanfa Yogananda

With the advancement of various imaging modalities, the diagnosis of malignant tumors has been improved. However, the extension of the tumor cannot always be assessed accurately by preoperative studies. Intraoperative evaluation, therefore, becomes critical in determining the stage and resectability of the tumor and in selecting the most appropriate operative procedure. During the operation, exploratory inspection and palpation are the essential means of evaluation for surgeons; however, intraoperative imaging methods can provide further valuable information. The use of intraoperative radiologic studies is limited in operations for tumors. On the other hand, intraoperative ultrasound (IOU) has wide applicability for various tumors.

Since the introduction of high-frequency high-resolution B-mode imaging in the late 1970s, IOU has been used in a variety of oncologic operations, including hepatobiliary pancreatic surgery, gastrointestinal surgery, neurosurgery, and endocrine surgery. We have performed IOU in more than 2,700 operations during the past 15 years (1–7). Of these operations, about 900 (33.6%) were for tumors (Table 1).

H. A. Zaren and J. H. Schwartz: Department of Surgery, The Mercy Hospital of Pittsburgh, Pittsburgh, Pennsylvania 15219.

B. Sigel: Allegheny University of the Health Sciences, Philadelphia, Pennsylvania 19102.

J. Machi: Department of Surgery, University of Hawaii at Manoa, Honolulu, Hawaii 96814.

In this chapter, we review our clinical experience and publications and summarize the instrumentation, techniques, indications, and specific organ uses of IOU in the general surgical oncology setting. Newer ultrasound imaging methods such as intraoperative color Doppler imaging and laparoscopic ultrasound are also discussed.

INSTRUMENTATION

With IOU, because the target organ is scanned directly, high-resolution real-time ultrasound is the equipment of choice (2,3,6). B-mode two-dimensional ultrasound has been most widely used; recently, color Doppler imaging has also been introduced. The latest innovation is the development of laparoscopic ultrasound, which is capable of B-mode or color Doppler imaging.

There are two transducer types: mechanical and electronic. Mechanical probes generally have a sector format. Electonic probes consist of phased-array transducers, which can be sector-, convex-, or linear-array formats. Transducer frequencies range from 5 to 10 MHz, with the 7.5-MHz transducer most frequently used. The depth of sound penetration with 7.5 MHz is about 6 to 8 cm, which is sufficient for scanning during most operations. The 5-MHz transducer is needed only when a target organ is markedly enlarged or a target lesion is deeply situated.

The size and shape of the ultrasound probe are important features for IOU scanning. The probe should be small enough to be manipulated in a small or narrow operative field. There are two principal shapes of probes: a flat T- or I-shaped probe (mostly side-viewing) and a cylindrical, pencillike probe (mostly front-viewing). The flat probe usually has a wider footprint (3 to 6 cm) and provides a wide near-field image. This probe is suitable for scanning relatively large, flat organs, such as the liver,

417

TABLE 1. *IOU of various organs and tumors*

Operated organ	No. of operations	Operations for tumors*
Liver	497	483
Biliary tract	772	44
Pancreas	240	68
Gastrointestinal tract	120	109
Other abdominal organs	48	8
Brain and spinal cord	102	65
Cardiovascular system	662	2
Endocrine system	69	66
Urinary system	109	5
Lung and mediastinum	70	64
Others	45	5
Total	2,734	919 (33.6%)

*Including both benign and malignant tumors

pancreas, and gastrointestinal tract. The pencillike probe is useful for scanning small target organs or structures, such as the extrahepatic biliary tract, that are located deep in the operative field.

Most probes can be cold-gas–sterilized. An alternative method is to place the probe in a sterile sheath before imaging. In the laparoscopic (intracorporeal) probe, the transducers are mounted at or near the tip of a long shaft, usually with a side-viewing capability. The shaft is 9 or 10 mm in diameter and is introduced into the peritoneal cavity through a 10-mm trocar. Recently, flexible probes have become available in addition to rigid probes.

TECHNIQUE

IOU can be performed at any time during the operation and, if necessary, can be safely repeated many times. There are some differences between IOU scanning and transcutaneous scanning. For IOU scanning, a contact gel (methylcellulose gel) is not needed, and sterile saline solution is used for acoustic coupling between the transducer surface and the tissue.

The two basic scanning techniques for IOU are contact scanning and probe-standoff scanning (2,3,6). In contact scanning, the probe is placed directly on the tissue or organ surface in a manner similar to transcutaneous ultrasound. In probe-standoff scanning, the probe is positioned 1 to 2 cm away from the surface of the structure. The probe-standoff technique using saline is unique to IOU. The distance from the probe to the target organ or the area of interest determines the choice of scanning technique. For example, contact scanning is chosen for the examination of the interior of organs such as the liver

and the pancreas, or for examination of target lesions located deep in the tissue. Probe-standoff scanning is essential for examination of the surface and the superficial area of organs or for examination of superficial structures, such as the extrahepatic biliary duct.

Another useful IOU scanning technique is compression scanning, in which the tissue is intentionally compressed by the probe. This method helps to displace air in tissue spaces and air in the gastrointestinal tract lumen. Compression can be also used to distinguish arteries from veins.

For complete evaluation, the organ should be systematically and thoroughly scanned—not only the area of interest, but the entire organ. Although the scanning method varies in different organs, it is usually important to obtain longitudinal and transverse views and, at times, oblique views of the target organ. In addition, IOU scanning can and should be performed from various positions and directions, using various probe manipulation techniques, including lateral movement, rotation, and angulation of the probe. By imaging the organ or the lesion in two-dimensional real-time, three-dimensional information can be obtained. During examination of malignant tumors, attention should be paid to surrounding structures, too. In particular, the major blood vessels should be followed and their relation to the tumor evaluated.

IOU is completed within a relatively short period. For example, screening of liver metastasis during laparotomy can be performed in 5 minutes. IOU evaluation of the extent of a malignant tumor usually requires 10 to 15 minutes.

Scanning techniques of intraoperative color Doppler imaging are basically the same as B-mode imaging. Laparoscopic ultrasound scanning is technically more demanding because the manipulation of the probe is obviously limited. However, with experience, complete laparoscopic ultrasound examinations of organs such as the liver, pancreas, and bile duct are possible (8–12).

INDICATIONS

Although IOU is one of the best methods for localizing islet cell tumors, parathyroid tumors, and other benign tumors, the major indication for the technique in surgical oncology is for malignant tumors. During surgery for malignant tumors, IOU is used to screen for metastases (mainly liver metastases), to localize nonpalpable tumors, to determine the extent of tumor and its resectability, and to guide surgical procedures.

IOU can be used to screen the liver for metastases whenever laparotomy is performed for malignant disease. Several studies have proven that IOU is more accurate in diagnosing liver metastases from colorectal cancer than preoperative studies and surgical exploration (13–18). During thoracotomy, the liver can be examined also from the thoracic cavity through the diaphragm (12).

Some tumors, even though diagnosed by preoperative studies, cannot be detected by inspection and palpation during the operation or until extensive tissue dissection has been performed. Such nonpalpable tumors include deep-seated liver tumors, small pancreatic cancers, and early gastric cancers. IOU can detect and localize these tumors early in the course of the operation.

The extent of malignant tumors can be assessed more accurately with IOU than with preoperative imaging methods. The depth of tumor invasion in esophagogastric cancers is determined by IOU. Vascular invasion by tumors such as hepatobiliary pancreatic cancers can be demonstrated. Color Doppler imaging that displays blood flow in real-time color within B-mode imaging facilitates the demonstration of the relation of blood vessels to the tumor (6,19). Detection of a tumor thrombus is also easier with intraoperative color Doppler imaging. Regional lymph nodes are delineated before tissue dissection. Although the final diagnosis of lymph node metastasis requires histologic examination, IOU can suggest the possible metastases based on the size, shape, and internal echo pattern of lymph nodes. By providing information on the local extent, lymph node status, and liver metastasis, IOU helps determine the stage of malignant tumors. Therefore, decisions about resectability and the selection of the most appropriate operative procedure can be facilitated by the IOU findings.

Surgical procedures guided by IOU are classified into two categories: first, intraoperative needle placement for fluid aspiration, agent injection, catheter or probe introduction, and biopsy, and second, surgical tissue dissection for incision or resection of organs (2,4,6,7). IOU-guided needle placement is especially valuable for nonpalpable deep lesions and helps avoid complications, including bleeding. Resection of some hepatocellular carcinomas cannot be completed without IOU guidance (4,20–22).

SPECIFIC ORGAN APPLICATIONS AND CLINICAL RESULTS

Liver

We have performed IOU of liver tumors in two major situations: screening for liver metastasis (n=371) during operations for 250 colorectal cancers and 121 other malignant tumors, and acquisition of beneficial information and guidance of operative procedures (n=112) during operations for 59 hepatocellular carcinomas, 40 colorectal metastases, eight other metastases, and five benign tumors.

IOU was routinely used during surgery for colorectal cancer in 250 patients, who were then followed more than 18 months postoperatively (2,13,17). Preoperative and intraoperative studies diagnosed a total of 147 metastatic liver tumors. In 25 patients (10%), IOU diagnosed 32 tumors that were not recognized by preoperative studies

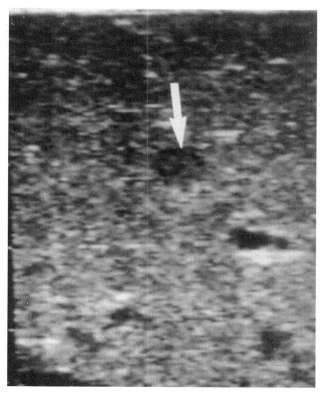

FIG. 1. A preoperatively unrecognized liver metastasis from a sigmoid colon cancer. Intraoperative ultrasound detected a 4×5-mm tumor *(arrow)* at the anterior inferior segment of the right lobe. The tumor was 2 cm from the liver surface and was not palpable.

and surgical exploration. These tumors were 4×4 mm to 15×18 mm in size, were located >1 cm from the liver surface, and were nonpalpable (Fig. 1). In the lesion-by-lesion analysis, the sensitivity, predictability of a negative test, and overall accuracy of IOU were significantly superior to those of preoperative ultrasound, computed tomography (CT), and surgical exploration (Table 2). During a median postoperative follow-up of 37 months, liver metastases that were not detected by any screening procedure, including IOU, were encountered in 18 patients (7.2% of total patients). Therefore, IOU appeared to diagnose 25 of 43 upstaged patients (58.1%) with occult liver metastasis (assuming that all these metachronous metastases were undetected but present at the time of surgery for colorectal cancer).

During 121 operations for other malignant tumors such as gastrointestinal cancers, sarcomas, and ovarian cancers, IOU screening for liver metastases was also conducted. In 14 of these operations (11.6%), preoperatively unrecognized nonpalpable metastatic liver tumors were diagnosed by IOU alone. Several reports have confirmed that IOU is more accurate than preoperative studies and that so-called occult metastasis can be detected by the routine use of IOU in about 5% to 15% of operations (13–18).

TABLE 2. *Accuracy (%) of four screening procedures in diagnosing liver metastasis from colorectal carcinoma*

	Preoperative ultrasound	Preoperative CT	Surgical exploration	IOU	p value
Sensitivity	40.8	49.0	66.0	93.8	<0.0001*
Specificity	95.8	94.4	89.3	94.4	—
Predictability of a positive test	87.0	85.7	80.8	92.0	<0.05†
Predictability of a negative test	70.2	72.9	79.2	95.7	<0.0001*
Overall accuracy	73.4	75.9	79.8	94.2	<0.0001*

*IOU versus each of the other three procedures
†IOU versus surgical exploration

When laparotomy is performed for hepatic resection for tumors, IOU provides various beneficial information (2,3,7,20–25). Hepatocellular carcinomas associated with cirrhosis are not palpable in more than half of these operations, and IOU readily localizes such nonpalpable tumors. Daughter nodules (intrahepatic metastases) and intravascular tumor thrombi of hepatocellular carcinomas that are often not identified preoperatively can be detected. IOU clearly delineates intrahepatic vascular and biliary structures in relation to liver tumors. In particular, IOU is more accurate than preoperative studies in diagnosing tumor invasion of vessels such as the portal vein or hepatic veins. These IOU findings of extension of malignant tumor can be obtained early in the operation, usually soon after laparotomy, and can help the surgeon determine the resectability and decide on the surgical procedure to be performed. In our experience, IOU provided beneficial information in 98 of 112 hepatic operations (87.5%). On the basis of IOU information, decisions on surgical procedures formed by preoperative studies and surgical exploration were changed in 44 of 112 operations (39.2%) (2,7). Others have also reported that IOU altered the surgical management of liver tumors, including primary and metastatic malignant tumors, in 30% to 50% of operations (20–25).

Laparoscopy was recently introduced for the evaluation of malignant liver tumors and for determining resectability. Although laparoscopy provides useful diagnostic information about tumor staging, an inherent disadvantage of laparoscopy is that it does not allow palpation. Laparoscopic ultrasound can compensate for this disadvantage and can become a new adjunct to laparoscopic examination. Our preliminary experience reveals the feasibility of laparoscopic ultrasound for the examination of primary and metastatic liver tumors (Fig. 2). One recent study on laparoscopic exploration of 50 malignant liver tumors demonstrated that laparoscopic ultrasound delineated tumors not visualized by the laparoscope in 33% of the cases and offered additional tumor staging information in 42% (26).

IOU provides not only diagnostic information but also therapeutic assistance in the form of IOU guidance during liver operations (2–7,20–22). This unique ability of real-time IOU cannot be matched by intraoperative radiography. IOU can be useful for intraoperative needle placement or hepatic tissue dissection. A needle is usually visualized well on B-mode imaging. When a very fine needle is used, its visualization is further enhanced by needle motion on color Doppler imaging (19,27). During tissue dissection for hepatic resection, the incision planes are delineated in relation to target lesions and vascular structures (Fig. 3). Small nonpalpable liver tumors can be biopsied or approached only with the assistance of IOU. Treatment of liver tumors by nonresectional techniques, such as cryosurgery, is also assisted by IOU guidance (28). Furthermore, new operative techniques such as IOU-guided systematic subsegmentectomy have been developed as a result of the utility of IOU (20–22).

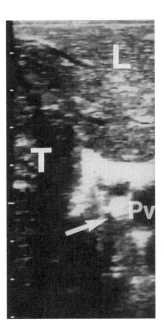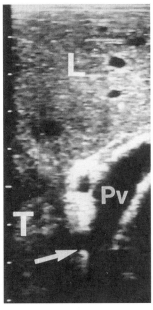

FIG. 2. Laparoscopic ultrasound examination of a hepatocellular carcinoma. Preoperative studies showed a large tumor of the right lobe, but the extent of the tumor was unclear. Laparoscopic ultrasound demonstrated that the tumor *(T)* was invading the main right portal vein *(arrow, PV)*. This finding indicated that the tumor was unresectable. *L,* normal liver parenchyma.

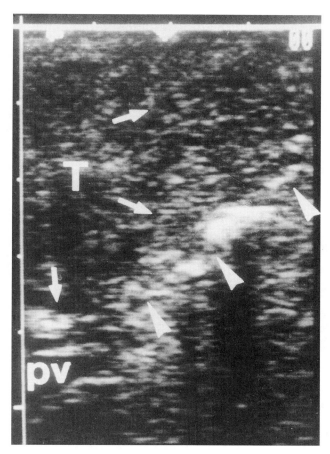

FIG. 3. Hepatic resection guided by IOU. A metastatic tumor *(T, arrows)* was at the anterior inferior segment of the right lobe, and a right portal vein branch *(pv)* was close to the tumor. The hepatic resection was underway, and IOU delineated the resection plane as a hyperechoic line *(arrowhead)*. It confirmed that the resection was proceeding appropriately toward the portion between the tumor and the vein. (Machi J. *Operative ultrasonography—fundamentals and clinical applications.* Tokyo: Life Science, 1987, with permission)

In our series, IOU-guided needle placement facilitated biopsy of the liver (n=36), especially for deeply situated nonpalpable tumors, injection of therapeutic agents (n=8) (Fig. 4), and catheterization of the intrahepatic biliary ducts (n=4). During 89 hepatic resections, which included anatomic subsegmentectomy, segmentectomy, and lobectomy, IOU guidance was used in 67 (75.3%) (2,4,6,7).

Biliary Tract

Although IOU has been used most frequently for biliary calculus disease, particularly screening for bile duct calculi, it can also be used for neoplastic biliary diseases (1–7). Benign gallbladder polyps as small as 1 to 2 mm are readily detected by high-resolution IOU. At times, dur-

ing cholecystectomy for gallstones or during other operations, gallbladder polyps are incidentally delineated.

The main indication for IOU of the biliary tract is to determine the extent of malignant tumors, including gallbladder cancer and bile duct cancer. With IOU, it is possible to assess precisely gallbladder cancer invasion into the liver parenchyma. Involvement of the portal vein and hepatic artery, regional lymph node status, and liver metastasis are evaluated without extensive tissue dissection. If the cause of obstructive jaundice is unknown preoperatively, IOU may detect bile duct calculi, thus excluding tumor, or may delineate a small bile duct cancer (Fig. 5). When the anatomy around the bile duct is distorted by large tumors, IOU facilitates localization of the obscured bile duct. In such situations, operative color Doppler imaging is especially helpful for localizing the duct by distinguishing it from blood vessels.

We have performed IOU of the biliary system in 44 operations: 18 for gallbladder cancer, 14 for bile duct cancer, and 12 for gallbladder polyps. Beneficial information was provided by IOU in 34 of the 44 operations (77.3%) (2,5–7).

IOU guides various procedures during biliary operations in a manner similar to hepatic operations. IOU facilitates the quick and precise placement of needles for tumor biopsy, aspiration of the bile duct, injection of contrast into the duct for intraoperative cholangiography, and catheterization of the intrahepatic bile duct. IOU guides operations for resection, which is most helpful when these operations include combined hepatic resection. During operations for malignant biliary tumors, we have used IOU guidance in needle placement for tumor resection (n=16), catheterization (n=10), biopsy (n=9), and bile duct aspiration or injection (n=8).

Pancreas

IOU is indicated during operations for pancreatic cancer as well as for pancreatitis (1–7,29,30). In pancreatic cancer, the purpose of IOU is to assess the intraoperative staging and thereby to determine the tumor's resectability. Main factors that influence the resectability of pancreatic cancer include vascular invasion, lymph node metastasis, liver metastasis, and peritoneal dissemination. IOU is valuable in evaluating all these factors except peritoneal dissemination, which is more accurately identified by surgical exploratory inspection and palpation. Tumor invasion of vascular structures such as the portal-mesenteric vein and the branches of the celiac artery can be evaluated more accurately by IOU than by preoperative studies. One advantage of IOU is that such an evaluation is performed immediately after laparotomy, without extensive tissue dissection. We have compared the accuracy of IOU in diagnosing portal vein invasion of 39 pancreatic cancers

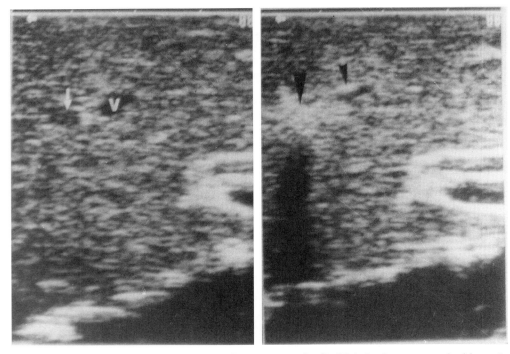

FIG. 4. IOU guidance of alcohol injection to a liver metastasis. **(Left)** A 4↔3-mm nonpalpable metastatic tumor *(arrow)* from a jejunal leiomyosarcoma detected by intraoperative ultrasound. *V*, a branch of the middle hepatic vein. **(Right)** After placement of a needle into the tumor under IOU guidance, 99.9% ethanol was injected into the tumor. Injected alcohol produced a hyperechoic area *(large black arrowhead)* with an acoustic shadow. Part of the alcohol was drained into the hepatic vein, seen as intraluminal flowing echoes *(small black arrowhead)*. (Machi J, Sigel B, Kurohiji T, Zaren HA, Sariego J. Operative ultrasound guidance for various surgical procedures. *Ultrasound Med Biol* 1990;16:37, with permission)

with preoperative studies including percutaneous ultrasound, CT, and the portal phase of superior mesenteric angiography (7). The final diagnosis was made by gross (surgical) and microscopic examination, which showed positive portal vein invasion in 22 cases and negative in 17. IOU demonstrated significantly better results than the combination of preoperative studies in terms of specificity and overall accuracy (Table 3; Fig. 6).

IOU delineates enlarged lymph nodes or lymph nodes suspicious for metastasis more readily than surgical palpation. These include regional lymph nodes such as para-aortic and periceliac nodes, which are often not easy to palpate before tissue dissection. Lymph nodes with possible metastasis identified by IOU are then submitted for frozen-section histologic examination in the early phase of the operation. The liver is also scanned quickly for liver metastasis.

Of 68 operations for pancreatic cancer in which we used IOU, it was considered beneficial in determining local tumor extension and in guiding surgical decisions in 49 (72.1%) (1–7,29). We recently introduced laparoscopic ultrasound for the examination of pancreatic cancer. It seemed that this new ultrasound method would provide similar information to IOU conducted at laparotomy. A few reports by others indicating the value of

laparoscopic ultrasound for staging pancreatic cancer were also published recently (10,11,31).

Gastrointestinal Tract

We have performed IOU during 109 operations on the gastrointestinal tract, including 63 for gastric cancer and 34 for esophageal cancer (2,5,6,32,33). IOU was used to evaluate the depth of tumor invasion in addition to vascular invasion, lymph node metastasis, and liver metastasis, all of which are important factors in determining the cancer stage.

On high-resolution ultrasound images, the wall of the gastrointestinal tract exhibits a five-layer appearance, which corresponds to the layered structures obtained on histologic examination. IOU can demonstrate distortion or destruction of the normal five-layer configuration as a result of cancer invasion. Thus, the depth of tumor invasion and intramural lateral tumor extension can be determined by IOU (Fig. 7). IOU can localize early gastric cancers that are sometimes not palpable during the operation. We investigated the accuracy of IOU in diagnosing the depth of tumor invasion in 31 gastric cancer operations by comparing IOU images with histologic examina-

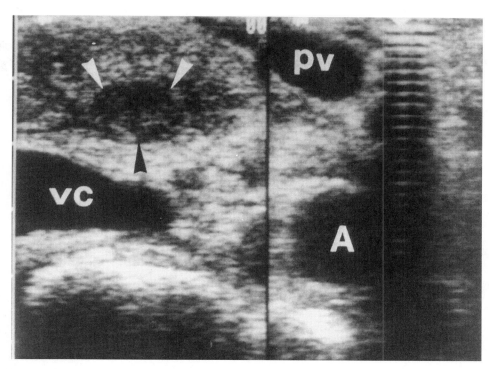

FIG. 5. A small nonpalpable distal bile duct cancer. Preoperative studies failed to demonstrate any tumor despite the presence of biliary obstruction. IOU performed immediately after laparotomy delineated an 8↔12-mm hypoechoic tumor *(arrowheads)* at the head of the pancreas near the ampulla. The tumor was away from the portal vein *(PV). VC,* vena cava; *A,* aorta. Pancreatoduodenectomy was performed, and histologic examination confirmed the bile duct cancer. (Machi J. *Operative ultrasonography—fundamentals and clinical applications.* Tokyo: Life Science, 1987, with permission)

tion of resected specimens (2,33). The layer-by-layer analysis revealed that the overall accuracy of IOU was 81% (Table 4).

During surgery for gastric cancer, dissection of perigastric lymph nodes is usually not difficult. However, dissection of lymph nodes remote to the stomach, in particular para-aortic lymph nodes, is technically more difficult and is time-consuming. Therefore, diagnosis of metastases to these lymph nodes by an imaging study is helpful for surgeons. For this reason, we evaluated the accuracy of IOU in diagnosing para-aortic lymph node metastasis in 30

TABLE 3. *Accuracy (%) of two procedures in diagnosing portal vein invasion of pancreatic carcinoma*

	Preoperative studies	IOU	p value
Sensitivity	76.5	94.1	—
Specificity	54.5	86.4	<0.05
Predictability of a positive test	56.5	84.2	—
Predictability of a negative test	75.0	95.0	—
Overall accuracy	64.1	89.7	<0.01

From Machi J, Sigel B, Zaren HA, Kurohiji T, Yamashita Y. Operative ultrasonography during hepatobiliary and pancreatic surgery. *World J Surg* 1993;17:640, with permission.

gastric cancer operations (33). The final diagnosis of the presence or absence of metastasis was made by histologic examination of dissected lymph nodes. In this study, lymph nodes detected by IOU were judged to be positive for metastasis when they satisfied the following criteria: the longest axis of node measured 7 mm or greater, the ratio of the shortest axis to the longest axis was 0.5 or greater, and the internal echo features were hypoechoic or mixed pattern. With these criteria, the sensitivity, specificity, and overall accuracy of IOU in diagnosing para-aortic lymph node metastasis were 100%, 84.6%, and 90.9%, respectively. IOU was significantly superior to preoperative ultrasound and CT (Table 5).

Esophageal cancer is often associated with extramural local invasion to such structures as blood vessels and the tracheobronchial tree. We examined aortic invasion of esophageal cancer by IOU in 34 operations (2,32). Preoperative studies included CT and magnetic resonance imaging. IOU was performed immediately after thoracotomy, before tissue dissection. The final diagnosis made by gross and microscopic examination revealed positive aortic invasion in four cases and negative in 30. Preoperative imaging tests had two false-positive and two false-negative results. On the other hand, IOU showed true results in all operations.

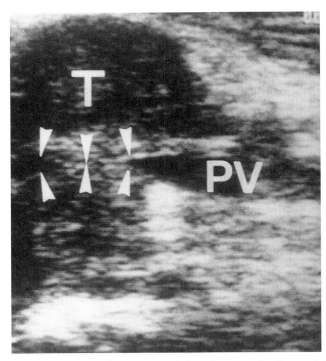

FIG. 6. Invasion of a pancreatic head cancer to the portal vein. IOU performed immediately after laparotomy and before tissue dissection demonstrated the invasion *(arrowheads)* of the tumor *(T)* to the portal vein *(PV)*. The vein was almost occluded by the tumor. This finding was later confirmed by surgical exploration with dissection. (Machi J. *Operative ultrasonography—fundamentals and clinical applications.* Tokyo: Life Science, 1987, with permission)

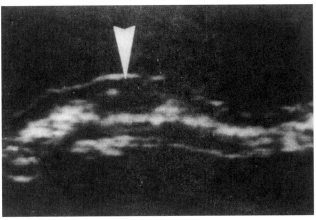

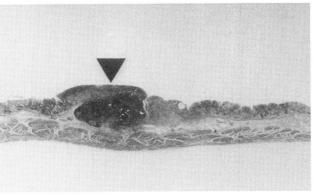

FIG. 7. An early gastric cancer. **(Upper)** IOU showing a small hypoechoic gastric cancer invading to the submucosa *(arrowhead)*. The third hyperechoic layer (submucosal layer) was partially destroyed by the tumor. Normal five-layer structures of the gastric wall are seen on both sides of the tumor. **(Lower)** The corresponding histology of the cancer after resection. (Machi J. *Operative ultrasonography—fundamentals and clinical applications.* Tokyo: Life Science, 1987, with permission)

These studies on gastric and esophageal cancer indicate that IOU may be a useful technique in determining the tumor extension early during surgery.

Endocrine System

Although IOU can be used for thyroid and adrenal tumors, its main indication is for islet cell tumors and parathyroid tumors (2,3,5,6,29). IOU is performed for precise localization and at times exclusion of endocrine tumors. For malignant endocrine tumors, IOU is performed to help in tumor staging.

More than half of insulinomas and gastrinomas cannot be localized preoperatively despite the use of various imaging methods; in addition, small islet cell tumors may be nonpalpable intraoperatively. Islet cell tumors are almost always hypoechoic relative to normal pancreatic tissue. Because of this characteristic ultrasound feature, tumors as small as 3 to 4 mm can be delineated by IOU (Fig. 8). IOU, therefore, has become an invaluable tool for intraoperative localization.

IOU also may diagnose multiple islet cell tumors or may exclude previously suspected multiple tumors. For

this reason, the entire pancreas should be completely scanned during surgery. Islet cell tumors within the pancreatic parenchyma can be detected by IOU with a high degree of accuracy; extrapancreatic tumors are more difficult to detect. Therefore, IOU is more effective for insulinoma than gastrinoma because most insulinomas are located within the pancreas. It was reported that the detectability of insulinoma by IOU was 83% to 100%, that of pancreatic gastrinoma was 95%, and that of extrapancreatic gastrinoma was 53% (34,35). Once a nonpalpable tumor is localized, extirpation of the tumor is facilitated with IOU guidance. For malignant islet cell tumors, IOU can be used to determine the extent of disease, particularly liver metastasis. In our experience on five insulinomas and three gastrinomas (including two malignant gastrinomas), IOU was able to localize all tumors, including two tumors otherwise undetectable (2,5,6).

TABLE 4. *Accuracy of IOU in diagnosing the depth of tumor invasion of gastric cancer*

Histologic examination	IOU						
	Undetected	M	SM	PM	SS	SE	Accuracy
M	1	4					4/5 (80%)
SM	1		7	2			7/10 (70%)
PM				5		1	5/6 (83%)
SS					4	1	4/5 (80%)
SE						5	5/5 (100%)
Total							25/31 (81%)

M, mucosa; SM, submucosa; PM, propria muscle; SS, subserosa; SE, extraserosa
From Kodama I, Machi J, Tanaka M, et al. The value of operative ultrasonography in diagnosing tumor extension of carcinoma of the stomach. *Surg Gynecol Obstet* 1992;174:479, with permission

For hyperparathyroidism, localization of the parathyroid tumor by imaging methods becomes especially important at the time of reoperation. Parathyroid adenoma and hyperplasia both exhibit hypoechogenicity. IOU helps localize these tumors early in the course of the operation and avoids extensive tissue dissection, which is difficult during reoperation. It was reported that during 39 reoperations for hyperparathyroidism, IOU accurately detected 33 of 41 tumors (80%). The sensitivity of IOU was 85%, and this was superior to that of the other modalities, such as CT and technetium/thallium scan (36). In particular, tumors in aberrant locations, such as undescended or intrathyroidal adenomas, were accurately delineated. In our experience, parathyroid tumors were localized by IOU in 10 of 18 operations (56%) (2,5,6).

CONCLUSION

We have performed IOU in more than 900 operations in the oncology setting. Benefits provided by IOU are twofold: acquisition of new information not available by preoperative studies and surgical exploration, and guidance of various surgical procedures. For malignant tumors, the extent of tumor spread such as local invasion and lymph node and liver metastasis can be assessed, thereby determining tumor resectability and the choice of operation. This helps avoid extensive surgical dissection and associated complications. IOU is indispensable during certain operations—for example, to detect occult tumors and to guide procedures such as accurate anatomic hepatic resection. IOU has multiple advantages as an intraoperative tool, including speed, safety, variety of imaging information, wide applicability, high accuracy, and guidance capability. In general surgical oncology, these advantages have a remarkable impact on management, especially during hepatobiliary pancreatic surgery for malignant disease. Newer IOU modalities—intraoperative color Doppler imaging and laparoscopic ultrasound—enhance the benefits and may widen the applications of IOU.

TABLE 5. *Accuracy (%) of three procedures in diagnosing metastasis of the para-aortic lymph nodes*

	Preoperative ultrasound	Preoperative CT	IOU	*p* value
Sensitivity	44.4	44.4	100	<0.01*
Specificity	92.3	69.2	84.6	—
Overall accuracy	72.7	59.1	90.9	<0.02†

*IOU versus each of the other two procedures
†IOU versus CT
From Kodama I, Machi J, Tanaka M, et al. The value of operative ultrasonography in diagnosing tumor extension of carcinoma of the stomach. *Surg Gynecol Obstet* 1992;174:479, with permission

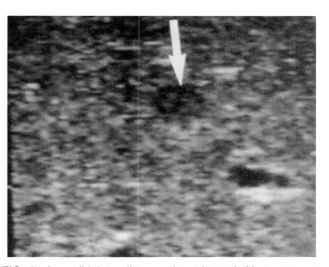

FIG. 8. A small islet cell tumor (gastrinoma). No tumor was detected by preoperative studies. IOU localized a 4×4-mm hypoechoic tumor in the pancreatic tail. (Sigel B, Machi J, Ramos JR, Duarte B, Donehue PE. The role of imaging ultrasound during pancreatic surgery. *Ann Surg* 1984; 200:486, with permission)

REFERENCES

1. Sigel B, Coelho JC, Machi J, et al. The application of real-time ultrasound imaging during surgical procedures. *Surg Gynecol Obstet* 1983; 157:33.
2. Machi J. *Operative ultrasonography—fundamentals and clinical applications.* Tokyo: Life Science, 1987 (in Japanese).
3. Sigel B. *Operative ultrasonography*, 2d ed. Philadelphia: Raven Press, 1988.
4. Machi J, Sigel B, Kurohiji T, Zaren HA, Sariego J. Operative ultrasound guidance for various surgical procedures. *Ultrasound Med Biol* 1990;16:37.
5. Machi J, Sigel B. Overview of benefits of operative ultrasonography during a ten-year period. *J Ultrasound Med* 1989;8:647.
6. Machi J, Sigel B. Intraoperative ultrasonography. *Radiol Clin North Am* 1992;30:1085.
7. Machi J, Sigel B, Zaren HA, Kurohiji T, Yamashita Y. Operative sonography during hepatobiliary and pancreatic surgery. *World J Surg* 1993;17:640.
8. Machi J, Sigel B, Zaren HA, et al. Technique of ultrasound examination during laparoscopic cholecystectomy. *Surg Endosc* 1993;7:544.
9. Yamamoto M, Stiegmann GV, Durham J, et al. Laparoscopy-guided intracorporeal ultrasound accurately delineates hepatobiliary anatomy. *Surg Endosc* 1993;7:325.
10. Jakimowicz JJ. Review: intraoperative ultrasonography during minimal access surgery. *J Roy Coll Surg Edinb* 1993;38:231.
11. Murugiah M, Paterson-Brown S, Windsor JA, Miles WFA, Garden OJ. Early experience of laparoscopic ultrasonography in the management of pancreatic carcinoma. *Surg Endosc* 1993;7:177.
12. Stiegmann GV, McIntyre RC, Pearlman NW. Laparoscopic intracorporeal ultrasound: an alternative to cholangiography? *Surg Endosc* 1994; 8:167.
13. Machi J, Isomoto H, Yamashita Y, et al. Intraoperative ultrasonography in screening for liver metastases from colorectal cancer: comparative accuracy with traditional procedures. *Surgery* 1987;101:678.
14. Russo A, Sparacino G, Plaja S, et al. Role of intraoperative ultrasound in the screening of liver metastases from colorectal carcinoma: initial experiences. *J Surg Oncol* 1989;42:249.
15. Olsen AK. Intraoperative ultrasonography and the detection of liver metastases in patients with colorectal cancer. *Br J Surg* 1990;77:998.
16. Stadler J, Holscher AH, Adolf J. Intraoperative ultrasonographic detection of occult liver metastases in colorectal cancer. *Surg Endosc* 1991; 5:36.
17. Machi J, Isomoto H, Kurohiji T, et al. Accuracy of intraoperative ultrasonography in diagnosing liver metastasis from colorectal cancer: evaluation with postoperative follow-up results. *World J Surg* 1991; 15:551.
18. Stone MD, Kane R, Bothe A Jr, et al. Intraoperative ultrasound imaging of the liver at the time of colorectal cancer resection. *Arch Surg* 1994;129:431.
19. Machi J, Sigel B, Kurohiji T, et al. Operative color Doppler imaging for general surgery. *J Ultrasound Med* 1993;12:455.
20. Makuuchi M, Hasegawa H, Yamazaki S. Ultrasonically guided subsegmentectomy. *Surg Gynecol Obstet* 1985;161:346.
21. Castaing D, Emond J, Kunstlinger F, Bismuth H. Utility of operative ultrasound in the surgical management of liver tumors. *Ann Surg* 1986; 204:600.
22. Makuuchi M, Hasegawa H, Yamazaki S, Takayasu K, Moriyama N. The use of operative ultrasound as an aid to liver resection in patients with hepatocellular carcinoma. *World J Surg* 1987;11:615.
23. Dunnington GL. Intraoperative ultrasonography in abdominal surgery. *Surg Ann* 1993;25:101.
24. Rifkin MD, Rosato FE, Branch HM, et al. Intraoperative ultrasound of the liver. An important adjunctive tool for decision making in the operating room. *Ann Surg* 1987;205:466.
25. Parker GA, Lawrence W Jr., Horsley JS, et al. Intraoperative ultrasound of the liver affects operative decision making. *Ann Surg* 1989;209:569.
26. John TG, Greig JD, Crosbie JL, Miles WFA, Garden OJ. Superior staging of liver tumors with laparoscopy and laparoscopic ultrasound. *Ann Surg* 1994;220:711.
27. Kurohiji T, Sigel B, Justin J, Machi J. Motion marking in color Doppler ultrasound needle and catheter visualization. *J Ultrasound Med* 1990; 9:243.
28. Onik GM, Atkinson D, Zemel R, Weaver ML. Cryosurgery of liver cancer. *Semin Surg Oncol* 1993;9:309.
29. Sigel B, Machi J, Ramos JR, Duarte B, Donehue PE. The role of imaging ultrasound during pancreatic surgery. *Ann Surg* 1984;200:486.
30. Plainfosse MC, Bouilot JL, Rivaton F, Vancamps P, Hernigon A, Alexandre JH. The use of operative sonography in carcinoma of the pancreas. *World J Surg* 1987;11:654.
31. John TG, Greig JD, Carter DC, Garden OJ. Carcinoma of the pancreatic head and periampullary region. Tumor staging with laparoscopy and laparoscopic ultrasonography. *Ann Surg* 1995;221:156.
32. Machi J, Takeda J, Kakegawa T, et al. The detection of gastric and esophageal tumor extension by high-resolution ultrasound during surgery. *World J Surg* 1987;11:664.
33. Kodama I, Machi J, Tanaka M, et al. The value of operative ultrasonography in diagnosing tumor extension of carcinoma of the stomach. *Surg Gynecol Obstet* 1992;174:479.
34. Zeiger MA, Shawker TH, Norton JA. Use of intraoperative ultrasonography to localize islet cell tumors. *World J Surg* 1993;17:448.
35. Klotter HJ, Ruckert K, Kummerle F, Rothmund M. The use of intraoperative sonography in endocrine tumors of the pancreas. *World J Surg* 1987;11:635.
36. Kern KA, Shawker TH, Doppman JL, et al. The use of high-resolution ultrasound to locate parathyroid tumors during reoperations for primary hyperparathyroidism. *World J Surg* 1987;11:579.

APPENDIX

Manufacturers of Specialized Equipment

All the contributors to this book were asked to list any specialized equipment and agents used in their procedures. The following was submitted. If any additional information is necessary regarding any of the procedures and protocols in this book, please send written requests to the following address and we will attempt to obtain the information for you.

Michael T. Lotze, M.D.
Joshua T. Rubin, M.D.
Suite 300, Kaufmann Building
3471 Fifth Avenue
Pittsburgh, PA 15213
Fax (412) 692-2520

CYTOREDUCTIVE SURGERY

Extended ball electrode: Olsen Electrosurgical Inc., Concord, CA

Quinton peritoneal catheter: Quinton Inc., Seattle, WA.

C.U.S.A. System 200, or the Macro: Cavitron, Stanford, CT

Electrosurgical unit: BARD, Englewood, CO

Hyper/hypothermia unit: Cincinnati Sub-Zero, Cincinnati, OH

Thompson retractor: Thompson Surgical Instrument, Inc., Barrington, IL

EEA-25, CEEA-31, and the Roticulator-55: Auto Suture, Norwalk, CT

GIA RCC75: Ethicon, Sommerville, NJ

St. Mark Stirrup: AMSCO, Erie, PA

Jackson-Pratt drain: Synder Hemovac (Zimmer), Dover, OH

Laser smoke filtration unit: W. Stackhouse Associates Inc., El Segunda, CA

CAPD solution transfer set: Travenol, Deerfield, IL

Neosporin GU irrigant: Burroughs Wellcome Inc., Research Triangle Park, NC

Argyle-Salem sump tube

Tenckhoff catheter transfer set: Travenol, Deerfield, IL

Chest tubes: Deknatel thoracic catheter, Deknatel Inc., Falls River, MA

Pleurevac: Deknatel Inc. Falls River, MA

Draneal 1.5%, PD-1 solution: Travenol, Deerfield, IL

Egg crate mattress

SCD compression boots: Kendall Co., Boston, MA

Bair Hugger upper body cover, Augustine Medical, Eden Praire, MN

INTRAPERITONEAL CHEMOTHERAPY

The catalog number and quantity needed are given.

Venous reservoir bag, 1,000 mL: Kol Biomedical, CXVRA1001TA; 1

Empty sterile split bag: Travenol, SC4462, 1

Cardioplegia delivery set: Electromedics, D1081A, 1

Morse stopcock with Luer lock: NAMIC, 70015003, 1

Sterile tubing $\frac{1}{4}''\times\frac{1}{16}''\times12'$: Kol Biomedical, SL5050, 2

Sterile tubing $\frac{3}{8}''\times\frac{3}{32}''\times2'$: Kol Biomedical, SL7100, 1

Connector reducer $\frac{3}{8}''\times\frac{1}{4}''$: Kol Biomedical, EC2175S, 2

Straight connector with Luer lock $\frac{3}{16}''\times\frac{3}{16}''$: Kol Biomedical, EC2154S, 1

Y connector $\frac{1}{4}''\times\frac{1}{4}''\times\frac{1}{4}''$: Kol Biomedical, EC2100S, 4

Blood bag spike 24'': Kol Biomedical, QPL36NU, 1

Quickie Prime Spike: Texas Medical Products, 301011, 2

Perfusion adapter: Texas Medical Products, 301022-000, 4

Closed suction catheter: Zimmer, 2567-000-10, 3

Tenckhoff curled peritoneal catheter: Quinton Instrument CO, 11313-010, 1

Esophageal temperature probe: Respiratory Support Products, ES400-18, 2

Cardiopulmonary pump: Sarns, 3500, 1

Heater/cooler: Sarns, 11160, 1

Labcraft digital thermometer: Curtin Matheson Scientific Inc., 084-541, 1

Temperature probe: Electromedics, 4700, 2

Temperature probe cable: Baxter Healthcare Products, 30703-409, 2

Smoke evacuator: Stackhouse, Inc., 1

Chemotherapy spill kit: Codan Medlon Inc., SK 200, 1

ABLATIVE PROCEDURES FOR CANCER PAIN

Radiofrequency generators and electrodes: Radionics, 22 Terry Ave., Burlington, MA 01803; (800) 466-6814

Implantable pumps and spinal cord stimulators: Medtronics, Inc., Neurological Division, 800 53rd Ave. NE, Minneapolis, MN 55421; (800) 328-0810

PERFUSIONAL THERAPY OF BRAIN METASTASES

These are available for use only with permission from the FDA or NIH. The Ommaya reservoir is available commercially for use from Baxter Heyer Schulte, Baxter Healthcare Corporation, Deerfield, IL. Drug-impregnated biodegradable polymers are undergoing a phase III trial. Interested researchers can contact Dr. Henry Brem, c/o Johns Hopkins University, Department of Neurosurgery, Baltimore, MD. Researchers interested in diastole-pulsed intra-arterial injections should contact Dr. John Doppman at the NIH.

ISOLATED PERFUSION

Perfusion pump: Cobe Cardiovascular, Arvada, CA
Atomlab 900 medical spectrometer: Biodex Medical Systems, Shirley, NY
Tumor necrosis factor: Knoll Pharmaceuticals, Whippany, NJ
Cannulae: DLP, Grand Rapids, MI
Perfusion packs: Baxter Bentley, Irvine, CA

Subject Index

Subject Index

A

Abdominal lymphadenopathy, 217
Abdominosacral resection, 235–246
  clinical results, 244–245
  five-year survival, 245
  functional impairments, 245
  methodology, 237–243
  morbidity and mortality, 236, 243–244
  pain relief objective, 245
  patient care considerations, 246
  preoperative evaluation, 236–237
  recurrence rates, 236
Ablation procedures, pain management,
    404–409, 427
Acetabulum lesions, surgery, 359–362
N-acetyl aspartate, 163
ACNU
  intra-carotid delivery, 200
  intrathecal delivery, 199
Acrometastases, 357
Activated NK cells, 7
Acyclovir, 387
Adeno-associated virus vectors, 376, 378
Adenocarcinoma, intraperitoneal chemotherapy,
    261–263, 265–267
Adenosine deaminase deficiency, 376, 380
Adenoviral vectors, 376–378
Adhesion, and tumor cell progression, 4–5
Adoptive cellular therapy, 397
Adrenal tumors
  imaging, 212–214
  laparoscopy, 230–231
Adriamycin. *See* Doxorubicin
Alcohol injection
  epidural neurolysis, 406
  hepatic cryoablation comparison, 137
  hepatic metastases, 103–104, 137–138
  intraoperative celiac neurolysis, 408
  intrathecal neurolysis, 405–406
  laser hyperthermia comparison, 138
Allogeneic bone marrow transplantation,
    384–385
Alpha-fetoprotein, 378
Alpha-interferon. *See* Interferon-alpha
Alternating pressure boots, 250
Altitude, and hepatic arterial chemotherapy, 125
Anaphylactic reactions, iodinated material, 156
Anastomotic recurrence, 235
Aneurysms, differential diagnosis, 167–168
Angiogenesis, 5
Angiography. *See also* CT-arteriography
  hypervascular bone metastases, 354
  pancreatic carcinoma, 211
Angiosarcoma, 344–345
Ankle lesions, surgery, 358
Anterior vertebral corpectomy, 363
Anticonvulsant drugs
  brain metastases, 178, 188

prophylactic use, 188
Anti-oncogenes, 386
Anti-TAG antibodies, 395
Antrectomy, 255–256
Aortoiliac nodes, dissection, 240
Appendiceal carcinomatosis
  intraperitoneal chemotherapy, 259–268
  peritonectomy, 249–258
  prognostic features, 267
Arrow Model 3000, 120
Arterial phase hepatic CT, 76–80, 85–86
Arteriovenous malformation, 167–168
Ascites. *See* Malignant ascites
Aspartate levels, 125
Ataxia, and intracranial metastases, 154
Autologous bone marrow transplants, 379
Axillary lymph node dissection, 296–298,
    314–316
  early mobilization role, 307
  extent of, controversy, 314–316
  history, 296
  and muscle resection, 307–308
  prophylactic versus therapeutic methods,
    315–316
  sampling accuracy, 297
  sentinel method, 297–298
  surgical procedure, 308

B

B16 melanoma metastases, 7
B72.3 antibody, 303
Bair Huggers, 132, 250
Basement membrane, tumor invasion, 3, 152
Batson's plexus, tumor seeding, 153
BCD-F9 antibody, 303
BCNU
  extracorporeal perfusion, 197
  intra-carotid therapy, 197
  microsphere delivery, 199
Bile duct carcinoma
  intraoperative radiation therapy, 287
  intraoperative ultrasound, 421, 423
Biliary cystadenocarcinoma, 79
Bio-Medicus centrifugal pump, 146
Bipedal lymphangiography, 302–303
Bispecific monoclonal antibodies, 197–198
Bladder cancer, lymphadenectomy, 321
Bleomycin, 59
"Block copolymers," 13
Blood-brain barrier
  pathophysiologic conditions, 196
  and regional perfusion, 197
Blood flow. *See* Tumor blood flow
Blood loss, pelvic exenteration, 243–244
Blood oxygen level-dependent method, 162–163
Blood pressure, and tumor blood flow, 6
Blood supply, pulmonary metastases, 38–39
BOLD method, brain metastases, 162–163

Bone grafts, 364
Bone metastases, 351–364
  evaluation, 352–354
  fracture risk, 354
  incidence, 351
  surgical treatment, 351–364
Bone scintigraphy, 352
  indications, 206
  multiple myeloma, 352
  sensitivity, 352
Bowel perforation, 268
Brachial vessel perfusion, 337
Brachytherapy, 182
Brain abscesses, 165–167
Brain atrophy, imaging, 170
Brain electrical stimulation, 402–403
Brain metastases, 151–171, 175–184, 187–193
  brachytherapy, 182
  clinical symptoms, 154
  computed tomography, 154–157
    disadvantages, 155–157
  conservative medical management, 188
  diagnostic imaging, 151–171
  differential diagnostic imaging, 164–168
  distribution, 195
  functional imaging, 162–163
  gene therapy, 383–384
  incidence, 151, 175, 187
  magnetic resonance imaging, 157–160, 178
  pathogenesis, 152–153
  pathology, 153–154
  patient assessment and care, 201
  perfusional therapy, 195–202
  positron emission tomography, 160–162
  post-treatment evaluation, 169–171
  radiosensitivity, 177
  radiosurgery, 187–193
  SPECT imaging, 160–162
  surgery, 175–184
    clinical results, 180–184
    indications, 176–178
    mortality and morbidity, 182, 184
  therapy rationale, 175–176
  treatment strategies, choice of, 192–193
Breast carcinoma
  nodal resection, 314–316
  sentinel nodal dissection, 296–298
Breast carcinoma metastases
  bone scintigraphy, 206
  brain recurrence, survival, 181
  intravenous contrast-enhancement, liver,
    77–78, 81
  noncontrast CT, liver, 85
  pulmonary metastasectomy, 46–47
Breslow thickness, 312
Bronchogenic carcinoma, brain metastasis, 179
Bronchoscopy, 32, 40
"Bystander effect," 383

C

Calcification
  computed tomography, brain, 155
  pulmonary metastases, 25–26, 39
Candela cryoprobes, 133
Carbon-11 PET, brain metastases, 161
Carbon suspensions, 17
Carcinoembryonic antigen
  hepatic metastases prognosis, 111
  and immunolymphoscintigraphy, 303
  monitoring use, 392
Carcinomatous meningitis, 200
Cavernous hemangiomas
  differential diagnosis, brain, 167
  dynamic contrast CT methods, 78–82
  magnetic resonance imaging, liver, 89–90
  ultrasonography, liver, 93–94
Cavitation
  post-therapy evaluation, brain, 169
  in pulmonary metastases, 27–28, 39
CC49 monoclonal antibody, 393, 395–397
CC83 monoclonal antibody, 396–397
CD4+ T-cells, 380–381, 388
CDDP. See Cisplatin
CEA levels. See Carcinoembryonic antigen
Celiac plexus neurolysis, 407–408
Central nervous system metastases. See Brain
    metastases
Cerebral atrophy, imaging, 170
Cerebral blood flow, functional imaging,
    162–163
Cerebral infarctions, 167
Cerebral metastases. See Brain metastases
Cerebral ventricles, metastases pathology,
    153–154
Cervical carcinomas, imaging, 214–216
Cervical lymph nodes
  esophageal carcinoma, 318
  imaging, 305
  sentinel identification, 294–295
Chemical shift imaging, 213–214
Chemoembolization, hepatic metastases, 104
Chemotherapy. See also Hepatic arterial
    chemotherapy; Intraperitoneal
    chemotherapy; Perfusional therapy
  brain imaging evaluation of, 169–170
  colorectal carcinoma, adjuvant use, 320–321
  head and neck cancer, adjuvant use, 313–314
  hepatic metastases, 100–102
  islet cell carcinoma, 368
  and peritonectomy, 256
  testicular cancer, 322–323
  and tumor blood flow, 6–7
Chest radiography
  computerized tomography comparison, 29
  indications, 206
  pulmonary metastases, 24–31
  solitary pulmonary nodules, 33
Cholecystectomy, 253, 256–257
Choline, and proton spectroscopy, brain, 163
Choroid plexus, imaging, 166
Chromosome 1 deletions, 18
Chromosome 18 deletions, 18
Chylous malignant ascites, 272
Cirrhosis, and isolated hepatic perfusion, 142
Cisplatin
  extracorporeal perfusion, 197
  intra-carotid perfusion, 197–200
  intraperitoneal administration, 259–268
  isolated limb perfusion, 343–344
  isolated lung perfusion, 65–66
  toxicity, 344
"Clamshell incision," 43
Cloquet's node, 303, 309, 321, 324

CMS Accuprobe, 133
Coagulation abnormalities, and surgery, 179–180
Cognitive impairment
  intracranial metastases symptom, 154
  radiotherapy side effect, 188
Coin lesion. See Solitary pulmonary nodules
Color Doppler ultrasound
  hepatocellular carcinoma, 94
  indications, 419
  needle placement guidance, 420
  pulmonary metastases, 32
Colorectal anastomosis, and peritonectomy, 255
Colorectal carcinoma. See also Recurrent
    colorectal carcinoma
  imaging, 208–210
  intraoperative radiation therapy, 285–287, 289
  laparoscopic resection, 221–229
  lymphadenectomy, 320–321
  nodal involvement, 320
  peritonectomy indications, 250
  surgery, 235–246, 391–398
Colorectal carcinomatosis
  intraperitoneal chemotherapy, 259–268
  peritonectomy, 249–258
  prognosis, 267
Colorectal metastases
  adoptive cellular therapy, 397–398
  CT-arterial portography, liver, 87
  hepatic resection, 110–113
  magnetic resonance imaging, liver, 88
  noncontrast CT, liver, 81, 83
  prognosis, 109–111
  pulmonary metastasectomy results, 45
  radioimmunoguided surgery, 391–398
  ultrasonography, liver, 93, 419–421
Commissural myelotomy, 409–410
Common femoral perfusion, 337
Common iliac nodes, 321–322
Compartment syndrome, 345
Complete axillary dissection, 314–315
Complete laparoscopic colectomy, 221–222
Compression ultrasound scanning, 418
Computed tomography. See also Contrast-
    enhanced CT; CT-arterial portography
  abdominopelvic imaging, 207–217
  brain metastases, 154–157
    disadvantages, 155–157
    post-therapy evaluation, 169–170
  colorectal carcinoma, 208–210, 236
  hepatic metastases, 76–87, 94
    screening use, 76, 81
    sensitivity, 76, 81
  lymph node metastases, 17, 304–305
  mucinous peritoneal adenocarcinoma, 263
  pancreatic carcinoma, 209–212
  pulmonary metastases, 26, 29–31, 33
    advantages, 29, 31
  solitary pulmonary nodules, 33
  spinal metastases, 354
Computed tomography-arterial portography. See
    CT-arterial portography
Contact ultrasound scanning, 418
Contrast-enhanced CT
  administration, 77
  brain metastases, 155–157
  cavernous hemangioma detection, 78–82
  cyst detection, 77–81
  hepatic metastases, 76–84
Corticosteroid therapy
  brain metastases management, 188
  preoperative use, 178
  side effects, 188
Craniopharyngiomas, 164–165
Cryosurgery. See Hepatic cryoablation

Cryotech system, 133
CT-arterial portography
  hepatic neoplasms, 76, 87, 132, 209
  MR-arterial portography comparison, 89
  sensitivity and specificity, 76, 87
CT-arteriography
  disadvantages, 86
  hepatic neoplasms, 85–87, 104
  in preoperative assessment, 104
CT-directed cordotomy, 411
CT-directed needle localization
  bone metastases, 353
  and fine-needle aspiration biopsy, 32, 306
  hepatic resection preoperative evaluation, 104
  pancreatic masses, 212
  and video-assisted thoracic surgery, 53–54
CT-peritoneography, 214
Cutaneous melanoma. See Melanoma
Cystic masses. See Hepatic cysts
CYT-356 antibody, 303
Cytokines
  dendritic cell maturation role, 15
  and gene therapy, 381–382
Cytosine arabinoside, 200
Cytosine deaminase gene, 385

D

Decompression laminectomy, 361–364
Deep brain electrical stimulation, 402–403
Deep venous thrombosis, 345
Delayed high-dose contrast CT
  disadvantages, 84
  hepatic neoplasms, 84–85
Dendritic cells
  gene delivery, 388
  infiltration of, and prognosis, 18–19
  maturation, cytokines role, 14–15
  migration, 16
Denver peritoneovenous shunt, 271–275
Denver pleuroperitoneal shunt, 277
2'-Deoxy-5-fluorouridine, 65–66
Deoxyhemoglobin, 162–163
Dermoid tumors, 165
Dexamethasone, preoperative use, 178
Dextran-coated supramagnetic iron oxide, 17
Diazoxide therapy, 372
Disease-free intervals
  hepatic metastases, 109–110
  pulmonary metastasectomy prognosis, 41–42
Disseminated intravascular coagulation, 275
Diuretic therapy
  malignant ascites, 272
  massive hepatic metastases, 272
DMRIE/DOPE, 378
Doppler ultrasound. See Color Doppler
    ultrasound
Dose intensity
  intraperitoneal chemotherapy, 249, 259
  and response rate, 119
"Double duct" sign, 211
Doxorubicin (adriamycin)
  intraperitoneal administration, 259–268
  islet carcinoma, 368, 372
  isolated lung perfusion, rats, 65
Drug delivery
  brain metastases, 196
  hepatic arterial chemotherapy, 125
Drug sensitivity genes, 382–384
Dural metastases, 178
Dural sac, 241–242
Dyspnea, and pulmonary metastases, 24

E

E48Ig, 303

Early motion exercises, 307
Early postoperative intraperitoneal chemotherapy, 265–266
Edema
    and brain metastases, 153
    isolated limb perfusion complication, 345
    magnetic resonance imaging, brain, 157–158, 170
Elbow lesions, 357–358
Elective nodal dissection. *See* Prophylactic nodal dissection
Electrical stimulation, 401–403
Electron beam radiation, 283
End-to-end anastomosis
    dehiscence, 244
    pelvic exenteration procedure, 239, 244
Endometrial carcinomas
    imaging, 214–216
    lymph node involvement, 323
Endorectal MR coils, 208
Endoscopic retrograde cholangiopancreatography, 210–211
Endoscopic ultrasound
    advantages, 206, 306
    colorectal staging use, 208–209
    nodal disease, 306
    sensitivity and specificity, 306
Endothelial cells
    activated NK cell interactions, 7
    adhesion molecules, 4–5
Enteroperineal fistula, 243–244
Epidermoid brain tumors, 165
Epidermoid oral carcinoma, 310, 313
Epidural neurolysis, 405–406
Epidural opiate administration, 403
Epigastric pain, 407–408
Equipment manufacturers, 427–428
c-erbB2, 18
Erythrocytes, lymph vessel output, 15–16
Esophageal carcinoma
    intraoperative ultrasound, 422–424
    lymph node involvement, 317–318
    three-field lymphadenectomy, 318
Ethanol injection. *See* Alcohol injection
Ethicon staplers, 255
Ethiodol, 302
ex vivo gene delivery, 381–382
External-beam radiation therapy
    hepatic metastases, 102–103
    intraoperative radiation comparison, 281
External iliac perfusion, 335–337
Extracorporal perfusion, 197
Extravasation, 2–4
Extremity melanoma
    isolated limb perfusion, 333–347
    prognosis, 293
    prophylactic versus therapeutic nodal dissection, 310–312
    sentinel node dissection, 294, 312
Extremity sarcoma, 335, 344–345

F
Fasting gastrin levels, 368, 371
Fat deposition, liver, 83
FDG-PET. *See* Fluorodeoxyglucose PET
Femoral head lesions, surgery, 359–362
Femoral shaft lesions, surgery, 355–356, 358
Fever, and tumor necrosis factor, 346
Fiberoptic bronchoscopy. *See* Bronchoscopy
Fibrinogen, peritoneovenous shunting, 275
Fibrolamellar hepatocellular carcinoma, 112
Fine-needle aspiration biopsy
    nodal disease, 306
    pitfalls, 306

pulmonary metastases, 32, 40
Fistula formation, 268
Five-year survival
    axillary nodal metastases, 314–316
    breast carcinoma, 314–316
    colorectal carcinoma, 320
    colorectal hepatic metastases, 100, 109–111
    gastric cancer nodal dissection, 319
    head and neck cancer, 312–313
    hepatic cryosurgery, 135
    intraoperative radiation therapy, 285
    islet metastesectomy, 369–371
    isolated limb perfusion, 341
    melanoma nodal metastases, 312
    pancreatic carcinoma, 317
    pelvic exenteration, 245
    prostate carcinoma, 322
    pulmonary metastasectomy, 44–47, 58
        as valid indicator, 58
    radical versus total mastectomy, 315
    radioimmunoguided surgery, 396
    three-field lymphadenectomy, 317
Fluorodeoxyglucose PET
    brain metastases, 161, 169
    colorectal metastases, liver, 209–210
    lymph nodes, 306
5-Fluorouracil
    colorectal carcinoma, 320
    hepatic arterial infusion, 122–123
    hepatic metastases, 100–101
    intraperitoneal administration, 259–268
    islet carcinoma, 368, 372
Focal fat deposition, 83
Focal fibrosis, 83–84
Foot melanoma
    isolated limb perfusion, 343
    prognosis, 293
Foot metastases, surgery, 358
Forearm metastases, surgery, 357
Fractionation radiation schedules, 189, 192
Fractures
    clinical guidelines, 354–355
    femoral shaft lesions, 358–359
Frameless stereotaxy, brain metastases, 178–179
Freeze-thaw cycles, hepatic cryoablation, 134
5-FU deoxyribonucleoside
    hepatic artery infusion, 101–102, 120–123
    toxicity, 124
Functional MRI, 162–163
Functional PET, 162
Furosemide therapy, 272
Fusion images, colorectal cancer, 209–210

G
Gadolinium enhancement
    hepatic metastases, 89
    intracranial metastases, 157
    lymph node metastases, 305
    safety, 157
1-3 Galactosyl transferase, 384
Gallbladder metastases, ultrasound, 92, 421
Gallium scanning
    abdominopelvic imagery, 206, 217
    indications, 206
    malignant melanoma, 217
Gamma detectors. *See* Radioimmunoguided surgery
Gamma knife radiosurgery, 189–193
Ganciclovir, 382–383
Gastric cancer
    intraoperative radiation therapy, 284–288

intraoperative ultrasound, 422–424
    lymphadenectomy, 318–320
    nodal involvement, 318–319
Gastric lymphoma, 324
Gastric ulcer, 124–125
Gastrin levels, 368, 371
Gastrinoma
    chemotherapy, 368
    diagnosis, 368
    intraoperative ultrasound, 424–425
    medical palliation, 369, 371–372
    metastasectomy, 367–373
    response rates, 369–370
    postoperative surveillance, 371
Gastritis, 124–125
Gastroduodenal artery
    catheterization, 121–122
    isolated hepatic perfusion, 143
Gastrointestinal carcinoid metastases, 142
Gastrointestinal neoplasms
    imaging, 208–210
    intraoperative ultrasound, 422–425
    laparoscopic resection, 212–232
Gender differences, melanoma metastasis, 292–293
Gene marking, 379–380
Gene targeting, 16
Gene therapy, 375–388
    adenovirus vectors, 377–378
    and allogeneic bone marrow transplantation, 384–385
    anti-oncogene approach, 386
    clinical protocols, 379–387
    delivery systems, 376–378
    drug sensitization method, 382–384
    glial tumors, 199
    radiation therapy combination, 387
    retrovirus vectors, 376–377
    tumor cell immunomodulation, 380–381
    and tumor suppressor genes, 385–386
    vaccine approach, 381–382
Genital tract tumors
    imaging, 212–214
    lymphadenectomy, 321–324
Germ cell tumors, 165
    differential diagnosis, brain, 165
    pulmonary metastasectomy results, 45–46
Giant cerebral aneurysms, 168
Glioblastoma, gene therapy, 382–384
Gliomas
    differential diagnosis, imaging, 165
    intra-carotid perfusion, 197–198
Glucagonoma, 368–369
    diagnosis, 368
    medical palliation, 369, 371–372
    metastasectomy, 367–373
Glucocorticoid therapy. *See* Corticosteroid therapy
Gluteus maximus muscle, 240–241, 243
GlyCAM-1, 16
GM-CSF, gene therapy, 381–382
Gradient echo images, 88–90
Graft-versus-host disease, 384–385
Granulation tissue, 169
Granulomata, differential diagnosis, 167
Granulocyte macrophage-colony stimulating factor, 381–382
Gray-white matter junction, 153
Greater omentectomy
    methodology, 250–251
    pretreatment evaluation, 250
    specimens, 256–257
Gynecologic neoplasms, imaging, 213–216

H

Hair loss
 radiosurgery, 190
 whole-brain radiation, 188
Hand metastases, surgery, 357
Harris-Oh protrusio shell, 360, 362
Head and neck melanoma
 preoperative lymphoscintigraphy, 293
 prognosis, 293, 312–313
 prophylactic versus therapeutic nodal
  dissection, 312–313
 sentinel node dissection, 294
Headache, 154
Heated intraperitoneal chemotherapy, 260–261
 benefits, 261
 methods, 264–265
Helical CT scanners
 abdominopelvic imaging, 207
 intravenous contrast-enhanced method, 77
 liver metastases, 81
Hemangiomas
 dynamic contrast Ct, 78–82
 magnetic resonance imaging, 89–90
 ultrasonography, 93–94
Hematogenous dissemination
 biology, 1–8
 pulmonary metastases, 38
Hemiarthroplasty, 358
Hemidiaphragm, peritonectomy, 251–253
Hemorrhage, and pelvic exenteration, 243–244
Hemorrhagic tumors
 computed tomography, brain, 155
 intraoperative precautions, brain, 179–180
 magnetic resonance imaging, 159, 167
 and radiosurgery, 192
Hemosiderin, 159
Hepatic arterial chemotherapy, 101–102,
  119–127
 adjuvant use, 123–124
 clinical results, 122–124
 drug delivery, 125
 implantable pumps, 120, 124–125
  complications, 124–125
 islet metastases, 372
 methods, 121–122
 morbidity and mortality, 124
 patient care considerations, 124–125
 patient selection, 120
 pretreatment evaluation, 120–121
 systemic chemotherapy comparison, 122–123
 toxicity, 124–125
Hepatic cryoablation, 103, 129–138
 advantages, 138
 alternative approaches comparison, 136–138
 clinical results, 134–135
 complications, 135–136
 ethanol injection comparison, 137
 islet metastases, 372
 laser photocoagulation comparison, 137–138
 methods, 132–134
 morbidity and mortality, 136
 patient care considerations, 136
 patient selection, 131
 pretreatment evaluation, 131–132
 ultrasound monitoring, 133–134
Hepatic cysts
 contrast-enhanced CT, 77–79
 magnetic resonance imaging, 89
 ultrasonography, 93–94
Hepatic metastases, 99–113
 alcohol injection, 103–104
 chemoembolization, 104
 complications, 111
 computed tomography, 76–87, 209

cryosurgery, 103, 129–138
hyperthermia, 103
imaging, 75–95, 209, 419–421
isolated perfusion, 141–149
magnetic resonance imaging, 87–90, 209
noncolorectal sources, surgery, 112
patient information, 113
prognosis, 109–111
radiation therapy, 102–103
regional chemotherapy, 101–102, 119–126
size and distribution, 110
staging, 111
surgery, 99–113
systemic chemotherapy, 100–101, 119
ultrasonography, 90–94, 227–228, 419–421
Hepatic perfusion. See Isolated hepatic perfusion
Hepatic resection, 99–113
 abdominal exploration, 105
 complications, 111
 failure patterns, 111–112
 history, 99
 intraoperative ultrasound guidance, 420–421
 lobar method, 105–108
 noncolorectal metastases, 112
 patient information, 113
 preparation, 104–105
 preoperative evaluation, 104
 results, 109–112
Hepatic transplantation, 112, 316
Hepatocellular carcinoma
 arterial phase contrast enhancement, 77, 82
 contrast-enhanced CT, 82–83, 92
 CT-arteriography, 86
 laparoscopic ultrasound, 420
 liver transplantation, 112, 316
 magnetic resonance imaging, 89–90
 mosaic sign, 82–83
 nodal involvement, 316
 ultrasonography, 92, 419–421
Hepatoma, 142
Herpes simplex thymidine kinase gene, 382–385
Hip metastases, surgery, 359–362
HLA-B7 gene, 386
HMB-45, 312
HMFG1 antibody, 303
Hodgkin's disease
 gallium scanning, 206
 laparoscopic evaluation, 231–232
 lymphangiography versus CT, 217
Human antimouse antibodies, 344, 392
Humeral head metastases, surgery, 358
Humeral shaft metastases, surgery, 357–358
Hyperdensity, brain metastases, CT, 154–155
Hyperparathyroidism, 425
Hypertension, and tumor blood flow, 6
Hyperthermia
 intraperitoneal chemotherapy, 260–261,
  264–265
 isolated hepatic perfusion, 147–148
 isolated limb perfusion, 337, 339–340
 isolated lung perfusion, 66–72
 laser guidance, liver, 103
 tumor necrosis factor augmentation, 66
Hypervascular tumors
 angiography, 354
 magnetic resonance imaging, 89
 noncontrast CT, 85–86
Hypointense tumors, MRI, brain, 157–158
Hypopharyngeal carcinoma, 313
Hypotension, and tumor necrosis factor, 346
Hypothermia, cryoablation complication, 136

I

Ileus, 268

Image-guided biopsy. See CT-directed needle
 localization
Imidazole carboxamide, 343
Immediate postoperative abdominal lavage, 264
Immunodepression, and nodal dissection, 308
Immunolymphoscintigraphy, 303–304
Implantable infusion opiate administration,
 403–404
Incontinence, and abdominosacral resection,
 245
Indium-111
 melanoma nodal identification, 303–304
 neuroendocrine tumors, 206–207
Induction intraperitoneal chemotherapy,
 266–267
Infections
 differential diagnosis, brain, 165–167
 temporal changes, 166
Infrahilar aortocaval dissection, 309
Infusaid Model 400, 120
Infusional chemotherapy. See Hepatic artery
 chemotherapy
Infusional systems, pain relief, 403–404
Inguinal nodes
 dissection technique, 309
 penile carcinoma, 323
 sentinel dissection, 294–295
Insulinoma
 chemotherapy, 368
 diagnosis, 368
 incidence and natural history, 367–368
 intraoperative ultrasound, 424
 medical palliation, 369, 371–372
 metastasectomy, 367–373
  response rates, 369–371
 postoperative surveillance, 371
Intercostal nerve blockade, 405
Interferon-alpha
 adjuvant therapy, 19, 312
 islet carcinoma, 372
Interferon-gamma
 gene therapy, 382
 isolated limb perfusion, 342–343
 isolated lung perfusion, 71–72
 T cell migration role, 16
 and tumor necrosis factor, perfusion, 66–67
Intergroup Melanoma Trial, 292, 310
Interleukin-2
 and 5-FU, hepatic metastases, 102
 gene therapy, 382
 glial neoplasms, 199
Interleukin-6
 and laparoscopic colectomy, 227
 stunned myocardium mediation, 69
Interleukin-7, gene therapy, 382
Interleukin-12, gene therapy, 382
Internal iliac arteries/veins, 240
Internal mammary nodes, 314
Interstitial laser hyperthermia. See Laser
 hyperthermia
Interstitial radiation therapy, 103
Interval abdominal paracentesis
 malignant ascites palliation, 272–273
 serum albumin levels, 276
Intestinal anastomosis
 dehiscence, 244
 pelvic exenteration procedure, 239, 244
Intestinal bypass procedure, 243–244
Intestinal obstruction, 243–244
Intra-arterial perfusion
 brain metastases, 196–202
  clinical results, 199–200
 hepatic metastases, 101–102, 119–127
Intracranial epidural space, 153

Intrahepatic artery chemotherapy. *See* Hepatic
    arterial chemotherapy
Intraoperative celiac neurolysis, 408
Intraoperative lymphatic mapping, 293–296
    breast cancer, 296–298
    clinical results, 294—296
    complications, 296
    melanoma, 293–296
Intraoperative radiation therapy, 281–289
    assessments, 289
    bile duct carcinoma, 287
    clinical evaluation, 284–288
    colorectal cancer, 285–287, 289
    complications, 288–289
    dual-arm trials, 287–288
    gastric cancer, 284–289
    methods, 281–284
    pancreatic cancer, 285–286, 288–289
Intraoperative ultrasound, 417–425
    biliary tract, 421, 423
    brain, 178
    clinical results, 419–425
    and cryoablation, 133–134
    gastrointestinal tract, 422–425
    indications, 418–419
    instrumentation, 417–418
    islet cell tumors, 424–425
    liver, 76, 91–92, 105, 133–134, 227–228,
        419–422
    needle guidance, 420–422
    pancreatic cancer, 421–424
    parathyroid tumors, 425
    technique, 418
Intraoperative ultrasound-guided needle
    placement, 420–422
Intraoperative ultrasound-guided systematic
    subsegmentectomy, 420
Intraperitoneal chemotherapy. 259–268, 427
    benefits, 260–261
    equipment manufacturers, 427
    indications, 261–262
    methods, 264–267
    morbidity and mortality, 268
    patient care considerations, 268
    patient information, 268
    patient selection, 261–263
    and peritonectomy, procedures, 256
    pretreatment evaluation, 263–264
    route and timing of, 260
Intraportal chemotherapy, 101
Intraspinal opiate administration, 403
Intrathecal chemotherapy, 198–199
    clinical results, 200
    complications, 200
    methods, 198–199
    patient information, 201
Intrathecal neurolysis, 405–406
Intrathecal opiate administration, 403–404
Intrathoracic metastases, 28
Intratumoral drug delivery, 199, 202–202
Intravenous contrast-enhanced CT. *See*
    Contrast-enhanced CT
Intraventricular opiate administration, 403–404
Iodinated contrast materials
    dose effects, brain CT, 155–156
    side effects and toxicity, 156–157
Iodine-125
    radioimmunoguided surgery, 393, 395
    side effects, 398
IODO-GEN method, 393
Iron oxide particles, 95
Ischemic events, brain, 167
Islet carcinoma, 367–373
    chemotherapy, 368

diagnosis, 368
hepatic therapies, 372
imaging, 211–212
incidence, 367
intraoperative ultrasound, 424–425
medical palliation, 369, 371–372
and MEN-1, 372–373
metastasectomy, 367–373
    response rates, 369–371
natural history, 367–368
postoperative surveillance, 371
subgroup analysis, 370
Isolated hepatic perfusion, 141–149
    alternative treatments, 148
    clinical trials, 146–147
    decannulation, 145
    equipment manufacturers, 428
    indications, 142
    instrumentation, 145–146
    magnetic resonance imaging, 148–149
    methodology, 142–145
    mortality and morbidity, 148
    patient assessment, 148
    patient information, 148–149
    patient selection, 146
    precautions, 146
    sequential steps, 144–145
Isolated limb perfusion, 333–347
    adjuvant melphalan response, 341–342
    alternative approaches, 346
    equipment manufacturers, 427
    history, 333–334
    indications, 334–335
    instrumentation, 337–338
    melphalan alone response, 339–341
    melphalan and tumor necrosis factor, 342–343
    methodology, 335–337
    morbidity and mortality, 345–346
    patient care considerations, 346–347
    patient information, 347
    and peripheral vascular system assessment,
        338
    rationale, 333–334
    response rates, 338–346
    soft tissue sarcoma, 344–345
    toxicity, 345–346
Isolated lung perfusion, 63–72
    clinical use, 66
    equipment manufacturers, 427
    experimental studies, 63–69
    hemodynamic changes, 67–68
    history, 63–64
    human studies, 69–72
    postoperative care, 72
    rat model, 65
    technique in humans, 69–70
Isosulfan blue vital dye, 293, 296, 302–303

J
Jaundice, 124

K
Knee joint lesions, surgery, 358

L
Lactate, proton spectroscopy, 163
Laminectomy
    abdominosacral resection, 241–242
    spinal metastases, 361–364
Langerhans cell histiocytosis, 164
Laparoscopic abdominoperineal resection, 229
Laparoscopic adrenalectomy, 230–231
Laparoscopic cholecystojejunostomy, 230
Laparoscopic colectomy, 221–232

advantages, 226–227
bowel function return time, 226
clinical results, 225–228
contraindications, 222
conversion rates, 226
cost evaluations, 226–227
indications, 222
lymph node harvest, 228
methodology, 222–225
mortality and morbidity, 224–225
open colectomy comparison, 225–228
operative times, 226
patient care considerations, 228–229
patient selection, 222
recurrence patterns, 228
surgical stress reduction, 227
Laparoscopic hepatic wedge biopsy, 231
Laparoscopic splenectomy, 231–232
Laparoscopic ultrasound, 227–228
    hepatocellular carcinoma, 420
    instrumentation, 418
    pancreatic cancer staging, 422
    technique, 418
Laparotomy, and ultrasound, 420
Large iron oxide particles, 95
Laser hyperthermia
    hepatic cryoablation comparison, 137–138
    hepatic metastases, 103, 137–138
Lateral thoracotomy, 42–43, 57
Left gastric artery, 250
Left hemicolectomy, 320
Left hemidiaphragm
    peritonectomy procedure, 251
    stripping specimens, 256–257
Left hepatic lobectomy, 107
Left segmental colectomy, 320
Left upper quadrant peritonectomy, 251–252
Lentigo maligna melanoma, 293
Leptomeningeal metastases
    computed tomography, 155–156
    differential diagnosis, infection, 167
    intrathecal drug delivery, 198–199
    magnetic resonance imaging, 159–160
    pathology, 153
    seeding, 153
    signs and symptoms, 177
    treatment, 177–178
Lesser omentectomy
    methodology, 253
    pretreatment evaluation, 250
    specimens, 256–257
Leucovorin, 100–101
Leukomalacia, 170
LeVeen shunt, 273, 275
"Light-bulb sign," 89
Linac radiosurgery, 189–193
Lipiodol CT, 86
Liposomal DNA vectors, 378
Liquid nitrogen cryoprobes, 130–131, 133–134
Liver cysts. *See* Hepatic cysts
Liver metastases. *See* Hepatic metastases
Liver mobilization, 105
Liver resection. *See* Hepatic resection
Liver transplantation, 112, 316
Lobar hepatic resection, 105–108
Longevity, and bone surgery, 355
Lower extremity bones, surgery, 355, 358–362
Lung metastases. *See also* Pulmonary
    metastases
Lymph node dissection, 301–325
    breast cancer, 296–298, 314–316
    complications, 307
    evaluation, 19, 307–325
    gallbladder carcinoma, 317

Lymph node dissection (*contd.*)
  gastrointestinal tract, 317–321
  general principles, 306–309
  genital tract, 321–324
  head and neck carcinoma, 313–314
  hepatocellular carcinoma, 316
  history, 301
  and immunodepression, 307
  laparoscopic sampling technique, 232
  lung neoplasms, 316
  melanoma, 291–293, 310–313
  pancreatic carcinoma, 316–317
  prophylactic versus therapeutic use, 291–292,
    307–325
  sentinel technique, 293–296, 312
  thyroid cancer, 314
  urinary tract, 321
Lymph node lymphocytes, 397
Lymph node metastases. *See also* Lymph node
    dissection
  abdominal imaging, 216–217
  biology, 11–19
  diagnosis, 291–298, 302–306
  elective regional dissection, 291–293
  frequency by tumor type, 306
  pathogenesis, 14
  surgical evaluation, 19
  therapeutic dissection, 307–325
Lymph nodes
  anatomy and organization, 12–14
  as cancer barrier, 11–12
  immune response role, 14–15
  and radioimmunoguided surgery, 397
Lymph system, biology, 11–19
Lymphadenectomy. *See* Lymph node dissection
Lymphangiography, 217, 302–303
  carbon particles, 17
  complications, 302
  computed tomography comparison, 217
  technical demands, 217
Lymphangitis metastases, 39
Lymphatic flow, 15–17
Lymphedema, 307
Lymphoceles, 307
Lymphocytes
  immunization effects on migration, 15–17
  lymph vessel output, 15–16
Lymphokine-activated killer cells, 199
Lymphoma. *See also* Hodgkin's disease; Non-
    Hodgkin's lymphoma
  laparoscopic staging, 231–232
  surgery and radiation, 324
Lymphoscintigraphy, 293, 296, 303

M

Magnetic resonance imaging
  abdominopelvic cancer, 208–217, 236–237
  brain metastases, 157–159, 162–163, 178
    post-therapy evaluation, 169–170
  hepatic hemangioma, 82
  hepatic metastases, 76, 87–90, 209
    sensitivity, 76, 88
  isolated hepatic perfusion assessment,
    148–149
  lymph node metastases, 17, 305
  pelvic exenteration evaluation, 236–237
  and radiofrequency cingulotomy, 412
  spine metastases, 353
Magnetic resonance spectroscopy, 163–164,
  169
Malignant ascites, 271–279
  diuretic therapy, 272
  interval abdominal paracentesis, 272
  palliative strategies, 272

shunting procedures, 271–279
Malignant melanoma. *See* Melanoma
Malignant pleural effusions, 277–278
Mannitol, 200
Margin resection
  hepatic metastases, 110–111
  pelvic exenteration, 242–243
Massive hepatic metastases, 272
Mayo Clinic melanoma trial, 292, 309–310
Median sternotomy, 42, 57
Mediastinal neoplasms, thoracoscopy, 59–60
Mediastinal nodes, esophageal carcinoma, 318
Medullary rod fixation, 357–359
Medullary thyroid carcinoma, 314
Melanoma
  anatomic sites, 292
  brain metastasis, hemorrhage, MRI, 159
  diagnosis, 291–296, 303–306
  gallium scanning, 206, 217
  gene therapy, 382, 388
  lymph node dissection, 291—293, 303–306
    sentinel method, 293–296, 312
  lymphoscintigraphy, 293, 296, 303
  prophylactic versus therapeutic dissection,
    310–313
  radiosurgery, 192
  recurrence in brain, survival, 181
  thickness of, 292
Melanoma-specific monoclonal antibody, 294
Melphalan
  intrathecal delivery, 199
  isolated hepatic perfusion, 147
  isolated limb perfusion, 339–344
  toxicity, 345
MEN-1, 367, 372–373
Meningeal carcinomatosis
  magnetic resonance imaging, 159–160
  meningiomas differential diagnosis, 164
  pathogenesis, 195–196
  perfusion therapy, 196, 198
Meningiomas, imaging, 164–165
Mesorectal nodal resection, 320
Mesothelioma, and peritonectomy, 249–258
Metallic cage vertebral body replacement,
  363–364
Metastatic melanoma. *See* Melanoma
Methotrexate, 199–200
Microenvironment, and metastasis, 4
Micrometastases
  nodal melanoma, 312
  sentinel nodal dissection, 312
Microspheres, 199
Mitomycin
  intra-carotid delivery, 200
  intraperitoneal administration, 259–268
  isolated hepatic perfusion, 147
  peritoneal-plasma barrier, 259–260
  toxicity, 148
Mn-DPDP, 89–90, 95
Monoclonal antibodies
  colorectal carcinoma imaging, 209–210
  drug delivery, brain, 197–199
  intrathecal delivery, 199
  melanoma nodal identification, 303–304
  in radioimmunoguided surgery, 394–398
Morphine, implantable infusion, 403–404
Mosaic sign, 82–83
Motor deficits, intracranial metastasis, 154
Motor strip, 178–179
Mouse monoclonal antibody R24, 344, 392,
  395–398
MR-arterial portography, 89
MUC 18 expression, 18
Mucinous adenocarcinoma

computed tomography, 262
intraperitoneal chemotherapy, 262–263
Multiple endocrine neoplasia type I, 367,
  372–373
Multiple myeloma, 352
Multiple metastases
  axillary nodes, prognosis, 314–316
  gastric cancer nodal involvement, 319
  liver cancer prognosis, 110–111
  prostate cancer nodal involvement, 322
  radiosurgery, brain, 192–193
  and surgery, brain, 177, 181–183
Multiple sclerosis, 168
Murine monoclonal antibodies
  melanoma response, 344
  in radioimmunoguided surgery, 392, 395–398
Murine retroviral vectors, 376–377
Mus dunni, 377
Myelomalacia, 170
Myoglobinuria, 136
Myonecrosis, 250
Myopathy, melphalan toxicity, 345

N

"Napkin ring" cord constriction, 362
Nasopharyngeal carcinoma, 313
Natural killer cells, 7
Nd:YAG laser, 53–54, 56, 137
Neck nodal dissection
  clinical results, 312–313
  muscle resection, 307, 310
  surgical procedure, 310
Necrotic brain metastases, 155–156, 158–159
Neodymium:yttrium-aluminum laser, 137
Neoprobe 1000 instrument, 391, 394
Nephrotoxicity, iodinated contrast, 156–157
Nerve root ablation procedures, 404–409
Neuroablative pain management, 404–409, 427
Neuroaxial block, 405–406
Neurolytic block procedures, 404–409
Neuromas, differential diagnosis, 165
Neuropathy, melphalan toxicity, 345
Neurosarcoidosis, 164
Neurostimulation, 401–403
Neutropenia, 345
Nitrogen mustard, 343
NKI/C3 monoclonal antibody, 294
Nodular melanoma, prognosis, 293
Noncontrast CT. *See* Unenhanced CT
Non-Hodgkin's lymphoma, 217
Number of metastases. *See* Multiple metastases

O

Obturator nodes, 321–322
Obesity, and laparoscopy conversion, 222, 226
Octreotide therapy, 372
Ocular melanoma metastases, 142
Oil-based contrast agents, 86
Omental bursa, stripping, 253–254
Omental "cake," 214–215
Omentectomy
  methodology, 250–253
  pretreatment evaluation, 250
Ommaya reservoir, 198
Oncogenes, 386
Onik-Cohen sets, 133
Onik introducer sets, 133
Operative ultrasonography. *See* Intraoperative
    ultrasonography
Opiates, implantable infusion, 403–404
Orchiectomy, 322
Organ microenvironment, and metastases, 4
Oropharyngeal carcinoma
  adjuvant therapy, 313

prophylactic versus therapeutic nodal
    dissection, 313–314
Orthotopic liver transplantation, 112
Osteosarcoma
    nodal metastases, 324
    pulmonary metastasectomy, 44–45
Ovarian carcinoma
    computed tomography, 214–215
    intraperitoneal chemotherapy, 263, 266
    lymph node dissection, 323–324
Oxygen-15 PET, 162

P

p53 gene therapy, 385–386
    biochemical functions, 385
    and radiation therapy, 387
Pain management, 401–413
    and abdominosacral resection
        implantable infusion systems, 403–404
    intracranial procedures, 412–413
    neuroablative procedures, 404–413
    neurostimulation, 401–403
    spinal cord stimulation, 401–402
    and spinal metastases, 364, 401–402
PAL-E staining, 13–14
Pancoast syndrome, 402
Pancreatic carcinoma
    computed tomography, 209–210
    imaging, 209–212
    intraoperative ultrasound, 421–424
    intraoperative radiation therapy, 285–286, 288
    laparoscopic procedures, 229–230
    nodal dissection, 316–317
    portal vein invasion, ultrasound, 422, 424
    prognosis, 317
    thin-needle biopsy, 212
Pancreatic cysts, 212
Pancreatic head cancer, 210–211
    computed tomography, 211
    endoscopic retrograde
        cholangiopancreatography, 210–211
    intraoperative radiation therapy, 288
    intraoperative ultrasound, 424
Para-aortic lymphadenectomy, 232
Para-aortic nodes
    computed tomography, 304
    intraoperative ultrasound, 423, 425
    prostate carcinoma, 321–322
Paracentesis
    intraperitoneal chemotherapy, 266
    malignant ascites, 272
Parathyroid tumors, ultrasound, 425
Paravertebral nerve block, 405
Paresthesias, 345
Parietal lobe metastases
    magnetic resonance imaging, 158, 176
    surgery indications, 176
Partial thromboplastin time, 275
Patient information
    brain perfusion therapy, 201–202
    hepatic resection, 113
    intraperitoneal carcinomatosis treatment, 268
    isolated hepatic perfusion, 148–149
    isolated limb perfusion, 347
    peritoneovenous shunts, 278–279
    pleuroperitoneal shunts, 279
    radioimmunoguided surgery, 398
Pelvic exenteration, 235–246
    blood loss, 244
    clinical results, 244–245
    five-year survival, 245
    functional impairments, 245
    methodology, 237–243
    morbidity and mortality, 236, 243–244

pain relief objective, 245
patient care considerations, 246
preoperative evaluation, 236–237
survival, 236
Pelvic nodes
    computed tomography, 304
    dissection, 307
    genital tract carcinomas, 321–324
Pelvic peritonectomy, 254–255
    gastric reconstruction, 255–256
    intraoperative chemotherapy, 256
    methodology, 254–255
    pretreatment evaluation, 250
    specimen, 257
Penile carcinoma, 323
Percutaneous CT-guided biopsy. *See* CT-directed
    needle localization
Percutaneous neuroaxial neurolysis, 405–406
Percutaneous peripheral somatic neurolysis,
    404–405
Percutaneous radiofrequency cordotomy,
    410–411
Percutaneous radiofrequency rhizotomy, 409
Percutaneous sympathetic ganglion neurolysis,
    406–409
Perflubron emulsions, 17
Perfusional therapy. *See* Intraperitoneal
    chemotherapy; Isolated hepatic perfusion;
    Isolated limb perfusion; Isolated lung
    perfusion
Peripheral neuropathy, melphalan, 345
Peripheral somatic neurolysis, 404–405
Peritoneal carcinomatosis, 249–258
    diuretic therapy, 272
    intraperitoneal chemotherapy, 256, 259–268
    malignant ascites, shunting, 271–277
    peritonectomy procedures, 249–258
    prevention, 262
    prognostic features, 261–264
    treatment options, 263
Peritoneal-plasma barrier, 259–260
Peritoneal reflection, 255
Peritonectomy
    and intraperitoneal chemotherapy, 256,
        259–268
    pretreatment evaluation, 249–250
    visceral and parietal procedures, 249–258
Peritoneovenous shunting, 271–277
    clinical results, 274–276
    complications, 274–275
    iatrogenic metastases, 276
    methods, 273–274
    morbidity and mortality, 276–277
    patient information, 278–279
    patient selection, 272–273
    pretreatment evaluation, 273
    shunt failure, 276–277
    tumor emboli, 276
PET scanning. *See* Positron emission tomography
Pharyngeal tumors, 313
Phenol neurolysis, 405–406, 408–409
Phosphorus spectroscopy
    brain metastases, 163, 169
    post-treatment evaluation use, brain, 169
Physical examination, axillary nodes, 314
Pineal tumors, diagnosis, 164–165
Pituitary adenomas, 164–165
Pituitary stalk tumors, 164
Plain radiography. *See also* Chest radiography
    bone metastases, 352–353
Plasmid DNA vectors, 378
Platelet count, peritoneovenous shunting, 275
Pleural effusions
    pleuroperitoneal shunts, 277–278

pulmonary metastases manifestation, 39–40
    and video-assisted thoracoscopy, 59
Pleurodesis, 59
Pleuroperitoneal shunts, 277–279
    clinical results, 278
    patient information, 278–279
Pneumothorax, 39
Polymethylmethacrylate bone cement, 355–357,
    362–364
Polymer microspheres, 199
Popliteal perfusion, 337–338
Portal vein
    chemotherapy infusion, 101, 123–124
    intraoperative ultrasound, 421–422, 424
Portal venous phase CT, 76–81, 85–86
Positron emission tomography
    brain metastases, 160–162, 169
    hepatic neoplasms, 95, 210
    lymph nodes, 17, 306
    pulmonary metastases, 31
    recurrent tumor diagnosis, 169
Posterior fossa, tumor seeding, 153
Posterior laminectomy, 362
Postirradiation injury/necrosis
    brain radiosurgery, 192
    diagnostic imaging, brain, 169–170
Post-operative radiation, brain, 176–178, 180–184
Preoperative lymphoscintigraphy, 293
Primary intracranial tumors, 164–165
Primary liver tumors, 142
Probe-standoff ultrasound, 418
Producer cells
    and brain tumors, 383
    gene delivery, 376
Prophylactic anticonvulsants, 188
Prophylactic nodal dissection
    axillary nodes, 315–316
    complications, 307
    head and neck cancer, 313–314
    melanoma, 291–292, 310–313
    patient selection, 292–293
    randomized studies, 308–310
    and survival, 291–292, 308–310
    therapeutic dissection comparison, 291–292,
        307–325
Prostacyclin analogs, 17–18
Prostate carcinoma
    computed tomography, 216
    diagnosis, 215–216
    lymphadenectomy, 322
    magnetic resonance imaging, 216
    nodal involvement, 3212–322
    transrectal ultrasound, 216
Prostatectomy, 322
Prothrombin time, 275
Proton spectroscopy, brain, 163–164
Protrusio shell, 360, 362
Pseudomyxoma peritonei, 261–262
Pulmonary metastasectomy, 41–44
    breast carcinoma metastases, 47
    colorectal metastases, 45
    eligibility criteria, 41, 57
    head and neck carcinoma metastases, 46
    osteogenic sarcoma, 44–45
    prognosis, 41–42, 44–47, 58
    renal cell carcinoma, 45
    soft-tissue sarcoma, 44
    technique, 42–43
    testicular carcinoma, 45–46
Pulmonary metastases, 23–33, 37–47
    computed tomography, 26, 29–31, 33
    diagnosis, 23–33, 40
    distribution, 39–40
    incidence, 38

Pulmonary metastases (*contd.*)
  isolated lung perfusion, 63–72
  pathogenesis, 23, 38
  positron emission tomography, 31
  preoperative assessment, 40–41
  radiology, 24–31, 33
  size and appearance, 26–27, 39–40
  surgery, 37–47
    eligibility, 41, 57
    prognosis, 41–42, 44–47
    thoracoscopy, 32–33
    vascular supply, 38–39
    video-assisted thoracoscopy, 44, 51–60
Pyelonephritis, 244

Q
Quality of life, 245

R
R24 monoclonal antibody, 344
Radiation necrosis. *See* Postirradiation injury/
    necrosis
Radiation therapy. *See also* Intraoperative
    radiation;
  brain imaging evaluation of, 169–170
  brain metastases, 176–178, 180–184,
    192–193
  dose-volume analysis, liver, 102
  gene therapy combination, 387
  hepatic metastases, 102–103
  radiosurgery comparison, 192–192
  spinal metastases, 361
Radical mastectomy, 315–316
Radical orchiectomy, 322
Radical prostatectomy, 322
Radiofrequency neuroablation, 409–412
Radioimmunoguided surgery, 391–398
  and adoptive cellular therapy, 397–398
  carrier substance, 394–395
  clinical results, 395–398
  history and rationale, 391–392
  indications, 392
  instrumentation, 394
  intraoperative survey sites, 394
  lymph node identification, 397
  metastatic colorectal carcinoma, 391–398
  methodology, 392
  patient information, 398
  preoperative considerations, 392
  safety, 398
Radiological Diagnostic Oncology Group, 205
Radiolymphoscintigraphic mapping, 296, 303
Radionuclide scintigraphy. *See also specific*
    techniques
  abdominopelvic imaging, 206
  lymph nodes, 296, 303
Radiosensitivity, brain metastases, 177
Radiosurgery, 187–193
  clinical results, 191–192
  indications, 192–193
  methodology, 189–190
  pain control, 412
  side effects, 190
  and survival, 192
  technique, 190
Reconstruction rods, 356, 358–359
Rectal carcinoma. *See also* Colorectal carcinoma
  endoscopic ultrasonography, 208–209
  intraoperative radiation therapy, 287
  laparoscopic resection, 229
  lymphadenectomy, 320–321
  positron emission tomography, 209
  recurrence of, surgery, 235–246
Rectal stalks, 238

Rectosigmoid colon resection, 255, 257
Recurrent colorectal carcinoma
  imaging, 208–209
  laparoscopy versus open colectomy, 228
  radioimmunoguided surgery, 391–398
  surgery, 235–246
Recurrent brain tumors
  post-treatment imaging, 169–170
  radiosurgery, 191–193
  radiotherapy outcome, 189
  resection, 177, 181
Renal cell carcinoma
  biopsy, 212
  gene therapy, 381–382
  hypervascular bone metastases, 354
  imaging, 212–213
  lymphadenectomy, 321
  pulmonary metastasectomy, 45
Reoperation, brain metastases, 181
Repeat abdominal paracentesis, 272–273
Repeat pulmonary metastasectomy, 44
Replication-competent viral vectors, 377,
    387–388
Retroperitoneal nodal dissection
    technique, 309
  testicular carcinoma, 322–323
Retroperitoneal sarcomas, 285, 288–289
Retroviral vectors, 376–377
  characteristics, 376–377
  production of, 377
Rib pain, 405
Right hemidiaphragm
    and peritonectomy, 252–253
    stripping of, 256–257
Right hepatic lobectomy, 106–107
Right laparoscopic colectomy, 222–224
Right trisegmentectomy, 108
Right upper quadrant peritonectomy, 253
Ring-like enhancement, 155–156, 158–159,
    161–162
Rosenmiller's node, 303
Rotter's nodes, 308

S
S-100 antiserum, 294, 312
Sacropelvic resection. *See* Abdominosacral
    resection
Sarcomas
    intraperitoneal chemotherapy, 266–267
    nodal metastases, 324–325
Scalp block, 188
Scapular lesions, 358
"Scar carcinoma," 25
Sciatic nerve, 240–241
Sclerosing cholangitis, 124
Secretin testing, 368, 371
"Seed and soil" theory, 38
Segmental resection, 108–109
Segmentation data analysis, 108–109
Seizures, 154
Seldinger technique, 133
L-selectin, 16
Seminoma. *See* Testicular cancer
Sentinel lymph node dissection, 293–296, 312
    breast cancer, 296–298
    clinical results, 294–296
    complications, 296
    melanoma metastases, 294–296, 312
    rationale, 293, 312
    technique, 293–294
Serial CT scanning, 30–31
Seromas, 307
Serum albumin levels, 276
Short bowel syndrome, 244

Shoulder metastases, surgery, 358
Shunt failures, 276–277
Shunting procedures
    malignant ascites, 271–279
    patient information, 278–279
    pleural effusions, 277–278
Side-to-side gastrojejunostomy, 255
Sigmoid colon, resection, 239–240
Sigmoid laparoscopic resection, 222–224
Simple mastectomy, 315–316
Single-photon emission computed tomography.
    See SPECT
Skeletal metastases
    evaluation, 352
    incidence, 351
    surgery, 354–364
Skin, lymphatic flow, 15
Skin toxicity, melphalan, 345
Skull metastases, surgery indications, 178
Small bowel fistula, 268
Soft-tissue sarcoma
    isolated limb perfusion, 344–345
    nodal metastases, 324–325
    pulmonary metastasectomy results, 44
Solitary brain metastases
    radiosurgery, 189, 192–193
    surgery indications, 176–178, 189
    surgery results, 180–184
    whole-brain radiotherapy, 189
Solitary pulmonary nodules
    diagnostic probability, 40
    metastasectomy prognosis, 58
    roentgenographic management, 33
    tissue diagnosis, 25–26
    video-assisted thoracoscopy, 52–53
SPECT
    brain metastases, 160–162
    colorectal carcinoma, 209–210
Speech centers, 178–179
Spin echo images, 88–89
Spinal cord compression, 361–364
Spinal cord metastases
    evaluation, 352–354
    incidence, 152, 351
    pain treatment, 364
    radiation therapy, 361
    surgery, 359–364
Spinal cord stimulation, 401–402
Spiral CT scanners. *See* Helical CT scanners
Spironolactone therapy, 272
Splenectomy
    Hodgkin's lymphoma staging, 231–232
    and peritonectomy, methodology, 250–251
Sputum cytology, 32
Starch microspheres, 125
Steinmann pin, 335–337
Stellate ganglia neurolysis, 406–407
Stereotactic cingulotomy, 412
Stereotactic mesencephalotomy, 412–413
Stereotactic surgery, 189–194
    clinical results, 191–193
    methodology, 189–190
    pain management, 412–413
    parenchymal metastases, 178–180
    side effects, 190
Steroid therapy. *See* Corticosteroid therapy
Stop-flow isolated lung perfusion, 65–66
Streptozocin, 368, 372
"Stunned myocardium," 69
Subarachnoid space, 198
Suicide gene therapy, 382–385
    in allo-bone marrow transplantation,
        384–385
    glioblastoma, 382–384

Superficial inguinal nodal dissection, 309
Superficial spreading melanoma, 293
Superior hypogastric plexus neurolysis, 408–409
Suprapubic prostatectomy, 322
Surgical margin. *See* Margin resection
Surgicel, 134
Survival. *See* Five-year survival
Susceptibility effect, 162
Sympatholysis, 406–409
Systemic chemotherapy, hepatic metastases, 100–101

T

T-cells, 15–17
T1-weighted images
    brain metastases, 157–159
    hepatic metastases, 88–89
    lymph node metastases, 305
T2-weighted images
    brain metastases, 157–159
    hepatic metastases, 88–89
TAG-72 antigen, 395
Technetium bone scan, 352
Technetium-labeled blue dye, 296, 303
Technetium-99m SPECT, 160
Ten-year survival
    colorectal liver metastases, 110
    radical versus total mastectomy, 315
Tenckhoff catheter, 256, 264–266
Testicular carcinoma
    chemotherapy, 310, 322–323
    lymph node metastases, 322
    nodal resection, 310, 322–323
    pulmonary metastasectomy results, 45–46
Tetracycline
    axillary space injections, 307
    and thoracoscopic talc pleurodesis, 59
TH1/TH2 cells, 380–381
Thallium-201 SPECT, 160
Therapeutic lymph node dissection. *See also*
        Lymph node dissection
    complications, 307
    elective dissection comparison, 291–292, 307–325
    melanoma, 291–292, 310–313
Thin-needle guided imaging. *See also* CT-directed needle localization
    nodal disease, 306
    pulmonary metastases, 32, 40
Thiotepa, intrathecal delivery, 199–200
Thompson Self-Retaining Retractor, 250
Thoracic esophageal carcinoma, 317–318
Thoracic spinal metastases
    bracing, 364
    incidence, 351
    radiography, 353
Thoracoscopic talc pleurodesis, 59

Thoracoscopy, 32–33, 43–44, 51–60. *See also*
        Video-assisted thoracoscopy
Thoracotomy, 42–43, 58–59
Three field lymphadenectomy, 318
Thrombosis. *See* Venous thrombosis
Thymidine kinase gene, 382–385
Thyroid cancer, 314
Tibial lesions, surgery, 358
Tonsillar fossa carcinoma, 313
Total hip arthroplasty, 359–362
Total knee arthroplasty, 358
Total mastectomy, 315–316
Total pancreatectomy, 317
Toxoplasmosis, differential diagnosis, 166
Transthoracic fine-needle aspiration biopsy, 32, 40
Trendelenburg traction, 223–224
Trisegmentectomy, 108
Truncal melanoma, 312
Tumor blood flow, 6–7
"Tumor cell entrapment" hypothesis, 259–260
Tumor doubling time, 41–42
Tumor embolization, 276
Tumor hemorrhage. *See* Hemorrhagic tumors
Tumor margin. *See* Margin resection
Tumor necrosis factor
    isolated hepatic perfusion, 147
    isolated lung perfusion, 65–72
        human trial, 71–72
        toxicity, 66–68
    and melphalan, limb perfusion, 342–344
    toxicity, 66–68, 345–346
Tumor necrosis factor-alpha, 16
Tumor size. *See* Tumor volume
Tumor spill, 262
Tumor suppressor genes, 385–386
Tumor thickness, melanoma, 292, 312
Tumor vaccines, 381–382
Tumor volume
    and intraperitoneal chemotherapy, 262–264
        survival factor, 264
    and radiosurgery, 192
Two-field lymphadenectomy, 318

U

Ultrasonic aspirator, 179–180
Ultrasound. *See also* Endoscopic ultrasound;
        Intraoperative ultrasound; Laparoscopic
        ultrasound
    abdominopelvic imaging, 206
    hemangioma, 82
    gynecologic neoplasms, 213–214
    hepatic cryoablation monitoring, 133–134
    hepatic metastases, 90–94
        sensitivity, 76, 91
    intraoperative use, 76, 91–92, 133–134, 178, 417–425
    nodal disease, 306

Ultrasound probe, 417–418
Unenhanced CT
    brain metastases, 154–155
    vascularized liver tumors, 84–85
Upper extremity bones, surgery, 355, 357–358
Ureteral anastomosis
    dehiscence, 244
    pelvic exenteration procedure, 239
Ureteral obstruction, 244
Urinary tract cancer, 45

V

Vaccine approach, 381–382
Vaginal closure, 255
Vascular malformations, 167–168
Vascular supply
    biology, 5–7
    pulmonary metastases, 38–39
Vasculopathy, 170
Vasoconstrictors, 125
Venous angiomas, 167
Venous thrombosis, 169–170
Vertebral metastases
    incidence, 351
    surgery, 361–364
Video-assisted thoracoscopy, 51–60
    candidate nodules, 52
    history, 51
    and malignant pleural processes, 59
    and mediastinal neoplasms, 59–60
    operative procedure, 53–55
    patient profile, 52
    preoperative strategies, 53–55
    and pulmonary metastasectomy, 32–33, 43–44, 51–60
    results, 55–57
    thoracotomy comparison, 58–59
VIPoma
    diagnosis, 368
    octreotide therapy, 372
VP-16, intra-carotid delivery, 200
Vulva carcinoma, 324

W

Wada test, 178
Wedge resection
    pulmonary metastases, 42–43
    and video-assisted thoracoscopy, 51–60
Whipple procedure, 317
White matter abnormalities, 170
WHO melanoma trials, 292, 308–309
Whole-brain irradiation
    post-treatment imaging, 170
    radiosurgery comparison, 188–189, 192–193
    side effects, 188
    and surgery, 176–178, 180–184
Wound infections, 243